Routledge Handbook of Global Public Health

At the beginning of the twenty-first century, key public health issues and challenges have taken centre stage. They range from arsenic in drinking water to asthma among children and adults; from the re-emergence of cholera, to increasing cancer rates and other chronic disease; from AIDS to malaria and hepatitis; from the crises faced by displaced or refugee populations to the new challenges that have emerged for reproductive health and rights.

Like most aspects of contemporary life, these problems have been impacted by globalisation. The issues that confront us are being shaped by evolving processes such as the growth of inequalities between the rich and the poor in countries around the world, the globalisation of trade and commerce, new patterns of travel and migration, as well as a reduction in resources for the development and sustainability of public health infrastructures.

The *Routledge Handbook of Global Public Health* explores this context and addresses both the emerging issues and conceptualisations of the notion of global health, along with expanding upon and highlighting the critical priorities in this rapidly evolving field. It will be organised in ten main sections. The topics covered include:

- The transition from international to global health
- Structural inequalities and global public health
- Ecological transformation and environmental health in the global system
- Population and reproductive health
- Conflict, violence and emergencies in global public health
- Global public health policy and practice
- Global public health and development
- Global mental health
- Global access to essential medicines
- Health systems, health capacity, and the politics of global public health.

This comprehensive handbook will provide an authoritative overview for students, practitioners, researchers, and policy makers working in or concerned with public health around the globe.

Richard Parker is Professor of Sociomedical Sciences and Anthropology in the Mailman School of Public Health at Columbia University in New York City, USA. He is also Director and President of the Brazilian Interdisciplinary AIDS Association (ABIA) in Rio de Janeiro, Brazil. He is the Editor-in-Chief of *Global Public Health* journal.

Marni Sommer is Assistant Professor of Sociomedical Sciences (SMS) and Director of the SMS Global Health Track in the Mailman School of Public Health at Columbia University. She is the Executive Editor of *Global Public Health* journal.

Routledge Handbook of Global Public Health

*Edited by Richard Parker
and Marni Sommer*

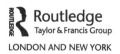

LONDON AND NEW YORK

First published 2011
by Routledge
2 Park Square, Milton Park, Abingdon, Oxfordshire OX14 4RN

Simultaneously published in the USA and Canada
by Routledge
711 Third Avenue, New York, NY 10017

Routledge is an imprint of the Taylor & Francis Group, an informa business

First issued in paperback 2012

Typeset in Goudy by Integra Software Services Pvt. Ltd, Pondicherry, India

British Library Cataloguing in Publication Data
A catalogue record for this book is available from the British Library

Library of Congress Cataloging in Publication Data
Routledge handbook of global public health / edited by Richard Parker and
Marni Sommer.
p. ; cm.
Other title: Handbook of global public health
Includes bibliographical references.
1. World health. 2. Public health. 3. International cooperation. I. Parker,
Richard G. (Richard Guy), 1956– II. Sommer, Marni. III. Title: Handbook
of global public health.
[DNLM: 1. Public Health. 2. World Health. 3. Health Policy. 4. International
Cooperation. WA 530.1]
RA441.R68 2011
362.1--dc22
2010029915

ISBN 13: 978-0-415-77848-0 (hbk)
ISBN 13: 978-0-415-81889-6 (pbk)
ISBN 13: 978-0-203-83272-1 (ebk)

Dedicated to the memory of Allan Rosenfield

Contents

Contents

PART V
Conflict, Violence, and Emergencies in Global
Public Health   227

PART VI
Global Public Health Policy and Practice   273

Contents

PART VII
Global Public Health and Development   **327**

PART VIII
Global Mental Health   **383**

List of figures and tables

Figures

Tables

Notes on contributors

Grace Adeya is a Senior Technical Manager for Maternal and Child Health for the Management Sciences for Health (MSH) Strengthening Pharmaceutical Systems (SPS) Program, USA.

Alastair Ager is Professor of Clinical Population and Family Health and Executive Director of the Global Health Initiative in the Mailman School of Public Health, Columbia University, USA.

Jill Astbury is Adjunct Principal Research Fellow in the School of Psychology and Psychiatry, Faculty of Medicine, Nursing and Health Sciences, Monash University, Australia.

José Ricardo Ayres is Professor of Preventive Medicine in the School of Medicine at the University of São Paulo, Brazil and frequently consults for the Brazilian Ministry of Health and the São Paulo State Health Department.

Florence Baingana is a psychiatrist working as a Research Fellow at Makerere University School of Public Health, Uganda, and the London School of Economics, UK. She previously worked as National Mental Health Coordinator with the Ugandan Ministry of Health and helped establish the Mental Health Unit.

Gary Barker is Director of the Gender, Rights and Violence portfolio at the International Center for Research on Women (ICRW), USA. Prior to joining ICRW, he was the founding Executive Director of Instituto Promundo, and is Co-Chair and Co-Founder of MenEngage, a global alliance of NGOs and UN agencies working to engage men and boys in gender equality.

Angela Beaton is a Research Fellow (Health Policy) and Ian Potter Fellow at the Menzies Centre for Health Policy, Sydney School of Public Health at the University of Sydney, Australia.

Sara Bennett is Associate Professor in the Health Systems Program of the International Health Department at the Johns Hopkins Bloomberg School of Public Health, USA.

Chantal Berger is project officer for capacity building at the Global Health Programme, Graduate Institute, Switzerland.

Jane T. Bertrand is Chair of the Department of Health Systems Management at Tulane University School of Public Health and Tropical Medicine, USA. Prior to this, Dr Bertrand was the Director of the Center for Communication Programs at the Johns Hopkins Bloomberg School of Public Health.

Neil Boothby is the Allan Rosenfield Professor of Clinical Forced Migration and Health at the Mailman School of Public Health, Columbia University, USA.

Jane Briggs is a Senior Program Associate for the Management Sciences for Health (MSH) Strengthening Pharmaceutical Systems (SPS) Program based in Guatemala.

Theodore M. Brown is Professor of History and of Community and Preventive Medicine and Medical Humanities at the University of Rochester, USA.

Gene Bukhman is Director of the Program in Non-Communicable Disease and Social Change at Harvard Medical School and the Chief of Cardiology for Partners in Health (PIH), USA.

Josh Busby is Assistant Professor of Public Affairs at the Lyndon B. Johnson School of Public Affairs and a Fellow in the RGK Center for Philanthropy and Community Service, as well as a Crook Distinguished Scholar at the Robert S. Strauss Center for International Security and Law, USA.

Colin D. Butler is Associate Professor at the National Centre for Epidemiology and Population Health, Australian National University, Australia.

Jacquelyn Campbell is the Anna D. Wolf Chair and Professor in the Johns Hopkins University School of Nursing, with a joint appointment in the Johns Hopkins Bloomberg School of Public Health, USA.

Fernando Chacón is Director General of Planning and Budgeting at the Ministry of Health of Mexico, Mexico.

Sarah Clement is a research psychologist and health services researcher at the Institute of Psychiatry, King's College London, UK.

Ruth Colagiuri is the Director of the Health and Sustainability Unit, Menzies Centre for Health Policy and an Associate Professor in the School of Public Health at the University of Sydney, Australia.

Anthony Costello is Professor of International Child Health and Head of the University College London (UCL) Centre for International Health and Development, and is the Director of the UCL Institute for Global Health, UK.

Joanne Csete is Associate Professor of Clinical Population and Family Health at the Mailman School of Public Health, Columbia University, USA.

Marcos Cueto is Director of the Institute of Peruvian Studies and a Professor of Sociomedical Sciences at the School of Public Health at the Peruana Cayetano Heredia University in Lima, Peru.

Haile T. Debas is Executive Director of Global Health Sciences at the University of California, San Francisco (UCSF), and founding Director of the University of California-wide Global Health

Institute. At UCSF, he served as Dean of Medicine, Vice Chancellor for Medical Affairs, and Chancellor.

Rebecca Dodd is a technical officer for Health Policy and Systems Research in the Western Pacific Regional Office of the World Health Organization, Philippines.

Andrew Ellner is Associate Physician in the Division of Global Health Equity at Brigham and Women's Hospital, an Instructor in Medicine at Harvard Medical School, and a faculty member of the Global Health Delivery Project, USA.

Martha Embrey is Senior Technical Writer for the Management Sciences for Health (MSH) Center for Pharmaceutical Management (CPM), USA.

Sara Evans-Lacko is a Postdoctoral Research Fellow at the Institute of Psychiatry, King's College London, UK.

Alex C. Ezeh is Executive Director of the African Population and Health Research Centre (APHRC) and Honorary Professor of Public Health at the University of the Witwatersrand, South Africa. Dr Ezeh is also the Director of the Consortium for Advanced Research Training in Africa (CARTA), Kenya.

Paul Farmer is the Presley Professor of Social Medicine and Chair of the Department of Global Health and Social Medicine at Harvard Medical School, Chief of the Division of Global Health Equity at Brigham and Women's Hospital, and the United Nations Deputy Special Envoy for Haiti, under Special Envoy Bill Clinton. He is a founding Director of Partners in Health (PIH), USA.

Laura Ferguson is Research Manager for the Program on International Health and Human Rights at the Harvard School of Public Health, USA.

Ivan França Jr. is Professor of Maternal and Child Health in the School of Public Health at the University of São Paulo, Brazil.

Maria C. Freire is President of the Albert and Mary Lasker Foundation, USA.

Julio Frenk is Dean of the Faculty at the Harvard School of Public Health and T & G Angelopoulos Professor of Public Health and International Development at the Harvard Kennedy School of Government, USA. He served as the Minister of Health of Mexico from 2000 to 2006 and was the founding Director-General of the National Institute of Public Health in Mexico.

Linda P. Fried is Dean and DeLamar Professor of the Mailman School of Public Health, Columbia University, and Professor of Epidemiology and Medicine, and Senior Vice President of Columbia University Medical Center, USA.

Sharon Friel is a Fellow at the National Centre for Epidemiology and Population Health at the Australian National University, and Principal Research Fellow at the Department of Epidemiology and Public Health at University College London, UK.

Laura J. Frost is Co-Founder and partner of Global Health Insights, USA.

Nancy Glass is Associate Professor in the Department of Community Public Health at the Johns Hopkins University School of Nursing and Associate Director of the Johns Hopkins Center for Global Health.

Octavio Gómez-Dantés, a physician, is a researcher at the Centre for Health Systems Research at the National Institute of Public Health of Mexico, and was previously Director General for performance evaluation at the Ministry of Health in Mexico.

Henry Greenberg is Associate Professor of Clinical Medicine at the College of Physicians and Surgeons and the Associate Director of Cardiology at St Luke's Roosevelt Hospital, USA.

Margaret E. Greene has worked at the Population Council, the Center for Health and Gender Equity and the International Center for Research on Women. She is Vice Chair of the Board of Advocates for Youth and Secretary of the Board of the Willows Foundation in Turkey.

Sofia Gruskin is Director of the Program on International Health and Human Rights and Associate Professor in the Department of Global Health and Population at the Harvard School of Public Health, USA, and is an Associate Editor for the *American Journal of Public Health*, *Global Public Health*, and *Reproductive Health Matters*.

Liz Hanna is a Fellow at the Centre for Epidemiology and Population Health at the Australian National University, and a Senior Research Fellow for the Climate Change Adaptation Research Network for Emergency Management hosted by the Royal Melbourne Institute of Technology, Australia.

Chris Holden is Lecturer in International and Comparative Social Policy at the University of York, UK.

Tanja A.J. Houweling is a Senior Research Associate at the University College London (UCL) Centre for International Health and Development, UK.

Rachel Jewkes is Director of the Medical Research Council Gender & Health Unit in Pretoria, South Africa.

Caroline W. Kabiru is Associate Research Scientist at the African Population and Health Research Centre (APHRC), Kenya.

Adam Kamradt-Scott is a Research Fellow in the Department of Global Health and Development at the London School of Hygiene & Tropical Medicine, UK.

Ethan B. Kapstein is Dennis O'Connor Regent's Professor of Business and Tom Slick Professor of International Affairs at the University of Texas, Austin, USA, and a Visiting Fellow at the Center for Global Development.

Gerald T. Keusch is Professor of International Health and Senior Advisor to the Center for Global Health and Development at Boston University School of Public Health, USA, and previously served as the Associate Director for International Research, and Director of the Fogarty International Center at the National Institutes of Health.

Ilona Kickbusch is Director of the Global Health Programme at the Graduate Institute of International and Development Studies in Geneva, Switzerland.

Mirja Koschorke is a psychiatrist and Wellcome Trust Clinical Research Fellow at the London School of Hygiene & Tropical Medicine, UK.

Margaret E. Kruk is Assistant Professor in Health Policy and Management at the Mailman School of Public Health, Columbia University, USA.

Ronald Labonté holds the Canada Research Chair in Globalization and Health Equity at the Institute of Population Health, Canada. He is Professor in the Faculty of Medicine at University of Ottawa, and Adjunct Professor at the Department of Community Health and Epidemiology, University of Saskatchewan, Canada.

Anne Langston is Health Coordinator for the International Rescue Committee (IRC), Rwanda.

Paul Lartey is President and CEO of LaGray Chemical Company, the first fully vertically integrated pharmaceutical manufacturer in West Africa and recipient of the 2009 African Excellence award in pharmaceutical innovation, Ghana.

Katie Leach-Kemon is one of the lead researchers on the Institute for Health Metrics and Evaluation's (IHME) annual global health financing report and has contributed to IHME's research on public financing of health in developing countries, USA.

Kelley Lee is Co-Director of the Centre on Global Change and Health at the London School of Hygiene & Tropical Medicine, UK. She has chaired the WHO Scientific Resource Group on Globalisation, Trade and Health, and co-chairs the health study group of the S. T. Lee Project on Asian Contributions to Global Governance based at the National University of Singapore.

Stephen Leeder is Professor of Public Health and Community Medicine at the University of Sydney and Director of the Menzies Centre for Health Policy, Australia.

Peter G. McCornick is Director for Water at the Nicholas Institute at Duke University, USA.

Therese McGinn is Associate Professor of Clinical Population and Family Health and the Director of the Reproductive Health Access, Information and Services in Emergencies (RAISE) Initiative at the Mailman School of Public Health, Columbia University, USA.

Anthony J. McMichael is Professor of Population Health at the Australian National University, currently holds an Australia Fellowship from the National Health and Medical Research Council, is Honorary Professor in Climate Change and Human Health at the University of Copenhagen, and is an Honorary Fellow of the London School of Hygiene & Tropical Medicine, UK.

Michael Marmot is Director of the International Institute for Society and Health and MRC Research Professor of Epidemiology and Public Health at University College London (UCL), UK. He chaired the Commission on Social Determinants of Health set up by the World Health Organization as well as the Strategic Review of Health Inequalities in England Post 2010 (Marmot Review).

Malebona Precious Matsoso is Director in Public Health Innovation and Intellectual Property (PHI) in the office of the Director General of the World Health Organization, Switzerland.

Ushma Mehta is on the Medicine Control Council at the National Adverse Drug Event Monitoring Centre at the University of Cape Town, South Africa.

Alice Payne Merritt is the Director of Global Programs, Center for Communication Programs at the Johns Hopkins Bloomberg School of Public Health, USA.

Marie Lynn Miranda is Associate Professor at Duke University in the Nicholas School of the Environment and the Department of Pediatrics and a member of the Integrated Toxicology and Environmental Health Program faculty and the Duke Global Health Institute faculty. She is the founding director of the Children's Environmental Health Initiative (CEHI) at Duke University, USA.

Eric Olawolu Moore is Director of Public Health at the Town of Winthrop, Massachusetts, USA.

Peter Muennig is Assistant Professor of Health Policy and Management at the Mailman School of Public Health, Columbia University, USA.

Jeffrey D. Mulvihill is an intern in the Department of Global Health Sciences at the University of California, San Francisco, USA.

Christopher J.L. Murray is Institute Director of the Institute for Health Metrics and Evaluation (IHME) and Professor of *Global Health* at the University of Washington, USA.

Marion Nestle is Paulette Goddard Professor in the Department of Nutrition, Food Studies, and Public Health at New York University, USA.

Veronica Njie-Carr is currently a Postdoctoral Fellow at the Johns Hopkins University School of Nursing, USA.

David Ofori-Adjei is a Professor at the University of Ghana Medical School, the former Director of the Noguchi Memorial Institute for Medical Research, Ghana, and Co-Founder of the International Network for the Rational Use of Drugs (INRUD).

David Osrin is a Wellcome Trust Fellow at the University College London (UCL) Centre for International Health and Development, UK.

Piroska Östlin is Adviser on Social Determinants of Health at the WHO Regional Office for Europe, and an Associate Professor in Public Health at the Karolinska Institutet, Sweden.

Vera Paiva is Professor of Social Psychology in the Institute of Psychology at the University of São Paulo, Brazil.

Richard Parker is Professor of Sociomedical Sciences and Director of the Center for Gender, Sexuality and Health in the Mailman School of Public Health at Columbia University, USA. He is the Editor-in-Chief of *Global Public Health*. In addition to his academic work, Dr Parker is Director and President of the Brazilian Interdisciplinary AIDS Association (ABIA), and Co-Chair of Sexuality Policy Watch (SPW).

John Pasch is a specialist in Water Resources Management and International Development, and engineer with the United States Agency for International Development (USAID), currently assigned to Cairo, Egypt.

Vikram Patel is Professor of International Mental Health and a Wellcome Trust Senior Clinical Research Fellow at the London School of Hygiene & Tropical Medicine, UK.

Christopher J. Paul is an Associate in Research at the Children's Environmental Health Initiative at Duke University, USA.

Martin Prince is Professor of Epidemiological Psychiatry at King's College London and Co-Director of the King's Health Partners/London School of Hygiene and Tropical Medicine Centre for Global Mental Health, UK.

Susan Purdin is Deputy Health Director of the International Rescue Committee (IRC), USA.

Jonathan D. Quick is President and CEO of Management Sciences for Health (MSH), USA. He was Director of Essential Drugs and Medicines Policy at the World Health Organization from 1996 to 2004.

Sharon A. Rachel is a Health Educator and Program Manager at the Centre of Excellence for Sexual Health in the Satcher Health Leadership Institute at Morehouse School of Medicine, USA.

Nirmala Ravishankar is an Associate Scientist at Abt Associates Inc, working in the areas of health resource tracking, monitoring and evaluation, and health governance.

Susan Raymond is Executive Vice President for Research, Evaluation, and Strategic Planning for Changing Our World, USA. She also serves as Chief Analyst for www.onPhilanthropy.com.

Michael R. Reich is the Taro Takemi Professor of International Health Policy at the Harvard School of Public Health, USA.

Nicolas Rüsch works as a consultant in General Adult Psychiatry and Research Fellow at the Department of Social Psychiatry, University of Zürich, Switzerland.

Gary Saffitz is Advocacy Manager at the Global Alliance for Improved Nutrition, USA.

Jonathan M. Samet is Professor and Flora L. Thornton Chair of the Department of Preventive Medicine at the Keck School of Medicine, as well as Director of the Institute for Global Health at the University of Southern California, USA.

David Satcher is Director of the Satcher Health Leadership Institute and the Centre of Excellence on Health Disparities at Morehouse School of Medicine, USA. He served as the 16th Surgeon General of the United States from 1998 to 2002, and as the Director of the Centers for Disease Control and Prevention and Administrator of the Agency for Toxic Substances and Disease Registry from 1993 to 1998.

Gita Sen is Professor of Public Policy at the Indian Institute of Management in Bangalore (IIMB), India, and Adjunct Professor of Global Health and Population, Harvard School of Public Health, USA. She was Co-Coordinator of the Knowledge Network on Women and Gender Equity for the WHO Commission on Social Determinants of Health.

Merrill Singer is Professor in the Department of Anthropology and a Senior Research Scientist at the Center for Health, Intervention and Prevention at the University of Connecticut, USA.

Alfred Sommer is Professor of Epidemiology, International Health, and Ophthalmology at Johns Hopkins University, USA, and Dean Emeritus of the Johns Hopkins Bloomberg School of Public Health, USA.

Marni Sommer is Assistant Professor of Sociomedical Sciences (SMS) and Director of the SMS Global Health Track at the Mailman School of Public Health, Columbia University, USA. She is also the Executive Editor for *Global Public Health*.

Celina Su is Associate Professor of Political Science at Brooklyn College of the City University of New York, USA.

Fatima Suleman is Head of the School of Pharmacy and Pharmacology at the University of KwaZulu-Natal in Durban, South Africa.

Daniel Tarantola is Professor of Health and Human Rights at the Faculty of Medicine of the University of New South Wales, Sydney, Australia.

Terri-Ann Thompson is a doctoral candidate in Reproductive, Perinatal and Women's Health at the Johns Hopkins Bloomberg School of Public Health, USA.

Graham Thornicroft is Professor of Community Psychiatry, and Head of the Health Services and Population Research Department at the Institute of Psychiatry, King's College London. He is Director of Research and Development at the South London and Maudsley NHS Foundation Trust, UK.

Chi-Chi Undie is an Associate in the Reproductive Health Services and Research program of the Population Council in Nairobi, Kenya.

Avner Vengosh is Professor of Earth and Ocean Sciences at Duke University, USA.

Ronald J. Waldman is Professor of Clinical Population and Family Health at the Mailman School of Public Health and Pandemic Preparedness/Humanitarian Response Team Leader in the Avian Influenza and other Emerging Threats Program of the United States Agency for International Development (USAID).

Erika Weinthal is Associate Professor of Environmental Policy at the Nicholas School of the Environment at Duke University, USA.

Heather Wipfli is Assistant Professor in Preventive Medicine and International Relations at the University of Southern California (USC) and the Associate Director of the USC Institute for Global Health, USA.

Ashley Wolfington is Reproductive Health Program Manager at the International Rescue Committee (IRC), USA.

Abdo Yazbeck is a Manager at the World Bank and a lead health economist, USA.

Helen Young is Research Director at the Feinstein International Center and a Professor at the Friedman School of Nutrition Science and Policy at Tufts University, USA.

Acknowledgements

The editors would particularly like to thank Margaret Bradley, who greatly assisted in preparing the manuscripts for publication, and Dulce Natividad and Alana Kolundzija at the Mailman School of Public Health, Columbia University, who liaised with contributors and assisted with related administrative support.

They would also like to thank:

Elsevier, for permission to reprint parts of 'Applying an Equity Lens to Child Health and Mortality: More of the Same is Not Enough' (2003) by C. Victora, A. Wagstaff, J. Schellenberg, D. Gwatkin, M. Claeson and J. Jabicht, *The Lancet*, 362/9387, 916–917.

Springer, for permission to reprint parts of 'Socioeconomic Inequalities in Diabetes Mellitus Across Europe at the Beginning of the 21st Century, (2008) by A. Espelt, *Diabetologia*, 51/11, 1971–1979.

American Public Health Association, for permission to reprint parts of 'The Widening Gap in Mortality by Educational Level in the Russian Federation' (2006) by M. Murphy, M. Bobak, A. Nicholson, R. Rose and M. Marmot, *American Journal of Public Health*, 96/7, 1293–1299.

Elsevier, for permission to reprint parts of 'The Role of Welfare State Principles and Generosity in Social Policy Programmes for Public health: An International Comparative Study' (2008) by O. Lundberg, M. Yngwe, M. Stjärne, J. Elstad, T. Ferrarini, O. Kangas, T. Norström, J. Palme and J. Fritzell, *The Lancet*, 372/9650, 1633–1640.

World Health Organization, for permission to reprint parts of 'Physical Status: The Use and Interpretation of Anthropometry (1995) by Expert Committee', from the *WHO Technical Report Series 854*.

World Health Organization, for permission to reprint the figure 'Age-standardized Death Rates from Chronic Disease for 2005 among Adults aged 30–69' (2005) from the report *Preventing Chronic Diseases: A Vital Investment*, available at: http://www.who.int/chp/chronic_disease_report/en/index.html.

World Health Organization, for permission to reprint the figure 'Median price (US$) of first-line antiretroviral drug regimens in low-income countries, 2004–2007' (2008) from the report *Towards Universal Access: Scaling up priority HIV/AIDS interventions in the health sector*, available online at http://www.who.int/hiv/pub/2008progressreport/en/.

World Health Organization, for permission to reprint the figure 'Non-communicable disease mortality among young adults. Age-standardized death rates from chronic disease for 2005 among adults aged 30–69' (2005) from the report *Preventing Chronic Diseases: a vital investment*, available online at http://www.who.int/chp/chronic_disease_report/en/index.html.

The Institute of Tropical Medicine, for permission to reprint the figure 'Dual pendulum swings of global health' by G. Ooms and J. Wenseleers.

Elsevier, for permission to reprint parts of 'Financing of Global Health: Tracking Development Assistance for Health from 1990 to 2007' (2009) by N. Ravishankar, P. Gubbins, R. Cooley, K. Leach-Kemon, C. Michaud, D. Jamison and C. Murray, *The Lancet*, 373, 9681, 2113–2124.

World Health Organization, for permission to reprint the figure 'Health Systems' (2007) from the report *Everybody's business: Strengthening health systems to improve health outcomes: WHO's framework for action*, Section 2, Page 3, available online at http://www.who.int/healthsystems/strategy/everybodys_business.pdf.

World Health Organization, for permission to reprint the figure 'WHO Framework for Equitable Access to Essential Medicines' (2004) from *Equitable Access to Essential Medicines: a Framework for Collective Action, WHO Policy Perspectives on Medicines Number 8*.

Organization for Economic Co-operation and Development, for permission to reprint the figure 'Aid Effectiveness Principles' (2005) from the *Development Co-operation Report* available online at http://masetto.sourceoecd.org/rpsv/dac05/.

1

Introduction

Richard Parker and Marni Sommer

At the beginning of the twenty-first century, key public health issues and challenges have taken centre stage on the global scene. Ranging from arsenic in drinking water to asthma among children and adults; from the re-emergence of cholera and diphtheria, to increasing rates of various forms of cancer; from HIV and AIDS to MDR-TB, malaria, and hepatitis; from the crises faced by displaced or refugee populations to the new challenges that have emerged for reproductive health and rights; from the experience of public health emergencies as the result of disasters such as tsunamis, earthquakes, and catastrophic storms to the growing spectre of potential global pandemics such as those linked to H5N1. The expansion of serious public health problems, increasingly taking shape on a global scale, has been one of the defining features of recent history.

Like most aspects of contemporary life, the range of key public health problems faced by specific countries has increasingly been affected by a range of factors associated with globalisation. The issues that confront us presently have been, and are being, shaped by evolving processes such as the growth of inequalities between the rich and the poor in countries around the world, the globalisation of trade and commerce, new patterns of travel and migration, as well as a significant reduction in available resources for the development and sustainability of public health infrastructures. The social, cultural, economic, and political transformations associated with globalisation have, in turn, increasingly intersected with the growing range of environmental threats produced by industrialisation, epidemics of newly emerging infectious diseases, and the rapid increase of chronic diseases linked to changing lifestyles.

The new public health challenges of the twenty-first century have taken place within the context of a rapidly changing political and institutional landscape. In recent decades the field that was initially described as *international health* involving sovereign states has increasingly been re-conceptualised as the field of *global health* within the global system. This change represents more than a simple shift in language. It stems from a fundamental transformation in the nature of health threats and in the kinds of solutions that must be posed to them. It recognises that many of the most serious health threats facing the world community today reach beyond the sovereign borders of nation-states and require the attention not only of governments but also of a range of non-state institutions and actors.

Just as we have witnessed remarkable changes in recent decades in the nature of the public health problems that challenge us globally, we have also witnessed an unprecedented period of growth in the field that has come to be known as *global health*. As is reported in a number of the contributions to this volume, there has been a massive increase in development assistance for health over the course of the past two years. A field once largely dominated by the agencies of the UN system and bilateral donor agencies in high-income countries has seen significant reorganisation with the entrance and rising importance of a growing range of new non-state or hybrid public/private agencies such as the Global Fund to Fight AIDS, Tuberculosis and Malaria (GFATM), the Global Alliance for Vaccines and Immunisation (GAVI), the Bill & Melinda Gates Foundation, and a wide range of international non-governmental organisations (NGOs). Multilateral institutions, bilateral agencies, private foundations, and universities and research institutes around the world have announced and begun to implement large-scale global health initiatives. These changes have been reflected, as well, on college and university campuses, where epidemiology, public health policy, and, in particular, global health have become among the fastest growing undergraduate and graduate courses of study for what has been described as the global generation.

As in any field undergoing such rapid and transformative change, the pace of events and the implementation of new initiatives often threaten to move more quickly than the capacity of the field to reflect upon its most basic assumptions, and to reorganise itself in order to provide the conceptual and structural foundations for its continued development. In the case of global health, key questions have emerged about the ways in which global transformations have affected the changing patterns of communicable and non-communicable disease (both North and South), about the impact of global inequalities on the social determinants of health and disease, about unresolved conflicts and contradictions in global health governance structures, and about the probable outcome and possible response to major environmental shifts such as global climate change, as well as to major economic events such as the global financial crisis. In turn, these questions have been linked to important, but largely unresolved, debates about both the possibilities and the potential limitations of technological advances aimed at confronting global health challenges and about the need for far-reaching changes to strengthen health systems and reorganise models of development cooperation to more effectively address global health priorities in the future. The very definition of *global health*, and the unique role of *public health* within this rapidly changing field, have both been questions that have been the focus of much recent attention and debate. The challenge of developing a vision for this field that will truly reflect the true extent of global diversity – inclusive as much of the voices and views of experts and policymakers from the global South as it is of those from the global North – continues as one of the key unmet objectives for a field that is still very much in a process of formation and transformation.

Within such a context, there is an increasingly urgent need to respond to these important questions and controversies by opening up new opportunities for meaningful intellectual dialogue, debate, and exchange about the key questions and challenges that currently confront the field of global health, and for critical reflection and increased awareness concerning the kinds of contributions that public health and population sciences can offer in relation to these challenges. This *Handbook* has emerged and taken shape within this context, and seeks to address both the emerging issues and conceptualisations of the notion of global public health, along with expanding upon and highlighting the critical priorities in this rapidly evolving field. While it has been developed with the goal of raising issues that are of importance for the field of global health broadly defined, it also prioritises an understanding of the special contributions that public health and population sciences can make within this field – an emphasis that we have sought to make explicit in choosing the title of the *Routledge Handbook of Global Public Health*. It seeks to offer in one location a broad introduction to key experts, key material, and key debates. All of the chapters take the form of original contributions, although a small number have been adapted in abridged form from elsewhere. Our goal is to offer readers a rich under-standing of the field of global public health, tracing the origins of big debates, describing the current state of play in particular fields, and hinting at where the future might be heading. The *Handbook* thus seeks to provide an authoritative overview for students, practitioners, research-ers, and policymakers working in or concerned with public health around the globe. It is organised into ten main sections (Parts I to X), which by no means exhaust the possible topics in such a vast field, but which do seek to map out some of the important areas of analysis and debate that are currently the focus of much of the most important attention in the field. In this Introduction to the volume, we will try to briefly describe the contents of each of these major sections, and to offer a sense of why these discussions are so central to the evolving field of global public health.

Part I of the *Handbook*, 'The Transition from International Health to Global Health', includes chapters about a number of the pioneering institutions and individuals in international health, with a key focus on exploring the conceptual transition to global health. It emphasises early efforts to build the field of international health, as well as more recent critique on the limited nature of conceiving health as international, rather than as operating within the global system. Contributions in this section explore the ways in which institutional structures, policies, and programmes have been shaped by broader social, economic, and political forces, and highlight the changing institutional architecture of the field as a growing range of intergovernmental agencies have become increasingly involved in health-related issues, and as the evolving field of global health has also become populated by private organisations and new hybrid public-private initiatives. They focus on the extent to which the major health issues confronting low-income countries are embedded in the global economic policies and practices that are articulated and controlled by wealthier countries, and describe the ways in which global health challenges have been framed through such policies in relation to health and security, health and development, health and global public goods, health and trade, health and human rights, and health and ethical reasoning.

Part II of the *Handbook*, 'Structural Inequalities and Global Public Health', examines the social patterning of health, including social exclusion, health disparities, and inequalities. Chapters in this section focus on the unequal distribution of power in society and its implications for the social determinants and the social distribution of health. They explore diverse strategies for eliminating inequities and disparities in health based on structural factors, including class, race and ethnicity, and gender, among other axes of inequality. They discuss the shift from public health approaches focused on behaviour change and individual agency, to the importance of utilising a structural approach in exploring public health challenges and devising realistic interventions for improving population health. Contributors emphasise the complex relationship that exists between diverse forms of power and the social distribution of health, highlighting the ways in which social exclusions translate into health disparities. They call our attention to the need for a fundamental re-conceptualisation in public health, in particular through a shift from a focus on what has been described as 'the natural history of disease' to a new emphasis on the 'social dimensions of vulnerability'. They offer key insights into the ways in which social transformations and the empowerment of disenfranchised communities and populations might be able to transform existing health inequalities – while also highlighting the very different conceptual and programmatic approaches that currently exist within global public health for how best to achieve such transformations. In different ways, all the chapters in this section of the *Handbook* thus call attention to the extent to which the most important challenges in the field of global public health are not merely technical but fundamentally political in nature, and highlight how the transformation of health systems will ultimately be possible only through the transformation of broader social, political, and economic systems that shape and determine health in highly specific ways.

Part III of the *Handbook*, 'Ecological Transformation and Environmental Health in the Global System', focuses on the transformative nature of the interactions occurring around the globe between populations and the environment, with significant ramifications for population health. The chapters in this section discuss the social dimensions of environmental health, including the long-term impact of climate change, the challenges of water and air pollution, and the synergy between environmental devastation and other health issues. The discussions here focus on the human-driven aspects of climate change and its profound implications for population health. Highlighting the ways in which rapid economic growth, if continuing to be driven by the burning of fossil fuels, will contribute to increasingly adverse health consequences, this analysis points to the need for more accelerated policy making linked to the actual rate of climate change occurrences. Climate-related health impacts discussed include those linked to temperature-related illness, extreme weather and sea level rise, air pollution, food security, and social upheaval. A full awareness of these issues highlights the need for public health alongside of responses from national governments, as well as an overdue linkage to be made in climate change advocacy – one that links the important relationship between climate change and health impacts. The chapters in this section also highlight the fragile nature of the world's existing water sources, and the potential responses to be utilised in protecting and managing the limited supply. Noting that as much as one-tenth of the global disease burden could be prevented by improving water supply, sanitation, hygiene, and management of water resources, they call attention to the importance of both quantity and quality of water supply, and the ways in which even water-scarce countries might be able to increase the availability of improved drinking water. They also focus on the interlinked nature of environmental factors and population health, such as the synergy that exists between vulnerable children's exposure to lead and their increased risk of morbidity and mortality from infectious disease, and the dangers of increasing air pollution for human health. Highlighting the challenges that exist in quantifying the health impacts of diverse forms of pollution, the analyses in this section also emphasise the need for increased public health attention to research and advocacy, in both high- and low-income countries.

Part IV of the *Handbook*, 'Population and Reproductive Health', examines the priority global health challenges in population studies, sexual and reproductive health and rights, and the health of young people, as well as the global challenges of ageing. The chapters in this section provide an overview of the important changes that have taken place in the field of population studies in recent decades, particularly through the process that led up to the International Conference on Population and Development (ICPD) held in Cairo in 1994 – and, in particular, the fundamental conceptual shift that took place as a field primarily focused on population control was gradually reinvented and reoriented to focus on reproductive health and reproductive rights. They highlight the impact of this transformation for the delivery of reproductive health services and for the diverse populations of women and men that must have access to these services. Within this broader context, the chapters highlight the importance of key areas that continue to be highly contested politically, such as the urgent priority of reducing death and disability from unsafe abortion, and the struggle to understand and confront challenges and barriers to recognising men and masculinity as important issues within reproductive health and public health more generally, highlighting the health risks that young men suffer in performing masculinities shaped by societal and cultural forces that make them vulnerable by virtue of their gender. Finally, this section emphasises the special vulnerability not only of children and young people, particularly in low-income countries and communities, but also the rapidly increasing populations of older adults even in resource-poor settings where ageing has not been considered a serious concern in the past. The concluding chapter in particular explores the implications of these major demographic changes for both country-specific and global public health approaches and solutions in the future.

Part V of the *Handbook*, 'Conflict, Violence, and Emergencies in Global Public Health', explores the current realities of conflict and health, including war, torture, civil disturbances, gender-based violence, and the public health challenges of displaced populations. Chapters in this section focus on the global dimensions of population-level violence, and the dispropor-tionate impact that violence has on the poor and disenfranchised within populations affected by conflict and disasters. They include an analysis of the ways in which armed conflict has changed in recent decades, and its implications for population health. Describing the emergence of humanitarian organisations over time, they emphasise that a disciplined public health response to post-conflict settings is a relatively recent development, and focus on the importance of developing public health responses within the often unstable political and social context of many countries. Also discussed is the global pervasiveness of violence against women; this challenge is examined within a human rights framework and an argument is made that such an approach is critical because of interrelated contextual factors (such as poverty and discrimination), which impact on women's lives and compound their vulnerability to violence. Related is an exploration of the need for protection of children as a population facing unique risks in conflict and post-conflict settings, with the presentation of eight fundamental elements of a framework for creating protected environments for vulnerable children, ranging from protective legislation and enforcement, to addressing relevant attitudes, traditions, customs, behaviours, and prac-tices. This section also presents a succinct guide to using nutritional indicators and reference levels in emergency-affected populations, and seeks to clarify a widely held myth that wars over water are imminent around the world, arguing that sub-national disputes over water are more the norm. It highlights challenges of access in relation to both nutrition and water deprivation in situations of conflict or emergency, emphasising the critical importance of addressing these issues, particularly in low-income countries where rapid population growth and urbanisation aggravate shortages caused by emergencies.

Part VI of the *Handbook*, 'Global Public Health Policy and Practice', focuses on the changing priorities in health policy within and between countries around the globe, with chapters addressing the crucial importance of global health diplomacy, and the roles of international agencies, governments, and civil society in fostering improved population health. It begins with an examination of what has come to be described as 'global health diplomacy', and emphasises that precisely because the trans-border health challenges that characterise the recent era of globalisation can only be resolved through joint action on the part of many countries working together, health more than many other fields has moved beyond the technical realm and is becoming a key element in foreign policy, trade relations, and security agreements between countries. The area of global health diplomacy recognises these tendencies and seeks to capture the multi-actor and multi-level negotiation processes that shape the global health policy environment and manage it through global governance systems. There is also an overview of the politics of global aid for development and health that examines the historical evolution of international aid efforts, particularly in relation to health and development. Chapters explore important trends and distinctions in relation to current patterns of international giving that are directly relevant for global public health policy and practice, as well as many of the key critiques that have been directed at dominant approaches to humanitarian assistance and development aid (and their impact, or lack of it, in relation to key global public health challenges). They also provide detailed case studies of two important areas of global public health policy: tobacco control and nutrition. They describe the process through which the WHO's Framework Convention on Tobacco Control (FCTC), a global public health treaty that seeks to incorporate best practices in terms of tobacco control, was developed and put into place, highlighting the extent to which the ongoing battle to control tobacco and the health impacts of smoking might provide a key case study offering insights that are relevant to global health diplomacy and global public health policy more broadly. The discussion of global nutrition includes a focus on the linkages between both undernutrition and overnutrition to poverty and economic exclusion, and signals the potential limitations of narrow technical solutions to the complex social, economic, and environmental challenges of global nutritional deprivation. This section also includes discussion of global health practice as well as policy, calling attention to the importance of health communication as a key to behaviour change aimed at reducing risk and vulnerability at both individual and population levels.

Part VII of the *Handbook*, 'Global Public Health and Development', examines the health effects of major economic development trends and the impact of key interventions aimed at responding to both long-term and emerging global health problems. It begins with a broad overview of the dramatic increase that has taken place in development assistance for health from 1990 to 2007. Following this overview, chapters provide detailed case studies of a number of key areas of intervention in global public health. The first focuses on addressing preventable blindness and visual impairment, and the strides that have been taken globally in combating cataract, trachoma, vitamin A deficiency, onchocerciasis, and other chronic causes of blindness, highlighting the ways in which visual impairment and economic development (or the lack of it) are intertwined globally. The next examines the importance of maternal and child survival for global health, highlighting the role of socio-economic inequalities in shaping both death rates and the success of interventions, providing an overview of the types of interventions that have been introduced to improve maternal and newborn survival, and giving attention to the importance of community-based interventions. The third case study outlines the emerging global crisis of chronic disease, highlighting the urgent need for action on what was once perceived to be a relatively low priority in resource-poor settings. This section also explores the challenges of creating access to health technologies in poor countries, emphasising that people's ability to obtain and use good-quality health technologies is far more than simply a technical issue involving the logistics of technology delivery. It focuses on the social values, economic interests, and political processes that influence access to technologies, and conceptualises access not as a single event but as a continuous process that involves a series of activities and actors over time.

Part VIII of the *Handbook*, 'Global Mental Health', explores the growing recognition of mental health as a significant health burden for populations in the global South as well as the global North. This section sounds a call for closing the global treatment gap in mental disorders. Chapters focus on the realities of populations living in low- and middle-income countries without adequate access to care and treatment for mental-health-related disorders. They highlight increasing evidence on the cost-effectiveness of many mental health interventions, and argue that increased investment in bringing such quality treatments to resource-poor settings is long overdue. Drawing on key case studies of the gap in mental health programmes in low- and middle-income countries, and emphasising the particular challenge of the human resources for health crisis, chapters in this section call attention to the fact that morbidity and mortality are not the only measures of relevance for a decision to increase investment in mental health services. They examine the ways in which mental disorders hinder individual and societal productivity, providing recommendations for integrating mental health into primary health care services, and the particular challenges to be addressed in conflict-affected settings, among others. They also highlight the unique importance of responding to sexual violence as a priority research area for global mental health, emphasising that the availability of quality health service interventions for women experiencing sexual violence remains inadequate, and underscoring the need for increased attention to this often overlooked contributor to women's poor mental health status globally.

Part IX of the *Handbook*, 'Global Access to Essential Medicines', focuses on the enormous challenge of ensuring that essential medicines are reaching populations around the globe, through improved pharmaceutical management systems, attention to counterfeit and poor quality drugs that are widespread within global and local markets, and the role of global powers in impacting the price and availability of medicines to populations in need. This section provides an introduction and overview to the field of global access to essential medicines. It reviews the early beginnings of pharmaceuticals, and the rise of the 'essential medicines' concept within the global health community, highlights the role of advocacy in widening access to essential medicines across the world, and emphasises the engagement of politicians, practitioners, international organisations, celebrities, and, most importantly, activists, in increasing access to AIDS medicines. While noting the enormous achievements in the provision of pharmaceuticals in the last 70 years, the analysis emphasises the significant challenges that remain, including a dearth of research and development for tropical diseases, unreliable supply systems in much of the world, and anti-microbial resistance. The chapters in this section take on different aspects of access to medicines, exploring the possibilities for local production of pharmaceuticals in improving access to medicines in low-income countries, and analysing current challenges in assuring medicine safety. They also focus on the unique essential medicine needs of children, highlighting the joint WHO and UNICEF approach to providing medicines to children, and emphasising the existing tools that public health has to improve childhood morbidity and mortality outcomes. This section of the *Handbook* also includes an analysis of the important impact of HIV treatment access campaigns, and the transformation of antiretroviral (ARV) medicines from 'private goods' – limited to the high-income world – into 'merit goods', thus stimulating action for universal access to treatment and transforming broader policy debates about access to essential medicines in resource-poor contexts.

Part X of the *Handbook*, 'Health Systems, Health Capacity, and the Politics of Global Public Health', examines the ongoing challenge of health system strengthening as well as the complicated politics of international development assistance in the changing context of the twenty-first century. It includes an historical overview, outlines current debates, looks at future challenges for health system strengthening in resource-poor settings, and highlights the ways in which dramatic increases in disease-specific funding, especially for HIV and AIDS, has placed huge pressures on weak health systems that in turn have made it impossible to reach the most ambitious goals of such initiatives. While the need for health system strengthening has increasingly become the focus of widespread agreement, there has been more disagreement about the means to achieve this objective, and about the most important challenges that will need to be addressed in the future as the existing problems of health systems in low-income countries are compounded by a range of issues such as globalisation, changes in technology, and the rise of chronic disease. This section also focuses on the increasing politicisation of aid for health and development. It argues that the field of global health is characterised by multiple inputs and agents – each with their own perspective and motivations. Ideological divisions in development discourse are typically played out in global public health policies, often resulting in major shifts in the health policies of large donors, just as non-state actors now have increasing power and influence, opening new possibilities for cooperation for the potential good of global public health. Some of these possibilities, such as public/private partnerships for drug development or other similar initiatives, offer an especially important set of opportunities with the potential to transform the field of global public health in profound ways. Yet significant hurdles also exist, and the chapters in this section of the *Handbook* also emphasise the difficulties of ensuring necessary financial resources and of sustaining commitment over time, as well as the complexities of building capacity, whether of researchers, health system personnel, policymakers, or advocates within a global public health system that continues to be characterised by serious inequities. They highlight dangers of unequal and unjust collaborative relations that accentuate the risks of 'brain drain' from the global South to the global North, and the continued inadequacy of resources, attention, and prioritisation of building strong health systems and cadres of effective health workers in the global South – as well as the role of long-term academic partnerships for building capacity and transferring technical expertise in resource-poor settings.

In bringing together the contributions that make up this *Handbook*, we have worked hard to ensure a text that will offer a scholarly yet accessible overview of the diverse and rapidly developing field of global public health today. In doing so, we have sought not to privilege any one particular perspective but rather to offer an up-to-date overview of the field. By describing past origins, present trends, and future possibilities, we want to offer readers insight into an area of work which has captured our own attention and imagination for many years now. We hope that you find this book helpful, and that it will be a useful source of reference for many years to come. We have selected the various contributions with a diverse readership in mind. Fundamentally, they aim to both describe and inform about the changing nature of global public health, along with advocating for new approaches to researching and addressing population health within the global system. Our hope is that the *Routledge Handbook of Global Public Health* will therefore appeal to a wide range of people working in health, human rights, and development, and that its potential readers will include trainee health professionals (including students in all fields of global public health), and graduates and undergraduates in the health-related social sciences, as well as public health educators, researchers, and policymakers. But we also hope that the book will appeal to activists, advocates, and practitioners around the globe who are working in the diverse fields of health policy, gender and health, sexual and reproductive health, infectious disease, environmental health, social work, and globalisation.

Part I

The Transition from International Health to Global Health

2

Global Health in Transition

Julio Frenk, Octavio Gómez-Dantés, and Fernando Chacón

Global health is experiencing a moment of unprecedented attention and expansion. Yet, despite its increasing importance, global health has developed in the absence of an academic tradition that can guide its efforts to generate knowledge and lead its practical applications. The purpose of this chapter is to present some ideas that may help build such a tradition on the basis of three elements (Frenk 1993): (1) a conceptual base, which serves to establish the limits of the specific areas for research, education, and action in global health; (2) a base for the production and reproduction of knowledge, which involves the creation of a critical mass of researchers, as well as academic initiatives, programmes, and institutions responsible for the generation of a body of specific knowledge and the construction of an intellectual field through the collaboration of several disciplines; and (3) a base for the utilisation of knowledge, which would translate evidence into technological developments, public policies, and global solidarity. The efforts to create an academic field for global health should respond to the interests of all countries, thus avoiding interpretations associated with a specific group of nations.

Conceptual base

Several definitions of global health have been proposed (Institute of Medicine 2008; Koplan *et al.* 2009; Fogarty International Center 2008). Some of them emphasise its object of analysis; others, its geographical focus; some others, its mission. However, as a field of public health, global health should be defined first of all by its population level of analysis (Frenk and Chacon 1991). Its distinctive feature is that it involves: the entire population of the world, along with the subjects of the international community, namely nations, with cultural and territorial identity; states, as the political organisations of these nations; and various bodies comprising multiple nations, such as economic and political blocs, multilateral organisations (public, private or mixed, profit or non-profit), and academic institutions charged with the production of knowledge-related global public goods.

These populations, as any population within a country, face health conditions for which social responses are developed. Thus, the concept of global health should include a component of global health conditions and a component of global health responses.

Global health conditions

The contents of the concept of global health needs should be distinguished from those traditionally attributed to 'international health' (Table 2.1). Coined around the creation of the International Health Commission in 1913 by the Rockefeller Foundation (Brown *et al.* 2006: 62), the term 'international health' was identified with the control of epidemics across borders and in sea ports, and with the health needs of poor countries, mostly communicable diseases, and maternal and child health (Godue 1992). In fact, before the creation of the International Health Commission, these activities were classified under the even more limited concept of 'tropical health', developed in Europe in the late nineteenth century, which has obvious colonial undertones (Wilkinson and Power 2008: 386).

The contents attributed to international health have been revitalised through the dissemination of the concept of 'global health'. In the media, in scientific literature, and in several of the main international health initiatives, global health is being identified with problems – respiratory infections, diarrhoeal diseases, HIV/AIDS, malaria, TB, maternal deaths – that are supposed to be characteristic of the developing world.

Global health, however, is not 'foreign health'. It should include those health conditions that affect most countries, regardless of their geographical position or stage of development, and should be centrally concerned with the distribution of those conditions around the world. Global health should not be identified with communicable diseases either. In the search for equity, public health professionals have disregarded a now well-documented reality: that *problems only of the poor*, like many common infections, malnutrition, and maternal deaths, are no longer the *only problems of the poor* (Frenk 2006). According to the WHO (2008), almost one-half of the disease burden in low- and middle-income countries is represented by non-communicable disorders. Salient among them are ischaemic heart disease, stroke, diabetes, and cancer.

In addition, the separation between communicable and non-communicable diseases is not as obvious as was once thought. Many diseases originally classified as non-communicable have been found to have an infectious cause. According to the WHO, one-fifth of all cancers worldwide are caused by chronic infections produced by agents such as the Epstein-Barr virus, human immunodeficiency virus, human papilloma virus, hepatitis B virus, and *Helicobacter pylori*. In addition, many non-communicable diseases or their treatments weaken the immune system, giving rise to associated infections that are often the precipitating cause of death. In

Table 2.1 Differences between international health and global health

Objects of analysis	International health	Global health
Health conditions	Health needs of poor nations, communicable diseases	Global transfer of health risks
	Dependence-oriented	Interdependence-oriented
	Unilateral	Bilateral and multilateral
Health responses	Technology-oriented	Considers behavioural, cultural, political, and economic determinants
	'Vertical' approach through disease-specific programmes	'Diagonal' approach to strengthen health systems through explicit priorities
	Assistance in health services	Cooperation in capacity strengthening
	Control of communicable diseases	Generation of public goods, management of externalities, and solidarity functions

sum, infectious diseases are not the exclusive domain of a primitive stage in the health transition, but rather a shifting component of every epidemiological pattern.

The concept that can best fit the notion of global health conditions is the 'global transfer of health risks', which occurs as a result of six basic processes: (1) the rise of global environmental threats; (2) the increasing movement of people; (3) the adoption of lifestyles; (4) the variance in environmental and occupational health and safety standards; (5) the trade in harmful legal and illegal products, and (6) the spread of medical technologies (Frenk *et al.* 1997: 1,405). At the heart of this concept lies the idea of the interdependence of the health of populations: the fact that many health problems spread mostly through processes created to support production, trade, and travel worldwide, and are common to developed and developing nations. Chen *et al.* (1996: 9) point to 'an era of global "health interdependence", the health parallel to economic interdependence'.

Global health response

As mentioned above, during most of the twentieth century, the actors of traditional international health – a few multilateral health organisations, a handful of international foundations, and the health branches of commercial and military institutions of developed nations – considered international health needs as alien and, very frequently, as threats. Consistent with these ideas, international health activities were identified as aid and defence, and implemented through unilateral perspectives.

International health activities were also influenced by the idea that health needs in developing countries could be fully addressed through technological interventions (Gómez-Dantés 2001). The corollary was the definition of health priorities in purely medical terms and the inclusion in the international health agenda of only those health challenges that seemed to lend themselves to technical solutions. This reflected the 1950s and 1960s conviction that Western science, technology, and managerial abilities could, on their own, transform the developing world (Tendler 1975). A similar approach is prevalent among various global health initiatives. According to Judith Rodin (2007), the temptation to pin all hope on the latest technology is every bit as powerful as it was in the near past. The new global health should recognise that most challenges have strong behavioural, cultural, political, and economic determinants, which demand comprehensive and not only technological, approaches.

International health also placed excessive emphasis on vertical programmes devoted to control specific diseases and paid limited attention to health systems. Disease-oriented programmes are again dominating the health arena. As Laurie Garret (2007: 23) puts it: 'HIV-positive mothers are given drugs to hold their infection at bay and prevent passage of the virus to their babies but still cannot obtain even the most rudimentary of obstetric and gynecological care or infant immunisations'. Furthermore, many of the patients that receive free antiretrovirals are cared for in clinics that have no physicians or nurses to guarantee their follow-up (Epstein and Chen 2002). We need 'magic bullets' it is true, but we also need 'magic guns' (Schellenberg 2005: 71), and those guns are health systems (Table 2.1).

The alternative, however, is not the classical 'horizontal' approach, which implies strengthening health systems without a clear sense of priorities, since in many developing countries this approach will end up catering mostly to the needs of the better off. The solution is a 'diagonal' approach, whereby explicit intervention priorities are used to drive improvements into the health system (Sepúlveda 2006: xv).

These priorities comprise all components of the *triple* burden of disease: first, the unfinished agenda of infections, malnutrition, and reproductive health problems; second, the emerging challenges represented by non-communicable diseases and injury; and third, the health risks associated with globalisation, including the threat of pandemics like HIV and influenza, the health consequences of climate change, and the trade in harmful products like tobacco and other drugs.

First of all, there is a need for stronger cooperation with those countries that are lagging in the attainment of the health-related Millennium Development Goals (MDGs). At the same time, a process must get started to enhance those goals by defining clear targets around the growing burden of non-communicable diseases and injury. In particular, obesity, diabetes, and cardiovascular diseases must be met head-on, or health systems in developing countries and economies in transition will be overwhelmed. Finally, surveillance and response capabilities must be enhanced everywhere so that each country is better prepared to meet global threats, while contributing to the international coordination necessary to deal with them.

Production and reproduction of knowledge

Having defined the conceptual foundations for the field of global health, it is necessary to develop the base for knowledge production (through research) and reproduction (through education). In accordance with the conceptual base, research and education must refer to the objects of analysis discussed earlier, namely, global health conditions and global health responses. Thus, the generation of knowledge and the education of human resources in this nascent field should focus on those conditions and interventions that go beyond country borders: the international transfer of health risks and the interventions designed to confront them.

The areas of application of global health include: (1) populations affected by global health problems (e.g., national populations affected by global health risks, migrants, displaced populations, victims of failed states, etc.); (2) problems related to the global transfer of health risks (pandemics, health impacts of global environmental threats, occupational health problems related to the exportation of occupational hazards, exportation of health products and services, etc.); and (3) national, bilateral, or multilateral interventions designed to deal with global health challenges (international epidemiological surveillance and response systems, programmes to prevent or control global health challenges, international occupational and environmental standards, etc.).

The comprehensiveness of global health problems and interventions requires the participation of the social sciences in this new academic field (Giovanni and Brownlee 1982). Among the social science disciplines, foreign relations and some related areas, such as political geography, international economy, and international law, should play major roles. It should be noted that this interdisciplinary collaboration represents a higher level of integration to the one already reached by public health, which brings together disciplines such as epidemiology, demography, biostatistics, life sciences, economics, sociology, administrative sciences, law, and ethics (Frenk *et al.* 1988).

Thus, global health becomes a meeting ground between the social sciences, including foreign relations, and the health sciences, especially those directly linked to public health. The body of knowledge and theoretical framework of foreign relations and its core disciplines provides the basis to explain the dynamics of the global society in relation to the economic, political, social, cultural, and ideological issues affecting the interactions among countries. Public health provides the theoretical, methodological, and technical elements to approach the study of the consequences of such interactions on the health status of the population, and on the organisation and functioning of health services.

Utilisation of knowledge

Knowledge produced through research must be translated into evidence that can then be utilised by global health actors to mobilise resources, formulate policy, implement programmes, develop advocacy activities, respond to natural or artificial disasters, and evaluate impact. The weakness of this utilisation base accounts for the knowledge-action gap in global health. In order to bridge such a gap, it is necessary to develop a better institutional architecture for global health based on the functions that each actor should perform.

The actors of global health now include, in addition to the specialised agencies and programmes of the United Nations system, multilateral development banks, bilateral aid agencies, international NGOs, multinational private corporations, academic institutions, philanthropic entities, and a set of novel public/private alliances resulting in 'quasi-multilateral' organisations, notably the Global Alliance for Vaccines and Immunisation and the Global Fund to Fight Aids, Tuberculosis and Malaria.

This increasing pluralism is a positive reflection of the growing importance of health in the global agenda. However, until now, the broad variety of actors has not been able to develop an effective global health system with the capacity for coordinated action. The identification of the essential functions of global health should help us determine 'who should do what' and what kind of institutional arrangements are needed to achieve the shared goal of better health for all.

In order to meet global health challenges, the members of the global health community should use the knowledge and evidence developed in this field to perform two major functions: (1) management of global public goods and externalities; and (2) mobilisation of global solidarity (Jamison *et al.* 1998).

The functions for which global health actors are better suited than any individual country are those related to the production of global public goods and the management of externalities that transcend national borders.

Salient among the public goods that global health organisations should produce are: databases, information, research, and comparative analyses that can generate evidence to inform national policies and stimulate a process of shared learning among countries; harmonised norms and standards for national use; and consensus-building on initiatives which can help mobilise political will within countries. The Alma-Ata Declaration and several efforts to control communicable diseases are good examples of the latter.

Actions against international externalities include epidemiological surveillance activities. These activities require warning systems to anticipate possible health crises, monitoring mechanisms to identify future needs, and efforts to control specific health challenges that spread across borders, from drug-resistant microbial threats to pandemics.

In addition to producing public goods and managing externalities, global collective action should mobilise solidarity with countries that have acute or chronic development needs, exhibit important capacity limitations, or house vulnerable populations. The broad concept of solidarity, which would seem to be a more enlightened and less asymmetrical term than 'aid', encompasses three major sub-functions: development financing, technical cooperation, and humanitarian assistance. In this last respect, human rights arguments dictate that the global community can become an agent for the dispossessed and act to protect certain populations in a variety of circumstances, as in the case of failed states that are chronically incapable of meeting the basic security needs of their own populations. A clear case for global solidarity occurs when public health preparedness in a country is insufficient or is overwhelmed by natural or artificial disasters.

Conclusions

Due to its links to security, sustainable development, and good governance, global health is occupying an increasingly visible space in the international agenda. This fact is associated with an expansion both of resources and initiatives directed to improve the health of populations worldwide. However, the large variation in the contents of these initiatives has created confusion as to what exactly the term 'global health' really means.

The efforts to define this term and establish the limits of the field that is being built around it have serious implications. First of all, they are crucial for those research centres interested in the production of knowledge on regional and global health problems, and on the interventions designed to confront them. Second, they are important to those academic institutions offering educational programmes in global health. Finally, they are vital for all bilateral, multilateral, and private organisations involved in activities that transcend national borders.

The gradual creation of a common language and an academic tradition for global health will undoubtedly help to mobilise additional resources, stimulate the production of new knowledge, improve educational programmes, clarify the functions and architecture of the global health system, generate consensus in the contents of the health agenda, determine the specific responsibilities of the actors of this field, and, most importantly, contribute to the improvement of the health of the world's population.

References

Brown, T.M., Cueto, M., and Fee, E. (2006) 'The World Health Organization and the Transition from International to Global Public Health', *American Journal of Public Health*, 96(1): 62–72.

Chen, L., Bell, D. and Bates, L. (1996) 'World Health and Institutional Change', in *Pocantico Retreat: Enhancing the Performance of International Health Institutions*, Cambridge, MA: The Rockefeller Foundation, Social Science Research Council, Harvard School of Public Health: 9–21.

Epstein, H. and Chen, L. (2002) '*Can AIDS be Stopped?*', available at http://www.nybooks.com/articles/15188 (accessed 21 August 2009).

Fogarty International Center (2008) 'Framework Programs for Global Health 2005', available at http://grants.nih.gov/grants/guide/pa-files/PAR-05-050.html (accessed 21 August 2009).

Frenk, J. (1993) 'The New Public Health', *Annual Review of Public Health*, 14: 469–89.

Frenk, J. (2006) 'Bridging the Divide: Global Lessons from Evidence-based Health Policy in Mexico', *The Lancet*, 368: 954–61.

Frenk, J. and Chacon, F. (1991) 'International Health in Transition', *Asia-Pacific Journal of Public Health*, 5(2): 170–5.

Frenk, J., Bobadilla, J.L., Sepúlveda, J., Rosenthal, J. and Ruelas, E. (1988) 'A Conceptual Model for Public Health Research', *Bulletin of the PAHO*, 22(1): 60–71.

Frenk, J., Sepúlveda, J., Gómez-Dantés, O., McGuinness, M.J., and Knaul, F. (1997) 'The Future of World Health: The New World Order and International Health', *British Medical Journal*, 314(7,091): 1,404–07.

Garret, L. (2007) 'The Challenge of Global Health', *Foreign Affairs*, 86(1): 14–38.

Giovanni, M. and Brownlee, A. (1982) 'The Contribution of Social Science to International Health Training', *Social Science and Medicine*, 16: 957–64.

Godue, C. (ed.) (1992) 'International Health and Schools of Public Health in the United States', in *International Health: A North-South Debate*, Washington, DC: Pan American Health Organisation: 113–26.

Gómez-Dantés, O. (2001) 'Health', in P.J. Simmons and C.De Jonge-Oudraat (eds) *Managing Global Issues: Lessons Learned*, Washington, DC: Carnegie Endowment for International Peace: 392–423.

Institute of Medicine (2008) 'The U.S. Commitment to Global Health: Recommendations for the New Administration', available at www.iom.edu/CMS/3783/51303/60714.aspx (accessed 20 August 2009).

Jamison, D., Frenk, J., and Knaul, F. (1998) 'International Collective Action in Health: Objectives, Functions, and Rationale', *The Lancet*, 351: 514–17.

Koplan, J., Bond, C.T., Merson, M.H., Reddy, K.S., Rodríguez, M.H., Sewankambo, N.K., and Wasserheit, J.N. (2009) 'Towards a Common Definition of Global Health', *The Lancet*, 373: 1,993–5.

Rodin, J. (2007) 'Navigating the Global American South: Global Health and Regional Solutions', plenary address presented at the University of North Carolina Center for Global Initiatives, Chapel Hill, 19 April.

Schellenberg, D. cited in M. Specter (2005) 'What Money can Buy', *The New Yorker*, 24 October: 57–71.

Sepúlveda, J. (2006) 'Foreword', in D.T. Jamison, J.G. Breman, A. Measham, G. Alleyne, M. Claeson, D.B. Evans, P. Jha, A. Mills, and P. Musgrove (eds) (2006) *Disease Control Priorities in Developing Countries*, Washington, DC: Oxford University Press: xiii–xv.

Tendler, J. (1975) *Inside Foreign Aid*, Baltimore, MD: Johns Hopkins University Press.

Wilkinson, L. and Power, H. cited in S.B. MacFarlane, M. Jacobs, and E.E. Kaaya (2008) 'In the Name of Global Health: Trends in Academic Institutions', *Public Health Policy*, 29(4): 383–401.

WHO (World Health Organization) (2008) *The Global Burden of Disease: 2004 Update*, Geneva: WHO: 40.

3

The World Health Organization and the World of Global Health

Theodore M. Brown and Marcos Cueto

Over the half century from 1948 to 1998, the World Health Organization (WHO) slipped from a commanding position as the unquestioned leader of international health to a much-diminished role in the crowded and contested world of global health. WHO began at a time of high idealism and heightened internationalist expectations, when visionary leaders saw the new organisation as the best hope for both health and peace in the post-war world (Fosdick 1944). That vision was glimpsed again at Alma-Ata in 1978, yet despite the dreams of many of its founders and early supporters, WHO was marked from its early days by political and diplomatic entanglements and budgetary constraints that, over five decades, compromised the organisation and restricted its operating capacity. Indeed, those entanglements and constraints eventually pushed WHO in the 1990s to try to reinvent itself as a coordinator of global health in a world with many new and powerful players.

The idea of a permanent, intergovernmental organisation for international health can be traced back to the creation in 1902 of the International Sanitary Office of the American Republics, which, some decades later, became the Pan American Health Organization (Cueto 2007a). Two European-based international health agencies also played critical historical roles. One was the Office Internationale d'Hygiène Publique (OIHP), which formally started functioning in Paris in 1907 and concentrated on the administration of negotiated international sanitary conventions and the exchange of information on reportable diseases (Abt 1933; Aykroyd 1968). The second agency, the League of Nations Health Organization (LNHO), began its work in 1920 (Balinska 1995; Dubin 1995). This organisation established its headquarters in Geneva, and over the course of the next decade and a half took on an increasingly ambitious range of activities (Borowy 2009; Weindling 2002). Although the LNHO was poorly budgeted by the League of Nations and faced opposition from some national health ministries and the OIHP, it received substantial support from the Rockefeller Foundation and was able to play an important and sometimes inspirational role in the inter-war period (Howard-Jones 1978; Weindling 1997). Both the OIHP and the LNHO survived through the Second World War, though barely, and were present at the critical post-war moment when the future of international health was defined (Borowy 2008).

WHO was planned and made operational by a series of international commissions which, working from 1946 to 1948 on a mandate voted in 1945 at the founding of the United Nations (UN), thrashed out a scope of work and basic administrative procedures (Goodman 1952). Country representatives were joined in this process by representatives of the Pan American Sanitary Bureau, OIHP, LNHO, and, until January 1947, of a well-funded and extremely powerful organisation new to the wartime and post-war 1940s, the UN Relief and Rehabilitation Administration (UNRRA), established in November 1943 (Sawyer 1947). For a brief few years, UNRRA played a crucial emergency role, working with a budget largely provided by the United States (US) and its the Second World War allies that far eclipsed the total resources of all other international health agencies. The first World Health Assembly convened in Geneva, Switzerland, in June 1948 and created the World Health Organization as a specialised agency of the UN, into which were formally merged the functions of OIHP, LNHO, and UNRRA. The Pan American Sanitary Bureau – then headed by former Rockefeller Foundation official Fred L. Soper – was allowed to retain semi-autonomous status as part of a regionalisation scheme, seen by many as forced upon WHO by the United States, that in the following years grew to a total of six WHO regional offices (in Africa, Europe, the Americas, south-east Asia, the eastern Mediterranean, and the western Pacific) (Howard-Jones 1981; Siddiqi 1995). The founding of WHO spanned post-war idealism and the hardening of the Cold War. Idealism was reflected in the preamble to its constitution (1948), in which health was defined as 'a state of complete physical, mental and social well-being and not merely the absence of disease and infirmity' (WHO 2006: 1).

The first director-general of WHO, Canadian psychiatrist George Brock Chisholm, tried to maintain these broad global ideals. But he was frustrated at almost every turn by the intrusion of the national self-interest of WHO's member countries, and especially by the rapidly intensifying politics of the Cold War (Farley 2008). The US played a contradictory role: on the one hand, it publicly supported the UN system and its broad worldwide goals and funded a significant portion of its budget, but on the other, it was insistent on its right to intervene unilaterally in the Americas and often elsewhere in the name of national security. As a main contributor to the WHO budget, the US threw around a lot of health policy weight.

As an intergovernmental agency, WHO was well-tuned to the larger political environment. The politics of the Cold War had an unmistakable impact on its policies and personnel. Thus, when the Soviet Union and other communist countries walked out of the UN system and, therefore, out of WHO in 1949, the US and its allies were easily able to exert a dominating influence. In 1953, Brock Chisholm, who had often testy relations with the US, completed his term as director-general and was replaced by the far more US-friendly Brazilian, Marcolino Candau. Candau had worked under Soper on malaria control in Brazil and was associated with the 'vertical' disease control programmes of the Rockefeller Foundation and their adoption by the Pan American Sanitary Bureau when Soper moved to that agency as director (Anonymous 1983). Candau would be director-general of WHO for over 20 years. During the period between 1949 and 1957 (when the Soviet Union returned to the UN and WHO), WHO was very closely allied with US interests.

In 1955, Candau was charged with overseeing WHO's campaign of malaria eradication, approved that year by the World Health Assembly. The ambitious goal of malaria eradication had been conceived and promoted in the context of unexamined optimism about the ability of DDT indoor spraying to kill mosquitoes, and of new anti-malarial drugs to kill or neutralise the *Plasmodium* parasite. WHO's malaria eradication programme was eagerly supported by another UN agency, UNICEF, and by the US State Department. The latter convinced the US Congress to fund the programme at a level of several million dollars (Cueto 2007b). Malaria eradication advocates concentrated on the growing awareness of mosquito resistance to DDT, arguing that only a comprehensive and relatively quick campaign would eliminate malaria before it spread all over the world.

As Randall Packard has shown, the US and its allies also believed that global malaria eradication could not only be achieved, but would usher in economic growth and create expanded overseas markets for US technology and manufactured goods (Packard 1997, 1998). Eradication efforts would also help win 'hearts and minds' in the battle against communism. The campaign reproduced the development strategies of the time by importing technologies brought in from outside while making no attempt to enlist the participation of local populations in planning or implementation (Packard and Brown 1997). This model of development assistance fitted neatly into US Cold War efforts to promote 'modernisation' with limited social reform.

But when the Soviet Union and other communist countries returned to WHO in the late 1950s, they made their presence felt almost immediately. The Soviet representative to the 11th World Health Assembly (1958), Viktor Zhdanov, was the deputy minister of health of the USSR, who argued that it was now scientifically feasible and economically desirable to attempt to eradicate smallpox worldwide (Fenner *et al.* 1988). The USSR obviously wanted to challenge US influence and make its own mark on world health policy. In 1959, the Assembly committed WHO to a global smallpox eradication programme (SEP), for which the USSR promised to provide 25 million doses of freeze-dried vaccine. Recognising the shifting balance in the World Health Assembly, director-general Candau felt the need to accommodate to changing political realities by backing WHO's smallpox eradication efforts. Yet for several years, WHO's smallpox programme remained modest and minimal while the US-backed malaria eradication programme lumbered forward on a much larger scale (Fenner *et al.* 1988). During the 1960s, however, malaria eradication encountered major difficulties in the field that ultimately led to colossal and embarrassing failures. In 1969, the World Health Assembly declared that it was not feasible to eradicate malaria in many parts of the world and began a process of returning once again to a malaria control agenda, while the SEP went forward on an expanded scale.

As the latter programme grew, smallpox eradication gained considerable momentum from technical improvements – jet injectors and bifurcated needles – which made the process of vaccination cheaper, easier, and more effective. Even more importantly, the US's interest in smallpox eradication sharply increased for foreign policy reasons (Manela 2010). The US did not want the USSR to gain unchallenged recognition for its global eradication efforts and thus felt the need to compete on the WHO stage. More positively, too, after a period of intensified tension in the early 1960s, both countries had begun to explore a more relaxed and collaborative détente phase of Cold War relations (Garthoff 1994). In 1965, the US pledged its support for a WHO-led programme to eradicate smallpox worldwide (Fenner *et al.* 1988). Candau was reluctant to commit WHO to a new US-endorsed global eradication campaign that might lead to another embarrassing failure, so insisted on US leadership to bear the blame if necessary (Henderson 1998a). At first disappointed that a Russian was not selected, the USSR agreed to the American choice of D. A. Henderson as head of the smallpox campaign, after deciding that he was both a good scientist and a person with whom they could work.

Thus began WHO's stunningly successful intensified smallpox eradication campaign built on US–USSR collaboration and later celebrated as a major 'cold war victory'. Henderson was an experienced and effective administrator who now proved himself also a masterful diplomat. He worked intimately and effectively with his Soviet counterparts to obtain the resources and personnel the programme needed, to smooth out problems when they inevitably occurred, and even to orchestrate diplomatic pressure to secure the cooperation of certain recalcitrant countries (Henderson 1987, 1998a). A good deal of his success depended on a de facto geopolitical understanding that the US would work primarily in Africa while the Soviet Union lent its major support to the Central Asian republics and the Indian subcontinent (Fenner et al. 1988). Even after Henderson left the programme and US–USSR tensions increased again in the late 1970s, WHO was able to bring the smallpox eradication programme to a successful conclusion (Fenner et al. 1988).

During the 1960s and 1970s, other major international events beyond US–USSR détente also influenced the course of WHO's history. These included the emergence of decolonised African nations, the spread of nationalist and socialist movements, and the dissemination of new theories of development that emphasised long-term socio-economic growth rather than short-term technological intervention. Rallying in organisations such as the Non-Aligned Movement, developing countries argued vigorously for fairer terms of trade and the more generous financing of development (Bhagwati 1977; Rothstein 1979). This changing political environment was reflected in corresponding shifts within WHO. In the 1960s, WHO acknowledged that a strengthened health infrastructure was a prerequisite to the success of its eradication and control programmes, especially in Africa. In 1968, Candau called for a comprehensive and integrated approach to curative and preventive care services. Soviet representatives called for the study of organisational methods for promoting basic health services (Litsios 2002). In January 1971, the executive board agreed to undertake an internal study, and the results of this study were presented to the full executive board in 1973 (WHO 1972, 1973). WHO was beginning to move from an older model of health service to what would become the 'primary health care' approach (Litsios 2002, 2004). The new model drew upon the thinking and experiences of non-governmental organisations (NGOs) and medical missionaries working in Africa, Asia, and Latin America at the grass-roots level. It also gained saliency from China's re-entry into the UN in 1973 and the widespread interest in Chinese 'barefoot doctors', who were reported to be transforming rural health conditions. These experiences underscored the urgency of a 'primary health care' perspective that included the training of community health workers, an emphasis on the creation of health outposts in underserved areas, and the tackling of basic economic and environmental problems (Bryant 1969; Newell 1975; Taylor 1976).

These new tendencies were embodied by Halfdan T. Mahler, a Dane, who served as WHO's director-general from 1973 to 1988. In 1975, the World Health Assembly reinforced the trend, declaring the construction of national programmes in primary care an urgent matter. In the World Health Assembly the following year, Mahler proposed the goal of 'Health for All by the Year 2000'. This slogan became an integral part of the primary health care movement. Mahler agreed to hold a major conference on the organisation of health services at Alma-Ata in the Soviet Union and to co-organise it with UNICEF. He was initially reluctant because he distrusted the Soviet Union's highly centralised and medicalised approach to the provision of health services (Litsios 2002). And although the Soviet Union succeeded in having the conference on its territory, the results reflected Mahler's views much more closely than it did those of the Soviets. The Alma-Ata Declaration of 1978 and the goal of 'Health for All in the Year 2000' advocated an inter-sectorial and multi-dimensional approach to health and socio-economic development, emphasised the use of 'appropriate' as opposed to excessive technology, and urged active community participation in health care and health education at every level (WHO 1978).

WHO now enjoyed considerable authority and esteem. Its smallpox eradication programme was in the final stages of successful completion, and Alma-Ata had added a sweeping vision and broad moral authority to WHO's reputation. But this peak also marked the high point from which decline rapidly set in. Some tried to strategise for the next disease eradication campaign by naïvely imagining it as a simple vertical assault, despite Henderson's strenuous objections (Henderson 1998b). Even more disturbingly, a number of governments, agencies, and influential individuals saw WHO's view of primary health care as overly idealistic, unrealistic, and unattainable (Henderson 1980; Tejada de Rivero 2003). The process of reducing Alma-Ata's idealism to a practical set of technical interventions that could be implemented more easily and assessed concretely began in 1979 at a small conference with a heavy US flavour held in Bellagio, Italy, and sponsored by the Rockefeller Foundation. Those in attendance included the president of the World Bank, the vice-president of the Ford Foundation, the administrator of USAID, and the new executive secretary of UNICEF (Black 1986, 1996). The Bellagio meeting focused on an alternative concept to that articulated at Alma-Ata – selective primary health care – which was built on the notion of pragmatic, low-cost interventions that were limited in scope and easy to monitor and evaluate. Pushed heavily by UNICEF, selective primary health care was soon operationalised under the acronym 'GOBI' (Growth monitoring to fight malnutrition in children, Oral rehydration techniques to defeat diarrhoeal diseases, Breastfeeding to protect children, and Immunisations) (Cueto 2004; UNICEF 1983).

In the 1980s, WHO also had to reckon with the rapidly growing influence of the World Bank. The Bank had initially been formed in 1946 to assist in the reconstruction of Europe and later expanded its mandate to provide loans, grants, and technical assistance to developing countries. At first, it funded large investments in physical capital and infrastructure, but then, in the 1970s, it began to invest in population control, health, and education, with the emphasis on population control (Ruger 2005). The World Bank approved its first loan for family planning in 1970. In 1979, the Bank created a population, health, and nutrition department and adopted a policy of funding both stand-alone health programmes and health components of other projects.

In its 1980 World Development Report, the Bank argued that both malnutrition and ill-health could be addressed by direct action with Bank assistance (World Bank 1980). It also suggested that improving health and nutrition could accelerate economic growth, thus providing a good argument for social sector spending. As the Bank began to make direct loans for health services, it called for the more 'efficient' use of available resources and discussed the roles of the private and public sectors in financing health care. Pushing a neo-liberal agenda that by the early 1980s the Bank and the International Monetary Fund had fully embraced, the Bank strongly promoted free markets and a diminished role for national governments (Harvey 2005; World Bank 1987). In the context of widespread developing-country indebtedness and increasingly scarce resources for health expenditures, the World Bank's insistence on 'structural adjustment' measures to fulfil the terms of its loans at the very time that the HIV/AIDS epidemic erupted drew angry criticism but also underscored the Bank's new influence.

In contrast to the World Bank's increasing authority, in the 1980s the prestige of the WHO was beginning to diminish. One sign of trouble was the 1982 vote by the World Health Assembly to freeze WHO's budget (Godlee 1994a). This was followed by the 1985 decision by the US to pay only 20 per cent of its assessed contribution to all UN agencies and to withhold its contribution to WHO's regular budget, in part as a protest against WHO's 'essential drug program', which was opposed by leading US-based pharmaceutical companies (Godlee 1994b). These events occurred amid growing tensions between WHO and UNICEF and other agencies, and the controversy over selective versus comprehensive primary health care. As part of a rancorous public debate conducted in the pages of *Social Science & Medicine* in 1988, Kenneth Newell, a highly placed WHO official and an architect of comprehensive primary health care, called selective primary health care a 'threat ... [that] can be thought of as a counter-revolution' (Newell 1988: 906).

Another symptom of WHO's problems in the late 1980s was the growth of extra-budgetary funding. As Gill Walt of the London School of Hygiene and Tropical Medicine noted, there was a crucial shift from predominant reliance on WHO's 'regular budget' – drawn from member states' contributions, based on population size and GNP – to greatly increased dependence on 'extra-budgetary' funding coming from donations by multilateral agencies or 'donor' nations (1993). By 1986–87, extra-budgetary funds of $437 million had almost caught up with the regular budget of $543 million. By the beginning of the 1990s, extra-budgetary funding had overtaken the regular budget by $21 million, thus contributing 54 per cent of WHO's overall budget. Major problems for the organisation followed from this budgetary shift. Priorities and policies were still ostensibly set by the World Health Assembly, which was made up of all member nations, but this Assembly, now dominated numerically by poor and developing countries, had authority only over the regular budget, which had been frozen since the early 1980s. Wealthy donor nations and multilateral agencies like the World Bank could largely call the shots on the use of the extra-budgetary funds they contributed. They thus created, in effect, a series of 'vertical' programmes more or less independent of the rest of the WHO's programmes and its decision-making structure. The dilemma for the organisation was that although the extra-budgetary funds added to the overall budget, 'they increase difficulties of coordination and continuity, cause unpredictability in finance, and a great deal of dependence on the satisfaction of particular donors' (Walt 1993: 129).

The growth of extra-budgetary funds and the embrace of selective primary health care resulted in some successful cases of disease control and new alliances between multinational agencies, NGOs, and the private sector. Two examples were the eradication of polio from the Americas and the control of onchocerciasis in Africa. In 1988, WHO and other multilateral agencies launched a campaign to eradicate polio by the year 2000, at a time when fewer than 50 per cent of the world's children were receiving the recommended three doses of oral polio vaccine. An important private partner, Rotary International, raised funds, provided a network of volunteers, and ensured political support for the 'Polio Plus' initiative. Polio Plus was instrumental in setting guidelines and vaccination schedules, organising national vaccination days, and using modern refrigeration systems (the cold chain) to preserve the vaccine's potency (Seytre and Shaffer 2005). Thanks to these activities, polio essentially disappeared from the Americas by 1991.

During the 1980s, onchocerciasis, a filarial disease causing wrinkling and depigmentation of the skin, eye lesions, and blindness, was brought under control thanks to WHO's Onchocerciasis Control Programme (OCP) in West and Central Africa (WHO 1985a). When OCP began its work, about one million individuals were suffering from onchocerciasis, and at least 100,000 persons were blind. OCP concentrated its work in seven countries of the savannah zone, covering an area of 640,000 square kilometres, and established its headquarters in the Upper Volta (WHO 1976). Partners in OCP were bilateral agencies in several industrial countries, the UN Development Programme, the World Bank, the Food and Agriculture Organization, and the Special Programme for Research and Training in Tropical Diseases (TDR), hosted at WHO. TDR's main goal was to identify new drugs for 'neglected' infectious diseases in poor nations (Morel 2000). Thanks to this broad partnership, the funding of OCP was significant.

Ebrahim M. Samba, a physician from Gambia, was appointed director of the OCP in 1980. In an unprecedented move, Samba travelled to the US and convinced Merck, Sharp & Dohme, which had developed and marketed ivermectin, an effective microfilaricide with few side effects, to provide the drug free of charge (Aziz et al. 1982). In addition, OCP used larvicides to destroy black fly vectors and produce a new biodegradable insecticide with no toxic effects for mammals and fish. By the late 1980s, it was estimated that 27,000 individuals were saved from going blind and about 3 million children born within the OCP programme area since the start of operations were safe from onchocerciasis (WHO 1985b).

Despite these successes, from the late 1980s to the late 1990s, WHO struggled through the most difficult decade in its history. A decline in operating budget, competition with new organisations for the leadership of international health, and confrontation with the governments of industrialised countries critical of the UN eroded the agency's former leadership position and created the perception that WHO was obsolete. This period coincided with Dr Hiroshi Nakajima's two terms as director-general (1988–98). Nakajima's critics blamed him for not doing enough to defend primary health care, for being incapable of adapting to new epidemiological and political realities, and for slowing the pace of institutional reform.

Particularly bitter criticism swirled around Nakajima because of his difficult relationship with Jonathan Mann, the controversial early leader in the fight against AIDS. Initially, WHO gave the disease low priority. Some changes occurred in 1985, when WHO co-sponsored the first international conference on AIDS in Atlanta, and in 1986 when the 39th World Health Assembly approved the creation of an AIDS programme within WHO. In February of the following year, the American physician Jonathan Mann became head of the Global Programme on AIDS (GPA) (Anonymous 1986). By the end of 1987, GPA was working with more than 90 countries, sending technical support missions to help design national AIDS programmes. In a 1987 briefing to the UN General Assembly, Mann sounded the alarm about the magnitude of the AIDS pandemic, and the danger of responses inspired by fear and discrimination. He argued that public health and human rights were fully compatible and that repressive policies endangered rather than protected public health (Altman 1987; Lewis 1987). Thus, in a short time, Mann was able to build GPA into the strongest and best-funded programme within WHO.

But Nakajima felt uncomfortable with the celebrity Mann enjoyed, the considerable independence with which he operated, and his expansive views on the importance of human rights for health. Nakajima also believed that the GPA had too much money and visibility and that attention needed to be paid to other diseases such as malaria and tuberculosis (Oestrich 2007). A study of all extra-budgetary funds for 1992 indicated that the GPA commanded over 25 per cent of these resources (Beigbeder 1998). Nakajima began to tighten control over Mann and restrict the operations of the GPA. In March 1990, after a series of angry exchanges in European newspapers, Mann resigned, citing his 'major disagreements' with the director-general. The US and many other industrial countries considered the event a major blow to the global campaign against AIDS and a black mark against Nakajima (Crosette 1997). The net result was that WHO lost its initial position in the world's response to AIDS, and the agency that emerged as the new multilateral leader was the UN Programme on HIV/AIDS (UNAIDS), created in the mid-1990s and outside the control of WHO.

In the mid-1990s, Fiona Godlee published a series of articles vigorously critical of WHO and its current leadership (Godlee 1994a, 1994b, 1995), and concluded with this dire assessment going well beyond WHO's bungled response to AIDS: 'WHO is caught in a cycle of decline, with donors expressing their lack of faith in its central management by placing funds outside the management's control. This has prevented WHO from [developing] … integrated responses to countries' long-term needs' (Godlee 1995: 182). As WHO lost credibility, the World Bank moved confidently into the vacuum. WHO officials were unable or unwilling to respond to the new international health economy structured around the Bank's neo-liberal approaches (Brown 1993 1997; Zwi 2000). The Bank maintained that, not only in the case of AIDS but more generally, existing health systems were often wasteful, inefficient, and ineffective, and argued in favour of greater reliance on the private sector with the corresponding reduction of public involvement in the delivery of health services (World Bank 1987).

Controversies surrounded the Bank's policies and practices, yet there was no doubt that it had become a dominant force in international health. The Bank's greatest comparative advantage lay in its ability to mobilise large financial resources; by 1990, the Bank's loans for health surpassed the total budget of WHO, and by the end of 1996, the Bank's cumulative lending portfolio in health, nutrition, and population had reached $13.5 billion. Yet the Bank recognised that, whereas it had great economic strength and influence, WHO still had considerable technical expertise in matters of health. This was clearly reflected in the Bank's widely influential 1993 World Development Report, 'Investing in Health', which gives credit to WHO, 'a full partner with the World Bank at every stage in the preparation of the Report' (World Bank 1993: iii–iv). Circumstances suggested that it was to the advantage of both parties for the Bank and WHO to work together.

This is the context in which WHO began to refashion itself as a coordinator, strategic planner, and leader of 'global health' initiatives. In January 1992, the 31-member executive board of the World Health Assembly decided to appoint a working group to recommend how WHO could be most effective in international health work in the light of the global change overtaking the world. The executive board may have been responding, in part, to the Children's Vaccine Initiative, perceived within WHO as an attempted coup by UNICEF, the World Bank, the UN Development Programme (UNDP), the Rockefeller Foundation, and several other players, who were seeking to wrest control of vaccine development (Muraskin 1998). The working group's final report of May 1993 recommended that WHO – if it were to maintain leadership of the health sector – must overhaul its fragmented management of global, regional, and country programmes, diminish competition between regular and extra-budgetary initiatives, and above all, increase the emphasis within WHO on global health issues and WHO's coordinating role in that domain (Stenson and Sterky 1994).

In 1998, the World Health Assembly reached outside the ranks of WHO for a leader who could restore credibility to the organisation and provide it with a new vision – to Gro Harlem Brundtland, a former prime minister of Norway and a physician and public health professional who brought formidable expertise to the task. In the 1980s, she had been chair of the UN World Commission on Environment and Development and had produced the 'Brundtland Report', which led to the Earth Summit of 1992. She was familiar with the global thinking of the environmental movement and had a broad and clear understanding of the links between health, environment, and development (McMichael et al. 1996; McMichael and Haines 1997).

Brundtland was determined to position WHO as an important player on the global stage, to move beyond ministries of health and gain a seat at the table when decisions were being made (Kickbusch 2000). She wanted to refashion WHO as a 'department of consequence' able to monitor and influence other actors on the global scene (Kickbusch 2000: 985). Brundtland established a Commission on Macroeconomics and Health, chaired by the economist Jeffrey Sachs, then of Harvard University, and including former ministers of finance, and officers from the World Bank, the International Monetary Fund, the World Trade Organization and the UNDP, as well as public health leaders. The Commission issued a report in 2001, which was criticised by many for condoning the global status quo, but which won praise from some because it drew attention to the argument that improving health in developing countries was essential to their economic development (Commission on Macroeconomics and Health 2001; Mills et al. 2002; Waitzkin 2003).

Brundtland also began to strengthen the WHO's financial position, largely by organising 'global partnerships' and 'global funds' to bring together 'stakeholders' – private donors, governments, and bilateral and multilateral agencies – to concentrate on specific targets (for example, Roll Back Malaria in 1998, GAVI in 1999, and Stop TB in 2001). These were semi-autonomous programmes bringing in substantial outside funding, often in the form of public/private partnerships (Buse and Walt 2001; Reid and Pearce 2003; Widdus 2001). A very significant player in these 'PPPs' was the Bill & Melinda Gates Foundation, which committed more than $1.7 billion between 1998 and 2000 to an international programme to prevent or eliminate diseases in the world's poorest nations, primarily through vaccines and immunisation programmes (McCarthy 2000). In 2002, the Gates Foundation donated $2.8 billion, $750 million of which went to GAVI (Maciocco 2008). But with the multiplication of PPPs came the multiplication of partners – Roll Back Malaria alone had more than 90 – which meant that leadership, management, and governance in global health had become extraordinarily complicated and confused (Yamey 2002c).

Brundtland's tenure as director-general drew other criticisms, as well. Some looked with considerable scepticism at her worrisome bias towards the private sector and, particularly, the seeming favouritism of the pharmaceutical industry in the Commission on Macroeconomics and Health and the PPPs (Katz 2005; Motchane 2002; Richter 2004). Some have claimed that other urgent issues did not receive sufficient attention (health promotion, health and human rights, and social and economic restructuring to achieve health improvement) (Mittelmark 2001). Still others were frustrated by the director-general's non-inclusive administrative style, the WHO's poor staff morale, and the large gap between the rhetoric of transformation and the realities of institutional inertia (Yamey 2002a, 2002b). Nonetheless, few disputed the assertion that Brundtland succeeded in achieving her principal objective, which was to reposition WHO or, at least, begin to reposition it as a credible contributor to the rapidly changing field of global health (Aitken 2003; Horton 2002).

Yet rapid and dramatic changes over which Brundtland had little control continued during her term as director-general and in the years following. Perhaps most notable was the emergence of the G8 nations (France, the US, the UK, Germany, Italy, Japan, Canada, and the Russian Federation) as a major collective force in global health. Health first became an important agenda item for summit meetings under French and US leadership in the late 1990s, when the focus was primarily diseases that affected the member nations themselves (Kirton *et al.* 2007). But when the Russian Federation became a full member, the G8 began to focus on HIV/AIDS. By 2000 the scope of health concern widened to include tuberculosis and malaria, and the G8 began to push for the creation of the 'Global Fund to Fight AIDS, Tuberculosis and Malaria', which was officially established in 2002 (The Global Fund to Fight AIDS, Tuberculosis and Malaria 2009; Labonte and Schrecker 2004). Since then the G8 has met regularly with African leaders, widened its agenda to include support for the health-related Millennium Development Goals, and broadened its approach still further to include health system strengthening (especially in developing nations) and maternal, newborn, and child health (Reich and Takemi 2009).

At recent G8 summits, increasing attention has been devoted to the reports and recommendations of a specially constituted G8 health experts group (G8 Health Experts Group 2008). But the G8 has also been listening to a group newly formed in July 2007 and calling itself the 'H8' (Health 8) – a self-appointed collaborative comprised of representatives from GAVI, the Global Fund, UNAIDS, the United Nations Population Fund (UNFPA), UNICEF, the World Bank, the Bill & Melinda Gates Foundation, and WHO (Reich and Takemi 2009; World Health Organization 2007). What is most notable about the H8 thus far is the World Bank's acknowledgement that its financing is becoming a smaller proportion of global health funds overall and WHO's new assertiveness in articulating a leadership role (Reich and Takemi 2009). WHO is only one of eight in the H8, but it is clearly jostling for recognition and authority as the global health leader with new energy and some success.

We thus return briefly to the issue with which this chapter began: what is WHO's role in 'global health'? The basic answer derives from the fact that WHO has had to work very hard to reinvent itself in order to maintain its authority in a new world that had initially bypassed it and declared it irrelevant. It had to find and keep a place on the rapidly evolving agenda it did not set and for which other, larger forces and stronger organisations were primarily responsible. But once in the mix, WHO contributed significantly to the dissemination of the new concepts and vocabulary of 'global health' and in that process gained recognition for what the organisation identified as a coordinating and leadership role (Yach and Bettcher 1998). Now many outside the organisation also promote this role for WHO, which suggests a brighter future on the basis of re-emerging legal, moral, and technical authority (Garrett 2007; Kickbusch 2000; Taylor 2002, 2004). Whether WHO's organisational repositioning will succeed in re-establishing it as the acknowledged steward of the health of the world's population remains an open question at this time.

References

Abt, G. (1933) *Vingt-Cinq Ans d'Activité de l'Office Internationale d'Hygiène Publique 1909–1933*, Paris: L'Office Internationale d'Hygiène Publique.

Aitken, D. (2003) 'WHO Responds', *British Medical Journal*, 326: 217–18.

Altman, L.K. (1987) 'Key World Health Official Warns of Epidemic of Prejudice on AIDS', *New York Times*, 3 June.

Anonymous (1983) 'In Memory of Sr. M.G. Candau', *WHO Chronicle*, 37: 144–7.

Anonymous (1986) 'WHO's Efforts to Contain AIDS', *The Lancet*, 1: 1,167.

Aykroyd, W.R. (1968) 'International Health: A Retrospective Memoir', *Perspectives in Biology and Medicine*, 11: 273–85.

Aziz, M.A., S. Diallo, I.M. Diop, M. Lariviere, and M. Porta (1982) 'Efficacy and Tolerance of Ivermectin in Human Onchocerciasis', *The Lancet*, 2: 171–3.

Balinska, M.A. (1995) 'Assistance and Not Mere Relief: The Epidemic Commission of the League of Nations, 1920–1923', in P. Weindling (ed.) *International Health Organisations and Movements, 1918–1939*, Cambridge: Cambridge University Press: 81–108.

Beigbeder, Y. (1998) *The World Health Organisation*, Dordrecht: Martinus Nijhoff.

Bhagwati, J.N. (ed.) (1977) *The New International Economic Order: The North South Debate*, Cambridge, MA: MIT Press.

Black, M. (1986) *The Children and the Nations: The Story of UNICEF*, New York: UNICEF.

Black, M. (1996) *Children First: The Story of UNICEF, Past and Present*, Oxford: Oxford University Press.

Borowy, I. (2008) 'Manoeuvring for Space: International Health Work of the League of Nations during World War II', in S.G. Solomon, L. Murard, and P. Zylberman (eds) *Shifting Boundaries of Public Health: Europe in the Twentieth Century*, Rochester, NY: University of Rochester Press.

Borowy, I. (2009) *Coming to Terms with World Health: The League of Nations Health Organisation 1921–1946*, Frankfurt am Main: Peter Lang.

Brown, P. (1993) 'Editorial: World Bank's Cure for Donor Fatigue', *The Lancet*, 342: 63–4.

Brown, P. (1997) 'The WHO Strikes Mid-life Crisis', *New Scientist*, 153: 12.

Bryant, J.H. (1969) *Health and the Developing World*, Ithaca, NY: Cornell University Press.

Buse, K. and Walt, G. (2000) 'Global Public-private Partnerships: Part I–A New Development in Health?', *Bulletin of the World Health Organisation*, 78: 549–61.

Commission on Macroeconomics and Health (2001) *Macroeconomics and Health: Investing in Health for Economic Development*, Geneva: World Health Organization.

Crosette, B. (1997) 'UN Health Official Opposed by US Won't Seek Re-election', *New York Times*, 30 April.

Cueto, M. (2004) 'The Origins of Primary Health Care and Selective Primary Health Care', *American Journal of Public Health*, 94: 1864–74.

Cueto, M. (2007a) *The Value of Health: A History of the Pan American Health Organization*, Washington, DC: Pan American Health Organization.

Cueto, M. (2007b) *Cold Wars, Deadly Fevers: Malaria Eradication in Mexico 1955–1975*, Baltimore, MD: Johns Hopkins University Press.

Dubin, M.D. (1995) 'The League of Nations Health Organisation', in P. Weindling (ed.) *International Health Organisations and Movements, 1918–1939*, Cambridge: Cambridge University Press.

Farley, J. (2008) *Brock Chisholm, the World Health Organisation, and the Cold War*, Vancouver: University of British Columbia Press.

Fenner, F., D.A. Henderson, I. Arita, Z. Jezek, and I.D. Ladnyi (1988) *Smallpox and Its Eradication*, Geneva: World Health Organization.

Fosdick, R.B. (1944) 'Public Health as an International Problem', *American Journal of Public Health*: 1133–8.

G8 Health Experts Group (2008) 'Toyako Framework for Action on Global Health', available at http://www.g8.utoronto.ca/summit/2008hokkaido/2008-healthexperts.pdf (accessed 15 October 2009).

Garrett, L. (2007) 'The Challenge of Global Health', *Foreign Affairs*, 86: 14.

Garthoff, R.L. (1994) *Détente and Confrontation: American-Soviet Relations form Nixon to Reagan*, Washington, DC: Brookings Institution Press.

Godlee, F. (1994a) 'WHO in Crisis', *British Medical Journal*, 309: 1,424–8.

Godlee, F. (1994b) 'WHO in Retreat: Is It Losing its Influence?', *British Medical Journal*, 309: 1,491–5.

Godlee, F. (1995) 'WHO's Special Programmes: Undermining from Above', *British Medical Journal*, 310: 178–82.

Goodman, N.M. (1952) *International Health Organisations and Their Work*, London: J&A Churchill Ltd.

Harvey, D. (2005) *A Brief History of Neoliberalism*, New York: Oxford University Press.

Henderson, D.A. (1980) 'Smallpox Eradication', *Public Health Reports*, 95: 426.

Henderson, D.A. (1987) 'Principles and Lessons from the Smallpox Eradication Program', *Bulletin of the World Health Organization*, 65: 535–46.

Henderson, D.A. (1998a) 'Smallpox Eradication: A Cold War Victory', *World Health Forum*: 115–18.

Henderson, D.A. (1998b) 'Eradication: Lessons from the Past', *Bulletin of the World Health Organization*, 76: 17.

Horton, R. (2002) 'WHO: The Casualties and Compromises of Renewal', *The Lancet*, 359: 1,605–11.

Howard-Jones, H. (1981) 'The World Health Organisation in Historical Perspective', *Perspectives in Biology and Medicine*, 24: 467–82.

Howard-Jones, N. (1978) *International Public Health Between the Two World Wars–The Organisational Problems*, Geneva: World Health Organization.

Katz, A. (2005) 'The Sachs Report: Investing in Health for Economic Development–or Increasing the Size of the Crumbs from the Rich Man's Table? Part II', *International Journal of Health Services*, 35: 171–88.

Kickbusch, I. (2000) 'The Development of International Health Priorities: Accountability Intact?', *Social Science & Medicine*, 51: 979–89.

Kirton, J.J., Roudev, N., and Sunderland, L. (2007) 'Making G8 Leaders Deliver: An Analysis of Compliance and Health Commitments, 1996–2006', *Bulletin of the World Health Organization*, 85: 193.

Labonte, R. and Schrecker, T. (2004) 'Committed to Health for All? How the G7/G8 Rate', *Social Science & Medicine*, 59: 1,666.

Lewis, P. (1987) 'UN Authority on AIDS Sees Up To 3 Million New Cases in 5 Years', *New York Times*, 21 October.

Litsios, S. (2002) 'The Long and Difficult Road to Alma-Ata: A Personal Reflection', *International Journal of Health Services*, 32: 709–32.

Litsios, S. (2004) 'The Christian Medical Commission and the Development of WHO's Primary Care Approach', *American Journal of Public Health*, 94: 1,884–93.

McCarthy, M. (2000) 'A Conversation with the Leaders of the Gates Foundation's Global Health Program: Gordon Perkin and William Foege', *The Lancet*, 356: 153–5.

Maciocco, G. (2008) 'From Alma Ata to the Global Fund: The History of International Health Policy', *Social Medicine*, 3: 41.

McMichael, A.J., and Haines, A.J. (1997) 'Global Climate Change: The Potential Effects on Health', *British Medical Journal*, 315: 805–809.

McMichael, A.J., Haines, A.J., Sloof, R., and Kovats, S. (1996) *Climate Change and Human Health*, Geneva: World Health Organization.

Manela, E. (2010) 'A Pox on Your Narrative: Writing Disease Control into Cold War History', *Diplomatic History*, 34(2): 299–323, available at http://isites.harvard.edu/fs/docs/icb.topic48666.files/Pox%20on%20your%20narrative-DH-post.pdf (accessed 16 October 2009).

Mills, A., Amoako, K.Y., and Kato, T. (2002) 'The Work of the Commission on Macroeconomics and Health', *Bulletin of the World Health Organization*, 80: 164–6.

Morel, C. (2000) 'Reaching Maturity: 25 Years of TDR', *Parasitology Today*, 16: 2–8.

Motchane, J.L. (2002) 'Health for All or Riches for Some: WHO's Responsible?', *Le Monde Diplomatique*, July.

Muraskin, W. (1998) *The Politics of International Health: The Children's Vaccine Initiative and the Struggle to Develop Vaccines for the Third World*, Albany, NY: State University of New York Press.

Newell, K.W. (1975) *Health by the People*, Geneva: World Health Organization.

Newell, K.W. (1988) 'Selective Primary Health Care: The Counter Revolution', *Social Science & Medicine*, 26: 903–906.

Oestrich, J.E. (2007) *Power and Principle: Human Rights Programming in International Organizations*, Washington, DC: Georgetown University Press.

Packard, R.M. (1997) 'Malaria Dreams: Postwar Visions of Health and Development in the Third World', *Medical Anthropology*, 17: 279–96.

Packard, R.M. (1998) '"No Other Logical Choice": Global Malaria Eradication and the Politics of International Health in the Post-war Era', *Parassitologia*, 40: 217–29.

Packard, R.M., and Brown, P.J. (1997) 'Rethinking Health, Development and Malaria: Historicizing a Cultural Model in International Health', *Medical Anthropology*, 17: 181–94.

Reich, M.R., and Takemi, K. (2009) 'G8 and Strengthening of Health Systems: Follow-up to the Toyako Summit', *The Lancet*, 373: 508–15.

Reid, M.A., and Pearce, E.J. (2003) 'Whither the World Health Organisation?', *Medical Journal of Australia*, 178: 9–12.

Richter, J. (2004) 'Public-private Partnerships for Health: A Trend with no Alternatives?', *Development*, 47: 43–8.

Rothstein, R.L. (1979) *Global Bargaining: UNCTAD and the Quest for a New International Economic Order*, Princeton, NJ: Princeton University Press.

Ruger, J.P. (2005) 'Changing Role of the World Bank in Global Health in Historical Perspective', *American Journal of Public Health*, 95: 60–70.

Sawyer, S. (1947) 'Achievements of UNRRA as an International Health Organisation', *American Journal of Public Health*, 37: 41–58.

Seytre, B. and M. Shaffer (2005) *The Death of a Disease: A History of the Eradication of Poliomyelitis*, New Brunswick, NJ: Rutgers University Press.

Siddiqi, J. (1995) *World Health and World Politics: The World Health Organisation and the UN System*, London: Hurst and Company.

Stenson, B. and G. Sterky (1994) 'What Future WHO?', *Health Policy*, 28: 235–56.

Taylor, A.L. (2002) 'Global Governance, International Health Law and WHO: Looking Towards the Future', *Bulletin of the World Health Organization*, 80: 975–80.

Taylor, A.L. (2004) 'Governing the Globalisation of Public Health', *Journal of Law, Medicine & Ethics*, 32: 500–8.

Taylor, C.E. (ed.) (1976) *Doctors for the Villages: Study of Rural Internships in Seven Indian Medical Colleges*, New York: Asia Publishing House.

Tejada de Rivero, D.A. (2003) 'Alma-Ata Revisited', *Perspectives in Health Magazine: The Magazine of the Pan American Health Organization*, 8: 1–6.

The Global Fund to Fight AIDS, Tuberculosis and Malaria (2009) *Fighting AIDS, Tuberculosis, and Malaria: Who We Are*, available at http://www.theglobalfund.org/en/fighting/?lang=en (accessed 15 October 2009).

UNICEF (United Nations Children's Fund) (1983) *The State of the World's Children: 1982/1983*, New York: Oxford University Press.

Waitzkin, H. (2003) 'Report of the WHO Commission on Macroeconomics and Health: A Summary and Critique', *The Lancet*, 361: 523–6.

Walt, G. (1993) 'WHO Under Stress: Implications for Health Policy', *Health Policy*, 24: 125–44.

Weindling, P.J. (1997) 'Philanthropy and World Health: The Rockefeller Foundation and the League of Nations Health Organisation', *Minerva*, 35: 269–81.

Weindling, P.J. (2002) 'From Moral Exhortation to the New Public Health, 1918–1945', in E. Rodriguez-Ocana (ed.) *The Politics of the Healthy Life: An International Perspective*, Sheffield: European Association for the History of Medicine.

Widdus, R. (2001) 'Public-private Partnerships for Health: Their Main Targets, Their Diversity, and Their Future Directions', *Bulletin of the World Health Organization*, 79: 713–20.

World Bank (1980) *World Development Report 1980*, Washington, DC: World Bank.

World Bank (1987) *Financing Health Services in Developing Countries: An Agenda for Reform*, Washington, DC: World Bank.

World Bank (1993) *World Development Report, 1993: Investing in Health*, Washington, DC: World Bank.

WHO (World Health Organization) (1972) *Organisational Study of the Executive Board on Methods of Promoting the Development of Basic Health Services*, Geneva: WHO.

WHO (World Health Organization) (1973) *Executive Board 49th Session*, Geneva: WHO.

WHO (World Health Organization) (1976) 'The Prevention of Blindness', *Chronicle of the World Health Organization*, 30: 391–7.

WHO (World Health Organization) (1978) 'Declaration of Alma-Ata', International Conference on Primary Health Care, Alma-Ata, USSR, 6–12 September 1978, available at http://www.who.int/publications/almaata_declaration_en.pdf (accessed 16 October 2009).

WHO (World Health Organization) (1985a) *Ten Years of Onchocerciasis Control in West Africa: Review of the Work of the Onchocerciasis Control Programme in the Volta River Basin Area from 1974 to 1984*, Geneva: WHO.

WHO (World Health Organization) (1985b) '*Onchocerciasis Control Programme in the Volta River Basin Area: Committee of Sponsoring Agencies, report of the twenty-fifth session*', Paris, 16–17 October.

WHO (World Health Organization) (2006) *Constitution of the World Health Organization*, available at http://www.who.int/governance/eb/who_constitution_en.pdf (accessed 15 October 2009).

WHO (World Health Organization) (2007) *Informal Meeting of Global Health Leaders*, available at http://www.unicef.org/health/files/Meeting_of_Global_Health_Leaders_-_Final_Summary.pdf (accessed 15 October 2009).

Yach, D. and Bettcher, D. (1988) 'The Globalisation of Public Health', *American Journal of Public Health*, 88: 735–41.

Yamey, G. (2002a) 'Have the Latest Reforms Reversed WHO's Decline?', *British Medical Journal*, 325: 1,107–12.

Yamey, G. (2002b) 'WHO's Management: Struggling to Transform a "Fossilised Bureaucracy"', *British Medical Journal*, 325: 1,170–73.

Yamey, G. (2002c) 'WHO in 2002: Faltering Steps Towards Partnerships', *British Medical Journal*, 325: 1,236–40.

Zwi, A. (2000) 'Introduction to Policy Forum: The World Bank and International Health', *Social Science & Medicine*, 50: 167.

4

The Shifting Landscape of Public Health

From International to Global Health[*]

Adam Kamradt-Scott, Chris Holden, and Kelley Lee

Introduction

Globalisation is fundamentally changing the nature of human interaction. Economic, political, technological, socio-cultural, and environmental changes are having a marked impact upon the nature and intensity of human relations, profoundly challenging many of the boundaries that previously separated us from each other. These boundaries, which include how we perceive and experience physical space and territory (spatial), how we perceive and experience time (temporal), and how we see ourselves and the world around us (cognitive) are being constantly eroded and redefined (Lee 2001). This is no more evident than in the realm of public health, where these changes are creating not only new threats but new opportunities as well. However, one of the key problems is that many of the existing institutions and structures that seek to govern human health remain firmly set within boundaries that derive from a previous era – for example, government ministries that artificially separate health from wider socio-economic considerations, and international organisations that continue to function on the basis of bargaining between nation states and which exclude civil society and non-governmental organisations (NGOs). Thus, even though in some contexts there has been a perceptible shift from international to global health (i.e. inclusive of actors other than governments alone), many of the existing institutions and structures are currently ill-equipped to respond effectively to these processes of change.

The changes arising from globalisation extend to the field of public health in three main ways. First, processes of global change are shaping the broad determinants of health. Aside from reshaping individual lifestyle factors, globalisation is also affecting such aspects as employment, housing, education, water and sanitation, as well as agriculture and food production. Second, there is growing evidence that health status and outcomes are being influenced by globalising processes, with different impacts on specific individuals and populations within and across countries. These in turn are giving rise to new patterns of health and disease. Third, as a

* This research has been made possible through funding from the European Research Council under the European Community's Seventh Framework Programme – Ideas Grant 230489 GHG, and the National Cancer Institute, US National Institutes of Health, Grant Number CA091021–08. All views expressed remain those of the authors.

consequence of the above, societies must adapt their collective responses to changing health determinants and outcomes – a challenge that remains largely unmet (Lee and Yach 2005). Indeed, national borders are being rendered increasingly permeable by globalising processes, and health policies pursued only on a national basis are becoming increasingly less relevant and effective. As this chapter explores, for example, the increasing power and ability of transnational corporations to operate outside the borders of their home countries is having a profoundly negative impact on health. Similarly, the low cost and speed of transport is facilitating growth in the numbers and frequency of international journeys, aiding and abetting the potential for the much more rapid spread of infectious diseases. The purpose of this chapter is to examine how globalisation is changing the structures and processes that govern health issues, demanding a change not only in how we perceive these issues, but also influencing how they are then addressed. To illustrate how globalisation is having an impact on public health, prompting a shift from international to global health, two case studies will be briefly examined – international tobacco control and influenza virus-sharing. These case studies demonstrate that globalising processes have altered spatial, temporal, and cognitive understandings of these issues, and this in turn has also shaped new attempts to regulate and govern them. As the case studies also reveal, understanding and responding effectively to these processes of change is unlikely to be achieved by a 'business as usual' approach.

Case study: tobacco control

The global epidemic of tobacco-related diseases has been a product of the restructuring of the industry into transnational tobacco companies (TTCs). Tobacco consumption in many countries began hundreds of years ago, yet the globalisation of the production of tobacco products is a relatively recent phenomenon. This process began with the development of the mass marketing of cigarettes by American and British tobacco companies, and their expansion abroad towards the end of the nineteenth century. British American Tobacco (BAT) was formed in 1902 as a joint company to run all business outside of the two home countries, but later became a solely British company as a result of anti-trust action in the US (Cox 2000). BAT has been prominent in a number of national markets since this time, but the current globalisation of the industry is the result of a renewed shift towards acquisition of foreign companies by American and British firms since the 1960s. In 1964, the US surgeon general published a milestone report identifying tobacco as the cause of a number of diseases, thus sparking the beginning of a period of substantial foreign investment by US tobacco companies, particularly in Latin America (Shepherd 1985). The decline of tobacco consumption in the 'mature' markets of the developed countries was further offset by the expansion of TTCs in East Asia during the 1980s, following the forced liberalisation of a number of markets by the United States Trade Representative (USTR) (Taylor et al. 2000), and in Eastern Europe and the former Soviet Union (FSU) in the 1990s following the collapse of communism (Gilmore and McKee 2004).

Consolidation in the industry through mergers and acquisitions has led to the global tobacco market being dominated today by a few large transnational corporations which compete with each other in an oligopolistic fashion in most countries, but which have also colluded when necessary to influence public policy and regulatory regimes in their favour. Today, the four major TTCs, ranked in order of magnitude of sales, are the Altria Group (which owns Philip Morris), BAT, Japan Tobacco, and Altadis/Imperial. In 2007, these four companies had a combined share of the global tobacco market (by volume) of 52.2 per cent (excluding China, which is dominated by the huge state monopoly CNTC) (Hedley 2007). In 2006, all four were large enough to be included in *Fortune* magazine's G500 list of the world's largest corporations by revenue (*Fortune* 2007), while Altria and BAT were transnational enough to appear in the United Nations Conference on Trade and Development's 'transnationality index' (UNCTAD 2008) of the 100 most transnational non-financial corporations in the world (Holden and Lee 2009).

The TTCs are thus a manifestation of the ways in which the spatial and temporal aspects of globalisation have affected the organisation of production systems, with calamitous consequences for health. The cognitive aspects of globalisation have been equally important to the TTCs, as they have launched massive advertising operations in order to create demand for their products (Shepherd 1985). The utilisation of global information and telecommunication networks has been a key tool, as they have attempted to create and promote 'global brands' which appeal to higher-income groups across the world. The exploitation of events which are broadcast across national borders, such as international sporting competitions, has been one mechanism to avoid the advertising restrictions that an increasing number of countries have imposed, with, for example, sponsored events in one country being televised in others through regional satellite networks (Collin 2003). The transnational nature of these companies and their operations has created an imperative for a global approach to tobacco control.

The Framework Convention on Tobacco Control (FCTC) entered into force in February 2005, as the result of a process in which the World Health Organization (WHO) utilised its treaty-making powers for the first time. As of July 2009, 165 countries had become party to it. The Convention embodies a deepening of global health governance in a number of ways. It recognises the activities of TTCs and tobacco use as a genuinely global problem that requires a coordinated global response from WHO member countries, and sets out the minimum international principles and guidelines for tobacco control that all state parties must adopt (WHO 2003). It has a governing body in the Conference of the Parties – which is composed of all state parties to the Convention and meets every two years to promote and review its implementation – and the facility to convene an Intergovernmental Negotiating Body to negotiate and agree on specific protocols to the Convention. The first potential protocol is the Protocol on Illicit Trade in Tobacco Products (PITTP), which was being negotiated at the time of writing. The negotiation process for the Convention facilitated the development of world–regional groupings of states to coordinate and give effective weight to the voices of developing countries, and permitted an unusual degree of formal participation in a multilateral negotiating process by civil society actors (Collin *et al.* 2005). The Framework Convention Alliance has played a particularly important role in bringing NGOs from around the world together in an umbrella organisation, which continues to monitor and have input into the Convention during the negotiations for the PITTP.

However, the WHO remains a state-based organisation, and the FCTC and whatever protocols may be agreed upon are the outcome of multilateral negotiations between these states. While the WHO and NGOs play a crucial role in monitoring the activities of the tobacco companies around the world, and in monitoring and supporting governments to implement the provisions of the FCTC, the commitments contained within the Convention must be legislated for and implemented at national level. TTCs will continue to exploit those regimes where the commitment or capacity to enforce effective tobacco control is weak, with dire consequences for the populations of such countries. The complicity of TTCs in smuggling, particularly as a means of accessing markets that remain relatively closed (such as that of China), remains a key problem, making the successful conclusion of negotiations for an effective PITTP vital (Lee and Collin 2006).

Case study: pandemic influenza virus-sharing

Influenza virus-sharing has been a well-established feature of the WHO's Influenza Programme for the better part of 60 years. Under this programme, which was established with the primary objective of preventing the reoccurrence of influenza pandemics, such as the 1918 Spanish Flu that killed approximately 50 million people worldwide (Kitler *et al.* 2002), WHO's Global Influenza Surveillance Network (GISN) has served as the primary vehicle in the international distribution of influenza viruses for scientific and research purposes. The network operates by receiving influenza virus samples from participating countries via national influenza centres (NICs). NICs then forward these samples to one of five WHO collaborating centres (WHO CCs), where the virus samples are analysed to identify which strains of the virus are currently circulating. This information is then used by pharmaceutical companies to inform the development of seasonal influenza vaccines and, in the event that a new strain of the virus emerges, a new pandemic-specific vaccine. Given that GISN also currently incorporates some 128 institutions throughout 99 countries (WHO 2009a), the network has considerable global reach.

Since 2005, however, both GISN and the WHO have come under heavy criticism from several lower- and middle-income countries (LMICs) over the network's virus-sharing practices. The denigration of the network's reputation was led by Indonesia and its then health minister, Siti Fadilah Supari. At the heart of the issue was the WHO's practice of passing the virus samples GISN receives from affected countries to pharmaceutical companies that use the samples to develop new vaccines, which are then patented and sold for profit. Like most pharmaceuticals, though, production capacity is limited (Lee and Fidler 2007), and given that the vaccine manufacturers seek to maximise their profits, the majority of vaccines are purchased by high-income countries who can afford to pay for them (Garrett and Fidler 2007). While this system has operated for decades, as the H5N1 avian influenza (AI) virus began to spread more widely from late 2003 onwards and there were legitimate fears that a new pandemic was imminent, issues surrounding the equitable access to influenza vaccines gained new significance (Fidler 2008). Indonesia, as one of the countries most severely affected by H5N1, began to question why their samples were being used (without their permission) to make vaccines that were unlikely to be affordable to Indonesia's citizens. Claiming several previous breaches of trust, in February 2007 Indonesia then announced that it would no longer be sharing its viruses with GISN after it was revealed that an Australian company had developed a new vaccine from an Indonesian H5N1 sample (Sedyaningsih *et al.* 2008).

Indonesia's decision to withhold samples sparked widespread alarm among the international community (Fidler 2008). The cause of this alarm was the sense of an impending pandemic and the recognition that no country would be immune from its effects. Invoking the Convention on Biological Diversity (CBD), however, Indonesia claimed that the samples were their sovereign property and that it was under no legal obligation to share the viruses with the international community. While the latter assertion was accurate due to the fact that, historically, participation in GISN has always been voluntary and the revised International Health Regulations (2005) – a new framework that requires countries to freely share all relevant information regarding public health emergencies of international concern – had yet to enter into force, Indonesia's claims of 'viral sovereignty' remained inconsistent with the object and purpose of the CBD treaty (Fidler 2008). Irrespective of the legal validity of Indonesia's claims, Health Minister Supari claimed in 2008 that as many as 112 countries have expressed their support for the stance taken by her government (Fedson 2009; Schnirring 2008).

In an attempt to resolve the impasse that had developed and address LMICs' concerns, in 2007 the WHO announced the creation of a global stockpile of pandemic vaccines that all countries would be able to access based on demonstrated need. In addition, a series of meetings were held throughout 2007 between WHO and Indonesian officials to address their specific concerns ahead of an intergovernmental working group that sought to negotiate a way through the diplomatic quagmire that had emerged (Fedson and Dunnill 2007). Representatives from 109 countries attended the 'Intergovernmental Meeting on Pandemic Influenza Preparedness: Sharing of Influenza Viruses and Access to Vaccines and Other Benefits' meeting, alongside representatives from various international and NGOs. Given that the outcome of the negotiations was also likely to have a bearing on pharmaceutical companies, a delegation from the International Federation of Pharmaceutical Manufacturers and Associations was also invited to attend (WHO 2007). Yet despite four rounds of talks being held between late 2007 and 2010, negotiations broke down over the nature and extent of benefits that LMICs should receive from participating in the WHO Influenza Programme. As such, no consensus was achieved on how the system could be made more equitable and accessible.

The diplomatic stand-off that has ensued at the time of writing highlights how globalising processes are having an adverse affect on the institutions and structures surrounding the global governance of pandemic influenza. It has revealed, for example, that the virus-sharing system that was designed and implemented in the early 1950s is no longer appropriate to meet the challenges and needs of global public health. While some attempt has been made to rebuild the system to ensure it is more equitable, transparent, and accountable, this is unable to be accomplished at present. In part, this is due to the multifaceted nature of the system that seeks to merge government services with private enterprise – two groups that often have competing and diametrically opposed goals. As the WHO director-general noted in her report to the fourth and final intergovernmental meeting on virus sharing:

> The relationship between the WHO network and the many related benefits is complex because some benefits, such as global risk assessment, are directly related to the work of the WHO network while other benefits, such as the production of potential pandemic vaccines, are done by entities outside of this network.
>
> (WHO 2009b: 27–8)

Aside from the fact that Indonesia continues to remain the most severely affected country by the H5N1 virus (163 human cases and 135 H5N1-related deaths as of 12 February 2010) (WHO 2010), the lack of a resolution on this issue is also disconcerting because it raises the prospect that other countries may seek to mimic Indonesia's actions in other health-related areas, perceiving them to be an acceptable negotiating tool. In short, Indonesia's decision has set a dangerous precedent that others may seek to emulate. The problem that remains, however, is that the criticisms levelled at the WHO and GISN do represent legitimate concerns, in that the profit-maximising practices of pharmaceutical companies do preclude many LMICs from purchasing vaccines to protect their populations. At the same time, by choosing to exercise the country's sovereign right to withhold samples, the entire world has now been effectively placed at risk. It is an unenviable situation and dilemma that only diplomacy of the highest order can resolve.

Conclusion

These brief case studies reveal that economic, political, technological, socio-cultural, and environmental changes are having a profound effect on contemporary human interaction. In the field of public health, globalising processes are creating new opportunities as well as threats, and these in turn are demanding that existing governance structures and institutions adapt to changing circumstances. At times, these opportunities and threats require innovative thinking to respond to the challenges they present. For example, the first case study explored contemporary international efforts to control tobacco usage, and how transnational tobacco companies have utilised technologies and production systems to adapt their business strategies over time to secure access to new worldwide markets. In response, this has prompted the development of new governance approaches in how to regulate and control their impact and thereby protect public health. Similarly, Indonesia's actions in relation to virus-sharing have caused much alarm among the international community due to the fact that it remains the most severely affected country from the H5N1 virus. The virus samples it collects, therefore, are perceived to be critical in developing an effective vaccine – a vaccine that will be crucial in preventing human deaths in a world where international trade and travel have undermined the spatial and temporal boundaries that once provided population groups with a measure of protection. While Indonesia's continued refusal to share viruses has not been resolved at the time of writing, it nevertheless highlights the fact that 'business as usual' approaches are insufficient to deal with the challenges globalisation presents and that innovative forms of governance and new ways of thinking are needed now more than ever.

References

Collin, J. (2003) 'Think Global, Smoke Local: Transnational Tobacco Companies and Cognitive Globalization', in K. Lee (ed.) *Health Impacts of Globalization: Towards Global Governance*, Basingstoke: Palgrave Macmillan.

Collin, J., Lee, K., and Bissell, K. (2005) 'Negotiating the Framework Convention on Tobacco Control: An Updated Politics of Global Health Governance', in R. Wilkinson (ed.) *The Global Governance Reader*, London: Routledge.

Cox, H. (2000) *The Global Cigarette: Origins and Evolution of British American Tobacco 1880–1945*, Oxford: Oxford University Press.

Fedson, D.S. (2009) 'Meeting the Challenge of Influenza Pandemic Preparedness in Developing Countries', *Emerging Infectious Diseases*, 15(3): 365–71.

Fedson, D.S. and Dunnill, P. (2007) 'From Scarcity to Abundance: Pandemic Vaccines and Other Agents for "Have Not" Countries', *Journal of Public Health Policy*, 28(3): 322–40.

Fidler, D. (2008) 'Influenza Virus Samples, International Law, and Global Health Diplomacy', *Emerging Infectious Diseases*, 14(1): 88–94.

Fortune (2007) *Fortune Global 500*, available at http://money.cnn.com/magazines/fortune/global500/2007/industries/27/1.html (accessed 26 June 2009).

Garrett, L. and Fidler, D. (2007) 'Sharing H5N1 Viruses to Stop a Global Influenza Pandemic', *PLoS Medicine*, 4(11): 1,712–14.

Gilmore, A.B. and McKee, M. (2004) 'Tobacco and Transition: An Overview of Industry Investments, Impact and Influence in the Former Soviet Union', *Tobacco Control*, 13: 136–42.

Hedley, D. (2007) 'Consolidation Endgame in Sight: But is There One More Big Throw of the Dice?', *Euromonitor*, 27 July, available at http://www.euromonitor.com/Consolidation_endgame_in_sight_but_is_there_one_more_big_throw_of_the_dice (accessed: 26 June 2009).

Holden, C. and Lee, K. (2009) 'Corporate Power and Social Policy: The Political Economy of the Transnational Tobacco Corporations', *Global Social Policy*, 9(3): 328–54.

Kitler, M.E., Gavinio, P., and Lavanchy, D. (2002) 'Influenza and the Work of the World Health Organization', *Vaccine*, 20 (Suppl 2): S5–S14.

Lee, K. (2001) 'Globalization: A New Agenda for Health?' in M. McKee, P. Garner, and R. Stott, (eds) *International Cooperation in Health*, Oxford: Oxford University Press

Lee, K. and Yach, D. (2005) 'Globalization and Health', in M. Merson, R. Black, and A. Mills (eds) *International Public Health: Diseases, Programs, Systems and Policies*, 2nd edn, New York: Jones & Bartlett.

Lee, K. and Collin, J. (2006) '"Key to the Future": British American Tobacco and Cigarette Smuggling in China', *PLoS Medicine*, 3(7): 1080–89.

Lee, K. and Fidler, D. (2007) 'Avian and Pandemic Influenza: Progress and Problems with Global Health Governance', *Global Public Health*, 2(3): 215–34.

Schnirring, L. (2008) 'Indonesia Claims Wide Support for Virus-sharing Stance', *Centre for Infectious Disease and Research Policy*, available at http://www.cidrap.umn.edu/cidrap/content/influenza/avianflu/news/may2708sharing.html (accessed 8 July 2009).

Sedyaningsih, E.R., Isfandari, S., Soendoro, T., and Supari, S.F. (2008) 'Towards Mutual Trust, Transparency and Equity in Virus Sharing Mechanism: The Avian Influenza Case of Indonesia', *Annals Academy of Medicine*, 37(6): 482–8.

Shepherd, P.L. (1985) 'Transnational Corporations and the International Cigarette Industry', in R.S. Newfarmer (ed.) *Profits, Progress and Poverty: Case Studies of International Industries in Latin America*, Notre Dame, IL: University of Notre Dame Press.

Taylor, A., Chaloupka, F.J., Guindon, E., and Corbett, M. (2000) 'The Impact of Trade Liberalization on Tobacco Consumption', in P. Jha and F. Chaloupka (eds) *Tobacco Control in Developing Countries*, Washington DC: World Bank.

UNCTAD (United Nations Conference on Trade and Development) (2008) *World Investment Report*, New York and Geneva: UNCTAD.

WHO (World Health Organization) (2003) *WHO Framework Convention on Tobacco Control*, Geneva: WHO.

WHO (World Health Organization) (2007) 'Intergovernmental Meeting on Pandemic Influenza Preparedness: Sharing of Influenza Viruses. List of Participants', available at http://apps.who.int/gb/pip/pdf_files/PIP_IGM_1Rev1-en.pdf (accessed 8 July 2009).

WHO (World Health Organization) (2009a) *WHO Global Influenza Surveillance Network*, available at http://www.who.int/csr/disease/influenza/surveillance/en (accessed 7 July 2009).

WHO (World Health Organization) (2009b) *Pandemic Influenza Preparedness: Sharing of Influenza Viruses and Access to Vaccines and other Benefits: Report by the Director-General*, available at http://apps.who.int/gb/pip/pdf_files/PIP_IGM_13-en.pdf (accessed 8 July 2009).

WHO (World Health Organization) (2010) *Avian Influenza – Situation in Indonesia*, available at http://www.who.int/csr/don/2010_02_12a/en/index.html (accessed 13 February 2010).

5

From International to Global

Framing Health in the New Millennium

Ronald Labonté

Introduction

In 2007, the foreign ministers of seven countries (Norway, France, Brazil, Indonesia, Senegal, South Africa, and Thailand) issued a declaration identifying global health as 'a pressing foreign policy issue of our time', one that is:

> ... deeply interconnected with the environment, trade, economic growth, social develop-
> ment, national security, human rights and dignity. In a globalised and interdependent
> world, the state of global health has a profound impact on all nations – developed and
> developing. Ensuring public health on a global scale is of benefit to all countries.
>
> (Ministers of Foreign Affairs of Brazil, France, Indonesia,
> Norway, Senegal, South Africa, and Thailand 2007: 1,373)

Other governments followed suit, with Switzerland releasing its health foreign policy document in 2006 and the UK launching its global health strategy two years later.

These statements formalise a decadal trend in which health became more prominent in global policy agendas. Demonstration of this was the dramatic rise in global financing for health, from US\$ 5.6 billion in 1990 to over US\$ 21.8 billion in 2007 (Ravishankar *et al.* 2009), accompanied by a proliferation of global health initiatives (such as the Global Fund), financing schemes (UNITAID, the airline tax that finances antiretroviral drugs for poor countries), and new private players (notably the Gates Foundation). Several of the Millennium Development Goals (MDGs), agreed to by all United Nations (UN) member states in 2000, refer specifically to health, and all address its social determinants (Table 5.1). Twice health has been identified as a global security issue by the UN Security Council with reference to HIV/AIDS, and concerns over pandemic disease (notably influenza) and bioterrorism retain health's position in the foreign policy agendas of many of the world's nations.

Table 5.1 Millennium Development Goals and health

Goal and targets	Health implications
Goal 1: Eradicate extreme poverty and hunger Target 1: Halve, between 1990 and 2015, the proportion of people whose income is less than one dollar a day Target 2: Halve, between 1990 and 2015, the proportion of people who suffer from hunger	Hunger target one of the specific health goals Poverty a major determinant of poor health and health inequities
Goal 2: Achieve universal primary education Target 3: Ensure that, by 2015, children everywhere, boys and girls alike, will be able to complete a full course of primary education	Education one of the most powerful predictors of health over the life-course
Goal 3: Promote gender equality and empower women Target 4: Eliminate gender disparity in primary and secondary education preferably by 2005, and to all levels of education no later than 2015	Gender empowerment one of the most powerful predictors of infant and child health and survival Patriarchal practices still a cause of violence against women in many countries, especially where education levels for both women and men are low
Goal 4: Reduce child mortality Target 5: Reduce by two-thirds, between 1990 and 2015, the under-5 mortality rate	One of the specific health goals
Goal 5: Improve maternal health Target 6: Reduce by three-quarters, between 1990 and 2015, the maternal mortality ratio	One of the specific health goals
Goal 6: Combat HIV/AIDS, malaria, and other diseases Target 7: Have halted by 2015, and begun to reverse, the spread of HIV/AIDS Target 8: Have halted by 2015, and begun to reverse, the incidence of malaria and other major diseases	One of the specific health goals
Goal 7: Ensure environmental sustainability Target 9: Integrate the principles of sustainable development into country policies and programmes and reverse the loss of environmental resources Target 10: Halve, by 2015, the proportion of people without sustainable access to safe drinking water Target 11: By 2020, to have achieved a significant improvement in the lives of at least 100 million slum dwellers	Scarcity of environmental resources increasingly a source of conflict, hunger, and subsequent poor health Unsafe or inaccessible drinking water a major cause of childhood morbidity and mortality, infectious disease, and health/safety risks for women Urban slums without sanitation, water, and sufficient food for good health likely to become sources of new and virulent infections
Goal 8: Develop a global partnership for development	Least-developed countries frequently experience the highest burden of disease, although most of the world's poor do not live in such countries

(continued on the next page)

Table 5.1 (continued)

Goal and targets	Health implications
Target 12: Address the special needs of least developed countries, landlocked countries, and small island developing states	Role of non-discriminatory open trade and finance system on health and development remains controversial; financial crises disproportionately hurt health of the poor
Target 13: Develop further an open, rule-based, predictable, non-discriminatory trading and financial system	
Target 14: Deal comprehensively with developing countries' debt	Debt servicing costs still crowd out health and education spending in many low-income countries; much debt should be considered odious and uncollectable
Target 15: In cooperation with pharmaceutical companies, provide access to affordable essential drugs	Role of extended patent protection in reducing access to essential drugs in many low-income countries remains contentious
Target 16: In cooperation with the private sector, make available benefits of new technologies, especially information and communications	

Inherently global health issues

Health's foreign policy continues to vacillate between two conceptual poles: international and global. The first is characterised by the concern of wealthier nations with the greater disease burden in poorer countries. Its origins extend back to medieval efforts to halt the spread of infection that accompanied the movement of goods and people. The twin triumphs of the germ theory and the first wave of globalisation in the mid- to late nineteenth century marked a formal approach to 'international health' in response to the spread of infectious disease, with many colonial governments and corporate philanthropies beginning to fund basic public health measures in developing countries (Birn 2006). Motivations were complex, embracing political and economic interests, reducing cross-border contagion or risks to nationals working abroad, and faith-based ideals of charity or missionary conversion.

Similar interests underpin the contemporary rise of health in foreign policy discourse, but with a shift in nomenclature to 'global health'. Kaplan and colleagues (2009) traced global health's 'fashionable' status to a combination of international health's disciplinary base in tropical medicine and public health's roots in population-wide intervention and social reform. Elsewhere Labonté and Torgerson (2005) argued that four world events have changed the landscape of 'international health' irrevocably:

1. The oil crisis of the 1970s, ensuing developing world debt, and the transformation of the international financial institutions into promulgators of a neo-liberal, structural adjustment economics then in favour with the wealthier countries that dominated their decision-making. These programmes effectively coerced many developing countries into a rapidly globalising economy.
2. The collapse of the Soviet Union and loss of a 'constitutive other' to market fundamentalism that had allowed post-colonial countries to experiment with mixed economies and a 'new international economic order'. The emergence of a human rights discourse on development has failed so far to occupy the same political imagination that socialism once held.

3. The rise of an environmental consciousness, imaged by earth photos from the first moon landing in 1969, advanced by social movement activists, endorsed by the world's nations at the 1992 UN Conference on Environment and Development, and driven now by climate change and the fearsome awareness of a finite world of declining life support capacities.
4. The suffusion of digital communication technologies. These assisted the post-1980s surge in international trade and were fundamental to the growth in unregulated financial instruments that globalised speculative investments divorced from the 'real' (production/ consumption) economy. The same technologies also increased the speed and scale with which a globalising civil society could analyse and mobilise responses to global capitalism's economic abuses.

This brief synopsis is neither definitive nor does it imply that acceptance of 'global health' means rejection of 'international health'. Notwithstanding the latter term's legacy in colonialism and charity, international health's concern with the disease conditions of poorer countries remains important since these conditions remain both different and more debilitating than those of wealthier ones. Whatever precise definition for global health sediments into common use, it will incorporate two axioms that distinguish it from its international predecessor: an understanding that heightened global economic interdependence ('globalisation') has become increasingly the cause and consequence of the (mal)distribution of global disease burdens; and that many of the pressing health issues facing nations are now inherently global (Table 5.2) not simply by dint of cross-border disease threats, but in the societal conditions that increase risk of and vulnerability to disease, and access to preventive and treatment services.

Globalisation's new health demands

Globalisation (notably its economic facets) underpins most of these 'inherently global health issues'. It is not a new phenomenon, with ancient empires, industrial colonialism, and

Table 5.2 Inherent global health issues

Environmental global degradation	1.	Greenhouse gas emissions (climate change)
	2.	Biodiversity loss
	3.	Water shortage
	4.	Decline in fisheries
	5.	Deforestation
Social /economic	1.	Increasing poverty
	2.	Financial instability (capital markets)
	3.	Digital divide
	4.	Taxation (tax havens, transfer pricing)
Cross-cutting	1.	Food (in) security
	2.	Trade in health-damaging products (tobacco, arms, toxic waste)
	3.	Governance
	4.	Tourism
	5.	Migration
	6.	War and conflict

Source: Adapted from Labonté and Torgerson 2005.

the post-industrial market liberalisation of Belle Époque marking earlier eras. Since the 1980s, globalisation has been characterised by the development of new multilateral institutions, enforceable trade rules, the creation of global production chains, and the increased financialisation of the world's economies (increasingly rendering it a singular economy) – shifts that distinguish this phase from its predecessors. These characteristics have also brought new health risks associated with asymmetries in economic gains and losses due to pre-globalisation differences in wealth, power, and productive assets. These differences, and the outsourcing of manufacturing production to (predominantly) China and South Asia, have increased wealth inequalities between countries, and between capital and labour; worsened labour market insecurities; precipitated financial crises due to volatility in prices and exchange rates; and accelerated environmental losses and climate change (Labonté *et al.* 2009).

Not all aspects of contemporary globalisation have been health-negative. Indeed, the global diffusion of new health knowledge and technologies did more to improve health status in developing countries in the last half of the past century than economic growth per se (Deaton 2006). This was attested to by the 'child health revolution', in which simple technologies and behavioural programmes (growth monitoring, oral rehydration, breastfeeding, immunisation, food fortification, family planning, and female education) led to dramatic declines in infant and under-five mortality. The employment opportunities afforded women in export industries, notably textiles, located in poor, patriarchal nations have played a role in gender empowerment and trickle-down health benefits (Kabeer 2004), albeit under adverse working conditions partly driven by retailers in high-income countries demanding low-cost, 'just-in-time' production. By the early 1990s, the global convergence in health reversed, with health inequities growing within and between most countries.

An econometric study, undertaken by Cornia and colleagues for the Globalisation Knowledge Network of the World Health Organisation's Commission on Social Determinants of Health, examined the role globalisation played in this reversal (Labonté *et al.* 2008). It compared life expectancy at birth (LEB) in 2005 against the counterfactual projection of LEB trends prior to the post-1980 onset of globalisation-related policies. It found that policy-driven aspects of globalisation reduced worldwide potential LEB gains by 1.53 years, due primarily to increases in income inequalities, economic instability, slowed improvements in the provision of health services, and stagnation in vaccination coverage. Regionally, OECD countries and nations in the Middle East and North Africa came out ahead; the transition countries (Eastern Europe) and those in sub-Saharan Africa (SSA) fared worst. In the latter case, globalisation-related policies contributed almost as much to the steep declines in LEB as did the HIV/AIDS pandemic.

HIV/AIDS: a global explanation

The HIV/AIDS pandemic in SSA itself has a partial explanation in the economics of globalisation, as is seen in this stylised story of a Zambian woman:

> … Chileshe waits painfully to die from AIDS. The global funds and antiretroviral programmes are too little and too late for her. She was infected by her now dead husband, who once worked in a textile plant along with thousands of others but lost his job when Zambia opened its borders to cheap, second-hand clothing. He moved to the city as a street vendor, selling cast-offs or donations from wealthier countries. He would get drunk and trade money for sex – often with women whose own husbands were somewhere else working, or dead, and who themselves desperately needed money for their children. Desperation, she thought, is what makes this disease move so swiftly…
>
> (Labonte *et al.* 2005: 1)

The facts behind this fiction involve the imposition of structural adjustment on Zambia in the early 1990s, which included the removal of tariffs on imported textiles. In what the World Bank later described as a 'regrettable mistake', most of Zambia's domestic textile 'infant industries' closed down within a few years, unable to compete for quality or cost with the used clothing that flooded the market. Privatisation of state enterprises, one of the conditions associated with structural adjustment loans, eliminated revenues that might have been used to support education and health care. To comply with wage and public sector spending ceilings, Zambia imposed user fees, cut health staff, and reduced the salaries of those who remained. These globally driven policy shifts occurred just as AIDS was gaining momentum. Zambia was not alone, and SSA's ill-timed and ideologically based adjustment policies are now widely regarded as fuelling an already festering pandemic (Commission for Africa 2005: 96–7).

It would be erroneous to blame HIV/AIDS in SSA simply on globalisation. Inadequate government responses, AIDS denialism, and cultural acceptance of multiple concurrent partners are all important factors. But globalisation played a role. It continues to do so as the poverty-induced 'survival sex' of Chileshe (Preston-Whyte *et al.* 2000; Wojcicki 2002) is joined by a new HIV risk: 'transactional sex', in which young women trade sex for cell phones, MP3 players, and Western fashion (Dunkle *et al.* 2007) as consumerism, its commodities, and its advertised images of success increasingly globalise.

Locating the global in the local

The implication of the HIV/AIDS example is that what happens within borders can no longer be isolated from global economic and political forces. Consider, first, a simple framework of influences on health, organised hierarchically by geographic and socio-political scale (Figure 5.1).

This framework argues that globalisation will have different health effects depending on the political history and resource endowments of different countries or regions: a point already made. It also identifies some of the key 'drivers' of global market integration: macroeconomic policies such as structural adjustment (now disappeared in name, if not always in content); trade and financial liberalisation agreements; multilateral institutions, such as UN agencies, but increasingly, global public/private partnerships, that provide global public goods under-supplied by the market; and development assistance as a crude system of global wealth redistribution.

Second, consider a typically 'international health' research question: What is the effectiveness of community health workers (CHWs) in improving maternal/child health? A typically sound approach to answering this question would be a pre-post study using a randomised, quasi-experimental or multiple case-study design where the number or skill-set of CHWs was the independent variable. Working down the framework (Figure 5.1) from the level of programme intervention, one would also ask: How are resources for health controlled within the home? How do household education and income levels interact with CHWs in explaining differences in outcomes? Working up, one would likely examine: Are CHWs distributed within and between rural and urban areas? Are policies for public provision of services adequate? Are there regional management structures in place to ensure quality and continuity?

But the global instantiates itself even in the local, and so working still further up the framework, one would need also to ask: What are the constraints on national government expenditures to ensure an adequate and equitable supply of community CHWs? What role do international aid agencies or multilateral institutions play in worsening or lessening these

Ronald Labonté

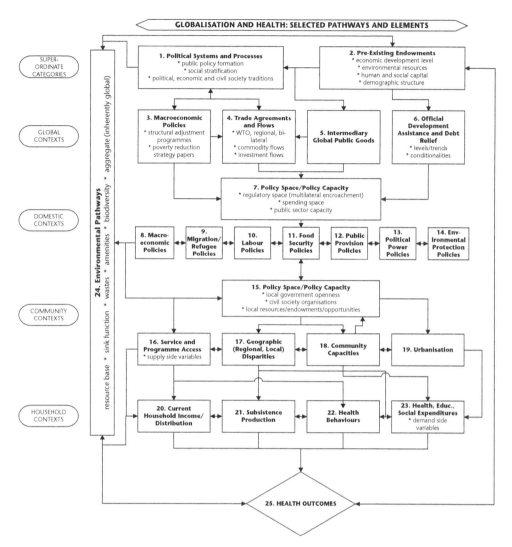

Figure 5.1   Globalisation and health: selected pathways and elements
Source: Labonté and Torgerson 2005.

constraints? How does the proliferation of siloed global health initiatives affect the development of a more integrated and effective public provision system? What role do trade agreements play, particularly in employment conditions or income generation that might affect household resource levels? How does the 'brain drain' of health professionals (internally from rural to urban, public to private, government to global health initiatives, and externally to higher-income nations) affect the supply of CHWs or, importantly, the supply of nurses and physicians needed as more highly skilled support? How does capital flight or the existence of offshore tax havens constrain expenditures, or promote corruption that, in turn, ripples down the public and private systems of delivery? No single evaluation or research study alone can address all of these questions. But ignoring them in an analysis or contextualisation of health programme effectiveness is likely to lead to partial and arguably mistaken conclusions.

Framing the right foreign policy response?

The two examples above describe how health issues in low-income countries are embedded within global economic policies and practices largely controlled by wealthier nations. A full explication of the adequacy or future potential of the foreign policies of wealthier nations to better address global health equity is beyond this chapter's capacity to address. What can be described is how global health has been framed in such policies. A limited number of such frames have been identified: security, development, global public good, trade, human rights, and ethical/moral reasoning (Labonté 2008). These frames are neither exclusive nor, importantly, congruent. How differences are reconciled, however, depends on which frame comes to predominate.[1]

Health and security

The most frequently encountered frame is that of security, with three major aspects: national (border protection), economic (growth and competitive advantage), and human (capacity for individual flourishing). There are some internal conflicts between all three, notably with respect to the arms trade, which brings economic advantage but which could threaten national and human security. There are also risks inherent in public health efforts to frame health in the 'high politics' of security.[2] One of these is that of a triage of global support for health based upon a country's self-interest and geopolitical strategic interests. Another is that such a triage reverses the historic concern with improving health equity as an ethical commitment, inherently 'good' in its own right. A third concern is that the securitisation of specific disease risks (such as HIV/ AIDS and pandemic influenza) has led to global financing of these disease risks disproportionate to the burden they represent. Evidence finally suggests that the self-interest of 'high politics' has not sustained foreign policy support for health in the past and is unlikely to do so in the future.

Health and development

Until recently, health improvements were seen primarily as positive externalities to economic growth. Over the past decade, a growing body of evidence has shown that improvements in health are associated with economic growth: health spending becomes as much an investment as a cost. While the development frame has attracted the greatest global health policy attention and documentation (now notably focused on the MDGs), it is weakened by persisting limitations in aid architecture, levels of support, unfulfilled commitments, disbursements based on donors' strategic interests rather than need, and a focus on aid to the exclusion of other foreign policies (such as trade) that affect countries' health and development potential. Instrumental arguments for health aid can also lead to a 'return on investment' ('results-based') approach, dispensing assistance by short-term or easier gains. Potential conflict exists between the development and security frames, when the constrained logic of national security (protection of national citizens) directs foreign policy away from global health equity as a public good in its own right. One important implication of the shift from 'international' to 'global', however, is the necessity to redefine development assistance from intermittent *noblesse oblige* to sustained obligation, based on political agreement (the MDGs) and their 'fundamental value' of 'solidarity: ... those who suffer or benefit least deserve help from those who benefit most' (UN General Assembly 2000: 2), legal requirements (found in human rights treaties), and ethical argument (notably the theory of relational justice, because evidence shows that global institutions and rules benefit those who dominate them, but imperils the health of others, and thus morally compels the former to acts of restitution).

Health and global public goods

Public good theory offers one of the strongest arguments for global health policy, but is rarely encountered in governments' foreign policy statements and may be more implied than explicit. Public goods arise from market failures that are only overcome by public provision or regulation that collectivises both costs and benefits. No consensus exists on the boundaries demarcating a 'global' public good from one that is international (a few nations only), regional (a geographic clustering of nations), club (a political clustering of nations), national, or local. However, peace, prevention of pandemics, financial stability, human rights, free access to knowledge, and a stable climate all have characteristics of such global public goods. While potentially powerful because of its origins in economic theory, a global public good frame has yet to lead to substantive action. As one example: climate stability, regarded as one of the most serious global public goods confronting the planet, is mired in equity issues, with inadequate financing (or lack of fulfilment of commitments) for assistance to low- and middle-income countries by high-income countries. A plausible reason is that climate change effects are not yet sufficiently serious to challenge the 'high politics' of national security and economic interest of today's wealthier, or rapidly growing, countries.

Health and trade

The trade frame is the most problematic, particularly from an equity vantage. While a rules-based global trading system is regarded as another global public good, the definition and enforcement of those rules is dependent upon countries' economic and political power and past development history. There is frequent evidence of conflict/incoherence between countries' trade policies (economic interests) and their foreign health and development policies. Even a successful completion of the so-called Doha Development Round of World Trade Organization (WTO) trade negotiations would disproportionately benefit OECD countries in economic gain, while costing developing countries substantially more in lost tariffs revenues. The global financial crisis both complicates and heightens the responsibilities for health-based arguments in trade negotiations – whether to avoid a protectionist spiral of uncertain environmental, social, and economic consequences, or to ensure that efforts to complete the Doha Development Round (now seen by some economists as a priority to avoid prolonging the global recession) is much more heavily influenced by health equity concerns and development outcomes aligned more closely to achievement of the MDGs.

Health and human rights

Human rights treaties are regarded by many international law experts as having primacy over other treaties when conflicts between the two sets of laws arise. UN special rapporteurs on several of these rights, notably the right to health, have pointed to existing and potential sources of conflict between trade treaties and health rights. Evidence suggests that the stronger the force of human rights is within domestic legislation, the more persuasive these rights become in foreign policy negotiations. But legal opinions on the argumentative value and policy effectiveness of human rights treaties obligations vary. There is no effective enforcement mechanism unless international treaty rights are written into national laws. Some scholars and civil society organisations argue against the present emphasis on human rights, which remain more *individual* than *collective* in application, for their lack of class and political economy analysis. At the same time, human rights have become the most globalised political value-statements of the new millennium.

Health and ethical/moral reasoning

States, the institutions they create, and the persons who function within them are moral actors. At present, moral or ethical arguments are largely absent in foreign policy, apart from reference to social justice as an overarching principle (though usually without definition). Equity is at the core of social justice theory, with two differing but non-exclusive conceptions: equality of opportunity (an emphasis on horizontal equity and procedural justice: all are treated the same) and equality of outcome (an emphasis on vertical equity and substantive justice: positive discrimination favouring the historically disadvantaged). In recent decades, an overemphasis on equality of opportunity has been used to argue for minimal state interventions into market economies for redistributive (social welfare) spending. Fairness in equality of opportunity, however, requires that all persons have the same initial capabilities, thus requiring redistributive measures to provide more 'capability' resources to historically least advantaged individuals and groups. This reasoning applies globally as well as nationally, with better-off countries having achieved the ability (if not always the will) for more generous redistributive welfare in part through past or ongoing economic exploitation of poorer nations.

Conclusion: advancing global health in an era of retreat

It is generally accepted in policy theory that the framing of an issue is critical, in path-dependent fashion, to the types of interventions that then fall within the negotiation space. If global health is seen principally as a matter of national security, negotiation space may be confined to prevention of pandemic disease or to strategic self-interest. If global health is approached primarily as an obligation under international human rights treaties, the negotiating space becomes much larger. Political contestation often revolves around how policy issues are framed. What does that mean for health advocates seeking to advance global health in foreign policy debate? Likely, it will mean a pragmatic infusion of arguments arising from each of these frames, as political moments arise (Table 5.3).

There are limitations with each frame: a moral language, while requisite, is insufficient in itself. It can too easily be invoked without consequence. Legal language is also needed and remains best provided in human rights covenants. But neither moral nor legal arguments (in the absence of enforcement mechanisms) are necessarily compelling as security or economic rationales, the two frames that continue to hold most sway in foreign policy actions. Economically, both the global public goods and development frames have some utility in positioning health in foreign policy debates, but only if they are located beneath a penumbra of ethical reasoning and legal obligation. Otherwise, the risk exists of a prioritisation of foreign policy or global governance decisions based on the interests of wealthier nations. The securitisation of health, even in its human rather than national or economic rendering, remains problematically premised in a conception of the individual made capable to function as a market actor; that is, it supports, rather than challenges, the social and economic assumptions that have driven the past three decades of neo-liberal globalisation.

The global financial crisis of 2008, itself a product of similar globalisation forces that first pushed health higher up in foreign policy debates, has led to speculation that health's moment in foreign policy may already be in retreat (Fidler 2008/2009). Wealthier nations are becoming less generous in development assistance and more protectionist in trade, and have failed (so far) to constrain through adequate regulation the ongoing financialisation of the global economy. The moral hazard created by bailouts for investment bankers is likely to precipitate more bubbles and collapses in the future. The UK and the USA (most

Table 5.3 Framing global health arguments

Policy frame	Health argument
Security	Gives global health interventions greater traction across a range of political classes than a rights-based argument alone. To the extent that this strengthens a base of public health expansion, securitisation of health may be a prerequisite to its eventual de-securitisation. But vigilance is needed to avoid national security from trumping human security.
Development	Remains the invitation to global governance debates. It provides a seat at the table. Risks inherent in its 'investing in health' instrumentalism can be tempered by continuously reminding decision-makers to distinguish which one is the objective (human development) and which one the tool (economic growth). The accountability advocacy of international NGOs continues to pressure rich nations to move beyond the inadequate patchwork of broken aid promises to a global system of taxation and redistribution.
Global public good	Provides a language by which economists of one market persuasion can convince economists of another that there is a sound rationale for a system of shared global financing and regulation.
Trade	Can improve health through global market integration, economic growth, and positive health externalities. However, present trade rules skew benefits towards more economically and politically powerful countries, and evidence of negative health externalities demands careful a priori assessments of trade treaties for their health, development, and human rights implications.
Human rights	Though weak in global enforcement, human rights have advocacy traction and legal potential within national boundaries. Such rights do not resolve embedded tensions between the individual and the collective, an issue to which human rights experts are now attending.
Moral/ethical reasoning	Suggested as a necessary addendum to the legalistic nature of human rights treaties. This has created scholarly momentum to articulate more rigorous arguments for a global health ethic based on moral reasoning. Competitors for such an ethic range from a liberal theory of assistive duties based on 'burdened societies' in need, to an emphasis on minimum capabilities needed for people to lead valued lives, to more recent arguments for relational justice, based on evidence that global institutional arrangements are disproportionately benefiting some and contributing to poverty of others and that those benefiting from/upholding these institutions are duty bound to rectify their inequities

Source: Adapted from Labonté and Gagnon 2010.

prominently, but not exclusively) face huge debts arising from these bailouts, and their countercyclical spending.

At the same time, many low- and middle-income countries are experiencing severe contractions in export-led growth, increases in poverty, and declines in all forms of capital flows (aid, remittances, and investment), with knock-on effects in lower health and social protection spending. The prospect that this will exacerbate cross-border health threats or worsen costly regional conflicts driven by disease and scarcity will ensure a role for health in global policy debate, even if not so high as previously.

The transition from international to global health, while episodic and perhaps incomplete, nonetheless follows a logic embedded in technology, economy, and ecology. We may increasingly see, hear, and view the world as a single human society (or witness its balkanisation). The world's economies may continue a global integration into a more singular one (or devolve into localism and conflict-ridden mercantilism). Climate change and the depletion of the environmental prerequisites to life will, of necessity, bind the world's populations (or lead to ecological wars of devastating consequence). Whichever of these dichotomous paths dominates the future, it will be global in scale, and an active promotion of 'global health' in foreign policy may be one important contribution to a path of least destruction.

Notes

1 The remainder of this chapter is adapted from Labonté and Gagnon (2010).
2 International relations theory ranks foreign policy objectives in a hierarchy of descending importance from national security (material interests/high politics) to economic interests to development to human dignity/humanitarian aid (normative values/low politics). The assumption is that 'high politics' framing is more likely to lead diplomacy and policy decision-making than 'low politics' framing.

References

Birn, A-E. (2006) *Marriage of Convenience: Rockefeller International Health and Revolutionary Mexico*, Rochester, NY: University of Rochester Press.

Commission for Africa (2005) *Our Common Interest: Report of the Commission for Africa*, London: Commission for Africa.

Deaton, A. (2006) 'Global Patterns of Income and Health', *WIDER Angle*, (2): 1–3.

Dunkle, K.L., Jewkes, R., Mzikazi, N., Nwabisa, J., Levin, J., Sikweyiya, Y., and Koss, M.P. (2007) 'Transactional Sex with Casual and Main Partners Among Young South African Men in the Rural Eastern Cape: Prevalence, Predictors, and Associations with Gender-based Violence', *Social Science & Medicine*, 65: 1,235–48.

Fidler, D. (2008/09) 'After the Revolution: Global Health Politics in a Time of Economic Crisis and Threatening Future Trends', *Global Health Governance*, II(2): 1–21.

Kabeer, N. (2004) 'Globalisation, Labour Standards and Women's Rights: Dilemmas of Collective (In) action in an Interdependent World', *Feminist Economics*, 10: 3–35.

Kaplan, J., Bond, C., Merson, M., Reddy, S., Rodriguez, M., Sewankambo, N., and Wasserheit, J.N. (2009) 'Towards a Common Definition of Global Health', *The Lancet*, 373(9,681): 1,993–5.

Labonté, R. (2008) 'Global Health in Public Policy: Finding the Right Frame?', *Critical Public Health*, 18 (4): 467–82.

Labonté, R. and Torgerson, R. (2005) 'Interrogating Globalization, Health and Development: Towards a Comprehensive Framework for Research, Policy and Political Action', *Critical Public Health*, 15(2): 157–79.

Labonté, R., Schrecker, T., Sen Gupta, A. (2005) *Health for Some: Death, Disease and Disparity in a Globalizing World*, Toronto: Centre for Social Justice.

Labonté, R., Blouin, C., Chopra, M., Lee, K., Packer, C., Rowson, M., Schrecker, T., Woodward, D., and *Globalization Knowledge Network* (2008) 'Towards Health-equitable Globalisation: Rights, Regulation and Distribution. Final Report of the Globalization Knowledge Network', Geneva: World Health Organisation Commission on Social Determinants of Health, available at http://www.globalhealthequity.ca/electronic%20library/GKN%20Final%20Jan%208%202008.pdf (accessed 30 August 2009).

Labonté, R., Schrecker, T., Packer, C., and Runnels, V. (eds) (2009) *Globalization and Health: Pathways, Evidence and Policy*, London: Routledge.

Labonté, R. and Gagnon, M. (2010) 'Framing Health and Foreign Policy: Lessons for Global Health Diplomacy', *Globalization and Health*, 6: 14.

Ministers of Foreign Affairs of Brazil, France, Indonesia, Norway, Senegal, South Africa, and Thailand (April 2007) 'Oslo Ministerial Declaration – Global Health: A Pressing Foreign Policy Issue of our Time', *The Lancet*, 369(9,570): 1,373–8.

Preston-Whyte, E., Varga, C., Oosthuizen, H., Roberts, R., and Blose, F. (2000) 'Survival Sex and HIV/AIDS in an African City', in R. Parker, R.M. Barbosa, and P. Aggleton (eds) *Framing the Sexual Subject: The Politics of Gender, Sexuality, and Power*, Berkeley, CA: University of California Press, 165–91.

Ravishankar, N., Gubbins, P., Cooley, R., Leach-Kemon, K., Michaud, C., Jamison, D., and Murray, C. (2009) 'Financing of Global Health: Tracking Development Assistance for Health from 1990 to 2007', *The Lancet*, 373(9,681): 2,113–24.

United Nations General Assembly (2000) 'United Nations Millennium Declaration', Resolution adopted by the General Assembly, 8th plenary meeting. 8 September 2000, available at http://www.un.org/millennium/declaration/ares552e.pdf (accessed 10 December 2009).

Wojcicki, J.M. (2002) '"She Drank His Money": Survival Sex and the Problem of Violence in Taverns in Gauteng Province, South Africa', *Medical Anthropology Quarterly*, 16(3): 267–93.

6

International Health, Global Health, and Human Rights

Daniel Tarantola, Laura Ferguson, and Sofia Gruskin

Introduction

Over the last four decades, international health and global health, terms often used interchangeably, have been gradually acquiring distinct meanings. Specifically, international and global health initiatives can increasingly be understood to be grounded in different motivations, to employ different mechanisms, and to be subjected to different modes of governance.

International health recognises the ability of nation states to participate fully as independent entities in the public discourse and action on health. International then becomes the sum of nations and their structured interactions through international fora and governance mechanisms relevant to health (Brown *et al.* 2006)[1]. Under this definition, nation states would be understood, under the auspices of the World Health Organization (WHO) or other United Nations (UN) entities, to define international health priorities, agree on international mechanisms of international cooperation, and take steps, within their realm of power, to fulfil their commitments towards common health goals.

Global health, on the other hand, considers health issues deemed of global relevance and magnitude, which attract interest, funding and, cooperation from not only the public sector but private actors including corporations, foundations, non-governmental organisations (NGOs), and civil society (Brown *et al.* 2006). While global *threats* can be recognised on the basis of epidemiological, social, and/or economic factors, global *programmes* are established for a mix of reasons, ranging from the need to draw attention to a threat of recognised magnitude, to the desire to avoid the cumbersome process of international consensus-building through the establishment of new governance structures. Determining whether a particular health issue is recognised to be global – rather than international – and how the response is constructed and governed, is strongly influenced by shifts in the distribution of political and financial power.

Human rights are referred to here as the set of norms and standards embodied in international human rights documents such as treaties, declarations, and other commitments resulting from the international negotiations between governments in the context of the UN system (UN 1948). Human rights represent the obligations of states towards people. These obligations include respecting rights (the state should not violate rights), protecting rights (the state should ensure that non-state actors do not violate rights and have redress mechanisms in place), and fulfilling rights (the state should establish structures and mechanisms to promote and protect rights including administrative, legal, and budgetary measures). The place of human rights in health efforts has evolved alongside increasing clarity about the definitions of international and global health, with attention to rights ranging from loose rhetorical concepts used to support a concern with inequality, to the application of specific human rights concepts and methods in the ways in which health programming is implemented.

The relationships between international health, global health, and human rights have differed across regions, health domains, and over time. Select large-scale public health ventures undertaken since the 1970s will be used to illustrate the intertwined, complex relationship of these approaches to evolving understanding of the role human rights can play in these efforts. These include: the eradication of smallpox; the evolution of primary health care and the Primary Health Care Movement; childhood immunisation, including the Expanded Programme on Immunization and creation of the Global Alliance for Vaccines and Immunisation; and the response to HIV/AIDS, including the creation of UNAIDS and the Global Fund to combat AIDS, Tuberculosis and Malaria (GFATM). The selection of examples is intended to capture some of the variety in approaches to health that we have witnessed in recent times – a vertical programme, a large-scale movement, the move towards public/private partnerships in the field of immunisation, and the truly global response to HIV.

Each – some of which overlap in time – sheds light on the shift from international health to global health and the potential role of human rights in such efforts. Of concern, however, core human rights principles, which began to permeate international health in the mid-1990s, including participation, non-discrimination, governmental obligations towards individuals and populations, as well as accountability, and are today challenged by the unclear division and risk of dilution of responsibility represented by current mechanisms of global health. The implications for rights, therefore, represent one of the determinants and outcomes to be watched in the transition from international to global health initiatives.

The central question this chapter will explore is how the rhetoric, concepts, and methods of human rights have been implicated in the transition from international health to global health, and how they can most usefully be employed moving forward. In order to anchor this analysis in large-scale health initiatives, the creation, life, and fortunate demise of the smallpox eradication programme – a historical success in international health – is recalled.

International health with a focus on disease eradication

It took over 150 years for vaccines to become safe and, in a freeze-dried presentation, fairly stable under different climatic conditions. In 1950, the Pan American Sanitary Organization embarked on a regional smallpox eradication campaign. Then, in 1958, in the midst of the Cold War, the USSR proposed to the World Health Assembly (WHA) to eradicate smallpox. Both East and West geopolitical blocs, in concert, engaged in the campaign, and, by 1977, the smallpox programme had achieved total success (Fenner *et al.* 1988). With a few notable exceptions, the smallpox eradication programme was conducted almost entirely by UN agencies, mostly WHO and government structures – in particular the then USSR and the US Centers for Disease Control and Prevention (CDC) – as well as those of affected countries.

The campaign's success can be attributed to a mix of humanitarian motives, desire to prevent the importation of smallpox into smallpox-free countries, and economics. The last ten years of the campaign cost less than US $300 million in total, of which $200 million came from affected countries themselves. The benefits of eradication to the world have been estimated at US $1.35

billion per year in 1980 dollars in treatment and prevention costs – a benefit which continues to accrue annually to the world economy.

Where were human rights in this effort? In the course of the eradication campaigns, human rights as such were barely visible. It should be recalled that the two treaties born out of the 1948 Universal Declaration of Human Rights (UN 1948) – the International Covenant on Civil Political Rights (ICCPR) (UN 1966a) and the International Covenant on Economic, Social and Cultural Rights (ICESCR) (UN 1966b) – did not come into force until 1976, as the smallpox eradication programme was coming to an end. It is worth noting that at this time, in the UN General Assembly, East and West were engaged in a bitter political confrontation on the value and meaning of social and economic human rights, including the right to the highest attainable standard of health. In those days, a common international health agenda governed by the WHA was in many ways the only opportunity for people from East and West, North and South to work together rather than argue with one another. The fact that nation states joined forces around a health theme was contributing to peace and security, and, therefore, to the realisation of human rights, even if this was never referred to as human rights per se.

The immediate benefits of the success of the eradication programme on international health were staggering, but there were also some unforeseen detrimental effects. In countries where the campaign had been intense, health systems were not prepared for a return to an integrated offer of services. On the positive side, however, the confidence of national health systems in international cooperation for health grew to a high point, culminating in the Alma-Ata conference in 1978, just as the smallpox campaign was ending.

Primary health care: the emergence of human rights and initial steps towards global health

The Alma-Ata conference followed a long evolution in thinking about basic health needs and how these could best be met. It was attended by delegations from 134 countries and by representatives of 67 UN agencies and NGOs. It set the goal of achieving health for all by the year 2000 through a *primary health care approach*. State, and for the first time, non-state actors, with the exception of commercial entities, came together to reset the international health agenda. The conference expressed 'the need for urgent action by all governments, all health and development workers, and the world community to protect and promote the health of the people of the world' (Litsios 2008: 308). The declaration which resulted from the conference affirmed that 'health … is a fundamental human right and that the attainment of the highest possible level of health is a most important world-wide social goal whose realisation requires the action of many other social and economic sectors in addition to the health sector' (UN 1978). The ICCPR and the ICESCR had entered into force only two years earlier so interest in rights language was high, even as rights concepts were not systematically considered or applied in what followed.

The Primary Health Care (PHC) movement started with much enthusiasm and a strong commitment on the part of state actors and gradually NGOs, many of which had by then embarked on health, social, and community development initiatives. The common goal was to reach out to the most underserved, vulnerable communities with a package of interventions that could be delivered with the active participation of community health workers and communities themselves. After Alma-Ata and into the early 1980s, genuine progress was made in some communities, but, too often, rhetoric gave rise only to dreams of utopian models of community participation, village self-management, and voluntary service providers.

Infant and childhood mortality rates, which had served as sensitive indicators of progress and had been gradually declining until then, began to show a tendency to level off or even re-ascend by the early 1980s (Hill and Yazbeck 1994; Hill *et al.* 1999). If progress was to be accelerated, or at least sustained, common wisdom suggested that the holistic vision of PHC had to create space for targeted programmes which brought back a certain amount of verticality, including narrow management systems, dedicated staff, and specifically assigned international resources. Several important actors in international health went on to promote, finance, and actively scale-up targeted programmes based on simple technology and universal delivery models intended (or stated) to support PHC. Packages of interventions targeted at specific diseases or health systems components were launched by UNICEF (GOBI: Growth monitoring, Oral rehydration, Breastfeeding and *I*mmunisations), USAID (CCCD: Combating Childhood Communicable Diseases), the World Bank (a basic health care initiative with emphasis on system-based service provision), and WHO, which noticeably erected and continues to maintain, within its own structure, individual programme entities dealing with each of the elements of PHC.

By the mid-1980s, a certain sense of disappointment with PHC had begun to spread. PHC had not shown convincing results, disease-targeted programmes had increased coverage but were unable to reach the 20 per cent of the population who needed services most, and financing remained largely dependent on international sources, raising concerns about long-term sustainability. In addition, both PHC and the intervention-based approaches that had been developed around it were seen as insufficiently connected to broader societal and environmental conditions impacting on health. By the end of the 1990s, it was apparent that the objectives of 'Health for All by the Year 2000' were not going to be achieved, and indeed they were not (Werner 2001). Summing up the outcome of a conference on PHC held in Spain in 2003, Bryant recalled that 'the insights at Alma Ata were strikingly accurate'. It had opened 'a critical place for human values – equity, fairness, gender sensitivity' (Bryant 2003: 1). It had underscored 'the importance of accurate information regarding the nature of problems and responses to them'. It had recognised the 'needs for building health system research, especially in relation to the poor' (Bryant 2003:2). But according to Bryant, the WHO and UNICEF-sponsored Alma-Ata conference had failed to recognise the 'limitations of governmental capacities to advance health care; the importance of health services interacting with other sectors; the importance of social and cultural parameters that are often locally unique; [and] the needs for health care reform in virtually every country' (Bryant 2003: 2). One could add to the factors impeding the success of PHC: the decline in international funding of PHC and related programmes in developing countries after the end of the Cold War in 1990; the gradual disengagement of such programmes as GOBI and CCCD; and the implementation by the World Bank and the IMF of counter-productive structural adjustment policies during the decade that followed; as well as the scarcity of funds set aside by developing country governments to offset the loss of international aid resulted in the weakening of health systems with devastating effects on PHC goals and, just as critically, to the ability to cope with the mounting HIV pandemic.

Yet PHC played a critical role in reorienting health thinking from a service orientation towards a population-centred focus. It contrasted strongly with the traditional medical and public health approach to health, which focused on investing most attention and resources in fixed medical facilities, in particular in hospitals serving urban populations. Further, even as the locus of decision-making remained fairly firmly with states and UN bodies, PHC illustrated some tentative steps towards global health with the inclusion of NGOs in its conceptualisation and communities in its implementation. PHC is now being revitalised as a key strategy for over-stressed health systems, and all regions and many countries, institutions, and professional groups are now engaged in this effort (WHO 2008).

While not articulated as governmental human rights obligations per se, the PHC movement was inspired by such principles as greater equality in the distribution of health, attention to vulnerable populations, enhanced access to health services, improved living conditions, and the need to ensure the underlying determinants of health including access to sanitation and clean water.

The evolution of the Expanded Programme on Immunization (EPI), from an international health construct inspired by smallpox eradication to the Global Alliance for Vaccines and Immunisation (GAVI), attests to the shift in what could be called the 'globalisation of international health', with implications for the ways in which human rights are engaged with the approach undertaken.

Childhood immunisation: from international to global health

The EPI was founded by WHO and UNICEF in 1974, and, over time, a mosaic of bilateral agencies and NGOs became actively involved. The distinct identity of EPI, rather than its inclusion as a routine activity of maternal and child health services, was due to international recognition of the persistently low immunisation coverage that existed around the world: less than 20 per cent of the world's children and less than 5 per cent of children in Asia and sub-Saharan Africa were actually immunised with the basic vaccines commonly available in industrialised countries (Bland and Clements 1998).

The programme had a dynamic start, applying management methods borrowed from the private sector, emphasising systematic planning and monitoring, skills-building, and logistic support. National plans were formulated and funded by a mix of national and external resources. Progress was rapid, although with wide variations across and within regions and countries. By 1990, 75 per cent of the world's infants were receiving the required three doses of vaccine against diphtheria, tetanus, and whooping cough, and this was improving every year with coverage ranging between a low 50 per cent in sub-Saharan Africa to over 80 per cent in industrialised countries. At the time, WHO and UNICEF claimed the goal of universal immunisation had been achieved (UN 1991) – a claim which failed to take into account whether the most vulnerable populations were receiving immunisation, and did not question the reported high immunisation rates in China, raising major doubts in the following years as better data became available (WHO 2002).

In 1990, 16 years into the programme, several factors not directly connected to the delivery of immunisation combined to stall this effort. First, donor fatigue occurred, combined with a refocusing of donor interest as East–West tensions subsided. Second, external financing had not been accompanied by increased financial commitments from recipient countries and, overall, funding became unsustainable. Third, structural adjustment programmes were detrimentally impacting the performance of health systems of developing countries, in particular the workforce and public investments in health. Lastly, other priorities such as the rising HIV/AIDS epidemics diverted attention away from immunisation programmes. The net result was the stall or decline of immunisation activities in most developing countries, and in particular in Africa.

An additional constraint was the lack of products that would provide immunity against a wider range of diseases at an affordable cost: new, more effective and stable vaccines, and new combinations of vaccines were needed. This called for greater investment in research and development, and a closer collaboration between intergovernmental agencies, foundations, and the corporate pharmaceutical sector, constituting another important step towards a global rather than an international response. The approach of choice was the creation in 1990 of a new initiative called the Children's Vaccine Initiative (CVI). UNICEF, WHO, the World Bank, the United Nations Development Programme (UNDP), and the Rockefeller Foundation formed a coalition dedicated to boosting the development and delivery of new, improved vaccines to the 140 million children born annually into the world. The CVI was launched on the occasion of the World Summit for Children in New York, which also served as the launching pad for the newly formulated UN Convention on the Rights of the Child – the most widely ratified human rights treaty of all time (UN 1989). The CVI survived over a decade, but it did not achieve its objectives. Limited funds, constant turf battles between agencies, unforeseen complexities in the technological challenges that were to be addressed, and lukewarm relationships between the various actors engaged in the initiative contributed to its premature demise.

In March 1998, the World Bank called a meeting bringing together WHO and UNICEF, industry leaders, and vaccine experts. The so-called Vaccine Summit was to rethink optional approaches to remedy the decline of childhood immunisation. The Bill & Melinda Gates Foundation had just announced a US $100 million grant in support of a newly created US-based group: the Child Vaccine Program. It was decided that, instead of the Child Vaccine Program, the lack of success in immunisation called for the creation of a new entity: GAVI, which would benefit from immediate funding of US $750 million. This was three times what the founders of the ailing CVI had estimated their annual requirement to be, and it was promised that billions of dollars would follow if the initiative showed signs of success. As of the end of 2008, the Alliance had received a total of US $3.8 billion in cash and pledges from public and private sector donors, and disbursed US $2.7 billion to eligible countries. Over the period up to 2015, the Alliance has an estimated US $3 billion funding gap out of the estimated US $8.1 billion total funding needed (WHO 2009).

GAVI is a vivid illustration of both the opportunities and the shortcomings of the globalisation of international health. Addressing what was then recognised as a global health issue and bringing together a wide array of stakeholders, the Alliance formed what is now called a Global Health Partnership. Launched in 2001, GAVI is governed by a board consisting of representatives of WHO, UNICEF, and the World Bank, foundations, official development agencies, NGOs, the vaccine industry, and selected developing and industrialised countries (GAVI 2009). The arrangement remains linked to fora, where global health policies are normally debated and resolved, in particular the WHA, where motions of support and periodic information on the progress of GAVI is shared with member states. Decisions on priority-setting, resource allocation, and directions for research and development, however, are determined by the GAVI board on the basis of expert advice and consulting firms on the basis of an 'investment case', which requires, in particular, robust operational and economic arguments. Conscious of the need for long-term financial sustainability, GAVI is concerned with ensuring a gradual increase of national financing of programmes and new schemes to generate external resources. While potentially useful with respect to funding, the locus of policy formation, decision-making, and accountability is increasingly drifting away from intergovernmental fora such as the WHA, where nations engage in a one-country one-voice debate, to a board which includes a mix of public and private interest with an unfavourable balance of power against developing countries and not-for-profit organisations.

From a human rights perspective, there are several implications of this approach for health, born coincidently, at the turn of this century, along with the Millennium Development Goals (MDGs) (UN MDG 2000). The EPI had been cast in the early 1990s by UNICEF as an important element of its strategy centred around the Convention on the Rights of the Child. In the early 2000s, however, under pressure from the US Administration, UNICEF began to de-emphasise the Rights of the Child as the backbone of its programming structure. GAVI policy and programme documents emphasise disease reduction outcomes with insufficient attention to human rights norms and standards even as some concepts, such as non-discrimination and participation, were incorporated as relevant to the achievement of programme goals (Hallgath and Tarantola 2008). Progress in health (through immunisation and other services such as vitamin A or bed net distribution, which can accompany the delivery of vaccines) is a contributor to progress towards child survival and development, and therefore towards the attainment of several of the MDGs. Undoubtedly, even if rights are not an explicit part of the framework, actions to improve the health of populations is fundamental to the advancement of children's rights and all human rights.

The emergence of GAVI as the forerunner of a series of global health partnerships born around the turn of this century also illustrates the tendency of global initiatives to cherry-pick select international legal frameworks, while ignoring others. International trade agreements and patent protection, for example, may be omnipresent in the mode of operations of such initiatives while international human rights treaties may not. Not all global health schemes, however, have turned a blind eye to human rights considerations, as illustrated by the emergence and evolution of the global response to HIV/AIDS.

The response to HIV/AIDS: a global effort rooted in human rights

A Special Programme on AIDS, the programme launched by WHO in 1987 and relabelled a few months later as the WHO Global Programme on AIDS, had as its aim to respond to the spreading HIV epidemics and mitigate their impact in the developing world (WHO 1987). Its strategy had something unique in that, from the very outset, it recognised the promotion and protection of human rights as integral to its public health approach.

Having built on a health promotion model to establish that a large and complex assembly of factors determines who is more likely to become HIV-infected or to cope with its impact, it drew attention to the links between the factors that come to play in HIV and civil, political, economic, social, and cultural rights (Gruskin and Tarantola 2001; Mann and Tarantola 1996). Human rights were seen to contribute to this analysis in three ways. First, they helped categorise determinants of HIV-related risks and vulnerability in a structured and logical way. Second, they opened avenues for action: not only did the determinants themselves need to be addressed, but possible underlying violations of human rights might call for specific remedial or preventive action. Third, as human rights are governmental obligations under international law and often entrenched in national law, a human rights approach was seen to provide additional leverage in inducing policy change through use of legal and accountability channels (Mann et al. 1994).

UNAIDS was founded in 1996 when it was realised that coordinating the efforts of UN agencies would help a more efficient response to the multiple roots and facets of the HIV epidemic. Its aim was, and remains, to support governments and civil society in mounting a more effective response to HIV.

Despite political commitment, the financial resources needed for this effort were not present. At a time when international funding in support of HIV programmes in developing countries did not exceed the US $1 billion mark, all estimates showed that six to ten times this amount was necessary. In response, the Global Fund to Combat AIDS, Tuberculosis, and Malaria (GFATM), originally called for by the-then UN Secretary General Kofi Annan, formed part of the negotiations between governments at the UN General Assembly Special

Session on AIDS in June of 2001, and was authorised by governments at the G8 summit in Genoa the following month. Launched in 2002, thanks to a major grant from the Bill & Melinda Gates Foundation, the Fund operates as a financing entity, not as an implementing entity.

As a global public/private partnership, the GFATM is governed by a board consisting of representatives of governments, civil society, the private sector, and affected communities. WHO and UNAIDS are observers, without voting rights (GFATM 2002). Several years after the awards of its first grants, the GFATM has resulted in important successes and continues to stimulate great expectations, even as concerns for the medium and long term remain (GFATM 2009)[2].

From a human rights perspective, the contribution of the Fund to increasing the likelihood that people with HIV, malaria, or TB have access to quality care is clear. While not explicitly rights-based, key components of a rights-based approach have been systematically integrated into the work of the Fund, including attention to non-discrimination, participation, transparency, and accountability. Several human rights concerns are, however, raised going forward. First and foremost, the sustainability of the GFATM is uncertain and even more so is the sustainability of funding for in-country HIV, malaria, and TB work, including in relation to treatment. In spite of the G8 support to the Fund, both in political and financial terms, insufficient debate has occurred on how beneficiary countries can fulfil their obligations to health in the event of the Fund having to scale down or interrupt its grants, if for no other reason than donor fatigue.

The relative successes of the GFATM and the US President's Emergency Plan for AIDS Relief (PEPFAR) also raise concerns in the ways the distribution of resources impact not only HIV, malaria, and TB, but also health and the realisation of human rights in countries more generally. Today, the flow of international aid resources is overwhelmingly dictated by the agendas of global entities taking precedence over other national priorities, whether they concern different emphases in HIV efforts, population mobility, climate change, education, or food security (PEPFAR 2009).

As both the GFATM and GAVI illustrate, informal monitoring mechanisms are not sufficient: international accountability mechanisms applicable to global health and to global partnerships are needed. How these might best be instituted is subject to debate involving nation states, civil society, and the private sector.

Discussion

The shift from international to global health brings with it new opportunities and challenges for the ways that human rights intersect with health efforts. With public/private partnerships increasingly replacing the one-country one-vote principle traditionally applied to the assemblies of nations presiding over international health, concerns around governance and accountability are paramount (Gostin 2007). It remains unclear, but worthy of continued scrutiny, whether the demand for governmental accountability is being stimulated or diluted by the broadening of the number and types of actors that take part not only in policy development but in the governance of global health. Moving beyond the selected use of international agreements and conventions by global initiatives, all such initiatives should be called on to examine the extent to which the accountability expected from beneficiary countries is in line with their human rights obligations under all relevant human rights instruments, and to consider also the implications for donor countries.

Although explicit to varying degrees, many initiatives do incorporate human rights concepts and principles into their policy and programming activities. Further, examples now abound within the realm of HIV where claims for the government to fulfil obligations have succeeded, as in the case of access to antiretroviral treatment in several Latin American countries or the formulation of laws prohibiting discrimination on the basis of HIV status or other related factors. And, adapting to the globalisation of health initiatives, some recent human rights-based advocacy efforts have targeted not only governments but also corporations, as was the case with the Campaign for Access to Essential Medicines (MSF 2009).

Yet, despite an upswing in the incorporation of human rights principles into global health, challenges remain. For example, with money driving the agenda of many health initiatives, concerns are raised when the primary sources of funding are foundations and corporations that fall outside the remit of human rights law, which was specifically designed to safeguard the interests of those who might least be able to demand such protection. What happens if the governmental responsibility to reach the most disadvantaged and to ensure the availability, accessibility, acceptability, and quality of all health services does not align with the priorities of a public/private partnership? This has been the case with some target-driven initiatives that focus on serving the easiest-to-reach populations, and raises questions of concern going forward.

Born out of the HIV response, the human-rights-based approach to public health reinforces and stimulates analyses and actions for the most disadvantaged population groups and across a widening array of fields including reproductive and sexual health, mental health, non-communicable diseases, tuberculosis, disability, and environmental health. But, for this approach to be effective, governments, while working with other partners, must remain squarely at the centre of the scene.

A frequently debated question in circles engaged in international and global health is: How explicit do references to human rights have to be for a public health strategy to be considered grounded in human rights? Several of the examples chosen for this chapter have illustrated that, although the semantics of human rights may be absent from policy and programme documents, it is still possible for them to be underpinned by, or at least consistent with, human rights principles. Nonetheless, the implicit incorporation of human rights in public health policy and programmes should be a minimum requirement for good public health. The explicit reference to human rights advances not only public health but a broad array of human rights in which many social determinants of health are firmly anchored.

Conclusions

In the last three decades, international health has opened promising avenues and made important strides in fostering international cooperation. Its successes have, however, been somewhat tempered by the inability of governments and intergovernmental organisations to sustain their commitments. Financial resources made available nationally and internationally have not been commensurate with the efforts needed to bridge the world's health gaps.

As the bipolar political division of the world subsided in the 1990s, and in the trail of the globalisation of the economy, international health and its ageing governance mechanisms proved inadequate to face large-scale world health threats. Global health has gradually come to overshadow international health by elevating health issues above nation states and inviting a greater role by civil society and private entities, in particular foundations and the health industry. There are now more than 70 global health partnerships on diverse aspects of health, including 45 on HIV, malaria, or tuberculosis alone. The competition for resources among these funds is an increasing concern, in particular as they are influenced by and respond to the will of donors. Further, the progress and impact of global partnerships on countries are acutely constrained by national-level systemic insufficiencies, which global partnerships are only beginning to address (Caines *et al.* 2004; Widdus 2001).

The role and responsibilities of governments remain crucial when the health and security of people are at stake. With emerging or re-emerging pandemics threatening the world, what is needed is a greater consciousness that international health is built by nation states with political interests, both within and outside their borders, and not by agendas set by some supra-governmental entity.

To help both international and global health initiatives as they move forward, the value of human rights for accountability, advocacy, and programming is increasingly understood. Human rights have been used to set priorities, examine and reshape processes, and promote participatory decision-making (including the participation of particular vulnerable groups living on the margins of health initiatives), monitor the impact of health work, and establish a system for the transparent accountability of all stakeholders. The current challenge for individual national governments is not only to further their obligations towards people in relation to health and to human rights, but to be able to truly speak on their behalf in international fora and as they engage in global schemes.

Notes

1 A broad definition of global health is given by the United States Institute of Medicine (1997) as 'health problems, issues, and concerns that transcend national boundaries, may be influenced by circumstances or experiences in other countries, and are best addressed by cooperative actions and solutions'.
2 See also for independent views: AVERT (2009) *The Global Fund to Fight AIDS, Tuberculosis and Malaria*, http://www.avert.org/global-fund.htm (accessed 27 November 2009), and Brown, H. (2007) 'Great Expectations', *British Medical Journal* 334: 874–6.

References

AVERT (2009) *The Global Fund to Fight AIDS, Tuberculosis and Malaria*, http://www.avert.org/global-fund.htm (accessed 27 November 2009).
Bland, J. and Clements, J. (1998) 'Protecting the world's children: the story of WHO's immunization programme', *World Health Forum*, 19(2): 162–73.
Brown, H. (2007) 'Great Expectations', *British Medical Journal*, 334: 874–6.
Brown, T., Marcos, C., and Fee, E. (2006) 'The World Health Organization and the transition from "international" to "global" public health', *American Journal of Public Health*, 96(1): 62–72.
Bryant, J. (2003) *Reflections on PHC, 25 Years after Alma Ata*, Global meeting on future strategic directions for primary health care, World Health Organization, 27–29 October 2003, Madrid, Spain.
Caines, K., Buse, K., Carlson, C., de Loor, R., Druce, N., Grace, C., Pearson, M., Sancho, J., and Sadanandan, R. (2004) *Assessing the Impact Of Global Health Partnerships: Synthesis of findings from the 2004 DFID Studies*, London: UK Department for International Development.
Fenner, F., Henderson, D.A., Arita, I., Jezek, A.Z., and Ladnyi, I.D. (eds) (1988) *Smallpox and Its Eradication*, Geneva: World Health Organization.
GAVI (2009), *The GAVI Alliance Board*, available at http://www.gavialliance.org/about/governance/boards/index.php (accessed 27 November 2009).
Global Fund to Fight AIDS, Tuberculosis, and Malaria (GFATM) (2002) *Framework Document on the Global Fund to Fight AIDS, Tuberculosis and Malaria*, Geneva: GFATM.
Global Fund to Fight AIDS, Tuberculosis, and Malaria (GFATM) (2009) *The Global Fund to Fight AIDS, Tuberculosis and Malaria*, http://www.theglobalfund.org (accessed 27 November 2009).
Gostin, L. (2007) 'Why Rich Countries Should Care, About the World's Least Healthy People', *Journal of the American Medical Association*, 298(1): 89–92.
Gruskin, S. and Tarantola, D. (2001) 'HIV/AIDS and human rights revisited', *Canadian HIV/AIDS Policy and Law Review*, 6(1–2): 24–9.
Hallgath, L. and Tarantola, D. (2008) 'A rights-based approach to the assessment of global health initiatives', *Australian Journal of Human Rights*, 13(2): 157–80.
Hill, K. and Yazbeck, A. (1994) *Trends in Under-Five Mortality, 1960–90: Estimates for 84 Developing Countries*, Washington, DC: World Bank.

Hill, K., Pande, R., Mahy, M., and Jones, G. (1999) *Trends in Child Mortality in the Developing World: 1960–1996*, New York: UNICEF.

Institute of Medicine (1997) *America's vital interest in global health: Protecting our people, enhancing our economy, and advancing our international interests*, Washington, DC: National Academy Press, available at http://books.nap.edu/openbook.php?record_id=5717&page=11 (accessed 27 November 2009).

Litsios, S. (2008) *The Third Ten Years of the World Health Organization: 1968–1977*, Geneva: WHO.

Mann, J. and Tarantola, D. (1996) 'From Vulnerability to Human Rights', in J. Mann and D. Tarantola (eds) *AIDS in the World II, Global dimensions, Social Roots and Responses*, New York: Oxford University Press.

Mann, J., Gostin, L., Gruskin, S., Brennan, T., Lazzarini, Z., and Fineberg, H.V. (1994) 'Health and human rights', *Health and Human Rights*, 1(1): 7–24.

Médecins Sans Frontières (MSF) (2009) *What is the Campaign? Campaign for Access to Essential Medicines*, available at http://www.msfaccess.org/about-us/ (accessed 27 November 2009).

PEPFAR (2009) *The US President's Emergency Plan for AIDS Relief*, available at http://www.pepfar.gov (accessed 27 November 2009).

UN (United Nations) (1948) *Universal Declaration of Human Rights*. Adopted and proclaimed by the United Nations General Assembly resolution 217 A (III) of 10 December 1948, New York: United Nations.

UN (United Nations) (1966a) *International Covenant on Civil Political Rights (ICCPR)*. Adopted and opened for signature, ratification and accession by the United Nations General Assembly resolution 2200A (XXI) of 16 December 1966, entry into force 23 March 1976, in accordance with Article 49.

UN (United Nations) (1966b) *International Covenant on Economic, Social and Cultural Rights (ICESCR)* Adopted and opened for signature, ratification and accession by United nations General Assembly resolution 2200A (XXI) of 16 December 1966, entry into force 3 January 1976, in accordance with Article 27.

UN (United Nations) (1978) *Declaration of Alma-Ata*. International Conference of Primary Health Care, 6–12 September 1978, Alma-Ata, USSR.

UN (United Nations) (1989) *Convention on the Right of the Child*. Adopted and opened for signature, ratification and accession by United Nations General Assembly resolution 44/25 of 20 November 1989.

UN (United Nations) (1991) *The Yearbook of the United Nations*, New York: United Nations.

UN MDG (UN Millennium Development Goals) (2000) 'About the Millennium Development Goals, United Nations Development Programme', available at http://www.undp.org/mdg/basics.shtml (accessed 27 November 2009).

Werner, D. (2001) 'Elusive promise, Whatever happened to "Health for All?"', *New Internationalist*, 331 (Jan/Feb).

Widdus, R. (2001) 'Public–private partnerships for health: their main targets, their diversity, and their future directions', *Bulletin of the World Health Organization*, 79(8): 713–20.

WHO (World Health Organization) (1987) 'The Global Strategy for AIDS Prevention and Control', Geneva: WHO (unpublished document SPA/INF/87.1).

WHO (World Health Organization) (2002) *State of the World Vaccines and Immunization*, 2nd edn, Geneva: WHO, available at http://www.who.int/vaccines-documents/DocsPDF02/www718.pdf (accessed 27 November 2009).

WHO (World Health Organization) (2008) *The World Health Report 2008: Primary Health Care (Now More Than Ever)*, Geneva: WHO, available at http://www.who.int/whr/2008/en/index.html (accessed 27 November 2009).

WHO (World Health Organization) (2009) *State of the World Vaccines and Immunization*, 3rd edn, Geneva: WHO, available at http://whqlibdoc.who.int/publications/2009/9789241563864_eng.pdf (accessed 27 November 2009).

Part II

Structural Inequalities and Global Public Health

7

Global Health Inequities

Structures, Power, and the Social Distribution of Health

Sharon Friel and Michael Marmot

The social distribution of health: health inequities within and between countries

Modern society has done much good for the health and well-being of people – the average global life expectancy has increased by more than two decades since 1950. However, not every group and nation experienced this to the same degree. Differences in health between countries have perpetuated and worsened, particularly over the last three decades (CSDH 2008). Life expectancy is often used as a marker of population health. Regionally, the health achievements enjoyed by the Organisation for Economic Co-operation and Development (OECD) countries have already started happening in South Asia and elsewhere (Figure 7.1) – but have considerable distance still to go. The lack of improvement in life expectancy in Central and Eastern Europe and the former Soviet Union is of concern. That life expectancy in sub-Saharan Africa showed almost no change in a 30-year period must be considered a failure of the global public health community.

The sub-regional level tells a story of marked inequalities between countries within the same region as well as across regions. Major differences exist in early death. Recent estimates from WHO suggest that living past the age of 60 is not the norm in 45 out of 195 countries (WHO 2006). The inequality is most pronounced among the male population – life expectancy at birth for males in 55 countries is 60 or less. The risk of dying at a very early age is higher today compared to almost 50 years ago among the poorest countries. Figure 7.2 illustrates how life expectancy at birth has deteriorated to less than 40 years in a number of African countries. High levels of infant mortality and HIV/AIDS in many of these countries continue to pull down the life expectancy.

Health gaps and gradients

Health within countries is markedly unequal. These differences in health occur along a number of axes of social stratification, including socio-economic, political, and cultural (Baum 2005; Labonte *et al.* 2005; Wilkinson and Pickett 2005). In developing countries, the emerging double burden of communicable and non-communicable disease (Choi *et al.* 2005; Ebrahim and Smeeth 2005; Ezzati *et al.* 2004) combined with pervasive poverty serves to compound the poor

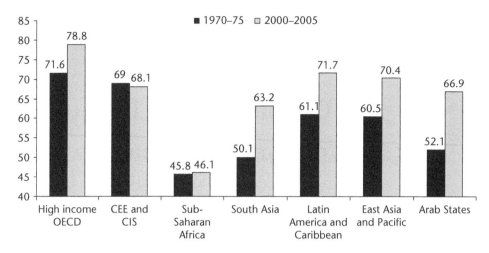

Figure 7.1 Life expectancy at birth by region, 1970–5 and 2000–5
Source: UNDP 2005.

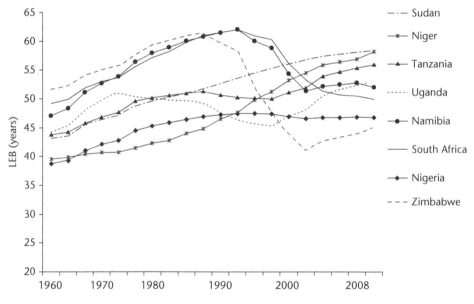

Figure 7.2 Life expectancy at birth, select African countries, 1960–2005
Source: World Bank 2005.

health opportunities for large sections of these populations. One way of describing the magnitude of health inequality is the gap between top and bottom socio-economic groups. In El Salvador, for example, if mothers have no education, their babies have 100 chances in 1,000 of dying in the first year of life; if mothers have at least secondary education, the infant death rate is a quarter of that (World Bank 2006). Such dramatic differences in health within countries are seen in rich as well as poor countries. In the early part of the twenty-first century, life expectancy of men in one of the most deprived neighbourhoods in Glasgow, Scotland, was 54 years, compared with 82 years in a most affluent area (Hanlon *et al.* 2006).

There is no doubt that poor people suffer from far higher levels of ill health and premature mortality than rich people, and addressing the health of poor people and poor nations must be a matter of concern for donors, policymakers, and service providers (Gwatkin *et al.* 2005). Indeed, the introduction of vertical initiatives to control major communicable diseases, such as the Global Fund to Fight Tuberculosis, AIDS, and Malaria (Global Fund), the WHO '3 by 5' Initiative (WHO n.d.-b) and the Roll Back Malaria Partnership (WHO n.d.-a), as well as horizontal initiatives to improve health systems, have substantially redressed the major infectious disease burden and improved average population health in developing countries. The Millennium Development Goals (MDGs) have focused much-needed attention on eliminating poverty in the world's poorest countries and put health clearly on the international and national development agendas (United Nations 2000).

However, poverty alone does not fully explain the observed inequalities in population health. It does not explain the variation in life expectancy and health status among poor people with different levels of education or from different ethnic backgrounds (Ezzati *et al.* 2004), nor why groups along the social spectrum differ in levels of mortality from, for example, cardiovascular diseases, cancers, and external causes (violence) (Wilkinson and Pickett 2005), nor why populations with different living and working conditions have differing health experiences (Bartley 2005; Christensen 2002; Marmot and Brunner 2005; Monden 2005). Focusing on the health gap between top and bottom fails to draw attention to a phenomenon that, in many countries, has increased over time: the social gradient in health (Marmot 2004). With few exceptions, the evidence shows that the lower an individual's socio-economic position, the worse their health – whether measured in life expectancy, morbidity, or under-five mortality (see Figures 7.3–Figures 7.5). This is a global phenomenon, seen in low-, middle-, and high-income countries alike (Victora *et al.* 2003).

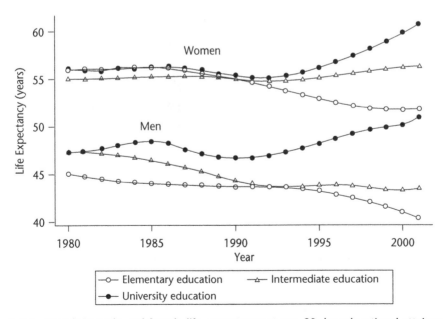

Figure 7.3 Trends in male and female life expectancy at age 20, by educational attainment, Russian Federation
Source: Murphy *et al.* 2006.

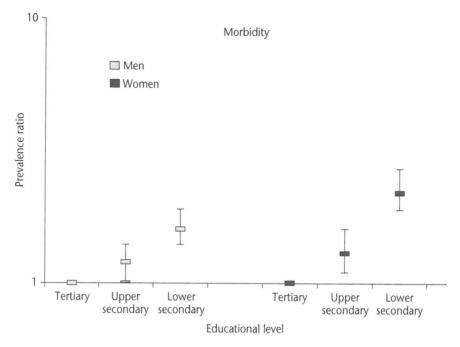

Figure 7.4 Prevalence ratio of diabetes mellitus, by educational level, age adjusted, men and women in 16 European countries
Source: Espelt *et al.* 2007.

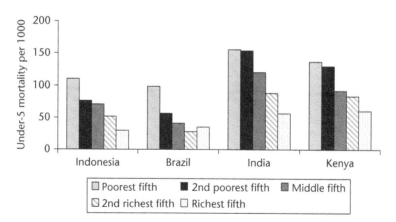

Figure 7.5 Under-five mortality rates, select countries, by household wealth
Source: Victora *et al.* 2003.

The social determinants of empowerment and global health inequity

Freedom, empowerment, and the social determinants

The existence of both the gap and social gradient in health suggests that having the freedom to live a long, healthy, and flourishing life is not the equal purview of every person, social group, or indeed nation. All societies have social hierarchies, manifesting across a range of intersecting social categories – class, education, gender, age, ethnicity, disability, and geography – in which economic and social resources, including power, money, and prestige, are distributed unequally. The unequal distribution of these resources impacts on people's freedom to lead lives they have reason to value (Sen 1999), and, arguably, manifests as the poor health of the poor, the social gradient in health within countries, and the health inequities between countries.

Pursuit of health equity recognises implicitly the need to redress the unequal distribution of opportunity to be healthy that is associated with membership of less privileged social groups (Ostlin et al. 2005). This requires empowerment of individuals, communities, and whole countries. Empowerment operates along three interconnected dimensions: material, psychosocial, and political. People need the basic material requisites for a decent life, they need to have control over their lives, and they need political voice and participation in decision-making processes.

And what lies behind empowerment and its social distribution are the social determinants – the fundamental socio-political, socio-economic, socio-environmental, and socio-cultural characteristics of contemporary human societies, which shape how people are born, grow, live, work, and age. That is, the economic and social policies that generate and distribute political power, income, goods, and services at global, national, and local levels also determine the immediate conditions of daily living – access to health care, schools, and education, conditions of work and leisure, the nature of homes, communities, towns, or cities, and the practices that different social groups follow (Marmot et al. 2008).

Technical and medical solutions such as disease control and medical care are, without doubt, necessary for health, but they are insufficient – medical and healthcare solutions do not exist for many of the problems that need to be addressed (Kickbusch 2008). At the 2004 World Health Assembly, the World Health Organisation's (WHO) former director-general, Dr Jong-wook Lee, announced the beginning of a process to act upon the social causes of global health inequities (Lee 2005). As a result, the Commission on Social Determinants of Health (CSDH) emerged in 2005 to build on previous and current United Nations (UN) efforts to work towards better health and greater health equity. The CSDH vision was a world where all people have the freedom to lead lives they have reason to value. Working towards this, the CSDH placed primary emphasis on the underlying factors that determine the social distribution of population health.

Material empowerment

Health equity relies on an adequate supply of and access to material resources and services, safe, health-promoting living and working conditions, and learning, working, and recreational opportunities. Money matters. Poverty and low living standards are powerful determinants of ill-health and health inequity. They have significant consequences for early child development and life-long trajectories through, for example, lack of basic amenities, crowded living conditions, parental stress, and lack of food security. In rich and poor countries, poverty means not participating fully in society, and having limits on leading the life one has reason to value.

Work

For most people in the world, living conditions are largely determined by economic opportunity afforded through the labour market. In 2007, there were 3 billion people aged 15 years and older in work – 1.3 billion of them did not earn above US$2 per day (ILO 2008). In 2009, the number of working poor may rise up to 1.4 billion, or 45 per cent of the world's employed (Benach *et al.* 2010).

In recent decades, the global labour market underwent significant changes, with growth in job insecurity and precarious employment arrangements (such as informal work, temporary work, part-time working, and piece work), job losses, and a weakening of regulatory protections. These labour market changes pose major health risks from the economic hazards associated with insecurity, lack of access to paid family leave, and unemployment (Bartley 2005; Benach and Muntaner 2007). Labour policy based on fair and decent employment and working conditions (Box 7.1) will help improve material conditions, empower workers, and increase global health equity.

Social protection

More equitable within-country distribution of resources and increased international financial transfers are necessary components of community empowerment, poverty reduction, and health improvement. Redistributive welfare systems, in combination with the extent to which people can make a healthy living through work, influence poverty levels (Lundberg *et al.* 2008). Studies in Latin America suggest that even a little redistribution of income through progressive taxation and targeted social programmes can go far in terms of poverty reduction (Paes de Barros 2002; Woodward and Simms 2006). In high-income countries, those with more generous social protection systems tend to have better population health outcomes (Lundberg *et al.* 2008). More generous family policies, for example, are associated with lower infant mortality levels (Figure 7.6). Nations also need sufficient material resources. For countries at all levels of economic development, increasing or reallocating public finance to fund action in child

---

Box 7.1 Minimum income for healthy living (Morris *et al.* 2000)

An assessment was made of the cost of living among single healthy men in the UK, aged 18 to 30, living away from their family and on their own. Based on consensual evidence, a basket of commodities considered necessary for healthy day-to-day living was priced, including food and physical activity, housing, household services, household goods, transport, clothing, and footwear, educational costs, personal costs, personal and medical care, savings and non-state pension contributions, leisure goods, and leisure activities. The total cost was considered indicative of the minimum disposable income that is now essential for health.

The minimum cost of healthy living was assessed at £131.86 per week (based on UK April 1999 prices). Component costs, especially those of housing (which represents around 40% of this total), depend on geographical region and on several assumptions. In today's society, the disposable income that could meet this minimal cost may be posited as a necessary pre-condition of health. Pay from the new national minimum wage (in April 1999), £3.00 an hour at 18–21 years and £3.60 at 22 years plus translates into disposable weekly incomes of £105.84 and £121.12, respectively, for a 38-hour working week, after statutory tax and social security deductions. At 18–21, 51 hours, and at 22 years plus, 42.5 hours, would have to be worked to earn the income needed to meet the assessed minimum costs of healthy living.

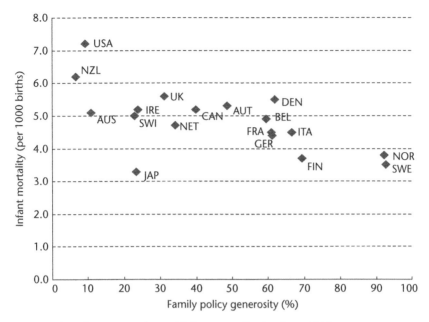

Figure 7.6 Family policy generosity and infant mortality levels, *c.* 2000
Source: Lundberg *et al.* 2008.

development and education, improve living and working conditions, and provide access to quality health care is fundamental to health equity.

Living environment

The social, economic, and physical make-up of the living environment is one of the most pressing issues for health equity. Urbanisation is reshaping population health problems, particularly among the urban poor, who are still struggling with the traditional health hazards of infectious and vector-borne diseases. They are also increasingly facing the challenges of noncommunicable diseases including diabetes, heart disease, overweight, and obesity (Figure 7.7), mental health problems, alcohol and drug abuse, and violence, injuries, and impact from ecological disaster. Socio-economic discrimination and exclusion in many places create higher health determinant exposures among disadvantaged population groups, and people living in slums are particularly affected.

Access to basic material resources such as clean water, sanitation, and shelter are essential for health equity. Current projections suggest that many countries are highly unlikely to reach the water-related targets of the MDGs (UNESCO 2006). Many cities in rich and poor countries alike are facing an affordable and quality housing crisis – a crisis that will worsen unless efforts to revitalise cities and manage development incorporate regional affordable housing measures. Equitable access to quality health care is vital for global health. Yet, with the exception of some rich industrialised countries, health care systems are frequently chronically under-resourced, and they are pervasively inequitable. Higher private-sector spending (relative to all health expenditure) is associated with worse health-adjusted life expectancy (Figure 7.8). The shift, globally, towards an emphasis on the individual management of risk has

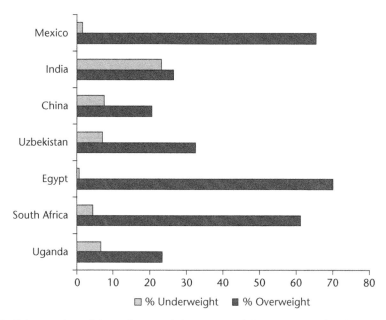

Figure 7.7 Urban underweight and overweight among adult women in select low- and middle-income countries
Source: Mendez *et al.* 2005.

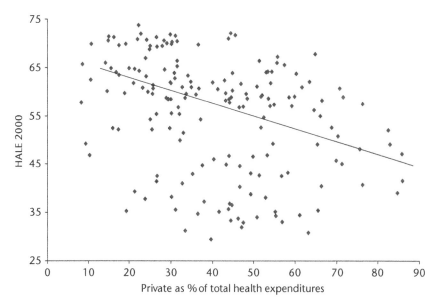

Figure 7.8 Healthy life expectancy (HALE) and private spending as a % of total health spending, 2000
Source: Koivusalo and Mackintosh 2005.

helped push upwards of 100 million people into poverty yearly through the catastrophic house-hold health costs that result from payments for access to services (Xu *et al.* 2007).

Psychosocial empowerment

Employees of the British government have clean water and bathrooms and shelter from the elements. Yet among these civil servants, men second from the top of the occupational hierarchy had a higher rate of death than men at the top. Men third from the top had a higher rate of death than those second from the top (Figure 7.9). Why, among men who are not poor in the usual sense of the word, should the risk of dying be intimately related to where they stand in the social hierarchy? (Marmot 2004) This social gradient in health suggests something other than, or in addition to, material security is important for health.

A range of different psychosocial factors have been posited as potential contributors to health inequities, including lack of control, support, social capital, and social cohesion. The combination of material disadvantage and reduced control over one's life among people lower down the social hierarchy limits people's freedom to lead the lives they have reason to value.

Work and control

Conditions of work are strongly related to psychosocial well-being, particularly aspects of individual demand and control. There is consistent evidence that low decision latitude, high work demands, low work social supports, work strain, and effort–reward imbalance – each associated with precarious work – are risk factors for subsequent mental and physical health problems (Artazcoz *et al.* 2005; Stansfeld and Candy 2006) and tend to be more prevalent among workers in lower social status occupations (Figure 7.10).

Early child development and empowerment

It is generally believed that the persistence and, in some cases, worsening of health inequities is transmitted from generation to generation through economic, social, and developmental

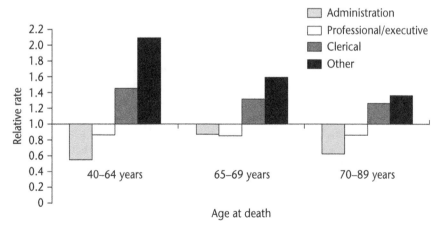

Figure 7.9 Mortality over 25 years according to level in the occupational hierarchy. First Whitehall study of British civil servants
Source: Marmot and Shipley 1996.

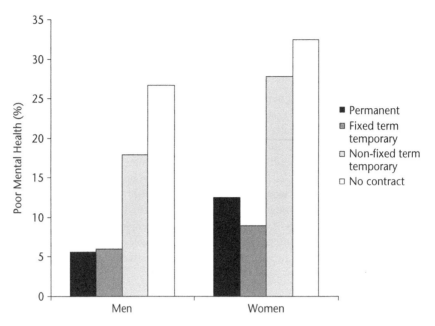

Figure 7.10 Poor mental health and precarious employment status among manual workers, Spain 2002
Source: Artazcoz *et al.* 2005.

processes, and that the advantages and disadvantages in early life are reinforced in adulthood. The Early Child Development Knowledge Network of the CSDH stressed the need for children's development to include attention to physical, cognitive/language, and social/ emotional components (Early Child Development Knowledge Network 2007). In addition to economic circumstance, each component of child development is dependent on the nature of the environments in which children exist. A child's early environment has a vital impact on the way the brain develops. The more stimulating the environment, the more connections are formed in the brain, and the better the child thrives in all aspects of life including basic learning, school success, economic participation, and social citizenry, each of which provides skills and resources that provide control over one's life and influence health.

One key factor that may mitigate adverse child development is education. Education and the associated high social standing in adult life may protect against health-damaging early life exposures. Children from disadvantaged backgrounds are more likely to do poorly in school and drop out early – and subsequently as adults are more likely to have lower incomes and be less empowered to provide good health care, nutrition, and stimulation to their own children, thus contributing to the intergenerational transmission of disadvantage (Grantham-McGregor *et al.* 2007). Early child development and quality education help equip people and communities with material security, resilience, and personal control.

Political empowerment

Health inequities flow from the systematically unequal distribution of power, prestige, and resources among different social groups, manifesting in inequities in both material and psychosocial conditions (Farmer 1999). Power exists in relationships between individuals and groups ('power over', or relational power), and power represents capabilities ('power to'). Inequity in power interacts across four main dimensions – political, economic, social, and cultural – together constituting a continuum along which groups are, to varying degrees, excluded or included. The *political dimension* comprises both formal rights embedded in legislation, constitutions, policies, and practices, and the conditions in which rights are exercised including access to safe water, sanitation, shelter, transport, energy, and services such as health care, education, and social protection. The *economic dimension* is constituted by access to and distribution of material resources necessary to sustain life (e.g. income, employment, housing, land, working conditions, livelihoods). The *social dimension* is constituted by proximal relationships of support and solidarity (e.g. friendship, kinship, family, clan, neighbourhood, community, social movements) and the *cultural dimension* relates to the extent to which a diversity of values, norms, and ways of living contribute to the health of all and are accepted and respected (Social Exclusion Knowledge Network 2007). Box 7.2 illustrates the way in which marked inequities in power between men and women have arguably led to, and perpetuated, the high prevalence of HIV/AIDS among women in southern Africa.

Addressing the distribution of power involves fostering a process of 'political empowerment', broadly defined as the process whereby people, or groups, gain control over the decisions that affect them and increase and release their 'capacity to act' (agency) in order to effect change in the areas that they define as important. Political empowerment, therefore, is a fundamental medium of social interaction, constituted both at the level of individuals – how much people can exercise control and decision-making over the course and content of their own lives – and of communities – how people can effectively apply their collective values and interests to the way societal resources are distributed.

Health equity depends vitally on the empowerment of individuals and groups to represent their needs and interests strongly and effectively and, in so doing, to challenge and change the unfair and steeply graded distribution of social resources (the conditions for health) to which all men and women, as citizens, have equal claim and rights (UN 2000). Any serious effort to reduce health inequities will involve changing the distribution of power within society and global regions.

Box 7.2 Gender inequity and disempowerment (Lewis 2005)

The differential status of men and women in almost every society across the globe is perhaps the single most pervasive and entrenched inequity and a pressing societal issue for health. Indeed, the feminisation of the AIDS epidemic in southern Africa is a clear demonstration of the lack of power of women to enjoy fundamental social freedoms. This marked health inequity encapsulates disempowerment at many levels – government and institutional incapacity to act on evidence of gendered impact, and the unequal participation of women in political institutions from village to international levels; unequal access to and control over property, economic assets, and inheritance; unequal restrictions on physical mobility, reproduction, and sexuality; sanctioned violation of women's and girls' bodily integrity; and accepted codes of social conduct that condone, and even reward, sexual violence against women.

A framework for policy and practice that goes beyond the individual

A focus on empowerment places attention not only on the relief of poverty but also on the structural determinants of health, including the global- and national-level social,

---

Box 7.3 Material, psychosocial and political empowerment: SEWA, The Self-Employed Women's Association, India

In India, 86 per cent of women and 83 per cent of men employed in areas outside the agricultural sector are in informal employment. In Ahmedabad, there are around 100,000 street vendors. They sell fruit, vegetables, flowers, fish, clothes, toys, footwear, and many other items for daily household use. Most vendors have been selling in the city's markets and streets for generations.

Vegetable sellers in Ahmedabad start work at dawn, when they buy their wares from merchants in the wholesale markets. The often borrow from the merchants at very high interest rates. They routinely face harassment and eviction from their sites by local authorities and traffic police. To support the livelihoods of the vegetable sellers, SEWA, together with the vegetable sellers and growers, set up its own wholesale vegetable shop in the main wholesale marketplace of Ahmedabad to link growers (all poor farmers and SEWA union members) directly to street vendors (also members), thereby cutting out exploitative middlemen. As a result, both vegetable growers and sellers are obtaining better prices for their produce.

As the vegetable sellers were routinely harassed by local authorities and evicted from their vending sites, they, together with SEWA, campaigned for licenses and identity cards, and representation in urban boards which formulate policies and laws for vendors and urban development in general. The SEWA vendors' campaign has been strengthened by nation-wide and international alliances.

SEWA Bank provides banking to poor self-employed women, including the vegetable sellers. Rather than facing the huge interest rates demanded by the middlemen, vegetable sellers can now apply for micro-credit from SEWA Bank. The Bank is owned by the self-employed women as shareholders, its policies are formulated by an elected board of women workers, and the Bank is professionally run by qualified managers accountable to the board.

SEWA also provides child care, running centres for infants and young children, which ensure that the vegetable sellers do not have to take their young children with them when they go out to sell vegetables on the streets. SEWA campaigns at the state and national level for child care as an entitlement for all women workers.

The vegetable sellers, like other poor self-employed women, live in poor areas of the city. SEWA is improving their living conditions through slum upgrading programmes to provide basic infrastructure such as water and sanitation. This happens in partnerships with government, people's organisations, and the corporate sector. Through the programmes, other services are provided to families, including financial services, insurance, health care, child care, and employment.

When the vegetable sellers or their family members fall ill, SEWA helps them obtain health care. They can use SEWA health insurance to pay for health care costs. In times of crisis (e.g. illness, widowhood, accidents, fire, floods), poor families not only lose work and income, but also sell their assets like land and houses, and even borrow money at very high rates. Hence, workers and their families are pushed further into the cycle of poverty and indebtedness.

Source: SEWA website (http://www.sewa.org/services/bank.asp)

---

environmental, and economic arrangements within which people live, plus the consequent conditions of daily living – access to health care, schools, and education, conditions of work and leisure, and the nature of homes, communities, towns, or cities. The work of SEWA (Self-Employed Women's Association) in India provides an example of integrated collective community action with national- and local-level policy, which operates on principles of empowerment (Box 7.3). The initiative aims to provide material resources, personal and community control, and voice to some of the most powerless groups in India, and in doing so, creates the conditions in which people have the opportunity to lead healthy and flourishing lives.

A social determinants approach to empowerment, health, and health equity has several advantages. It bridges the artificial distinction between technical and social interventions, and demonstrates how both are necessary aspects of action. It seeks to redress the imbalance between curative and preventive action and individualised and population-based interventions. Also, by acting on structural conditions in society, a social determinants approach offers better hope for sustainable and equitable outcomes (CSDH 2008).

References

Artazcoz, L., Benach, J., Borrell, C., and Cortès, I. (2005) 'Social Inequalities in the Impact of Flexible Employment on Different Domains of Psychosocial Health', *Journal of Epidemiology and Community Health*, 59: 761–7.

Bartley, M. (2005) 'Job Insecurity and its Effect on Health', *Journal of Epidemiology and Community Health*, 59: 718–19.

Baum, F. (2005) 'Who Cares about Health for All in the 21st Century?', *Journal of Epidemiology and Community Health*, 59: 714–15.

Benach, J. and Muntaner, C. (2007) 'Precarious Employment and Health: Developing a Research Agenda', *Journal of Epidemiology and Community Health*, 61: 276–7.

Benach, J., Muntaner, C., Chung, H., Solar, O., Santana, V., Friel, S., Houweling, S., and Marmot, M. (2010) 'Health Inequalities: The Importance of Government Policies in Reducing Employment Related Health Inequalities', *British Medical Journal*, 340: c2154.

Choi, B.C.K., Hunter, D.J., Tsou, W., and Sainsbury, P. (2005) 'Diseases of Comfort: Primary Cause of Death in the 22nd Century', *Journal of Epidemiology and Community Health*, 59: 1,030–34.

Christensen, C. (2002) 'World Hunger: A Structural Approach', *International Organisation*, 32: 745–74.

CSDH (Commission on Social Determinants of Health) (2008) *Closing the Gap in a Generation: Health Equity through Action on the Social Determinants of Health. Final Report of the Commission on Social Determinants of Health*, Geneva: World Health Organization.

Early Child Development Knowledge Network (2007) *Early Child Development: A Powerful Equalizer. Final Report of the Early Child Development Knowledge Network of the Commission on Social Determinants of Health*, Geneva: World Health Organization.

Ebrahim, S. and Smeeth, L. (2005) 'Non-communicable Diseases in Low and Middle-income Countries: A Priority or a Distraction?', *International Journal of Epidemiology*, 34: 961–6.

Espelt, A., Borrell, B., Rodrigeuz-Sanz, M., Raskam, A.J., Dalmau, A., Mackenbach, J.P., and Kunst, A.E. (2007) 'Socioeconomic Inequalities in Diabetes Mellitus across Europe at the Turn of the Century', in Erasmus MC – University Medical Centre Rotterdam (eds) *Tackling Health Inequalities in Europe: An Integrated Approach*, Rotterdam: Erasmus University.

Ezzati, M., Lopez, A., Rodgers, A., and Murray, C. (2004) *Comparative Quantification of Health Risks: Global and Regional Burden of Disease Attributable to Selected Major Risk Factors*, Geneva: World Health Organization.

Farmer, P (1999) 'Pathologies of Power: Rethinking Health and Human Rights', *American Journal of Public Health*, 89: 1,486–96.

Grantham-McGregor, S., Cheung, Y.B., Cueto, S., Glewwe, P., Richter, L., and Strupp, B. (2007) 'Developmental Potential in the First 5 Years for Children in Developing Countries', *The Lancet*, 369: 60–70.

Gwatkin, D., Wagstaff, A., and Yazbeck, A. (2005) *Reaching the Poor with Health, Nutrition and Population Services*, Washington, DC: The World Bank.

Hanlon, P., Walsh, D., and Whyte, B. (2006) *Let Glasgow Flourish*, Glasgow: Glasgow Centre for Population Health.

ILO (International Labour Organization) (2008) *Global Employment Trends*, Geneva: International Labour Organization.

Kickbusch, I. (2008) 'Health in All Policies: Setting the Scene', *Public Health Bulletin*, 5: 3–5.

Koivusalo, M. and Mackintosh, M. (2005) *Health Systems and Commercialisation: In Search of Good Sense*, Basingstoke: Palgrave Macmillan.

Labonte, R., Schrecker, T., and Gupta, A. (2005) *Health for Some: Death, Disease and Disparity in a Globalising Era*, Toronto: Centre for Social Justice.

Lee, J.W. (2005) 'Public Health is a Social Issue', *The Lancet*, 365: 1,005–06.

Lewis, S. (2005) *Race against Time*, Toronto: House of Anansi Press.

Lundberg, O., Yngwe, M.A., Stjärne, M.K., Elstad, J.I., Ferrarini, T., Kangas, O., Norström, T., Palme, J., Fritzell, J., and NEWS Nordic Expert Group (2008) 'The Role of Welfare State Principles and Generosity in Social Policy Programmes for Public Health: An International Comparative Study', *The Lancet*, 372: 1,633–40.

Marmot, M. (2004) *Status Syndrome*, London: Bloomsbury.

Marmot, M. and Shipley, M. (1996) 'Do Socioeconomic Differences in Mortality Persist after Retirement? 25 Year Follow Up of Civil Servants from the First Whitehall Study', *British Medical Journal*, 313: 1,177–80.

Marmot, M. and Brunner, E. (2005) 'Cohort Profile: The Whitehall II Study', *International Journal of Epidemiology*, 34: 251–6.

Marmot, M., Friel, S., Bell, R., Houweling, A., and Taylor, S. (2008) 'Closing the Gap in a Generation: Health Equity through Action on the Social Determinants of Health', *The Lancet*, 372: 1,661–9.

Mendez, M., Monteiro, C., and Popkin, B. (2005) 'Overweight Exceeds Underweight among Women in Most Developing Countries', *American Journal of Clinical Nutrition*, 81: 714–21.

Monden, C. (2005) 'Current and Lifetime Exposure to Working Conditions: Do They Explain Educational Differences in Subjective Health?', *Social Science & Medicine*, 60: 2,465–76.

Morris, J., Donkin, A., Wonderling, D., Wilkinson, P., and Dowler, E. (2000) 'A Minimum Income for Healthy Living', *Journal of Epidemiology and Community Health*, 54: 885–9.

Murphy, M., Bobak, M., Nicholson, A., Rose, R., and Marmot, M. (2006) 'The Widening Gap in Mortality by Educational Level in the Russian Federation, 1980–2001', *American Journal of Public Health*, 96(7): 1,293–9.

Ostlin, P., Braveman, P., and Dachs, N. (2005) 'Priorities for Research to Take Forward the Health Equity Policy Agenda', *Bulletin of the World Health Organization*, 83: 948–53.

Paes de Barros, R. (2002) *Meeting the Millennium Poverty Reduction Targets in Latin America and the Caribbean*, Santiago: United Nations Economic Commission for Latin America and the Caribbean.

Sen, A. (1999) *Development as Freedom*, New York: Alfred A. Knopf, Inc.

Social Exclusion Knowledge Network (2007) *Understanding and Tackling Social Exclusion: Final Report of the Social Exclusion Knowledge Network of the Commission on Social Determinants of Health*, Geneva: World Health Organization.

Stansfeld, S. and Candy, B. (2006) 'Psychosocial Work Environment and Mental Health: A Meta-Analytic Review', *Scandinavian Journal of Work and Environmental Health*, 32: 443–62.

UN (United Nations) (2000) *General Comment 14: The Right to the Highest Attainable Standard of Health*, Geneva: Office of the United Nations High Commissioner for Human Rights.

UNDP (United Nations Development Programme) (2005) *Human Development Report 2005: International Cooperation at a Crossroads. Aid, Trade and Security in an Unequal World*, New York: UNDP.

UNESCO (United Nations Educational, Scientific, and Cultural Organisation) (2006) *Water: A Shared Responsibility: The United Nations World Water Development Report 2*, Paris: UNESCO.

Victora, C., Wagstaff, A., Schellenberg, J., Gwatkin, D., Claeson, M., and Habicht, J. (2003) 'Applying an Equity Lens to Child Health and Mortality: More of the Same is Not Enough', *The Lancet*, 362: 233–41.

Wilkinson, R. and Pickett, K. (2005) 'Income Inequality and Health: A Review and Explanation of the Evidence', *Social Science & Medicine*, 62(7): 1,768–84.

Woodward, D. and Simms, A. (2006) *Growth isn't Working: The Unbalanced Distribution of Benefits and Costs from Economic Growth*, London: New Economics Foundation.

World Bank (2005) *World Development Report 2006: Equity and Development*, Washington, DC: World Bank.

World Bank (2006) *World Development Report 2006: Equity and Development*, New York: World Bank and OUP.

WHO (World Health Organization) (2006) *WHOSIS: Statistical Information System*, Geneva: WHO.

WHO (World Health Organization) (n.d.-a) *Roll Back Malaria Partnership*, available at http://rbm.who.int/ (accessed 2 September 2010).

WHO (World Health Organization) (n.d.-b) *WHO 3 by 5 Initiative*, available at http://www.who.int/3by5/ en/ (accessed 2 September 2010).

Xu, K., Evans, D., Carrin, G., Aguilar-Rivera, A., Musgrove, P., and Evans, T. (2007) 'Protecting Households from Catastrophic Health Spending', *Health Affairs*, 26: 972–83.

8

Eliminating Global Health Inequities

Bridging the Gap

David Satcher and Sharon A. Rachel

Introduction

In the year 2000, through *Healthy People 2010*, the United States committed to the goal of eliminating disparities in health. In 2008, the World Health Organization committed to working towards the elimination of global health inequities in response to recommendations from the Commission on Social Determinants of Health. Health inequities are the unfair and avoidable differences in health status seen within and between countries (WHO 2008). Health inequities grow out of conditions that are largely beyond an individual's control, such as the conditions one is born into and in which one lives. Focusing on the social determinants of health as a means of reducing health inequities emphasises the importance of the overall environment where people live and work (Wilensky and Satcher 2009).

Healthy People 2010 describes the determinants of health as an array of critical influences that determine the health of individuals and communities. These determinants include biology, environment, individual behaviour, access to care, and overriding social, economic, health, and other policies (Figure 8.1).

More specific to the determinants of health of populations are *social determinants of health*. The World Health Organization defines social determinants of health as 'the conditions in which people are born, grow, live, work and age, including the health system' (WHO 2009), and which are largely responsible for health inequities both between and within nations. These conditions include, but are not limited to, income and socio-economic status (SES), access to care, culture, access to education, and environment. Human behaviour is influenced by the social environment but also controlled at the individual level and contributes to both favourable and poor health outcomes. All of these determinants are overridden and heavily influenced by policy, within and beyond the health system.

In short, social determinants of health are the 'causes of the causes' (WHO 2008: 42) of health inequities and outcomes. This chapter examines the social determinants of health and how they influence health outcomes and health inequities. It provides an overview of how access to care, individual behaviour, culture, education, the environment, and socio-economic status affect health on a global scale. A close examination of the social determinants of health is essential to devise health strategies and interventions that will be effective within existing social, political, and

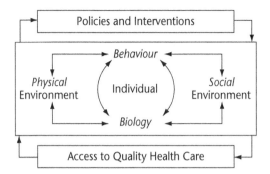

Figure 8.1   Determinants of health
Source: Healthy People 2010.

cultural structures in reducing inequities in health outcomes between (and within) rich and poor nations and improving health for all people (Wilensky and Satcher 2009).

Access to care

Access to health and medical care is based on several factors. First, the ratio of providers[1] to patients varies from country to country, and region to region within countries. In North America, Europe, Russia, and Australia, we generally see an average ratio of 300–500 inhabitants to each provider (300–500:1). Countries with critical shortages of providers include India and Papua New Guinea (20,000:1), Ethiopia, Burundi and Mozambique (33,500:1), and Tanzania and Malawi (50,000:1) (WHO 2006a).

Availability of an appropriate provider is often a barrier for people with rare health conditions requiring specialised care or for people living in remote areas. Lack of skilled care is largely responsible for over half a million maternal deaths worldwide from complications of pregnancy and childbirth and for around 4 million infant deaths within the first four weeks of life (UNICEF 2008). Lack of availability of appropriate treatments further exasperates global health inequities. For instance, over 90 per cent of children infected with HIV are infected through mother-to-child (vertical) transmission (UNAIDS 2007) – usually during labour and delivery or through breastfeeding. While prevention of vertical transmission of HIV through use of prenatal antiretroviral therapy (ARV) reduces the risk of HIV transmission to only 2 per cent of babies born to infected mothers in developed nations (Cooper *et al.* 2002), in the poorest nations, an HIV-positive pregnant woman has up to a 45 per cent risk of transmitting the virus to her infant given the absence of preventive care (UNICEF n.d.).

Other barriers to access include distance required to travel from place of residence to a provider's location, cultural barriers, language, and affordability. Distance is often reported as a major barrier for which people prolong seeking care. Even in countries with lower provider-to-patient ratios, major metropolitan areas have far more providers per inhabitant than rural and sparsely populated 'frontier' areas (Farley *et al.* 2002).

However, even when access is available, cultural and language barriers may still exist in obtaining care. Patients may not have access to a provider who speaks their language, or limited health literacy may affect patients' abilities to understand what they are being told, and fear and embarrassment may keep the patients from asking providers important questions. Patients also may not trust individual providers or the overall healthcare system. Stigma may surround the condition for which treatment is sought, such as in cases of mental or sexual health. Hospitals and clinics may not be accessible to people with disabilities, including mobility, vision, or hearing impairments. Providers may not be equipped with the skills to treat patients in a culturally sensitive way, and in many instances women are not empowered to advocate on their own behalf for their health.

Finally, affordability can be an underlying barrier to accessing care: socio-economic status accounts for a marked connection between poverty, access to care, and health inequities. Cost of care increases as treatments and technology become more sophisticated and complex, particularly in profit-driven healthcare systems. For those with limited financial resources who must pay for part or all of the cost of health services like routine checkups, tests, treatments, and medications, competing priorities such as food, childcare, and housing may take precedence over healthcare.

Culture

People's behaviours, attitudes, beliefs, and approaches to health are greatly shaped by culture. When considering health interventions, it is important to consider values, attitudes, and beliefs, and approach culture and health carefully and respectfully, employing cultural sensitivity and competence. Culture permeates the health of communities in many distinct and underlying ways. Generally, a community's health can be predicted by the status of women's health, and maternal and child health. Examining the status of women in various cultures allows us to draw correlations with overall health.

One example of a women's health issue that has received increased global attention since the 1990s is the effects of female genital cutting (FGC).[2] This practice – partial or complete excision of the clitoris and labia – has many cultural and health implications and has become a focal point of the international women's rights movement. Cutting is usually done by untrained practitioners under unsanitary circumstances. It is highly associated with infection and death. Sexual intercourse is painful for circumcised women and, when they become pregnant, maternal morbidity and mortality problems arise, such as haemorrhage, the need for Caesarian deliveries, longer recovery post-delivery, episiotomy, perineal tearing, and maternal death. Infants born to circumcised mothers are at higher risk for low birth weight and stillbirth (WHO 2006b).

While the practice is officially illegal in most countries, it still persists. In some ethnic groups, FGC is seen as an important tradition, a rite of passage into womanhood, and a means for preserving virginity and marital fidelity by curbing women's sexual desire and pleasure. FGC is considered necessary for women in these cultures to attain marriage and motherhood, which are essential for women's economic security, and often mere survival, within their communities. While overcoming cultural barriers is challenging, international women's and human rights movements have called for an end to this practice out of concern for women's physical, mental, and sexual health.

Another relevant example of cultural importance relates to the strong relationship that exists between maternal and child health, decreased fertility rates, and community health. Research has shown that women who have fewer babies encounter fewer of the risks associated with pregnancy, labour, and delivery (Callister 2005), and are able to devote more resources to fewer children. Increased access to contraception has effectively lowered fertility rates, which ameliorates poor health outcomes associated with poverty by promoting economic growth due to improved health, education, and productivity. However, cultural values, for example among Palestinian women, pressure them to bear many (male) children and perpetuate their culture, and in places like sub-Saharan Africa, women may refuse to use contraception because of persistent rumours that they cause HIV infection (Callister 2005). Culture often presents a significant barrier to implementing interventions that may otherwise succeed in reducing health inequities.

Education

Literacy is one of many basic measures of education and, worldwide, more than one in eight adults lacks basic literacy skills (Callister 2007). Two-thirds of the world's illiterate adults are women, and 50 million girls do not attend school (UNESCO 2009). Research has shown a strong positive relationship between education and health, particularly for women and girls. Improved maternal and child health outcomes associated with education include greater earning potential, increased age at first marriage, decreased fertility rates, delayed childbearing, and lower infant, child and maternal mortality (Callister 2007). Furthermore, the more education a mother attains, the more likely her children are to receive an education (WHO 2008). Conversely, adults who lacked access to education or did poorly in school tend to earn less income, have more children, and have less access to health care for themselves and their children (WHO 2008).

A study by Jukes and others (2008) that examined the association between girls' education and HIV infection in sub-Saharan Africa found that the higher the educational attainment, most notably secondary education, the lower the HIV prevalence. This finding proposed that education decreases HIV infection by increasing cognitive ability to respond to prevention messages, by building social capital and networks that reinforce protective behaviours, and by increasing access to learning about the biological transmission of the disease.

An intervention described by McGinn and Allen (2006) reached even the most transient and vulnerable populations when a non-profit conglomerate worked on a reproductive and sexual health literacy project for illiterate and semi-literate women in a refugee settlement in West Africa. The content included safe motherhood, family planning, HIV/AIDS, sexually transmitted diseases, and violence against women. Despite the instability of the population, the women who participated reported increased literacy skills and reproductive health knowledge, increased contraceptive use, healthier behaviour, and increased sense of empowerment.

Despite the overwhelming evidence that improved education mitigates health inequities and promotes upward socio-economic mobility, millions of adults and children worldwide lack access to formal education, and many children continue to perform poorly in school.

Environment

A person's health is greatly affected by their surrounding environment. A healthy physical environment includes safe access to areas where one may enjoy physical activity, such as adequate urban 'green space' like parks and other landscaped areas, while the social environment includes where and how people interact with one another within a social community. A healthy ecological environment is dependent on air and water quality, as well as sanitation infrastructure and waste management. However, physical, social, and ecological environments in both developed and developing nations often lack ideally livable conditions.

Nearly half the world's population lives in urban areas, with cities continuing to grow due to natural population growth and in-migration from rural areas (WHO 2008). Opportunities for healthy living in cities include access to parks, paved paths, and trails for exercise, which encourages physical activity among city residents and also benefits the ecological health. However, parks, trails, and pavements are typically found in more affluent and safer areas of cities, and those living in poor urban conditions prone to violence and disease do not have the same access to healthy city living. Additionally, urban infrastructure like pavements, paved paths, pedestrian crossings, recreational parks, and trails are not always accessible to people with disabilities. For example, kerbs need ramps to provide safe access for people with mobility impairments and pedestrian crossings need audio signals for the visually impaired, indicating when it is safe to cross streets.

Worldwide, nearly a billion people live in urban slums and face daily struggles with conditions like poor sanitation, overcrowding, violence, and poor infrastructure, which lead to the spread of disease and premature death. Rates of child mortality and tuberculosis infection are greater than twice the national averages in slums like those in Nairobi, Kenya, and Manila, Philippines (WHO 2008). In addition, a study on children in Chicago who were exposed to severe violence in their neighbourhoods, including murder, found that the children were much more likely to become victims or perpetrators of violence later in life than children who did not witness such violence (Bingenheimer *et al.* 2005). Conversely, in-migration from rural to urban areas results in diminished investment in rural sustainability and agriculture, impacting the ecology and health of the land itself.

A major ecological health issue is global climate change and pollution of the air, land, and water, and the significant impact these have had on health. Climate change affects where and how people live, how people can support themselves and their families occupationally, people's diets, access to safe and clean water supplies, and choices in physical activity[3] (US DHHS 2009a). In many regions of the developing world, access to clean water is only available to those who are able to pay for it. And even in developed nations, such as the United States, minority children are more likely to grow up living near toxic waste disposal sites (Satcher and Higginbotham 2008), which thus contributes to racial and ethnic disparities in health. Natural disasters and disaster preparedness and management have also impacted public health, as was seen in the aftermath of these disasters:

- The 2004 Indian Ocean earthquake and tsunami, which killed over 200,000 people
- Hurricane Katrina, which caused over $100 billion in damage to New Orleans and the United States Gulf Coast in 2005
- The 2008 earthquake in the Sichuan province of China, which caused nearly 90,000 deaths
- The 2010 earthquake in Port-au-Prince, Haiti, which claimed over 200,000 lives, left over 2 million people homeless and hundreds of thousands of people without any access to medical treatment for their injuries.

Health is enhanced when the physical environment is conducive to safe physical activity, the social environment is free from violence and danger, and the ecology – particularly air and water quality – is safe and sanitary.

Behaviour

Human behaviour, arguably the most salient of the determinants of health, is particularly influenced by the social determinants of health, and accounts in large part for the variations seen in health outcomes. It is the determinant of health over which an individual has the most control, though it is highly dependent upon factors such as the environment, education, and personal income. Such behaviours include alcohol, drug, and tobacco use, physical activity, nutritional habits, and sexual behaviour (Satcher and Higginbotham 2008). Only recently, however, are we targeting the social determinants that influence health behaviours.

More than one in five people worldwide smoke cigarettes, and the prevalence of men who smoke is four times that of women. The health outcomes associated with smoking – cancer, heart and lung disease, to name a few – cost national health systems billions each year (WHO 2008). The WHO Commission also found that the number of alcohol-related deaths each year rivals that of deaths from HIV/AIDS worldwide. Poverty is a strong predictor of smoking and excessive alcohol use. Undernutrition is still a problem in many impoverished parts of the world, but now overnutrition and physical inactivity are the main reasons for the worldwide obesity pandemic. There are now more overweight and obese children and adults than ever before. This is due in large part to lifestyles that have become increasingly sedentary and to living in environments that are not conducive to exercise and outdoor recreation.

Human sexuality is personally intimate and has the potential for positive, life-affirming outcomes. But the negative consequences of irresponsible and/or forced or nonconsensual sexual behaviour may be life-long, and affect individuals, families, communities, and nations (US DHHS 2001). Sexual behaviours associated with poor health outcomes include unprotected sex, sexual coercion, rape and incest, intimate partner violence, and global sex trafficking. Some of the outcomes include unintended pregnancy, unsafe abortion and maternal death, STD and HIV infection, depression, sexual dysfunction, and decreased or altogether lost capacity to form and sustain healthy intimate relationships.

Many sexual health inequities occur among women, minorities, people of colour, and people with disabilities. In the United States, nearly half of both newly diagnosed AIDS cases and AIDS deaths are among African Americans, even though African Americans account for only about 12 per cent of the population (US DHHS 2009b). HIV is the leading cause of death for African American women ages 25–34 (US DHHS 2008). An analysis of data from the 2002 National Survey of Family Growth in the United States found that people with disabilities were more likely to have had forced heterosexual or homosexual experiences, more likely to have an STD, and more likely to have had ten or more lifetime sexual partners than people without disabilities. Women with disabilities were twice as likely as women without disabilities to report having experienced forced penis-in-vagina intercourse (Kurki *et al.* 2007).

Behaviour change is a challenge to improving health, and therefore public health practitioners must understand the challenges faced by interventions that aim for behaviour change to protect the health of all people.

Overriding policies

Community, local, regional, and national policies affect health outcomes at all levels. In order to promote health, leaders must support policies that address the social determinants of health. While many policy areas may not appear to address health, they still have ramifications on people's well-being. Hence, education, labour, zoning, and environmental policies all become health policies.

Health suffers in times and places of political unrest and instability. Guerilla warfare in sub-Saharan Africa, such as the 1994 Rwandan genocide, and the war that has ravaged the Darfur region of Sudan since 2003, has killed millions and forced millions more into refugee settlements with little to no access to health care, and where people still live with the daily threat of violence, rape, torture, and murder. Myanmar (formerly Burma) suffered a devastating cyclone in 2008, after which the de facto military leadership refused to allow foreign aid into the country. The ensuing lack of access to critical care contributed to the 140,000 deaths that followed the disaster. The 2009 coup that removed the president of Honduras from power resulted in the closure of government-funded hospitals and clinics due to the loss of funding for supplies and personnel needed to treat patients in violent, remote areas.

Policies that support education are likely to improve the health of communities given the positive association between literacy, education, and favourable health outcomes. Egypt, Bangladesh, and Cameroon, for example, all implemented policies that committed to building schools and providing scholarships and other funds to poor families to send their daughters to school (Callister 2007). Chile promotes education for children in poor families that integrates quality education, healthy eating habits, care for the children, and social attention for families (WHO 2008). Swedish school systems integrated a comprehensive approach to physical activity and playtime that enhanced children's development and natural learning strategies (WHO 2008).

Policies are also enacted that directly address health. In 2003, the WHO passed a global tobacco treaty, which has already dramatically reduced smoking prevalence and smoking-related deaths. In the 1990s, the United States began requiring fortification of grain products with folic acid for its known effects on preventing neural tube defects. As a result, incidence in defects like spina bifida decreased considerably in just a little over a decade. The Global Alliance for Vaccines and Immunisations (GAVI) was launched in 2000 to provide support for making vaccines available to those most in need. Since then, national policies around vaccination have been enacted, vaccinations have increased notably, and rates of many vaccine-preventable diseases have been dramatically reduced (François *et al.* 2008).

Conclusion

The WHO Commission's final report (2008) made three overarching recommendations:

- Improve daily living conditions
- Tackle the inequitable distribution of power, money, and resources
- Measure and understand the problem and assess the impact of action.

Social determinants of health are a complex and interrelated set of conditions. All people must have access to health care and take personal accountability for health. Providers must use cultural competency and sensitivity to address and resolve health inequities. Governments must 'provide quality education that pays attention to children's physical, social/emotional, and language/cognitive development, starting in pre-primary school' (WHO 2008: 57). The health of people with disabilities must not be overlooked. Investment in urban infrastructure and rural sustainability should prioritise environmental health along with promoting outdoor activity, preventing violence, preparedness for disasters, and addressing climate change.

The WHO Commission's report addresses the goal of 'closing the gap in a generation'. A goal is an aspiration with specific strategies and plans to move towards a result. The aspiration to lay out a finite time frame to bridge the gap of inequities between wealthy and developing countries, as well as disparities in health within countries, is an asset as well as a detriment. In 2001, the US surgeon general decreed, 'doing nothing is unacceptable' (US DHHS 2001: iii). While the task of eliminating global health inequities is overwhelming, public health leaders must be cognisant of these needs and take action. Governments and grant-making foundations must be encouraged to direct resources to replicating and sustaining successful health programmes, and make healthy living a top priority.

Notes

1 The *World Health Report 2006* categorises *health service providers* inclusive of physicians, nurses, mid-wives, traditional medicine practitioners, and faith healers.
2 Also referred to as female circumcision or 'female genital mutilation' (FGM).
3 For example, climate change affects physical activity by way of limiting safe outdoor time based on temperature, sun and harmful UV exposure, and breathing unsafe, polluted air. Exposure to these and other toxins increase risk for heart and lung disease, while lack of physical activity is also a predictor of poor health. The very young and very old are especially vulnerable to poor health resulting from exposure to environmental hazards.

References

Bingenheimer, J.B., Brennan, R.T., and Earles, F.J. (2005) 'Firearm violence exposure and serious violent behavior', *Science*, 308: 1,323–6.

Callister, L.C. (2005) 'Global maternal mortality: Contributing factors and strategies for change', *American Journal of Maternal/Child Nursing*, 30(3): 184–92.

Callister, L.C. (2007) 'Improving literacy in women and girls globally', *Global Health and Nursing*, 32(3): 194.

Cooper, E.R., Charurat, M., Mofenson, L., Hanson, I.C., Pitt, J., Diaz, C., Hyani, K., Handelsman, E., Smerigilo, V., Hoff, R. and Blattner, W. (2002) 'Combination antiretroviral strategies for the treatment of pregnant HIV-1-infected women and prevention of perinatal HIV-1 transmission', *JAIDS*, 29 (5): 484–94.

Farley, D., Shugarman, L., Taylor, P., Inkelas, M., Ashwood, J.S., Zeng, F. and Harris, K.M. (2002) *Trends in Special Medicare Payments and Service Utilization for Rural Areas in the 1990s*, Santa Monica, CA: The Rand Corporation.

François, G., Dochez, C., Mphalele, M.J., Burnett, R., Van Hal, G. and Mehaus, A. (2008) 'Hepatitis B vaccination in Africa: mission accomplished?', *The Southern African Journal of Epidemiology and Infection*, 23(1): 24–8.

Jukes, M., Simmons, S. and Bundy, D. (2008) 'Education and vulnerability: The role of schools in protecting young women and girls from HIV in southern Africa', *AIDS*, 22(S4): S41–S56.

Kurki, A., Hendershot, G. and Tepper, M. (2007) 'Sexually transmitted infections, sexuality, and disability: data from national surveys', in American Public Health Association, '135th Annual Meeting and Expo', Washington, DC, 3–7 November 2007, Washington, DC: American Public Health Association.

McGinn, T. and Allen, K. (2006) 'Improving refugees' reproductive health through literacy in Guinea', *Global Public Health*, 1(3): 229–48.

Satcher, D. and Higginbotham, E.H. (2008) 'The public health approach to eliminating disparities in health', *American Journal of Public Health*, 98(3): 400–403.

UNAIDS (2007) *07 AIDS Epidemic Update*, Geneva: Joint United Nations Programme on HIV/AIDS and World Health Organization.

UNESCO (2009) *Literacy*, available at http://cms01.unesco.org/en/education_ar/themes/learning-throughout-life/literacy/ (accessed 11 August 2009).

UNICEF (United Nations Children's Fund) (n.d.) *Goal: Improve Maternal Health*, available at http://www.unicef.org/mdg/maternal.html (accessed 13 August 2009).

UNICEF (United Nations Children's Fund) (2008) *State of the World's Children 2009*, New York: UNICEF.

US DHHS (US Department of Health and Human Services), (2001) *The Surgeon General's Call to Action to Promote Sexual Health and Responsible Sexual Behavior*, Washington, DC: US Government Printing Office.

US DHHS (US Department of Health and Human Services), Centers for Disease Control and Prevention (CDC) (2008) *HIV/AIDS Among Women*, Washington, DC: US Government Printing Office.

US DHHS (US Department of Health and Human Services), and National Institutes of Health (NIH), (2009a), *Fact Sheet: Health Effects of Climate Change*, Washington, DC: US Government Printing Office.

US DHHS (US Department of Health and Human Services), Centers for Disease Control and Prevention (CDC) (2009b) *HIV/AIDS Among African Americans*, Washington, DC: US Government Printing Office.

Wilensky, G.R. and Satcher, D. (2009) 'Don't forget about the social determinants of health', *Health Affairs*, 28(2): w194–w198.

WHO (World Health Organization) (2006a) *The World Health Report 2006: Working Together for Health*, Geneva: WHO.

WHO (World Health Organization) (2006b) 'Female genital mutilation and obstetric outcome: WHO collaborative prospective study in six African countries', *The Lancet*, 367: 1,835–41.

WHO (World Health Organization) Commission on Social Determinants of Health (2008) *Closing the Gap in a Generation: Health Equity through Action on the Social Determinants of Health*, Geneva: WHO.

WHO (World Health Organization) (2009) *Social Determinants of Health*, available at http://www.who.int/social_determinants/en/ (accessed 9 December 2009).

9

Gender-Based Inequities in Global Public Health

Gita Sen and Piroska Östlin

Introduction

In no field of scientific enquiry does the challenge of distinguishing the relative importance of biological versus environmental factors confront researchers as starkly as in the field of public health. To what extent and in what ways is our health affected by our environment, and how much is it due to more intrinsic characteristics that are imprinted in our genetic coding and our chromosomes? The problem of 'nature' versus 'nurture' is an old problem in health research, and one for which researchers have developed a variety of analytical methods. We know now that both matter and, what is more, interact with each other in complex ways. During the last few decades, there has been an emerging recognition among health professionals that environmental factors are not only physical but also social. As women and men, for example, our experiences of health are profoundly affected by a wide range of differences in access to and control over resources and knowledge, decision-making power in the family and community, and divisions of labour, as well as the roles and responsibilities that society assigns to us.

Gender, as a socially constructed distinction, can reinforce, counteract, or work independently of biological sex to affect our health. For example, evidence suggests that women's lower social autonomy and economic disadvantages exacerbate their biological susceptibility to HIV and other diseases. Together, gender and sex influence exposure to health risks, access to health information and services, health outcomes, and the social and economic consequences of ill health. Gender inequities in health arise (1) when the biologically specific health needs of women and men are not fairly addressed, and (2) as a result of unfair gender power relations between women and men (Östlin *et al.* 2001).

The dynamics of gender power relations that govern hierarchy, authority, and decisions are, together with biological vulnerabilities, of profound importance to the health of both women and men worldwide.[1] These dynamics flow through several pathways in which different factors interact, at the individual and collective levels, to generate gender-based inequities in global public health. Understanding these pathways helps us address a number of questions. How do biological sex differences and gendered social determinants combine to affect women's and men's health? How do they affect women's and men's differential exposure and vulnerability to health risks? How do gendered norms in health manifest in households and communities, and how can these norms, values, and practices be challenged? Why are women's and men's experience of health systems so different, and how can we minimise gender bias in health systems? What mechanisms and policies need to be developed to ensure that gender imbalances in health research are avoided and corrected? How can we overcome the organisational rigidities and lacunae that hinder the implementation of gender-equal policies both within and outside the health sector? What is required for building effective leadership, creating well-designed organisational mandates, structures, incentives, and accountability mechanisms that would ensure gender equitable laws, policies, and programmes?

The role of gender as a social determinant of health: a framework

Gender affects health by four major pathways leading from gendered structural determinants to inequitable health outcomes through (1) discriminatory values, norms, practices, and behaviours, (2) differential exposures and vulnerabilities to disease, disability, and injuries, (3) biases in health systems, and (4) biased health research. Such outcomes can, in turn, have serious economic and social consequences for girls and boys, women and men, for their families and communities, and for their countries. Feedback effects from outcomes and consequences to the structural determinants or to intermediary factors can also be important (Sen *et al.* 2007). Figure 9.1 summarises these relationships.

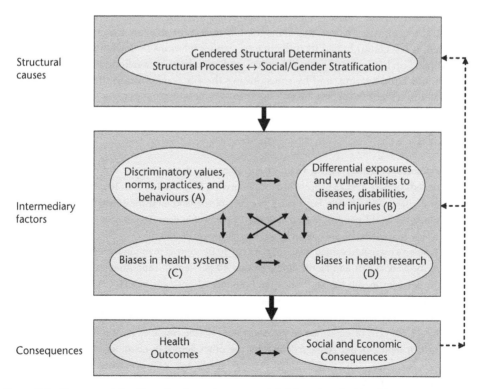

Figure 9.1   Framework for the role of gender as a social determinant of health
Note: The dashed lines represent feedback effects.
Source: Sen, Östlin and George 2007.

Gita Sen and Piroska Östlin

Gendered structural determinants and processes

Gender relations of power constitute the root causes of gender inequality and are among the most influential of the social determinants of health. Women have less land, wealth, and property in almost all societies, and their participation in decision-making is low at all levels (Box 9.1). Girls in some contexts are fed less, educated less, and more physically restricted; and women are typically employed and segregated in lower-paid, less secure, and 'informal' occupations. At the same time, women and young girls have higher burdens of work in ensuring the survival, reproduction and security of people, young and old. Men, on the other hand, have greater wealth, better jobs, more education, greater political power, and fewer restrictions on behaviour. Moreover, men in many parts of the world often exercise power over women, making decisions on their behalf, regulating and constraining their access to resources and personal agency, and sanctioning and enforcing their behaviour through socially condoned violence or the threat of violence (Garcia-Moreno *et al.* 2006). The unequal power relationships between women and men place women in subordinate social positions in a systematic manner and have a profound impact not only on the physical and mental health of girls and women, but also of boys and men (Barker and Ricardo 2005). Although men typically enjoy many tangible benefits from their superior position in society through resources, power, authority, and control, social norms of masculinity often translate into risky and unhealthy behaviours, and premature mortality.

Although gender hierarchies are pervasive and persistent, they are not immutable, even if not all changes may be positive. First, the gender gap in primary education has been narrowed significantly in almost all countries, although there is still a significant gap in parts of sub-Saharan Africa.

Second, in countries where the demographic transition towards lower fertility has been completed, it has certainly had its influence on gender relations by lowering the time women have to spend on bearing and raising children, and on culture by weakening the links between sexuality and child-bearing, and by transforming the size, composition of, and relationships within families (Presser and Sen 2000).

Box 9.1

- In Cameroon, Kenya, Nigeria, Tanzania, and other countries in sub-Saharan Africa, while women undertake more than 75 per cent of agricultural work, they own less than 10 per cent of the land. In Pakistan, women own less than 3 per cent of the land, and the situation is no better in the Americas: 11 per cent of land in Brazil, 13 per cent in Peru, 16 per cent in Nicaragua, and 22 per cent in Mexico are owned by women (Grown *et al.* 2005).
- Women's estimated earned income is around 30 per cent of men's in the countries surveyed in the Middle East and North Africa, around 40 per cent in Latin America and South Asia, 50 per cent in sub-Saharan Africa, and around 60 per cent in CEE/CIS, East Asian, and industrialised countries (ILO 2006, cited in UNICEF 2007).
- Women are under-represented in all national parliaments. In June 2008, they accounted for 18 per cent of parliamentarians worldwide. Nordic countries have the highest rates of participation (41 per cent), followed by the other European countries and the Americas (21 per cent), sub-Saharan Africa (17 per cent), Asia (16 per cent), and the Pacific (13 per cent). Arab states rank lowest, with a regional average of less than 10 per cent (Inter-Parliament Database 2008).

Third, some aspects of globalisation are of particular significance for our focus on gender relations. For example, feminisation of work-forces has gone hand-in-hand with increased casualisation of work. The resulting job insecurity, coupled with continuing burdens for unpaid work in the household, has had serious implications for women's health (Messing and Östlin 2006). A second gendered consequence of globalisation is through its narrowing of national policy space that has resulted in reducing funds for health and education in some of the poorest countries, with negative impacts on girls' and women's access (Herz and Sperling 2004). A third aspect of globalisation with consequences for women's health is the rise in violence linked to the changing political economy of nation states in the international order (Laurie and Petchesky 2008). Importantly, gendered violence does not only affect girls and women but includes violence against boys and men, as well as transgender and intersex persons and all those who do not meet heterosexual norms.

Fourth, on the positive side, global and national recognition of the human rights frame-work for health has led to hitherto poorly understood dimensions of inequality and inequity – gender, sexual orientation, ethnicity, race, caste, and disability – being debated in various fora. The explicit recognition of 'lived' realities – for example, of rape as a violation of women's human rights (United Nations 1993), or racism as a violation of the human rights of specific racial or ethnic groups (United Nations 2001) – has been critical to their being acknowledged as needing legal and policy remedies. A further important way in which the human rights framework has been deepened is through interpreting the right to health to include reproductive and sexual health and reproductive rights (United Nations 1994) and sexual rights (United Nations 1995). In 2007, a distinguished group of international human rights experts launched the Yogyakarta Principles on the application of international human rights law to sexual orientation and gender identity (see http://www.yogyakarta principles. org/docs/File/Yogyakarta_Principles_EN.pdf). Of particular note are Principles 17 (the right to the highest attainable standard of health) and 18 (the right to protection from medical abuses).

Structural changes such as these affect gender equity in health through four distinct pathways discussed below.

Intermediary factors: understanding the pathways

Discriminatory values, norms, practices, and behaviours

Gendered norms in health manifest in households and communities on the basis of values and attitudes about the relative worth or importance of girls versus boys and men versus women: about who has responsibility for different household/community needs and roles, about mascu-linity and femininity, about who has the right to make different decisions, about who ensures that household/community order is maintained and deviance is appropriately sanctioned or punished, and about who has final authority in relation to the inner world of the family/ community and its outer relations with society (Keleher and Franklin 2008; Quisumbing and Maluccio 1999). Norms around masculinity not only affect the health of girls and women but also of boys and men (Barker and Ricardo 2005).

Gender-biased values translate into practices and behaviour that affect people's daily lives, as well as key determinants of wellness and equity such as nutrition, hygiene, acknowledgement of health problems, health-seeking behaviour, and access to health services to the extent that the latter are in the hands of communities. Many of these practices are in the area of sexuality, biological reproduction, and the life cycle: son preference, female genital mutilation and ritual,

---

Box 9.2

- It is estimated that 60 million girls are missing in Asia (UNFPA 2006).
- In Africa, 3 million girls are at risk every year for female genital mutilation. In some 28 countries, 135 million girls and women have undergone FGM (WHO 2006).
- Recent findings from the WHO multi-country study on women's health and domestic violence, conducted in Bangladesh, Brazil, Ethiopia, Japan, Namibia, Peru, Samoa, Serbia and Montenegro, Thailand, and Tanzania, found that the reported lifetime prevalence of physical or sexual partner violence, or both, varied from 15 per cent to 71 per cent, with two sites having a prevalence of less than 25 per cent, seven from 25 per cent to 50 per cent, and six from 50 per cent and 75 per cent. Between 4 per cent and 54 per cent of respondents reported physical or sexual partner violence, or both, in past year (Garcia-Moreno *et al.* 2006).

(and painful) 'deflowering' of brides represent only a few examples of practices that seriously affect women's and girls' physical and mental health (Box 9.2).

Specific norms related to masculinity may place both women and men at risk. Men and boys may view risk-taking behaviours, including substance use, unsafe sex, and unsafe driving as ways to affirm their manhood (Barker *et al.* 2007).

Differential exposures and vulnerabilities to diseases, disabilities, and injuries

Male–female differences in health vary in magnitude across different health conditions (Box 9.3). Some health conditions are determined primarily by biological sex differences. Others are the result of how societies socialise women and men into gender roles supported by norms about masculinity and femininity, and power relations that accord privileges to men, but which adversely affect the health of both women and men. Risk and vulnerability have to be understood, not only in bio-medical terms, but in social terms (Snow 2008). For example,

---

Box 9.3

- The Global Burden of Disease estimates for 2002 indicate that 68 out of the 126 health conditions have at least a 20 per cent difference between women and men (Snow 2008).
- Young women worldwide between the ages of 15 and 24 are 1.6 times as likely as young men to be HIV-positive. In sub-Saharan Africa, approximately 6.2 million young people are infected, 76 per cent of whom are females (UNAIDS 2006). In sub-Saharan Africa and the Caribbean, young women are 3 times and 2.4 times, respectively, more likely than men to be HIV-positive. In Trinidad and Tobago, the number of women between 15 and 19 years old with HIV is 5 times higher than among adolescent males (UNICEF 2006).
- In developing countries, nearly 2 million poor women and children die annually from exposure to indoor air pollution caused by smoke from cooking fuels. Many more suffer from acute and chronic respiratory infections (Smith and Maeusezahl-Feuz 2004).
- Globally, 2.7 times as many men as women die from road traffic injuries (Snow 2002).

---

how much of women's greater vulnerability to HIV infection is due to female biology, and how much can be attributed to girls' and women's lack of power in sexual relationships? The biological factors involved include: the nature of vaginal mucous membranes and reproductive lifecycles (Forrest 1991), the infectiveness of semen (UNAIDS 1999), and women's higher rates of sexually transmitted infections (STIs). However, equally significant are the power relations that influence sexual behaviour and constrain health-seeking behaviour and social support. Excess female blindness (150 blind women for every 100 blind men) offers another compelling example of a health outcome attributable to a combination of sex and gendered causes. The greater global burden of blindness among women is due to the (hypothesised) sex-linked inherent risks of cataract for women, a gendered risk of trachoma (women having more contact with infected children), and a gendered distribution of eye-care services (greater access to cataract surgery for men) (Lewallen and Courtright 2002; Snow 2008).

Biases in health systems

Gender inequities are endemic in health care systems globally (Box 9.4). Women and men often have different needs due to both biological and social factors, but health care systems do not always take these into account. When health services are provided to meet women's health needs, they tend in some contexts to focus on women's reproductive functions, neglecting all their other functions (Sen et al. 2007). In addition, gender inequalities in society can lead to inequitable access to health care services. For example, health insurance schemes provided by employers may cover women to a lesser extent, as they are more likely to work at home or in the informal labour market (Messing and Östlin 2006).

Health systems also tend to ignore women's crucial role as health providers, both within the formal health system (at its lower levels) and as informal providers and unpaid carers in the home (George 2008). Health sector reforms introduced during the last two decades have had limited success in achieving improved gender equity in health. The most obvious and striking expression of the failure to adequately address women's biologically specific health needs is the persistence of extremely high rates of maternal mortality in many parts of the world. Between 350,000 and 550,000 women are estimated to die each year from maternal causes (Hogan et al. 2010). Minimising gender bias in health systems requires systematic approaches to building awareness and transforming values among service providers, steps to improve access to health services, and effective mechanisms for accountability.

Box 9.4

- In ten OECD countries and the Russian Federation between 1993 and 1997, women made up between 62 to 85 per cent of the health labour force. In the United States, frontline health workers are 79 per cent female (George 2008).
- It is estimated that up to 80 per cent of all health care and 90 per cent of HIV/AIDS- related illness care is provided in the home (Uys 2003).
- In many African countries, such as Burkina Faso, Senegal, Nigeria, Malawi, Cameroon, Morocco, Ethiopia, Zambia, and Lesotho, more than half of the women are not allowed to make decisions about their own health care (CSDH 2008).

Biases in health research

Gender discrimination and bias not only affect differentials in health needs, health-seeking behaviour, treatment, and outcomes, but also permeate the content and the process of health research (Östlin et al. 2004) (see Box 9.5). Gender imbalances in research processes include: non-collection of sex-disaggregated data in individual research projects or larger data systems; research methodologies that are not sensitive to the different dimensions and health implications of social inequality; methods used in medical research and clinical trials for new drugs that lack a gender perspective and exclude female subjects from study populations; gender imbalance in ethical committees, research funding, and advisory bodies; and discriminatory treatment of women researchers and scientists.

Box 9.5

- Female applicants for post-doctoral fellowships in Sweden had to be 2.5 times more productive than their male colleagues to get the same peer review rating for scientific competence (Wennerås and Wold 1997).
- In 2004, only 21 per cent of the members of WHO's expert and advisory committees were women (Östlin et al. 2004).

Conclusion

As discussed above, gender power is a key social determinant of inequity in health. However, insufficient resources, weak organisational mechanisms, and poor political commitment have resulted in fragmented efforts, significant mismatches between stated gender policy and programme efforts, and serious gaps between political rhetoric and actual practice. Working towards gender equality and equity challenges long-standing male-dominated power structures, and patriarchal social capital (old boys' networks) within organisations. Resistance to gender-equal policies may take the form of trivialisation, dilution, subversion, or outright resistance, and can lead to the evaporation of gender equitable laws, policies, or programmes.

Despite this less than cheerful situation, and although gender inequity in health is pervasive and persistent, it *can* be changed through effective political leadership, well-designed policies and programmes, institutional incentives, and strong accountability mechanisms. Sweden's new public health policy, which came into force in 2003, is an excellent example of integrating gender within the framework of an existing equity-oriented public health policy (Östlin and Diderichsen 2001). While there are still only a few countries that have taken such comprehensive, multisectoral action backed by policies and legislation and supported by civil society actions, there are many smaller cases and examples from which all actors can learn, and which can be the basis for moving forward.

The Final Report of Women and Gender Equity Knowledge Network (Sen et al. 2007) of the WHO Commission on Social Determinants of Health, identifies seven critical areas for action:

1. Addressing the essential structural dimensions of gender inequality
2. Challenging gender stereotypes, norms, and practices that directly harm women's and men's health

3. Reducing the health risks of being women and men by tackling gendered exposures and vulnerabilities
4. Transforming the gendered politics of health systems by improving their awareness and handling of women's problems as both producers and consumers of health care, improving women's access to health care, and making health systems more accountable to women
5. Taking action to improve the evidence base for policies by changing gender imbalances in both the content and the processes of health research bodies
6. Making organisations at all levels function more effectively to mainstream gender equality and equity, and empower women for health by creating supportive structures, incentives, and accountability mechanisms
7. Supporting women's organisations that are critical to ensuring that women have voice and agency, that are often at the forefront of identifying problems and experimenting with innovative solutions, and that prioritise demands for accountability from all actors, both public and private.

Note

1. More recently, emerging research in the gender and health equity field has called for a more systematic examination of how gender intersects with economic inequality, racial or ethnic hierarchy, caste domination, differences based on sexual orientation, and a number of other social markers in the social patterning of health (Iyer *et al.* 2008; Schulz and Mullings 2006). For example, studies confirm that socio-economic status measures cannot fully account for gender inequalities in health: both gender and class may affect the way in which risk factors are translated into health outcomes (Annandale and Hunt 2000). Other studies indicate that responses to unaffordable health care often vary by the gender and class location of sick individuals and their households (Iyer 2005). They strongly suggest that economic class should not be analysed by itself, and that apparent class differences can be misinterpreted without gender analysis.

References

Annandale, E. and Hunt, K. (2000) 'Gender inequalities in health: Research at the crossroads', in E. Annandale and K. Hunt (eds) *Gender Inequalities in Health*, Buckingham and Philadelphia, PA: Open University Press.

Barker, G. and Ricardo, C. (2005) *Young Men and the Construction of Masculinity in Sub-Saharan Africa*, Washington, DC: World Bank.

Barker, G., Ricardo, C., and Nascimento, M. (2007) *Engaging Men and Boys to Transform Gender-Based Health Inequities: Is There Evidence of Impact?* Geneva: The World Health Organisation and Instituto Promundo in collaboration with the MenEngage Alliance.

Commission on Social Determinants of Health (CSDH) (2008) *Closing the Gap in a Generation: Health Equity Through Action on the Social Determinants of Health* (Final Report), Geneva: World Health Organization.

Forrest, B.D. (1991) 'Women, HIV, and mucosal immunity', *The Lancet*, 337: 835–6.

Garcia-Moreno, C., Jansen, H., Ellsberg, M., Heise, L., and Watts, C.H. (2006) 'Prevalence of intimate partner violence: Findings from the WHO multi-country study on women's health and domestic violence', *The Lancet*, 368: 1260–69.

George, A. (2008) 'Nurses, community health workers, and home carers: gendered human resources compensating for skewed health systems', *Global Public Health*, Supplement 1, 3(2): 75–89.

Grown C., Rao Gupta, G., and Kes, A. (2005) *Taking Action: Achieving Gender Equality and Empowering Women. Report of the UN Millennium Project Taskforce on Education and Gender Equality*, London and Virginia: Earthscan.

Herz, B., and Sperling, D. (2004) *What Works in Girl's Education: Evidence and Policies from the Developing World*, New York: Council on Foreign Relations.

Hogan, M. C., Foreman, K.J., Naghavi, M., Ahn, S.Y., Wang, M., Makela, S.M., Lopez, A.D., Lozano, R., and Murray, C.J.L. (2010) 'Maternal mortality for 181 countries, 1980–2008: A systematic analysis of progress towards Millennium Development Goal 5', *The Lancet*, 375(9726): 1609–23.

ILO (International Labour Organization) (n.d.) *LABORSTA Internet Database*, available at http://laborsta. ilo.org (accessed March 2006), cited in UNICEF (2007) *The State of the World's Children 2007. Women and Children: The Double Dividend of Gender Equality*, New York: UNICEF.

Inter-Parliament Union (2008) *Women in Parliaments: World and Regional Averages*, available at http://www.ipu.org/wmn-e/world.htm (accessed 31 July 2008).

Iyer, A. (2005) *Gender, Caste, Class, and Health Care Access: Experiences of Rural Households in Koppal District, Karnataka*, Trivandrum: Achutha Menon Centre for Health Science Studies, Sree Chitra Tirunal Institute for Medical Sciences and Technology.

Iyer, A., Sen, G., and Östlin, P. (2008) 'The intersections of gender and class in health status and health care', *Global Public Health*, Supplement 1, 3(2): 13–24.

Keleher, H., and Franklin, L. (2008) 'Changing gendered norms about women and girls at the level of household and community: A review of the evidence', *Global Public Health*, Supplement 1, 3(2): 42–57.

Laurie, M., and Petchesky, R.P. (2008) 'Gender, health and human rights in sites of political exclusion', *Global Public Health*, Supplement 1, 3(2): 25–41.

Lewallen, S., and Courtright, P. (2002) 'Gender and use of cataract surgical services in developing countries', *Bulletin of the World Health Organization*, 80: 300–303.

Messing, K., and Östlin, P. (2006) *Gender Equality, Work and Health: A Review of the Evidence*, Geneva: World Health Organization.

Östlin, P., and Diderichsen, F. (2001) 'Equity-oriented national strategy for public health in Sweden: A case study', in A. Ritsatakis, *Policy Learning Curve Series*, Brussels: European Centre for Health Policy, World Health Organization.

Östlin, P., George A., and Sen, G. (2001) 'Gender, health, and equity: The intersections', in T. Evans, M. Whitehead, F. Diderichsen, A. Bhuiya, and M. Wirth (eds) *Challenging Inequities in Health: From Ethics to Action*, New York: Oxford University Press.

Östlin, P., Sen, G., and George, A. (2004) 'Paying attention to gender and poverty in health research: Content and process issues', *Bulletin of the World Health Organization* 82(10): 740–5.

Presser, H., and Sen, G. (2000) *Women's Empowerment and Demographic Processes: Moving Beyond Cairo*, New York: Oxford University Press/IUSSP.

Quisumbing, A.R., and Maluccio, J.A. (1999) 'Intrahousehold allocation and gender relations: New empirical evidence', The World Bank Development Research Group/Poverty Reduction and Economic Management Network, Policy Research Report on Gender and Development, Working Paper Series, No. 2, Washington, DC: World Bank.

Schulz, A.J., and Mullings, L. (eds) (2006) *Gender, Race, Class and Health: Intersectional Approaches*, San Francisco, CA: Jossey-Bass.

Sen, G., Östlin, P., and George, A. (2007) *Unequal, Unfair, Ineffective and Inefficient – Gender Inequity in Health: Why It Exists and How We Can Change It, Final report of the Women and Gender Equity Knowledge Network to the WHO Commission on Social Determinants of Health*, Bangalore and Stockholm: Indian Institute of Management Bangalore and Karolinska Institutet.

Smith, K.M., and Maeusezahl-Feuz, M. (2004) 'Indoor air pollution from household use of solid fuels', in M. Ezzati, A.D. Lopez, A. Rodgers, and C.J.L. Murray, *Comparative Quantification of Health Risks: The Global and Regional Burden of Disease Due to Selected Major Risk Factors*, Geneva: World Health Organization.

Snow, R. (2002) *Sex, Gender and Traffic Accidents: Addressing Male Risk Behavior*, Geneva: World Health Organization.

Snow, R. (2008) 'Sex, gender, and vulnerability', *Global Public Health*, Supplement 1, 3(2): 58–74.

UNAIDS (1999) *HIV/AIDS Prevention in the Context of New Therapies*, Geneva: UNAIDS.

UNAIDS (2006) *Report on the Global AIDS Epidemic 2006*, Geneva: UNAIDS.

UN (United Nations) (1993) *The Report of the UN World Human Rights Conference in Vienna*, Vienna: UN.

UN (United Nations) (1994) *Report of the United Nations International Conference on Population and Development (ICPD)*, Cairo, Egypt, 5–13 September 1994, New York: UN.

UN (United Nations) (1995) *Report of the Fourth World Conference on Women, United Nations World Conference on Women*, Beijing, China, 4–15 September 1995, New York: UN.

UN (United Nations) (2001) Report of the World Conference against Racism, Racial Discrimination, Xenophobia, and Related Intolerance, Durban, South Africa, 31 August–7 September 2001, New York: UN.

UNFPA (United Nations Population Fund) (2006) *State of World Population 2006. A Passage to Hope: Women and International Migration*, New York: United Nations Population Fund.

UNICEF (United Nations Children's Fund) (2006) *The State of the World's Children: Excluded and Invisible*, New York: UNICEF.

Uys, L. (2003) 'Guest editorial: Longer-term aid to combat AIDS', *Journal of Advanced Nursing*, 44: 1–2.

Wennerås, C. and Wold, A. (1997) 'Nepotism and sexism in peer-review', *Nature*, 387: 341–3.

WHO (World Health Organization) (2006) *The World Health Report 2006: Working Together for Better Health*, Geneva: WHO.

10

From Natural History of Disease to Vulnerability

Changing Concepts and Practices in Contemporary Public Health

José Ricardo Ayres, Vera Paiva, and Ivan França Jr.

A fundamental resource for public health intervention is its theory. Concepts are tools we use to respond to social needs, which demand that we possess knowledge to support our action. This knowledge is based on the material resources, the science and technologies available, as well as the political and ideological conditions, and ethical and moral values existing at a given place and time.

The aim of this chapter is to review three main conceptual frameworks that guide preventive actions in contemporary public health: (1) natural history of disease/levels of prevention, (2) health promotion, and (3) vulnerability.

Natural history of disease and levels of prevention

The concept of natural history of disease (NHD) evolved from a seminal concept in the development of modern epidemiology: the concept of *epidemic constitution*. Originally formulated by Hippocrates and rediscovered in the seventeenth century by the British physician Thomas Sydenham, the concept referred to a set of conditions which determined that some diseases would become more prevalent in certain places and times and that they would assume, under such circumstances, specific characteristics – becoming more or less intense, showing stronger or more attenuated signs and symptoms, etc. (Creighton 1894). The concept remained almost forgotten for approximately 200 years until it was recovered by epidemiologists at the Royal Society of Medicine, in London. These epidemiologists saw in the concept of epidemic constitution a comprehensive way to study, in modern scientific bases, the epidemic behaviour of diseases. They named this method 'the natural history of disease' (Hamer 1929).

The idea of epidemic constitution offered the possibility to relate the diseases' behaviour to the observations of diverse environmental conditions, based on exhaustive compilation, inter-relation, and systematic comparison of data referred to diverse places, times, seasons, geographical characteristics, population features, etc.

In spite of being controversial for its time (Goodall 1927), this concept was shown to be crucial for the development of epidemiology as a modern science, delimiting the specificity of its field of knowledge in contrast with other related disciplines, such as bacteriology and medical statistics (Amsterdanka 2005; Ayres 2005). Investigations on epidemic constitutions demonstrated that the study of infectious agents, focused on the bacteriological approach to epidemic phenomena since the 1870s, was not sufficient to explain the epidemic behaviour of diseases. They indicated the relevance of integrating several areas of science in order to produce knowledge about the occurrence and distribution of diseases. During the first decades of the twentieth century, the concept of epidemic constitution was largely criticised and modified until it was completely transformed into what is now referred to as 'the natural history of disease' (Gordon 1953).

In the United States, William Perkins (1938) defined NHD as the causal chain resulting from the interaction between environment, aggressor agents, and the human organism. Perkins defended and systematised the proposal that one should extend causal investigations to periods and spaces prior to the anatomical and physiological affliction, and that preventive action should be developed during the whole course of the disease, from its causal factors to the different moments of its clinical course and its consequences. Following such developments, Edwin Clark from Columbia University and Hugh Leavell from the Harvard School of Public Health proposed, in the 1950s, a model of NHD which became the definitive reference (Leavell and Clark 1958).

With the concept of NHD, Leavell and Clark postulated the overcoming of rigid distinctions between medicine and public health and between curative and preventive measures. They demonstrated that prevention should be present at every moment that there was a possibility that an intervention could prevent the disease or its consequences. An intervention, therefore, is composed of different *levels of prevention* (LP), ranging from the transformation of environmental and social conditions that influence the appearance of the disease to the reduction of worse effects of the disease in those that are already ill. To support this viewpoint, they adopted the thesis of the multiple causation of disease. According to this thesis, the intervention and the knowledge about the factors that determine the disease require an interdisciplinary framework construction, with the technologies of bio-medical and human sciences mediated by the epidemiological method and statistical analysis.

The NHD/LP model allows us to analytically distinguish two stages involved in the genesis and development of ailments: the pre-pathogenic period, during which the determinants that enhance the appearance of the disease occur, and the pathogenic period, which refers to the evolution of the disease as it runs its course. The pre-pathogenic period distinguishes the determinants related to the agent, the host, and the environment, and the pathogenic is subdivided into three stages: early pathogenesis, advanced disease, and outcome. During the diverse periods and stages, different prevention strategies may be considered, any of which may be initiated at any time during the evolution of the disease. These prevention strategies can be grouped in three phases and five levels of prevention (Figure 10.1).

Primary prevention aims to prevent the pathogenic processes from being initiated (pre-pathogenic period). It has two levels: (1) *health promotion*, which refers to actions taken to improve the living conditions of individuals, families, and communities, promote health and quality of life in general, and increase barriers to different pathogenic processes through health education, sanitation, and improved living and working conditions, etc.; and (2) *specific protection*, which refers to actions turned towards preventing specific diseases (e.g. vaccination).

Secondary prevention is employed during the pathogenic period, for example in situations where the health–disease process has already been established. It aims to achieve a favourable clinical evolution and the best attainable outcomes for the affected individuals. It also aims to interrupt or reduce the spread of the disease to other people. To achieve these goals, two other levels are defined: *early diagnosis and prompt treatment*, and *disability limitation*.

José Ricardo Ayres, Vera Paiva, and Ivan França Jr.

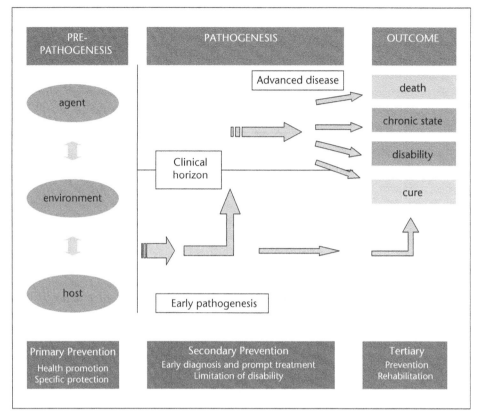

Figure 10.1   Diagram of the natural history of disease and corresponding levels of prevention
Source: Adapted from Leavell and Clark 1958.

Finally, *tertiary prevention* refers to the moment in which the health–disease process has reached a cure or progressed to a chronic state or irreversible defect or disability. The goal here is to minimise harm to the affected people and to protect their quality of life.

Health promotion

Since the 1970s, the term 'health promotion' has captured a powerful movement of ideas and actions for the renewal of health practices. It is related to Leavell and Clark's classic primary level of prevention, but introduces significant changes. This new version of health promotion expanded   the range of actions originally associated with the primary level and changed its conceptual basis and practical methods.

This 'new health promotion' (NHP) has its origin in the renowned 1974 Lalonde Report, which was issued by Canada's former minister of health. The report questioned the health care model of that country, which was expensive and had little effect on enhancing the population's health. It concluded that health actions were excessively centred in hospital practices and in the biological determinants of ailments, and required that greater attention be given to the role of environment and lifestyles in people's health (Lalonde 2009).

In 1978, the first Conference on Primary Health Care, summoned by the World Health Organization (WHO) and the United Nations Children's Fund (UNICEF), highlighted the importance of prevention and primary care practices, especially regarding the different levels of health promotion, which was emphasised in the conference's 'Declaration of Alma-Ata' (WHO/UNICEF 1978). The NHP proposals were then stimulated by the subsequent International Conferences on Health Promotion – Ottawa, 1986; Adelaide, 1988; Sundsvall, 1991; Jakarta, 1997; Mexico, 2000; and Bangkok, 2005. These conferences, which gathered technicians, managers, politicians, and activists, consolidated concepts and strategies oriented towards enhancing the health conditions of populations throughout the world, especially the poor.

The result of these conferences can be summarised in seven health-policy orientations (Sícoli and Nascimento 2007):

1. *Comprehensive approach.* The concept of health as the physical, mental, social, and spiritual well-being of individuals and the population as a whole needs to consider people's daily well-being, and not only their medical issues.
2. *Intersectorality.* To respond to health needs in their comprehensive conception, it is necessary to articulate different sectors of social activity, involving the action of legislation, education, housing, social services, health care, employment, nutrition, leisure, agriculture, transportation, and urban planning, among others.
3. *Empowerment.* It is necessary for individuals to have the power to transform diverse social situations that restrict or threaten their health, and address matters of civil and social rights, juridical support, psycho-social support, etc.
4. *Social participation.* By means of articulating empowerment, it is expected that collective discussion and action be a necessary ingredient in defining priorities in health promotion and the means by which to obtain it. This requires a democratic production and circulation of information, and the development of accessible channels of political participation.
5. *Equity.* Goals and methods to obtain good health are not universal, but require policies that recognise inequity in order to achieve justice in terms of distribution of resources for health.
6. *Multi-strategic actions.* It is assumed that knowledge and actions of different natures contribute to interfere in health–disease processes. For the NHP, the different disciplines involved in health promotion and the role of each are not pre-established. Rather, these depend on political processes that influence the choice of solutions to concrete health needs.
7. *Sustainability.* On one hand, this refers to the need that health promotion policies be synergic with the principle of sustainable economic development, for example a productive development which will not consume in a predatory way the natural and socio-cultural resources of the population. On the other hand, it points to the efforts to create long-lasting material resources and to build legitimate and manageable proposals that guarantee their continuity and effectiveness.

In short, health promotion is no longer seen as a moment of technical organisation of primary prevention actions, rather it is now seen as a political proposal which integrates all the phases and levels of prevention defined in the NHD/LP model. This reconstruction can be summarised as the search for an intensified dialogue between available diverse scientific and technical knowledge, on one hand, and the values of individuals and communities, on the other hand, in a way that progressively increases people's control over health–disease processes, the health care system, and the overall quality of their lives.

NHP still faces challenges to its consolidation. Polland (2007) analysed its successes and failures during the almost 20 years since the policy was adopted in Canada. Polland points to the successes of health promotion: the reduction in smoking; the decentralisation and regionalisation of health planning, with higher autonomy of district participation; a deeper concern for health promotion in hospitals; and the training of a significant number of health professionals in the field. Failures, on the other hand, include the increasing gap between the rich and the poor in terms of economic, social, and health indicators; the deterioration of housing conditions in the marginal social segments; the increase of juvenile diabetes and obesity in poor youngsters; and the progressive erosion of funds for social programmes. While reflecting on the reasons for such failures, Polland stresses the continued individualised focus of health care and the fact that health promotion strategies still centre on bio-medical knowledge and the personal behaviour change education model.

One may add to Polland's analysis the need to strengthen the interdisciplinary and intersectoral approach to technical propositions, as well as the active and autonomous participation based on the solidarity of individuals and communities in defining the aims and methods of health actions (Campos *et al.* 2004). It is in this direction that we face another innovation of the world's public health scenario at the end of the twentieth century: the development of the concept of *vulnerability*.

Vulnerability

The concept of *vulnerability* refers to a set of conditions that render individuals and communities more susceptible to disease or disability. Inextricably linked to this is the lack of resources that could protect these individuals and communities from disease and/or disability (Ayres *et al.* 2006; Mann and Tarantola 1996). While the notion of vulnerability is not exactly new, its conceptual emergence in the field of public health is relatively recent, as it is related to the construction of the responses to the HIV/AIDS epidemic, as described below.

The outbreak of AIDS in the 1980s and the panic surrounding it generated the search for explanations using epidemiological instruments to identify the causes of this unknown disease, that is, the search for identifying population subgroups in which there was a significantly higher chance of finding people with AIDS, rather than in the so-called 'general population'. Epidemiological studies were then fundamental tools for the aetiological elucidation of AIDS. From the point of view of prevention and health care, however, this approach proved to be limited and even damaging.

Risk, which was merely a probability measure in epidemiological studies, was translated by preventive practices into a concrete condition, a true social identity: the so-called *risk groups*. Thus, the 'sanitary isolation' of such groups frequently became the sole or main proposal for prevention. The supposed members of risk groups should abstain (or be prevented) from having sexual intercourse, donating blood, or injecting drugs. The media and public opinion extended this 'quarantine', of indefinite duration, to other aspects of social life – people identified as members of risk groups faced severe limitations as they could potentially lose their jobs, access to school, family life, and health services, etc.

In summary, risk analysis allowed epidemiology to quickly identify groups that would be more susceptible to the disease, but gave little information as to the meaning of such distribution of cases. As far as prevention was concerned, the language of 'high risk' groups increased stigma and discrimination, making the social and clinical situation of people affected by AIDS even more difficult, and leaving populations even more unprotected. The laboratory isolation of HIV in 1983 and the diagnostic test produced in 1985 opened new possibilities for health prevention and care. The identification of the pandemic characteristic of the disease was also fundamental in changing the scenario, as it showed several patterns in the distribution of cases in the population. In Africa, for example, there was a generalised epidemic affecting women, with predominantly heterosexual transmission. These developments contributed to a decreased use of the concept of 'risk groups'. It was, nevertheless, the intense reaction of the gay movement, especially in North America, that established new directions for prevention strategies, with the emphasis on condom use as a key asset in AIDS prevention policies.

Abstinence and isolation were progressively substituted for broader strategies of reducing risk and promoting safer practices, such as universal information dissemination, blood bank control, advancing the use of condoms and the practice of 'safer sex', testing, and counselling and harm reduction strategies for injecting drug users. Prevention strategies thus began to emphasise the concept of *risk behaviour*, whether in terms of actions or research. Field research moved towards a positive interaction between clinical and epidemiological investigation and the fields of human sciences.

The main advantage of the risk behaviour approach was the development of a universal commitment to active involvement in prevention and to increasing initiatives that mitigate the stigma associated with affected groups. Yet a negative aspect of the approach was its tendency to hold individuals exclusively responsible for changing their behaviour, which made people easily fall into situations of 'guilt': infected individuals were responsible for what happened to them, for supposedly not having 'adhered' to a safe behaviour, and for having 'failed' in prevention. Again, organised movements, such as women's movements and homosexual rights movements, criticised such behaviourist and individualised models, emphasising that a significant part of the prevention strategies, such as the use of condoms, did not depend solely on personal information and will, but were constructed by other social and inter-subjective conditions. How can we deal with the differences in social power and in the access to condoms? How can a woman carry a condom and propose its use in sexist societies in which she is expected to be chaste, ignorant about sex, and passive? Questions such as these challenged researchers, professionals, and activists. Seeking to understand the political and social bases of risk behaviour and the ethical–political implications of risk reduction policies, the fertile discussions on *vulnerability* emerged.

The concept of vulnerability is in line with several aspects of the NHP movement, since they both seek to understand and transform, through a socio-political perspective, the processes and determinants uncritically described in the NHD/LP classical model. The focus on vulnerability also promotes a significant rearrangement of the analytical moments in the latter model.

First, in the context of vulnerability, it is assumed that mutual interactions between agent, host, and environment are not limited to pre-pathogenesis, but they determine the health–disease process throughout the course of the disease, including its outcomes.

Secondly, the vulnerability approach assumes that health care and promotion are inextricable pieces in the analysis of the health–disease processes. In other words, the characteristics of these processes are directly determined by the set of knowledge, technology, and services which are already in force. The intervention – prevention, treatment, and rehabilitation – already constitutes a part of the determination of health–disease processes by virtue of its accessibility, technical organisation, moral orientation, etc. Health services are not merely a solution – they are also part of the problem to be considered. The health–disease processes are, therefore, always *health-disease-care* processes.

A third aspect to remember in the vulnerability perspective is that there is no aggressor agent per se. Any agent – biological, physical, or chemical – is only perceived as such when faced by the specificity of the physical, cognitive, affective, and behavioural characteristics of its host,

José Ricardo Ayres, Vera Paiva, and Ivan França Jr.

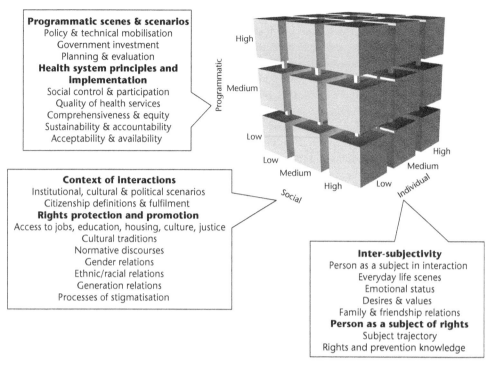

Figure 10.2 Vulnerability and human rights framework: individual, social, and programmatic dimensions
Source: Adapted from Paiva et al. 2010.

which in turn depend on the cultural and socio-political environment, as well as on the inter-subjective context in which people live and interact.

Finally, the vulnerability framework assumes that there is not a natural history of disease but a *social history of disease*. This is not only because the biological content of this history is at the same time social and historical, rather, this history is also 'told' in a social and historical way. As the response to AIDS has shown, there is not one single and necessary way to describe the determinants, distribution, and developments of a health-disease-care process. The history of a disease and of the interventions to it admit different evaluations, based on the perspective of whoever is describing them, what scientific and technological resources are available, and what knowledge can be used.

Vulnerability analyses involve three inextricable dimensions: individual, social, and programmatic. A starting point for an analysis of the *individual dimension* of vulnerability is the concept of the individual as (inter)subjectivity. When individuals experience or protect themselves from a certain ailment, aspects ranging from their physical constitution to their way of dealing with the changes in their daily routine will be involved. It is this experience of daily life which challenges the way we comprehend the different intensities and forms of vulnerability. Without ignoring the knowledge and importance of the biological aspects of disease, the focus of the individual dimension of vulnerability is the totality of psycho-social dynamics, expressed in the amount and quality of information that people make use of, the way they elaborate on this information, and their power to incorporate it in daily practice.

Unlike more traditional epidemiological and socio-cognitive approaches, the aspects considered here are not to be reduced to individual attributes, such as motives, attitudes, knowledge, and practices. In understanding the context of an individual's vulnerability, the individual has to be understood as *inter-subjectivity*, as an active participant in social constructions, neither a mere 'result' nor an independent creator of social relations.

In analysing the individual dimension of vulnerability, it is also understood that this dimension deals with the realm of the citizen-rights holder. The individual's psycho-social trajectory depends on inter-subjective contexts and power relations that can only be understood in terms of their local meanings and structural contexts – cultural, institutional, and legal contexts. In other words, people in their daily scenes continuously face conflicting discourses, values, and personal desires, constructed throughout the socialisation process, accessed through social networks, community and family relations, friendship, and professional worlds, and dependent as well on local definitions of rights protection and fulfilment.

As seen above, the analysis of the individual aspects of vulnerability calls for the evaluation of other processes which cannot be addressed exclusively at the individual dimension. Access to information, the meaning of such information in relation to people's values and experiences, the chances of using this information in practice, all remits to the social relations within which they occur and are shaped. The *social dimension* of the vulnerability analysis seeks specifically to focus such contextual aspects that are 'of the same substance' with individual vulnerabilities. In this dimension, the synergy of various aspects have to be taken into consideration, such as economic, gender, ethnic, racial, and generation relations, as well as religious beliefs, poverty, social exclusion, and others.

Do health services take into account that people's health needs are embedded in their diverse social contexts? How do health services enable people to identify the inter-subjective relations and contexts that increase their vulnerability to disease and disability? Do they provide ways by which individuals and communities can respond to contexts of vulnerability? These are the questions that the *programmatic dimension* of the vulnerability analysis seeks to answer. It is necessary to know how the policies and institutions, especially regarding health, education, social well-being, justice, and culture, act as elements that reduce, reproduce, or increase the vulnerability conditions of individuals and communities in their contexts.

Fundamental to the vulnerability approach, and involving its three analytic dimensions, is the *human rights* perspective (Gruskin and Tarantola 2002), covering civil and political, economic, social, and cultural aspects. The analysis of human rights violations or protections addresses social relations and programmatic conditions that increase or mitigate inequities in health-disease-care processes. In order to identify and overcome vulnerabilities, it is necessary to examine to what extent and in what ways the state regulates, respects, protects, and fulfils human rights, which represents the institutional mark of social relations and the horizon towards possible transformation. In employing a rights perspective, health care professionals will be in a more favourable position to positively identify socially disadvantageous situations and to find legitimate ways to overcome the same (Ayres *et al.* 2006; Paiva 2005; Paiva *et al.* 2007).

The diagram in Figure 10.2 synthesises key elements for identifying and understanding the vulnerability of individuals and social groups to disease and disability. The tridimensional layout highlights the inseparability of the three analytical dimensions of vulnerability discussed above and how in each concrete situation there are different ways and intensities that individual, social, and programmatic aspects may combine. The ever-changing and dynamic synergy of these dimensions must be considered to make prevention and health promotion more realistic, pragmatic, and ethically oriented. The knowledge required for action to cope with vulnerability situations in public health, on each analytical dimension, is also dependent on inputs from different scientific disciplines and on available practical knowledge, especially knowledge produced by people directly affected by the disease and disability.

Final considerations

It has become clear, at the end of our journey, how complex our knowledge needs to be in order to develop good public health practices. We have seen that health-disease-care are dynamic processes, involving biological and psychosocial, technical, and socio-political determinants which influence the conditions that enable the emergence of ailments, and their clinical evolution and outcomes, including the different means by which we respond to them.

The NHD/LP was the result of a series of conceptual efforts to systematise and articulate the scientific knowledge on the multiple dimensions involved in the health and disease, improving our capability to identify the disease determinants and strategic points by which to act on it preventively.

The NHP has reinforced the important idea that the task of public health is not only the prevention of disease but also the enhancement of the individual's quality of life, including both personal and social well-being. As such, the individuals and the community, in general, and policymakers and health care providers, in particular, must actively participate in identifying priorities for health and in constructing effective proposals to achieve these goals. The health care sector also needs to articulate its actions and knowledge to other sectors to promote the creation of a healthy society.

In conclusion, the concept of vulnerability points to the perspective of subjects and the contexts of inter-subjectivity as bases for identifying and transforming social relations that create both illness and the means to overcome it. It emphasises social policies and the technical and social organisation of health care practices as inextricable parts of the vulnerability analysis and actions, thus reinforcing human rights and citizenship as fundamental references.

As human *constructo*, deriving from ever-changing social experiences, all of the foregoing concepts need to be understood in their historicity, limitations, and range; a 'noble legacy', which, in the words of George Rosen (1958: 495), 'we must strive to enhance and hand on'. In this sense, it is crucial to critically examine their historical development and relation to concrete health practices, so that we may adequately use them, even transform them, to achieve more effective, equitable, and democratic public health.

References

Amsterdanka, O. (2005) 'Demarcating epidemiology', *Science Technology Human Values*, 30(1): 17–51.

Ayres, J.R.C.M. (2005) *Acerca del riesgo: para comprender la epidemiología*, Buenos Aires: Lugar.

Ayres, J.R.C.M., França Jr., I., Calazans, G.J., and Saletti Fo., H.C. (2006) 'El concepto de vulnerabilidad y las prácticas de salud', in D. Czeresnia and C.M. Freitas (eds) *Promoción de la salud: conceptos, reflexiones, tendencias*, Buenos Aires: Lugar, 135–62.

Ayres, J.R.C.M., Paiva, V., França Jr., I., Gravato, N., Lacerda, R., Della Negra, M., Marques, H.H.S., Galano, E., Lecussan, P., and Segurado, A.A.C. (2006) 'Vulnerability, human rights, and comprehensive care needs of young people living with HIV/AIDS', *American Journal of Public Health*, 96(6): 1001–6.

Campos, G.W., Barros, R.B., and Castro, A.M. (2004) 'Avaliação de política nacional de promoção da saúde', *Revista Ciência & Saúde Coletiva*, 9(3): 745–9.

Creighton, C. (1894) *A History of Epidemics in Britain*, vol. 2, London: Cambridge.

Goodall, E.W. (1927) 'The epidemic constitution', *Proceedings of the Royal Society of Medicine*, 21: 119–27

Gordon, J. E. (1953) 'Evolution of an epidemiology of health I–III', in I. Galdston (ed.) *The Epidemiology of Health*, New York: Health Education Council, 24–73.

Gruskin, S. and Tarantola, D. (2002) 'Health and human rights', in R. Detels, J. McEwen, R. Beaglehole, H. Tanaka (eds) *Oxford Textbook of Public Health*, New York: Oxford University Press, 311–14.

Hamer, W. H. (1929) *Epidemiology, Old and New*, New York: Macmillan.

Lalonde, M. (2009) 'A new perspective on the Health of Canadians: a working document', Ottawa: Government of Canada, available at www.hc-sc.gc.ca/hcs-sss/alt_formats/hpb-dgps/pdf/pubs/1974-la-londe/lalonde_e.pdf (accessed 24 September 2009).

Leavell, H. R. and Clark, E. G. (1958) *Textbook of Preventive Medicine*, New York: McGraw-Hill.

Mann, J. and Tarantola, D. J. M. (eds) (1996) *AIDS in the World II*, New York: Oxford University Press.

Paiva, V. (2005) 'Analysing sexual experiences through "scenes": a framework for the evaluation of sexuality education', *Sex Education*, 5(4): 345–59.

Paiva, V., Santos, N., França Jr., I., Filipe, E., Ayres, J.R., and Segurado, A.C. (2007) 'Desire to have children, gender and reproductive rights of men and women living with HIV: a challenge to health care in Brazil', *AIDS Patient Care STDs*, 21(4): 268–77.

Paiva, V., Ayres, J.R.C.M., and Gruskin, S. (2010) 'Being young and living with HIV: the double neglect of sexual citizenship', in P. Aggleton and R. Parker (eds) *The Routledge Handbook of Sexuality, Health and Rights*, New York: Routledge and Taylor and Francis: 422–30.

Perkins, W. H. (1938) *Cause and Prevention of Disease*, Philadelphia, PA: Lea and Febiger.

Polland, B. (2007) 'Health promotion in Canada: perspectives and future prospects', *Revista Brasileira em Promoção da Saúde*, 20(1): 3–11.

Rosen, G. (1958) *A History of Public Health*, New York: MD Publications.

Sícoli, J.L. and Nascimento, P.R. (2007) 'Promoção da saúde: concepções, princípios e operacionalização', *Interface*, 7(12): 101–22.

WHO (World Health Organization) and UNICEF (United Nations Children's Fund) (1978), *Primary Health Care: Report of the International Conference on PHC, Alma-Ata*, Geneva: WHO.

11

Attacking Inequality in Health
A Challenging but Winnable War

Abdo Yazbeck

This chapter reviews the growing body of literature on tackling inequality in the health sector,[1] with a specific focus on inequality in the use of health services, and on the evidence to date of successful policies addressing health inequalities in low- and middle-income countries (LMIC).

Data and assumptions

The development of an innovation in calculating proxy measures of wealth (Filmer and Pritchett 2001) resulted in a flood of data and research on health sector inequalities (Goldman *et al.* 2009; Gwatkins *et al.* 2007). While some of what the data revealed is not surprising, the consistent nature of inequalities across 56 LMIC (representing over 2.8 billion in population), and the size of the gap between the poorest and wealthiest in most countries, is sobering. This is exemplified in Figure 11.1, which captures the gaps in infant mortality rates (IMR) between the richest and poorest segments of the population across six regions. The data shows a consistent and sizable gap in IMR between the richest and poorest 20 per cent of the populations. Latin America and East Asia show the largest levels of inequality in IMRs, as measured by the concentration index, despite having, on average, lower levels of mortality than regions like Africa and South Asia.

Large gaps in health outcomes between the rich and poor are also found for other mortality-, morbidity-, and fertility-related outcomes (Gwatkin *et al.* 2007; Yazbeck 2009), reflecting the vulnerability of the poor due to factors like education levels, living and working conditions, and lack of access to resources. Given this vulnerability, we would expect health services to be targeted at the neediest and poorest populations within a country. In fact, many countries and international agencies implicitly assume that spending on health services is mainly justified by the health-related needs of the poor. The assumed redistributive effect (the transfer of resources from the better-off to the poor) of public spending on health is an often-cited justification in policy documents. What the data on public spending actually showed, however, was the exact opposite. Publicly financed or delivered health services are far from pro-poor. Naïve assumptions like 'spending on health is spending on the poor' and 'universal programmes in low- and middle-income settings serve the poor' have been proven completely wrong by the

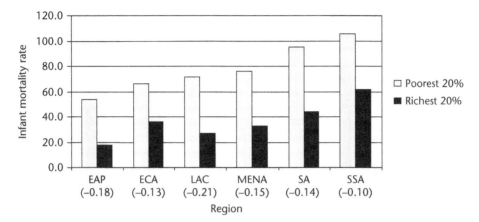

Figure 11.1 Infant mortality gaps in LMIC

Notes: EAP: East Asia and the Pacific; ECA: Europe and Central Asia; LAC: Latin America and the Caribbean; MENA: Middle East and North Africa; SA: South Asia; SSA: sub-Saharan Africa. The concentration index, which measures inequality, for each region is listed in parentheses.
Source: Yazbeck 2009.

overwhelming wave of data on inequality in health services use. To this effect, the data on basic services (Figures 11.2a and 11.2b) is unambiguous and alarming. Even when publicly funded or delivered, health services in the majority of LMIC are not pro-poor.

As Figure 11.2a shows, even the most basic of health services, like immunisation and deliveries attended by training professionals, appears to favour the rich over the poor. Figure 11.2b presents the same information as odds ratios, which allow comparisons across services. What stands out in addition to the consistent pro-rich picture is that health services seem to especially fail poor women, since the most lopsided distribution is for attended deliveries and use of contraception by women.

A complex and contextual problem

The available evidence from the increasing volume of literature on inequality in health service utilisation points to two general themes that are critical to understanding the underlying causes of the problem, and for fashioning successful policy responses. The first theme is the complex and persistent nature of the problem, reflecting a situation with multiple and interactive determinants of inequality. An example of such multiple causes is looking at possible supply-side constraints faced by the poor, like lack of geographic access to services, that can be made worse by demand-side constraints, like limited knowledge of, and demand for, preventive services due to low levels of education and access to basic information. Simplistic policy responses to such complex scenarios are likely to fail.

A second critical general theme relates to the fact that poverty, and the resulting inequality in use of services, is highly contextual. The dominant causes of inequality in service use tend to be different between LMIC, across different countries of the same development level, and even across different parts of large countries. If the driving causes of inequality are different from place to place, then policy responses will probably need to be different in order to best address the underlying causes.

Since the data tells us that the problem of inequality in health service utilisation is both complex and contextual, policy responses need to reflect an understanding of the main

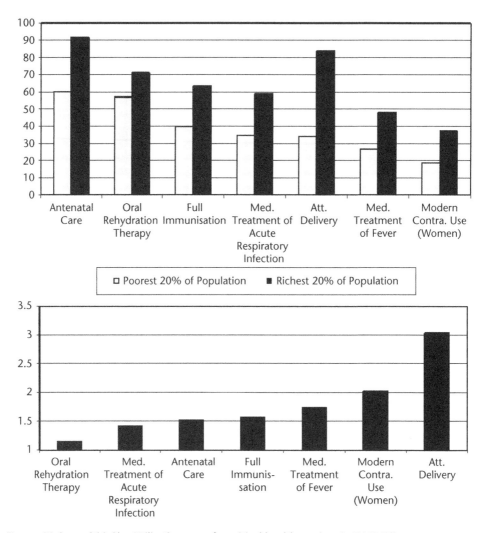

Figures 11.2a and 11.2b Utilisation gaps for critical health services in 56 LMIC
Source: Gwatkin *et al.* 2005; Yazbeck 2009.

constraints faced by the poor. Such constraints could be the result of geographic barriers, financial barriers, cultural factors, a lack of information, a lack of support, or a combination of a number of these and other factors. The best way to capture this understanding for different population groups in different countries is to actually listen to the poor before formulating policy answers. Moreover, it is important to keep listening after the policies have been implemented, to ensure that the expected results are being achieved. Integrating the poor into the policy process at all stages is not easy or without cost, but evidence now exists, such as the cases summarised in this chapter, that it can be done in a variety of ways that strengthen the process and increase the likelihood of successful outcomes.

A recently published book on the topic of inequality in health (Yazbeck 2009) includes a menu of diagnostic tools that have been used in a number of countries to answer the difficult question of the main causes of inequality in the use of health services in any context. Chapter 3,

'The Importance of Listening', lays out the different tools, and the analytical questions the tools can be used to answer. One way to think of the menu of tools is to categorise them as qualitative and quantitative, or active and passive. There are clear trade-offs in the decision to use an active versus a passive listening tool. One trade-off relates to the extent to which we can get answers that are representative of the population but superficial (with quantitative or active tools), versus getting sufficiently deep answers that only facture the views of small group (with qualitative or passive tools).

We can get representative, or statistically significant, answers if we use *quantitative* survey methods that ask the same questions of a representative sample of people from our target population. For such surveys to work, however, the same and limited number of questions needs to be asked in the same way to all respondents. Such approaches limit active interactions and can give us a representative picture that may be superficial in nature. The alternative approach, *qualitative* data collection, requires more active listening through focus group discussions or informant interviews using more flexible instruments. The downside of active listening is that a much smaller number of respondents are heard from, and the richness of the conversations usually means that the questions are not identical. Both factors, limited number and different lines of questioning, make it very hard to draw representative or statistically significant answers for the whole population. The gold standard, subject to available resources and time, is combining active and passive listening in order to get representative answers with appropriate depth.

A menu of proven pro-poor health-sector policies

The increase in evidence of inequalities in the health sector has renewed interest in identifying, documenting, and learning from successes in tackling the problem. The Reaching the Poor Program[2] (RPP) was initiated in 2001 to respond to the need for evidence-based policies for attacking inequality in the use of health services. Through a series of evaluations, conferences, and publications, RPP assembled a number of programmes that successfully and positively impacted inequality. The remainder of this chapter summarises briefly the pro-poor policy menu that emerged from RPP, including a generic list of process actions that have proved to be effective in successful programmes. The recurring themes from successful programmes include the following.

Analysing the causes of inequality

Consistent with the main message of the last section, listening to the poor – through passive or active tools – allows policy design to tackle the most pressing constraints faced by the poor.

Customising answers to address local constraints and capacities

The contextual nature of poverty refers not only to the different types of constraints faced by different populations, but also to the different capacity of local or national authorities to implement policy solutions. Successful programmes adapt answers to local capacity to implement.

Trying out new ways of doing business

Successful programmes often include innovations in how services are delivered and financed in order to address long-term problems and constraints. Trying out new ways of doing business while monitoring results and constraints is a proven approach for tackling inequalities.

Improving the results over time by learning from pilots and experimentation

Many of the successful programmes require mid-course adjustments as new policies are implemented.

Verifying that the use of services by the poor is improving, and bottlenecks are being eliminated

Almost all the successful programmes include a strong monitoring programme that tracks service utilisation, and also the extent to which the programmes eliminate bottlenecks.

Beyond the process, however, there are six rules of thumb that appear to be effective in making services more pro-poor (described below). Each of the six rules of thumb relate to one of the six reform levers in the health sector,[3] the latter of which include: Revenue Generation, Resource Allocation, Provider Payment Mechanisms, Organisation of Service Delivery, Regulation of Services, and Behaviour Change/Persuasion.

The six rules of thumb as related to the six reform levers are as follows:

Revenue generation: delink payment by the poor from use of services

An important deterrent to service utilisation by the poor is the financial barrier faced when seeking care at facilities. A number of successful programmes have tackled this barrier in two different ways. One approach is to provide poor households with health insurance coverage, and the second is to protect the poor from high fees through well-designed exemptions. In the case of Colombia's 1993 health sector reform programme and Mexico's Seguro Popular programme, policymakers extended health insurance to poor populations by heavily subsidising the premiums (Ecsobar 2005; Frenk *et al.* 2006). Both programmes resulted in well-targeted subsidies for insurance programmes, leading to increases in the utilisation of health services by the poor. Another type of extension of health insurance to the poor took place in Rwanda in the form of community-based voluntary health insurance. The latter increased coverage of the poor, and consequently the utilisation of health services (Diop and Butera 2005).

User fees or cost recovery at health facilities have been found to deter health service utilisation by poor households. Therefore, systems that exempt the poor from paying for care, while simultaneously compensating facilities for serving the poor, can help to mitigate this problem. Two evaluated programmes were shown to successfully increase utilisation of health services by the poor, by the programmes providing fee exemptions and alternative sources of financing for the health facilities. One, the Cambodia Health Equity Fund, financed by a donor agency, used non-governmental organisations (NGOs) to identify the poor who were seeking hospital care, exempt them from paying hospital fees, and provide payments to reimburse hospitals for the services provided to the poor (Noirhomme *et al.* 2007). The second, the health card programme in Indonesia, was developed to help cushion the impact of the financial crisis in 1998. The programme provided exemptions to card holders seeking care at public facilities, while also providing additional resources to facilities to compensate for the loss of revenue from the exemptions (Saadah *et al.* 2001).

Resource allocation: make the money follow the poor

Resource allocation in the health sector, especially in LMIC, tends to be strongly linked to fixed facilities such as hospitals. However, hospitals have repeatedly been found to serve the rich more than the poor, in part due to their locations, which are typically in urban areas or in areas where the better-off live. To help change the resource allocation inequality, a number of approaches have been evaluated and found to be successful. One approach aims to improve geographic targeting of investments in health programmes by implementing a phased national plan that focuses investments on the localities where the poor live. The Brazil Family Health Programme reorganised and strengthened primary health care throughout the country, and did so by first targeting the locations where the poor live (Barros *et al.* 2005). The programme included other pro-poor elements, which will be addressed later in this chapter.

A radically different approach to resource allocation is to have resources follow the poor and be conditioned according to the poor's demand for health care. Two examples of what are called conditional cash transfers (CCTs) were extensively evaluated and found to disproportionately benefit the poor. The best-known example of health CCTs is the Mexico Progresa/Oportunidades programme, which provided monthly payments to poor families if children and pregnant women received preventive care (Coady *et al.* 2005). CCTs are also an important part of Chile's Solidario programme, where poor families received financial support if progress was made in implementing an agreed-upon family health plan (Government of Chile 2004; Galasso 2006; Palma and Urzua 2005).

Provider payment mechanisms: link provider payment to utilisation by the poor

An important dimension of health financing reform relates to how providers are paid, and the incentives that the different payment mechanisms create. A repeated theme in the literature on inequality is the perception of bad treatment of the poor by health providers. A typical explanation given is that facilities and providers have limited financial incentives to provide quality treatment to the poor since the poor often cannot pay. Successful pro-poor reforms seek to reverse these negative incentives by linking provider payment to the utilisation of their health services by the poor. The three successful examples of provider payment reforms that have been evaluated structured incentives at very different levels of decision-making. The Brazil Family Health Programme described earlier included an incentive structure that provided financial incentives to municipalities that increased utilisation by the poor.

In Cambodia, two different programmes successfully used incentives in how providers are paid in order to change utilisation of health services in favour of the poor. The Cambodia NGO contracting project, financed by an Asia Development Bank loan, included explicit language in the contract about serving the poorest 50 per cent of the population, and structured independent evaluations to ensure that the contractors were effective in increasing utilisation of critical services by the poor (Schwartz and Bhushan 2005). The project piloted two forms of contracting, management-only and full-control, and both performed much better in increasing utilisation by the poor than control areas with no contracting. The second Cambodian project described earlier (the Health Equity Fund) created an environment where hospitals were guaranteed payment if they served the poor. This made the poor financially attractive and a sought-after population.

Organisational reforms: close the distance between the poor and services

Whether poor households seek care in facilities is strongly influenced by what is offered and how services are organised. Moreover, the role the community plays in the organisation and delivery of health services can have a positive impact on utilisation rates. One of the most frequently utilised technical interventions in programmes that have successfully decreased inequality is the definition of a new benefits package that takes into account the needs of poor households. This took place in the Brazil Family Health Programme, the Cambodia NGO contracting project, the Colombia and Mexico expansion of health insurance reforms, the Nepal Adolescent Reproductive Health project (described later), and the Rwanda Community Based Health Insurance programme.

Another important determinant of demand by the poor is the social distance between the poorest among the population and those providing services. An example of a successful programme that brings service provision closer to the poor, both physically and socially, is the Self-Employed Women's Association (SEWA) health programme in the Indian state of Gujarat (Ranson *et al.* 2005). SEWA is a trade union that includes a programme to deliver critical health services through mobile clinics and by using the trust of the community. Another example of strong community ownership that closes the social distance between providers and the poor is the Rwanda Community Based Health Insurance programme partially described earlier. A critical element that ensures the success of the Rwanda programme is the degree of trust the community has in the scheme, which is built through strong community ownership and management of the funds and facilities delivering care.

Regulation reforms: amplify the voice of the poor

Poor households suffer not only from a lack of market power, but also from limited political representation or voice. Programme reform efforts that strengthen the voice of the poor in health systems have been found to successfully decrease inequality in the use of health services. How voice is amplified can take a number of different forms. In the Nepal Adolescent Reproductive Health project, poor adolescents played a critical role in planning the health programme, which led to a large decrease in inequality of access (Malhotra *et al.* 2005). A different form of voice is that of community oversight of a programme, as was used in the Rwanda Community Based Health Insurance programme.

Another way that voice can be amplified is to directly listen to the poor, to better understand their needs and preferences. One such example is the successful social marketing approach employed in Tanzania to ensure the poor have access to and use impregnated bed nets to prevent malaria (Hanson *et al.* 2003). Successful social marketing invested in research to understand what would make the poor demand the service. The Chile Solidario programme described earlier takes an even more direct approach to listening to the poor by developing household-specific programmes that reflect household needs and preferences. Finally, another successful approach that includes community participation is the use of community mobilisation in health-related campaigns, as was the case in the immunisation campaigns for measles in Kenya (Vijayaraghavan *et al.* 2002).

Persuasion/behaviour change: close the gap between need and demand by the poor

The evidence on the causes of inequalities in utilisation points to a lower demand for care by poor households. The gap between what the poor need and demand is driven by factors that can range from lack of knowledge to cultural influences. Increasing utilisation by the poor, therefore, requires an understanding of the dominant causes for the low demand in the targeted population, programmes to decrease the need–demand gap. Successful programmes have used a variety of means including information, persuasion, and incentives to increase demand by the poor. Examples include the conditional cash transfers in Chile and Mexico, which create incentives for poor families to seek preventive care. Information and education can also play a role in increasing demand, as was the case through outreach for health education in the successful programmes in Brazil, Cambodia, Chile, and Kenya. Finally, a social marketing programme in Tanzania also included successful marketing of (or making more attractive) an important preventive service.

Hope and hard work

In an ocean of inequality, there are islands of hope. But the lessons of hope point to an end to arrogance about ideological or elegant solutions that are not built on a foundation of empiricism. The evidence assembled from evaluated, successful programmes guides efforts for attacking inequality that are based on the hard work of documenting the problem, analysing its causes, and learning from the successes of others by selecting the relevant policy tools that match local needs and capacity. The overwhelming evidence on inequality cannot be ignored and should warn us that attacking inequality will be hard work. However, proven analytical and policy tools do now exist and can be used to effectively change the conditions for the poor and vulnerable.

Notes

1 For more in-depth reading on this topic the following books are recommended: Gwatkin *et al.* 2005 and Yazbeck 2009.
2 The Reaching the Poor Program was financed by the World Bank, the Bill & Melinda Gates Foundation, and the governments of the Netherlands and Sweden.
3 Roberts *et al.* (2004) describe five policy levers in the health sector. Yazbeck (2009) extended the first lever, financing of care, by dividing it into two levers, revenue generation and resource allocation.

References

Barros, A.J.D., Victora, C.G., Cesar, J.A., Neumann, N.A., and Bertoldi, A.D. (2005) 'Brazil: Are Health and Nutrition Programs Reaching the Neediest?', in R. Gwatkin, A. Wagstaff, and A. Yazbeck (eds) *Reaching the Poor with Health, Nutrition, and Population Services: What Works, What Doesn't, and Why*, Washington, DC: World Bank: 281–306.

Coady, D.P., Filmer, D.P., and Gwatkin, D.R. (2005) 'PROGRESA for Progress: Mexico's Health, Nutrition, and Education Program', *Development Outreach*, 7(2): 10–12.

Diop, F.P. and Butera, J.D. (2005) 'Community-Based Health Insurance in Rwanda', *Development Outreach*, 7(2): 19–22.

Escobar, M.L. (2005) 'Health Sector Reform in Colombia', *Development Outreach*, 7(2): 6–9.

Filmer, D. and Pritchett, L.H. (2001) 'Estimating Wealth Effects without Expenditure Data – or Tears: An Application to Educational Enrollments in States of India', *Demography*, 38(1): 115–32.

Frenk, J., González-Pier, E., Gómez-Dantés, O., Lezana, M., and Knaul, F. (2006) 'Comprehensive Reform to Improve Health System Performance in Mexico', *The Lancet*, 368(9,546): 1,524–34.

Galasso, E. (2006) *With Their Effort and One Opportunity: Eliminating Extreme Poverty in Chile*, Washington, DC: World Bank.

Goldman, A., Azcona, G., Crawford, R., and Yazbeck, A. (2009) 'Health Inequalities in Developing Countries: An Annotated Bibliography', World Bank Institute (working paper).

Government of Chile (2004) 'An Introduction to Chile Solidario and El Programa Puente' prepared for the World Bank International Conference on Local Development, Washington, DC, 16–19 June, available at http://www1.worldbank.org/sp/LDConference/Materials/Parallel/PS2/PS2_S13_bm1.pdf (accessed 27 February 2008).

Gwatkin, D., Rutstein, S., Johnson, K., Suliman, E., Wagstaff, A., and Amouzou, A. (2007) *Socio-Economic Differences in Health, Nutrition, and Population*, Washington, DC: World Bank.

Gwatkin, R., Wagstaff, A., and Yazbeck, A. (eds) (2005) *Reaching the Poor with Health, Nutrition, and Population Services: What Works, What Doesn't, and Why*, Washington, DC: World Bank.

Hanson, K., Kikumbih, N., Armstrong Schellenberg, J., Mponda, H., Nathan, R., Lake, S., Mills, A., Tanner, M., and Lengeler, C. (2003) 'Cost-Effectiveness of Social Marketing of Insecticide-Treated Nets for Malaria Control in the United Republic of Tanzania', *Bulletin of the World Health Organization*, 81(4): 269–76.

Malhotra, A., Mathur, S., Pande, R., and Roca, E. (2005) 'Do Participatory Programs Work? Improving Reproductive Health for Disadvantaged Youth in Nepal', *Development Outreach*, 7(2): 32–5.

Noirhomme, M., Meessen, B., Griffiths, F., Jacobs, P. Ir, B., Thor, R., Criel, B., and Van Damme, W. (2007) 'Improving Access to Hospital Care for the Poor: Comparative Analysis of Four Health Equity Funds in Cambodia', *Health Policy and Planning*, 22(4): 246–62.

Palma, J., and Urzúa, R. (2005) *Anti-Poverty Policies and Citizenry: The Chile 'Solidario' Experience*, Management of Social Transitions Policy Paper No. 12, Paris: UNESCO.

Ranson, M.K., Joshi, P., Shah, M., and Shaikh, Y. (2005) 'India: Assessing the Reach of Three SEWA Health Services among the Poor', in R. Gwatkin, A. Wagstaff, and A. Yazbeck (eds) *Reaching the Poor with Health, Nutrition, and Population Services: What Works, What Doesn't, and Why*, Washington, DC: World Bank: 163–88.

Roberts, M., Hsiao, W., Berman, P., and Reich, M. (2004) *Getting Reform Right: A Guide to Improving Performance and Equity*, New York: Oxford University Press.

Saadah, F., Pradhan, M., and Sparrow, R. (2001) 'The Effectiveness of the Health Card as an Instrument to Ensure Access to Medical Care for the Poor during the Crisis', prepared for the Third Annual Conference of the Global Development Network, Rio de Janeiro, Brazil, 9–12 December.

Schwartz, J. and Bhushan, I. (2005) 'Cambodia: Using Contracting to Reduce Inequity in Primary Health Care Delivery', in R. Gwatkin, A. Wagstaff, and A. Yazbeck (eds) *Reaching the Poor with Health, Nutrition, and Population Services: What Works, What Doesn't, and Why*, Washington, DC: World Bank: 137–62.

Vijayaraghavan, M., Martin, R., Sangrujee, N., Kimani, G., Oyombe, S., Kalu, A., Runyago, A., Wanjau, G., Cairns, L., and Muchiri, S. (2002) 'Measles Supplemental Immunization Activities Improve Measles Vaccine Coverage and Equity: Evidence from Kenya', *Health Policy*, 83(1): 27–36.

Yazbeck, A. (2009) *Attacking Inequality in the Health Sector: A Synthesis of Evidence and Tools*, Washington, DC: World Bank.

12

Pathways to Health Systems Strengthening for the Bottom Billion

Andrew Ellner, Gene Bukhman, and Paul Farmer

At 4.53 p.m. on 12 January 2010, an earthquake measuring 7.0 on the Richter scale struck 16 miles from the centre of Port-au-Prince, Haiti. The quake's shocks devastated the capital's vulnerable infrastructure, crumbling buildings as grand as the President's Palace and National Assembly, as well as countless humble homes. As of April 2010, the disaster had claimed the lives of more than 220,000 Haitians through crush injury, starvation, and the lack of basic medical care for communicable and non-communicable disease, and had profoundly and irrevocably impacted the lives of millions more through displacement and both physical and mental trauma (Government of Haiti 2010).

If Haiti's earthquake exacted an unprecedented toll on a nation's people and infrastructure, the global response to the quake has also exceeded most previous humanitarian efforts. Almost instantaneously, CNN and other major media outlets broadcasted the disaster's worst images worldwide, making the present and profound human suffering nearly unavoidable for anyone with access to a television. Within 48 hours, the first planeload of trauma surgeons, nurses, and medical supplies departed from Boston hospitals to staff operating rooms and other medical facilities both in and outside Port-au-Prince. These much-needed specialists saved many lives, but came to realise, as so many had before them, that for Haitians to enjoy improved health care it would be necessary to strengthen, rebuild, or build stronger health systems – a task complicated by the loss of the country's chief training institutions (see Figure 12.1). To build back better requires not only stronger and safer facilities, but also significant investment in human capital. At an international donor conference on 31 March 2010, the global community pledged over $5 billion towards reconstruction and recovery efforts in Haiti during the following 18 months (Charles 2010).

While certainly welcome, such an outpouring of global goodwill in response to a specific disaster is in some ways dissonant with the reality that thousands of humans die unaided and unpublicised every day from starvation and preventable, treatable disease. Haiti's trauma, devastating in its own right, is also a metaphor for the daily injustice visited on the world's poorest billion citizens, who have been left vulnerable by historical legacy, unprotected by adequate social safety nets, destabilised by unpredictable environmental shocks, and who, ultimately, far too often meet an untimely demise that extends poverty's legacy and its accompanying instability

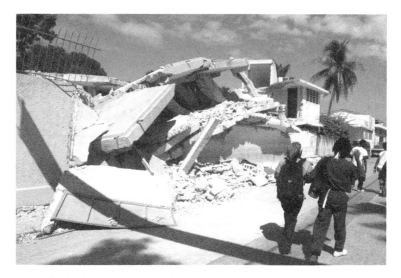

Figure 12.1 Haiti's chief public nursing school destroyed, 12 January 2010
Source: Courtesy of Andrew Marx; © Partners In Health, 2010.

and despair to another generation (Farmer 2010a, 2010b). And, although the world's initial response to Haiti is in many ways admirable, it has also been largely reactive and inadequate.

One can, nonetheless, hope, and we will argue that the disaster presents an opportunity for continued progress towards a new paradigm in global health – one that is proactive and strategic, and that affords a greater degree of stability, prosperity, and justice for all of us. Far from being a charitable response to crisis, we must begin to see global health as a critical set of activities which not only promote global security, but which also, by bringing together creative minds from across the world, enable us to redesign the delivery of life-saving technologies and health interventions to improve the performance of health systems in low- and high-income countries alike.[1]

Recent themes in global health

The Haiti earthquake struck at an inflection point in the trajectory of the global response to the health needs of the poor. For centuries, wealthier nations have concerned themselves with the conditions of nations 'less developed' than themselves. What began as unabashed conquest and exploitation gave way to slightly more benign colonial occupation, and has evolved over the last half-century into a more organised international response to alleviating suffering and promoting health and well-being. The creation of the World Health Organization (WHO) in 1948 as one of the original United Nations institutions was surely a milestone in this process, as were the Alma-Ata Declaration of 1978 and the launch of the Global Fund to Fight AIDS, Tuberculosis and Malaria ('The Global Fund') in 2002 (Behrman 2004; Cueto 2004; Siddiqi 1995). Crucial changes in global epidemiology (for instance, the emergence of HIV/AIDS and resurgence of tuberculosis (TB) and malaria in the 1980s and 1990s) provide key contexts to this evolution (Behrman 2004).

Over the last half-century, two major dialectics have emerged in global health. The first is between the 'horizontal' approach, which connotes a broad-based attempt to strengthen countries' capacities to deliver services to comprehensively meet their populations' primary health needs, and the 'vertical' approach, whereby the global community and/or individual countries selectively target specific diseases for eradication or control. The successful WHO-led smallpox eradication campaign, launched in 1967 and consummated in 1977, stands out as a paradigmatic example of the latter (Brilliant 1985). In contradistinction, the approach outlined in the Alma-Ata Declaration to guarantee 'Health for All' by 2000, through universal access to primary health care, is a quintessential example of the horizontal approach (WHO 1978). More recently, the WHO's 2008 World Health Report, *Primary Health Care: Now More than Ever*, appears to represent an attempted return to Alma-Ata principles.

Alma-Ata also defines one pole of the other major dialectic, which is between responses that emphasise collective, global responsibility for guaranteeing basic health care to all as a universal human right (and the implied responsibility of wealthier nations to provide for poorer ones) and responses that emphasise individual nations' responsibility for the welfare of their own citizens.[2] The 'structural adjustment' policies promulgated by the World Bank and the International Monetary Fund during the late 1980s and 1990s are a defining example of the latter approach (Kim *et al.* 2000; Ruger 2005).

Accompanying the pendulum swings between these poles are several interrelated constants and trends. The first constant is the reality of profound resource scarcity for the majority of the world's nations and people – and a daily struggle for survival for the 'bottom billion'. The second is that nations always act in their own perceived self-interest – even if, among the more enlightened ones (such as Norway), this involves strategic investments in promoting

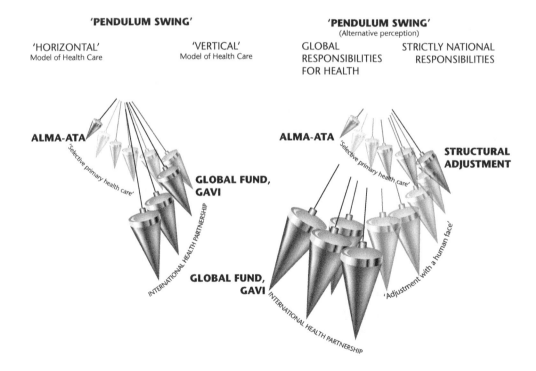

Figure 12.2 Pendulum swing
Source: 'Dual Pendulum Swings of Global Health' by Gorik Ooms and Jean-Pierre Wenseleers, courtesy of the Institute of Tropical Medicine.

development in the poorest countries, in order to promote long-term global stability (Homme 2009). China takes a different approach, investing in massive physical infrastructure improvements in Africa, which serves the dual purpose of helping African nations and of establishing Chinese access to the natural energy resources that will provide its lifeblood for the next century (French 2010; Webb and Mathiason 2008). For the United States, aid to developing countries is increasingly characterised as a means to prevent the establishment of breeding grounds for terrorists, and a tactic of the military doctrine of 'counter-insurgency'.[3]

A key trend is that, while conditions for the world's poorest citizens have remained relatively stagnant over the last half-century, there has been significant global economic growth, so that the gap between the world's very wealthiest and very poorest people continues to widen (UNDP 2003: Box 2.2). An interrelated global trend is towards increasing scientific and technological sophistication, which in the health sector manifests as continued progress in our capacity to characterise, prevent, diagnose, and treat disease – a trend that has revolutionised our ability to care for individuals with specific diseases (including HIV), but strained our ability to equitably and efficiently provide for the health of populations (as best evidenced by the current challenges confronting the US health care system). The final important trend – referred to most commonly as 'globalisation' – involves the ever-increasing interconnectedness of the world's citizens via technologies for communication and travel.

For global health, the confluence of these trends – and particularly the attempt to leverage rich-world technologies to address health needs in areas of scarcity – has necessitated approaches prioritising the technological interventions developed to address different diseases. Cost-effectiveness analysis (CEA), typified by the 1993 World Bank Report, *Investing in Health*, is a major development in priority-setting: the report's authors used novel (at the time) econometric analyses to estimate the global burden of different diseases, in terms of the cumulative toll they take on the length and quality of human life, and quantitatively compared the cost-effectiveness of various interventions at alleviating this burden. While a potentially useful tool in the panoply of implements in the policymaking shed, CEA has at times been used in an overly deterministic way that under-appreciates its methodological limitations as well as the possibility of major changes in the policy environment and interrelated fluctuations in the price of technologies.[4]

The relatively recent construct of the 'health system' provides another useful analytic tool for thinking about organised global and national health responses. Murray and Frenk (2000) have defined the health system to include 'the resources, actors and institutions related to the financing, regulation and provision of 'health actions', where 'health actions' are 'any set of activities whose primary intent is to improve or maintain health'. In its most recent iteration, the WHO (2006) identified the health system's building blocks as Service Delivery, Leadership/Governance, Financing, Health Workforce, Information, and Medical Products, Vaccines, and Technologies; WHO has designated 'improved health (outcomes and equity)', 'social and financial risk protection', 'responsiveness', and 'improved efficiencies' as the desired outcomes of the health system.

An NGO's experience

The experiences of Partners In Health (PIH) over the last three decades illustrate many of these themes in global health. A Boston-based non-governmental organisation (NGO), PIH's mission is to provide a preferential option for the poor. The organisation's genesis was in rural Haiti in the early 1980s, where (co-author) Paul Farmer lived as a medical and anthropology student. Haiti at the time was still in the grips of the Duvalier family's brutal, dynastic dictatorship and was hobbled by centuries of deleterious foreign intervention by the United States and other nations. Haiti's health system governance and financing (and all the other health system

THE WHO HEALTH SYSTEM FRAMEWORK

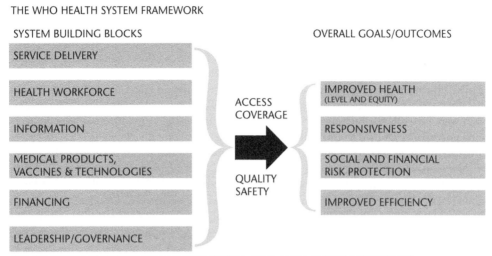

Figure 12.3   The WHO health system framework

Source: Reprinted from WHO, *Everybody's Business: Strengthening Health Systems to Improve Health Outcomes: WHO's Framework for Action*, section 2, p. 3, copyright 2007, with permission.

building blocks) were poor to non-existent, and Haitians in rural areas were suffering from, and dying of, easily preventable and treatable diseases. Struck by the dissonance between this reality and his experiences as a student doctor in Boston hospitals, Farmer, along with Ophelia Dahl and fellow student Jim Kim, co-founded PIH to partner with Haitians to establish meaningful access to health care in Haiti's Central Plateau.

Financed for its first decade almost exclusively by private philanthropy, PIH has tended to set priorities based on the manifested and expressed needs of local communities – what might be considered a 'bottom-up' as opposed to a 'top-down' approach to health planning (Farmer and Gastineau-Campos 2010). Indeed, the NGO's initial design was largely determined by a community needs assessment conducted by Farmer and Dahl in partnership with Haitian colleagues. In solidarity with rural Haitians, and out of a shared belief in the universal right to health, PIH employees have tended to 'do whatever it takes' to meet patients' health needs, up to and including flying patients to Boston for technologically sophisticated medical care – an approach that would seem to fly in the face of CEA. Such ostensibly cost-ineffective tactics have comfortably co-existed in the NGO alongside highly cost-conscious approaches, such as the use of community health workers (CHWs) to deliver directly observed therapy (DOT) for TB and HIV.

Confluent with, and perhaps in some ways as a consequence of the 'do whatever it takes' approach, the context for global health has dramatically changed over the last two decades. PIH's efforts around multidrug resistant (MDR) TB are a case in point. In the mid-1990s, the prevailing wisdom was that treating MDR-TB was not cost-effective and too complex, and therefore should not be incorporated into TB control strategies in poor countries; for a patient, developing resistance to the standard four-drug TB regimen was a death sentence (a very similar dialogue would emerge later in the decade around the care and treatment of HIV).

After a personal brush with the tragic consequences of MDR-TB, Kim and Farmer set out to prove that the disease could in fact be treated, even in the most desperate places. PIH expanded its operations to urban Lima, Peru, establishing a sister NGO, Socios En Salud, in partnership with Peruvian doctors and public health specialists. Using a network of CHWs to deliver DOT of drugs, which Farmer and Kim had procured at premium cost in the United States, Socios demonstrated that MDR-TB could in fact be treated with efficacy rates similar to those of non-resistant strains (Farmer and Kim 1998). Armed with this evidence, Kim and Farmer challenged global TB experts to re-think their strategy. The WHO Green Light Committee was formed, helping to pool global demand for drugs that treat MDR, allowing pharmaceutical companies to shift from low-volume, high-margin to high-volume, low-margin production, drastically reducing prices for drugs used to treat MDR-TB, and thus fundamentally changing CEA equations and making MDR-TB treatment a viable part of global TB strategy (Gupta *et al.* 2001).

Not long after PIH engaged in a similar process with HIV treatment (Farmer *et al.* 2001) – and within a one-year span – G8 leaders announced the multi-billion dollar Global Fund, and President George W. Bush announced the five-year, $15 billion US President's Emergency Plan for AIDS Relief (PEPFAR).[5] These new funding sources, which drastically increased the availability of funds to NGOs as 'implementing partners' of governments, and new private funds enabled PIH to significantly expand its operations. The NGO's support and revenue increased from $36.1 million in fiscal year (FY) 2005 to $53.9 million in FY 2008, and it professionalised many of its operations.[6]

PIH is increasingly operating according to the strategic plans of the democratically elected governments in countries where it serves, including Haiti and Rwanda. It has used HIV and TB funding to work with local and national governments to build local capacity to deliver comprehensive, primary health care services (including HIV and TB prevention, care, and treatment) (Porter *et al.* 2009; Walton *et al.* 2004). The vast majority of PIH's employees are citizens of the nations where they work, and the vast majority of its operating budget flows into the economies of those countries. PIH has continued to work closely with local government partners in an iterative and expanding effort to meet the primary health needs of the rural communities where it operates, including attempts to mitigate the social and economic determinants of the health of local communities through nutrition, housing, and employment assistance. PIH has at times been criticised for having a 'gold-plated' care delivery model that could not be reproduced (Gilks *et al.* 2001), but PIH employees often feel remorse for not being able to do nearly enough, and for regularly losing patients to disease processes which are entirely manageable in the health systems of developed economies.

Shifts in global health architecture

To understand the changing global health paradigm, it is critical to appreciate the recent seismic shift in the 'architecture' of institutions supporting these efforts. Prior to the 1990s, the majority of development assistance for health (DAH) was administered through bilateral (i.e. directly from donor to recipient nation), or multilateral mechanisms (i.e. pooled funding between donor nations, typically channelled through UN institutions or development banks like the World Bank). The formation of the Bill & Melinda Gates Foundation, along with the Global Fund and PEPFAR, has resulted in two major trends over the last decade: a significant increase in the overall DAH budgetary envelope, from $5.6 billion in 1990 to $21.8 billion in 2007 (Ravishankar *et al.* 2009), and a major shift in global health financing from the traditional bilateral and multilateral arrangements to funding that often derives from private philanthropic sources and which is channelled through the recently established 'Global Health Initiatives' (GHIs), which include PEPFAR and the Global Fund, as well as the Gates-funded Global Alliance for Vaccines and Immunisations (GAVI). Of the quantifiable,

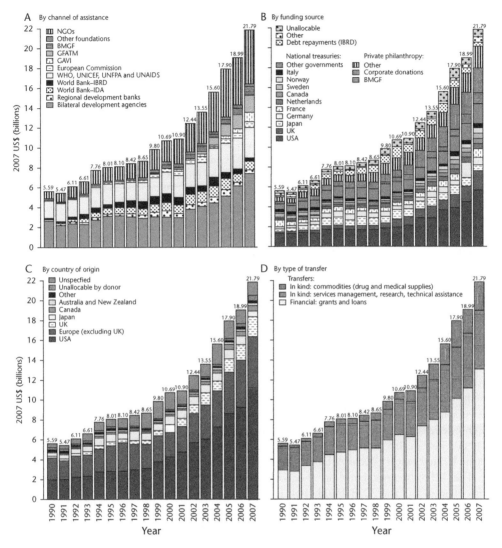

Figure 12.4 Direct assistance for health

Source: Reprinted from *The Lancet*, vol.373, Ravishankar, N. *et al.*, *Financing of Global Health: Tracking Development Assistance for Health from 1990 to 2007*, pp. 2, 113–24, copyright 2009, with permission from Elsevier.

project-level information available in 2007, $5.1 billion was for HIV/AIDS, whereas $0.9 billion was directly attributable to 'health sector support' as opposed to a specific disease (Ravishankar *et al.* 2009).

Accompanying this trend in financing is increased involvement of NGOs, like PIH or Médecins Sans Frontières (MSF), which implement the scale-up of health services, in varying degrees of collaboration with local governments, as well as non-implementing NGOs, such as the US-based Health GAP or GROOTS Kenya, the mission of which is to advocate for increased government accountability to citizens – a set of non-governmental actors that is considered part of 'civil society' (for a more complete definition of civil society, see London School of Economics 2004). While the increasing involvement of civil society organisations

(CSOs) has been seen as a positive development for enhancing government accountability in both donor and recipient countries – and particularly for responding to the unique needs of the marginalised, impoverished, voiceless communities that are often hardest hit by diseases such as HIV and TB (Biesma *et al.* 2009; Global HIV/AIDS Initiatives Network 2009) – the proliferation in number and diversity of CSOs has also further complexified and fragmented the global health space. There are now more than 50,000 NGOs running global programmes (Keane 2003: 5) – and 10,000 NGOs in Haiti alone (Daniel 2009) – not all of which are effective or accountable, or acting in coordination with governments and one another.

This shift in the balance of power has spawned attempts to conceptually and practically reconcile the traditional dialectical poles of global health – the vertical with the horizontal – and the commitment to universal human rights with the empowering of national governments to adequately and responsibly meet the needs of their citizens. The 2008–09 WHO Maximizing Positive Synergies Initiative (MPS), which brought together representatives of governments, CSOs, and academia to address how GHI funding could best be used to simultaneously meet disease-specific objectives and strengthen countries' health systems, was one such effort.

MPS participants concluded that, while there is a tremendous amount of variability between different GHIs and between and within countries, the available evidence supports that GHI funding does, on balance, strengthen health systems, particularly in the realm of service delivery; and that there are key areas of 'synergy', roughly corresponding to the WHO building blocks, which may be seen as focal areas for enabling both GHIs and countries to meet their complementary objectives (Atun *et al.* 2009; Kim 2008; WHO MPS Collaborative Group 2009). Vertical programmes, when strategically designed, can in fact strengthen the delivery of primary health care (Walton *et al.* 2004). A particularly notable area of synergy is in health workforce: the global community must emergently address the number and strategic deployment of health care workers if there is any hope of meeting the health-related Millennium Development Goals (WHO MPS Collaborative Group 2009)[7] – a reality that is notably acknowledged in PEPFAR's recent commitment to support the training and retention of 140,000 new health care workers in partner countries between FY 2010 and FY 2014 (Office of the United States Global AIDS Coordinator 2009).

The MPS findings built on the conclusions of the 2005 Paris Declaration on Aid Effectiveness and the 2008 Third High Level Forum on Aid Effectiveness in Accra, Ghana, which emphasised the importance of donor harmonisation and alignment with country planning, recipient-country ownership, and mutual accountability towards agreed-upon development goals (OECD 2005, 2008). The recently established International Health Partnership Plus (IHP+) aims to actualise these principles by establishing formal pacts between donor and recipient nations around one national health plan, one health budget, and one evaluation framework in each country (Norad-AHHA 2009).

Perspectives on sustainability

A final important theme in the political economy of global health is concern for programme 'sustainability'. In simplistic terms, observers have demonstrated concern that health programmes serving the world's poorest citizens are almost entirely reliant on external funding sources and will cease when this funding dries up; and that recipient countries will become 'dependent' on foreign aid, which is ultimately detrimental to their national growth and development (see Collier 1999). While in the short term, the former is manifestly true, the latter is, at best, a matter of opinion – and at worst, at least in the case of many countries, such as Rwanda and Ethiopia, empirically wrong.[8] Taken together and to their extreme, these concerns amount to a Malthusian or social Darwinist worldview that, despite the ample availability of life-saving resources and medicines, we should accept that many of the poorest sixth will prematurely die for the good of the species.

There is indeed no short-term alternative to external funding for providing essential health care to the bottom billion. The health financing strategy of instituting user fees and requiring other out-of-pocket expenses results in the poorest citizens – who are thus forced to choose between purchasing medicines and other commodities such as food, education for their children, and investments to enhance their economic livelihood – foregoing medically necessary treatments (McIntyre *et al.* 2006; Newhouse 1993). A very limited private health care sector has emerged in many developing countries, but this is inaccessible to the vast majority of their citizens, who live on less than $2 per day. At a national level, governments with limited budgets must choose between investments in the health sector (which they may, in some cases, have actively been encouraged to constrain (Ooms *et al.* 2010)) and investments in other sectors that are equally critical to their national growth and sovereignty (Ooms *et al.* 2006).

It bears explicit acknowledgment that despite substantive, often ideologically motivated disagreement on short-term tactics, most organisations engaged in global health have the same long-term strategic goal: that developing countries experience the economic, social, and political growth that will enable them to ably provide essential health care to their own citizens in the future, without external assistance. Long-term sustainability, then, is a common goal, but we must be realistic about what this will require.

Achieving true sustainability will require dramatic capacity building across all of the health system's building blocks, and is inherently a long-term endeavour – closing the massive gap in the health workforce alone will take a generation or more, as it requires building many more schools and training many more workers (Beaglehole and Dal Pos 2003). In the interim, given a financing gap for attaining the health-related MDGs that experts estimate at between $36 and 45 billion per annum, there is an emergent need for continued, additional external assistance for health, if we are to adequately address even the most basic, essential health needs of the bottom billion (High Level Task Force on Innovative International Financing for Health Systems Working Group 1, 2009). Recent efforts to broaden the scope of health sector capacity building in developing countries will imperil the gains made in addressing epidemic diseases over the last decade if the amount of overall health sector investment is not increased (McNeil 2010).

Innovative financing mechanisms, such as the UNITAID levy on airfare in 15 countries, are needed to fill this gap, and we must be creative about identifying others (High Level Task Force on Innovative International Financing for Health Systems Working Group 2, 2009). Additional efforts are also necessary to ensure that a greater proportion of DAH actually reaches its ostensible target, given evidence that as little as 24 and 9 per cent of bilateral aid in low- and middle-income countries, respectively, 'can actually finance real MDG-based development investments on the ground', 'after one subtracts the money counted as official development assistance that is actually interest payments on debt, technical cooperation payments to consultants from developed countries, food aid (emergency and nonemergency), and debt forgiveness' (UN Millennium Project 2005: 197–8).

A changing paradigm

Our natural tendency, when confronted with catastrophe and suffering on the Haiti earthquake's scale, is to believe that this was a unique event that could not possibly happen again – or to us or our families. Of course, we are deceiving ourselves, if only to cope effectively with the human condition. As the earth's climate changes, disasters will continue to happen, likely on an accelerated scale, and although these disasters will take a greater proportional toll on the less developed countries that are most geographically vulnerable and least prepared,[9] they will also strike rich countries – as those in the US discovered with Hurricane Katrina in 2005. Even in wealthy nations, with reasonable coverage for screening and preventative care, disease processes, such as cancer – which might also be construed as unanticipated natural shocks that devastate individuals and families – strike at people from across the socio-economic and geographic spectrum. As bubonic plague (the Black Death) emerged in the 1400s, HIV and obesity in the 1980s and 1990s, and swine flu in 2009, humanity will continually be confronted with new epidemics of varying and often deadly virulence (Morens *et al.* 2004).

Political disagreements pertaining to global health often relate to fundamental ideological disagreements, which themselves relate to differences in belief about human nature. To vastly oversimplify, those on the modern left tend to believe that humans are or should strive to be fundamentally altruistic, and that the common good is best achieved through collective, public action; those on the right tend to believe that humans are inherently self-interested, and that the common good is best achieved through competition and struggle by private actors. If we have learned anything from the last 150 years of human history, surely it is that neither view is completely true; and if we have made any progress in global health over the last two decades, surely it is by finding a path between.

A prevailing approach to responding to natural or man-made disasters of late has been to use them as an opportunity to rapidly introduce radical, free market reforms – what has been identified as the 'shock doctrine' (Klein 2007). For better or worse, Haiti is unlikely to be seen by the purveyors of this particular line of thought and action as a desirable target. The health sector, too, can be a particularly problematic arena for the application of free market principles, as outlined by the seminal health economist and Nobel Prize winner, Kenneth Arrow (1963). We therefore believe that, rather than free market reform, the Haiti earthquake presents an opportunity to rapidly actualise an alternative paradigm for global health.

The staggering explosion in technologies for diagnosing and treating human disease over the last three decades has provided those of us in the medical profession with an amazing armamentarium for helping people; the majority of this innovation has happened in the US and Europe, probably due to a combination of major investment in basic science research and the commercialisation of health technologies. Those who believe that the right to health is completely at odds with market-based approaches would do well to remember that this rapid innovation made life possible for millions of HIV-infected people the world over.

This explosion in technology has also brought the US to the brink of what experts have termed 'financial Armageddon' as increases in health expenditure far outpace overall economic growth (Chernew *et al.* 2010). Other OECD countries lag behind the US in this regard, but not by much. From the global health perspective, technological advancement has made the health inequalities between nations and between people all the more stark.

As technological advancement is thus the key driver of both uncontrolled growth in health expenditure in wealthy nations and the increasingly evident health inequality between nations, a major option would seem to be taking steps to curb this innovation – but, as doctors confronted every day with people suffering from diseases we do not yet know how to treat well, we are biased against this approach. We believe in addition to ongoing technological innovation, we need rapid, disruptive innovation in the organisation and delivery of health care, in order to create more efficient and equitable health systems on both national and global levels – and that joining both types of innovation is the true pathway to finally achieving the right to health for all.

Mexico City's 1985 earthquake proved an opportunity for Mexico to introduce a series of innovative health sector reforms – culminating with the Seguro Popular in 2004 – which guaranteed social protection and health care access to the entire population, and provided 'conditional cash transfers' to the poorest citizens to reward health-promoting behaviours such as vaccinating children (Frenk *et al.* 2006). The leaders of the Mexican health sector reform have characterised their innovation as a 'diagonal' approach to health systems strengthening (Sepulveda *et al.* 2006). Confronted with the potentially existential challenge of the HIV epidemic, Brazil made a courageous and controversial decision to actualise its constitutional commitment to the right to health by striving to rapidly achieve universal access to HIV care and treatment; its national strategy of committing to universal access, negotiating large-volume price discounts from pharmaceutical companies, and partnering with CSOs has been widely imitated and is considered global best practice. Brazil now has an HIV prevalence on par with that of the US, and has experienced excellent economic growth over the last decade. Both Mexico and Brazil benefitted from initial external investment in their health sectors, but are now largely independent of this assistance (WHO, n.d.).

In the US, we must respond to the Haiti earthquake with significant federal and private investment to enable our major research universities to partner with Haiti and nations with similar socio-economic indicators to engage in primary health care systems innovation. We should openly acknowledge that this investment is in our own self-interest – not only to promote stability and security and control the spread of epidemic disease, but also to help all of us creatively re-think the organisation and delivery of health care in settings less encumbered by payment models, professional norms, and legal and regulatory frameworks that strangle innovation. This closely mirrors an argument that Nigel Crisp – the former head of the UK's single-payer National Health Service – has made for a new paradigm in thinking about global health (Crisp 2010). The *Harvard Business Review* recently recognised 'Reverse Innovation' – the global dissemination of technological innovations developed through research and development investment in resource-poor settings – as one of the 12 'most influential management ideas of the millennium' (Immelt *et al.* 2009; GE Reports 2010). We must now apply this approach to the redesign of health care delivery systems that *all* countries in the world desperately need.

We must help Haiti build back better in the health sector, in solidarity and close collaboration with Haitian government officials, health care workers, and entrepreneurs; but we should also frankly and explicitly acknowledge to our Haitian colleagues that we have our own interests as well as theirs at heart: we help them 'build' capacity in Haiti in order to bolster our own, and we have the highest expectations from the endeavour. We must understand and fully acknowledge that health systems strengthening for the bottom billion is truly for the good of all of us – not merely from a moral perspective, but also from a strictly pragmatic one.

Notes

1 Lord Nigel Crisp (2010), the former head of the UK's National Health Service, has elegantly described this necessary paradigm shift in thinking about global health.

2 For an example of the collective responsibility to ensuring access to health care, see Ooms and Van Damme (2009).

3 See, for instance, the US military counter insurgency manual, which names economic development and the provision of essential services to the population as essential goals of any campaign to establish support for a national government during a counterinsurgency operation (United States Department of the Army 2007).

4 For example, Marseille *et al.* (2002: 1,851) claimed that HIV prevention was '28 times more cost-effective than HAART'. For a critique of the logic of CEA, see chapter 9, 'Rethinking Health and Human Rights: Time for a Paradigm Shift' in Farmer (2005).

5 For more on the genesis of PEPFAR and the GFATM, see Behrman (2004).
6 See 'Partners In Health: Historical Data' on CharityNavigator.org: http://www.charitynavigator.org/index.cfm?bay=search.history&orgid=4884 (accessed 4 June 2010).
7 Also in 2009, the High Level Task Force on Innovative International Financing for Health Systems – formed in response to a call by world leaders for an additional US $30 billion to save 10 million mother and child lives, and chaired by UK Prime Minister Gordon Brown and World Bank President Robert Zoellick – released two reports. The report of Working Group 1 (2009) is entitled 'Constraints to Scaling Up and Costs'. The report of Working Group 2 (2009) is entitled 'Raising and Channelling Funds'.
8 In response to critics of aid, Jeffrey Sachs (2009) points to Rwanda as an example of a nation where aid has been integral to growth.
9 Haiti is consistently cited as a nation that is particularly vulnerable to the deleterious effects of climate change (Swarup 2009).

References

Arrow, K. (1963) 'Uncertainty and the welfare economics of medical care', *American Economic Review*, 53: 941–73.
Atun, R., Dybul, M., Evans, T., Kim, J.Y., Moatti, J.P., Nishtar, S., and Russell, A. (2009) 'Venice Statement on global health initiatives and health systems', *The Lancet*, 374: 783–4.
Beaglehole, R. and Dal Pos, M. (2003) 'Public health workforce: Challenges and policy issues', *Human Resources for Health*, 1: 4.
Behrman, G. (2004) *The Invisible People: How the U.S. Has Slept through the Global AIDS Pandemic, the Greatest Humanitarian Catastrophe of Our Time*, New York: Free Press.
Biesma, R., Brugha, R., Harmer, A. Walsh, A., Spicer, N., and Walt, G. (2009) 'The effects of global health initiatives on country health systems: A review of the evidence from HIV/AIDS control', *Health Policy and Planning*, 24: 239–52.
Brilliant, L. (1985) *The Management of Smallpox Eradication in India*, Ann Arbor: The University of Michigan Press.
Charles, J. (2010) 'Haiti receives $5 billion in aid pledges', *Miami Herald*, 31 March.
Chernew, M.E., Baicker, K., and Hsu, J. (2010) 'The specter of financial Armageddon: health care and the federal debt in the United States', *New England Journal of Medicine*, 362: 1,166–8.
Collier, P. (1999) 'Aid "Dependency": A Critique', *Journal of African Economies*, 8: 528–45.
Crisp, N. (2010) *Turning the World Upside Down: The Search for Global Health in the Twenty-First Century*, London: The Royal Society of Medicine Press.
Cueto, M. (2004) 'The origins of primary health care and selective primary health care', *American Journal of Public Health*, 94: 1,864–74.
Daniel, T. (2009) 'Bill Clinton tells diaspora: "Haiti needs you now"', *Miami Herald*, 9 August, available at http://www.miamiherald.com/2009/08/09/1179067/bill-clinton-tells-diaspora-haiti.html (accessed 2 June 2010).
Farmer, P. (2005) *Pathologies of Power: Health, Human Rights, and the New War on the Poor*, Berkeley, CA: University of California Press.
Farmer, P. (2010a) 'An anthropology of structural violence', in H. Saussy (ed.) *Partner to the Poor: A Paul Farmer Reader*, Berkeley, CA: University of California Press: 350–75.
Farmer, P. (2010b) 'On suffering and structural violence: Social and economic rights in the global era', in H. Saussy (ed.) *Partner to the Poor: A Paul Farmer Reader*, Berkeley, CA: University of California Press: 328–49.
Farmer, P.E. and Kim, J.Y. (1998) 'Community-based approaches to the control of multidrug-resistant tuberculosis: Introducing "DOTS-plus"', *British Medical Journal*, 317: 671–4.
Farmer, P. and Gastineau Campos, N. (2010) 'Rethinking Medical Ethics: A View from Below', in H. Sauss (ed.) *Partner to the Poor: A Paul Farmer Reader*, Berkeley, CA: University of California Press, 471–86.
Farmer, P., Léandre, F., Mukherjee, J., Gupta, R., Tarter, L., and Kim, J.Y. (2001) 'Community-based treatment of advanced HIV disease: Introducing DOTHAART (directly observed therapy with highly active antiretroviral therapy)', *Bulletin of the World Health Organization*, 79: 1,145–51.
French, H. (2010) 'The Next Empire', *The Atlantic Magazine*, May, available at http://www.theatlantic.com/magazine/archive/2010/05/the-next-empire/8018/ (accessed 15 April 2010).
Frenk, J., Gonzalez-Pier, E., Gomez-Dantes, O., Lezana, M.A., and Knaul, F.M. (2006) 'Comprehensive reform to improve health system performance in Mexico', *The Lancet*, 368: 1,524–34.

GE Reports (2010) 'Reverse Innovation Hits Harvard's Most Influential List', available at http://www.gereports.com/reverse-innovation-hits-harvards-most-influential-list/ (accessed 16 April 2010).

Gilks, C., AbouZahr, C., and Turmen, T. (2001) 'HAART in Haiti: evidence needed', *Bulletin of the World Health Organization*, 79: 1154–5.

Global HIV/AIDS Initiatives Network (2009) 'The Impact of Global Health Initiatives in Kyrgyzstan: July 2009 Policy Brief', available at http://www.ghinet.org/downloads/Kyrgyzstan_policy_brief.pdf (accessed 15 April 2010).

Government of the Republic of Haiti with support from the International Community. (2010) 'Haiti Earthquake PDNA: Assessment of Damage, Losses, General and Sectoral Needs; Annex to the Action Plan for National Recovery and Development of Haiti', available at http://gfdrr.org/docs/PDNA_Haiti-2010_Working_Document_EN.pdf (accessed 15 April 2010).

Gupta, R., Kim, J.Y., Espinal, M., Caudron, J.M., Pecoul, B., Farmer, P.E., and Raviglione, M. (2001) 'Responding to market failures in tuberculosis control', *Science*, 293: 1,049–51.

High Level Task Force on Innovative International Financing for Health Systems Working Group 1 (2009) 'Constraints to Scaling Up and Costs', available at http://www.who.int/pmnch/media/membernews/2009/htltf_wg1_report_EN.pdf (accessed 16 April 2010).

High Level Task Force on Innovative International Financing for Health Systems Working Group 2 (2009) 'Raising and Channeling Funds', available at http://www.who.int/pmnch/media/membernews/2009/20090319_tfwg2.pdf (accessed 16 April 2010).

Homme, E.S. (2009) *Health as Foreign Policy*, 3 October, Policy Analysis and Development Agency, Department of Foreign Affairs, Indonesia, available at http://www.norway.or.id/Norway_in_Indonesia/Society--Policy/Health-as-Foreign-Policy/ (accessed 15 April 2010).

Immelt, J.R., Govindarajan, V., and Trimble, C. (2009) 'How GE Is Disrupting Itself', *Harvard Business Review*, 87: 56–65.

Keane, J. (2003) *Global Civil Society?* Cambridge: Cambridge University Press.

Kim, J.Y. (2008) 'Health systems and Global Health Initiatives: the status of affairs', Presentation during the expert consultation on positive synergies between health systems and Global Health Initiatives, World Health Organization, Geneva, 29–30 May.

Kim, J.Y., Millen, J., Irwin, A., and Gershman, J. (2000) *Dying for Growth: Global Inequality and the Health of the Poor*, Monroe: Common Courage Press.

Klein, N. (2007) *The Shock Doctrine: The Rise of Disaster Capitalism*, New York: Henry Holt and Company.

London School of Economics (2004) 'What is Civil Society?', Centre for Civil Society, London School of Economics, available at http://www.lse.ac.uk/collections/CCS/what_is_civil_society.htm (accessed 2 June 2010).

McIntyre, D., Thiede, M., Dahlgren, G., and Whitehead, M. (2006) 'What are the economic consequences for households of illness and of paying for health care in middle-income country contexts?' *Social Science & Medicine*, 62: 858–65.

McNeil, D. (2010) 'At Front Lines, AIDS War is Falling Apart', *New York Times*, 10 May.

Marseille, E., Homann, P.B., and Kahn, J.G. (2002) 'HIV Prevention before HAART in sub-Saharan Africa', *The Lancet*, 359: 1,851–6.

Morens, D.M., Folkers, G.K., and Fauci, A.S. (2004) 'The challenge of emerging and re-emerging infectious diseases', *Nature*, 430: 242–9.

Murray, C. and Frenk, J. (2000) 'A framework for assessing the performance of health systems', *Bulletin of the World Health Organization*, 78: 717–31.

Newhouse, J.P. (1993) *Free for All? Lessons from the RAND Health Insurance Experiment*, Cambridge, MA: Harvard University Press.

Norad-AHHA (2009) 'The Global Health Landscape and Innovative International Financing for Health Systems: Trends and Issues', available at http://www.internationalhealthpartnership.net/pdf/TF_Background_paper_HLTF_Norad%203Nov08.pdf (accessed 18 April 2010).

Office of the United States Global AIDS Coordinator (2009) 'The U.S. President's Emergency Plan for AIDS Relief: Five-Year Strategy', available at http://www.pepfar.gov/documents/organization/133035.pdf (accessed 16 April 2010).

Ooms, G. and Van Damme, W. (2009) 'Global responsibilities for global health rights', *The Lancet*, 74: 607.

Ooms, G., Derderian, K., and Melody, D. (2006) 'Do we need a World Health Insurance to realize the right to health?' *PLoS Medicine*, 3: e530.

Ooms, G., Decoster, K., Miti, K., Rens, S., Leemput, L.V., Vermeiren, P., and Van Damme, W. (2010) 'Crowding out: are relations between international health aid and government health funding too complex to be captured in averages only?' *The Lancet*, 375: 1,403–5.

Organisation for Economic Cooperation and Development (OECD) (2005, 2008) 'The Paris Declaration on Aid Effectiveness and the Accra Agenda for Action', available at http://www.oecd.org/dataoecd/11/41/34428351.pdf (accessed 16 April 2010).

Porter, M.E., Lee, S., Rhatigan, J., and Kim, J. (2009) *HIV Care in Rwanda*, HBS Case # 709474, Boston, MA: Harvard Business Press.

Ravishankar, N., Gubbins, P., Cooley, R., Leach-Kemon, K., Michaud, C.M., Jamison, D.T., and Murray, C.J. (2009) 'Financing of global health: Tracking development assistance for health from 1990 to 2007', *The Lancet*, 373: 2,113–24.

Ruger, J. (2005) 'The changing role of the World Bank in global health', *American Journal of Public Health*, 95: 60.

Sachs, J. (2009) 'Without aid, Rwanda's investment programmes would have collapsed', *FT.com*, 27 May.

Sepúlveda, J., Bustreo, F., Tapia, R., Riera, J., Lozano, R., Oláiz, G., Partida, V., García-García, L., and Valdespino, J. (2006) 'Improvement of child survival in Mexico: The diagonal approach', *The Lancet*, 368: 2,017–27.

Siddiqi, J. (1995) *World Health and World Politics: The World Health Organization and the UN System*, Chapel Hill: University of North Carolina Press.

Swarup, A. (2009) *Haiti*: ' "A Gathering Storm": Climate Change and Poverty', Oxfam Research Reports, available at http://www.oxfam.org.uk/resources/policy/climate_change/climate-change-poverty-haiti.html (accessed 16 April 2010).

UNDP (United Nations Development Programme) (2003) *Human Development Report 2003: Millennium Development Goals: A Compact among Nations to End Human Poverty*, New York: Oxford University Press.

UN Millennium Project (2005) 'Investing in Development: A Practical Plan to Achieve the Millennium Development Goals', London: United Nations Development Programme, available at http://www.unmillenniumproject.org/documents/MainReportComplete-lowres.pdf (accessed 16 April 2010).

United States Department of the Army (2007) *The U.S. Army/Marine Corps Counterinsurgency Field Manual: U.S. Army field manual no. 3–24: Marine Corps Warfighting* Publication No. 3–33.5, Chicago, IL: University of Chicago Press.

Walton, D., Farmer, P., Lambert, W., Léandre, F., Koenig, S.P., and Mukherjee, J.S. (2004) 'Integrated HIV prevention and care strengthens primary health care: Lessons from rural Haiti', *Journal of Public Health Policy*, 25: 137–58.

Webb, T. and Mathiason, N. (2008) 'China buys its future from Africa', *The Observer*, 10 February, available at http://www.guardian.co.uk/business/2008/feb/10/mining.china (accessed 15 April 2010).

World Bank (1993) *World Development Report 1993: Investing in Health*, New York: Oxford University Press.

WHO (World Health Organization) (1978) 'Declaration of Alma Ata. International Conference on Primary Health Care, Alma-Ata, USSR, 6–12 September 1978', Geneva: World Health Organization, available at www.who.int/hpr/NPH/docs/declaration_almaata.pdf (accessed 15 April 2010).

WHO (World Health Organization) (2006) *The World Health Report 2006: Working Together for Health*, Geneva: WHO.

WHO (World Health Organization) (2007) *Everybody's Business: Strengthening Health Systems to Improve Health Outcomes: WHO's Framework for Action*, Geneva: WHO.

WHO (World Health Organization) (2008) *The World Health Report 2008: Primary Health Care; Now More than Ever*, Geneva: WHO.

WHO (World Health Organization) (n.d.) 'National Health Accounts', available at http://www.who.int/nha/en/ (accessed 2 June 2010).

WHO (World Health Organization) Maximising Positive Synergies Collaborative Group (2009) 'An assessment of interactions between global health initiatives and country health systems', *The Lancet*, 373: 2,137–69.

Part III

Ecological Transformation and Environmental Health in the Global System

13

Climate Change and Global Public Health

Impacts, Research, and Actions

Elizabeth G. Hanna, Anthony J. McMichael, and Colin D. Butler

Introduction

Human-driven climate change – now deemed by international climate science to be real and, indeed, accelerating – reflects the mounting pressures of human numbers and economic activity. Melting ice, higher temperatures, more intense weather variability, and rising sea levels, predicted by climate scientists to appear in coming decades, have been increasingly observed during this first decade of the twenty-first century. This unexpected steepening in the trajectory of change heightens the urgency for a coordinated global response. While climate change will have some positive consequences in some regions, the continuation of rapid global economic growth – if substantially driven by the burning of fossil fuels (the 'business-as-usual' approach), plus forest clearance – will cause increasingly serious adverse impacts.

Humans have the knowledge and potential capacity to limit, even reverse, these changes, thus preventing serious and increasing risks to human health and well-being – and perhaps averting a potentially catastrophic decline in Earth's capacity to support civilisation. Achieving this is primarily a matter of will, combined with new forms of international governance. Unless, however, the policymaking response accelerates at a rate commensurate with that of climate change, then even a greatly invigorated public health system is unlikely to be able to manage the attendant risks to population health. This chapter describes those risks, and the needed public health research and action. Beyond that professional task, health researchers must also communicate information about health risks into the mainstream of public discourse on averting ('mitigating') climate change – thus stimulating national and global action.

Climate change

About 17 per cent of the incoming solar energy passing through the troposphere (the lower atmosphere) is prevented from re-radiating from Earth's surface back to space by several gases that exist at trace concentrations. This capture of energy warms Earth's surface, creating a 'greenhouse effect' (Weart 2003). Without it, the average global temperature would be about 35 °C cooler than it is today (Richardson *et al.* 2009), and unsuitable for human habitation.

Naturally occurring 'greenhouse gases' (GHGs) include water vapour, carbon dioxide (CO_2), methane (CH_4), and nitrous oxide (NO_2). Human activity, power generation, industry, agriculture, and transportation have also generated halocarbons and black carbon, releasing billions of tonnes of GHGs into the air every year. The Kyoto Protocol (1997), forged within the UN Framework Convention on Climate Change (1992), sought to reduce GHG emissions. However, governments and citizenry have not yet understood the full import of climate change; mitigation policies are seriously lagging and GHG emissions continue to rise – along with global temperatures (Richardson *et al.* 2009). Further inaction risks feedbacks, which will liberate additional billions of tonnes of GHGs, currently sequestered/stored in the ocean, permafrost, and forests.

Recent observations on climate

In March 2009, the Climate Change Congress in Copenhagen distilled six key messages from the latest research findings (summarised in Box 13.1) (Richardson *et al.* 2009). Global climate model simulations project that, if 'business-as-usual' is maintained, then by the end of the twenty-first century the global surface mean temperature will increase by at least 2.8 °C, with an average warming of 3.5 °C on land and up to 7 °C in the Arctic (IPCC 2007a). These changes would have substantial effects on the physical-chemical-biological-hydrological systems that drive life on this planet. The rate of sea-level rise (SLR) has already doubled to over 3 mm/yr, and there is growing consensus that sea-level rise will reach one metre by 2100, compared with 1990 (Rahmstorf 2009).

Wind speeds in storms increase exponentially as temperature rises. The reinsurance[1] industry has reported a recent shift towards Category 5 storms, estimated to have doubled in frequency since 1851. Whether or not the recent trend to stronger storms is confirmed, storm surges

---

Box 13.1 Climate change: Global Risks, Challenges, and Decisions Congress

Climatic trends – Worst-case Intergovernmental Panel on Climate Change (IPCC) scenario trajectories are being realised. There is significant risk that the trends will accelerate, leading to an increasing risk of abrupt and irreversible climatic shifts.

Social disruption – Societies are highly vulnerable to even modest levels of climate change, and temperature rises above 2 °C will be very difficult for contemporary societies to cope with.

Long-term strategy – Rapid, sustained, and effective mitigation based on coordinated global and regional action is required to avoid 'dangerous climate change', regardless of how it is defined.

Equity dimension – Climate change is having, and will have, strongly differential effects on people within and between countries and regions, on this generation and future generations, and on human societies and the natural world.

Inaction is inexcusable – There is no excuse for inaction.

Meeting the challenge – To achieve the societal transformation required, we must overcome a number of significant constraints and seize critical opportunities.

(*Source*: http://climatecongress.ku.dk/pdf/synthesisreport/)

---

combined with rising sea levels will threaten millions of people living in low-lying areas. Meanwhile, other forms of extreme climatic events such as heat waves, droughts, and bushfires are also increasing.

Impacts of climate change: elucidating the health risks

Regional differences in climate change manifestations, along with the geographic and cultural diversity of human populations, mean that climate change will have diverse health consequences. Climate change, however, is not a new and separate environmental risk factor for human health, rather, it is a complex and evolving systemic change that extends and amplifies many existing risks to health. In general, it will impinge more severely on vulnerable and poor populations in low-income countries (i.e. those who have contributed least to global warming over past decades). Climate change will thus tend to amplify existing health inequalities, including those related to weather disaster impacts, food and water shortages, diarrhoeal disease, and various other infectious diseases.

In addition to various direct impacts of changes in meteorological conditions, climate change will have some important, indirect effects. In 2007, the IPCC concluded that an average global temperature rise of 1.5 to 2.5 °C would eliminate 20 to 30 per cent of the world's species, leading to major changes in ecosystem structure and function (IPCC 2007b). Such loss and disruption would greatly harm human health and well-being by contributing to reduced food and water security (Butler 2009).

An understanding of likely regional health impacts is therefore crucial for governments to develop appropriate national adaptation policies. Climate adaptation is defined as 'adjustment in natural or human systems in response to actual or predicted climatic stimuli or their effects, which moderates harm or exploits beneficial opportunities' (IPCC 2001). In the public health domain, adaptation spans changes to various social, physical, and institutional systems, plus strategies to increase the resilience of communities to adverse health impacts.

Effective adaptation requires knowledge of the main locally relevant climate-related health risks (current and future) in the population, and ascertains who is most vulnerable. The appropriate sequence of research and health risk assessment tasks to acquire that knowledge is as follows.

The first task is to learn more about the 'baseline' relations between climatic conditions and health outcomes (a topic that has received minimal attention during the past half-century of 'modern epidemiology' research). Such research clarifies the extent and form of the sensitivity of each specified health outcome to variations in climatic conditions. Second, there is already a need and opportunity to seek evidence of ongoing changes in health risks and outcomes that are linked to climate change – a complex task that is subject to all the usual difficulties of multivariate influences, confounding effects, and making causal attribution. Third, it is reasonable and useful to estimate statistically the proportions of the current global, regional, and national burdens of disease that are attributable to the climate change that has already occurred.

Fourth, there is the task of estimating future risks to health. Such risks can be modelled by applying the information gleaned from the first task above to geocoded and time-specific scenarios of future climate change, as generated by climate science. This necessarily entails new collaborations with climate scientists, mathematical modellers, and others. Indeed, extended collaborations with social scientists, economists, and others will enrich this predictive exercise by factoring in reasonable estimations of how other modulating factors are likely to change concurrently with future climate change.

Finally, there are the research and assessment tasks that relate to the prevention of adverse health outcomes by: (i) avoiding future unmanageable risks via mitigation of climate change – and assessing the immediate collateral (hopefully beneficial) local health effects of those mitigation actions; and (ii), in the interim, managing unavoidable risks to health via adaptation actions, especially in the most vulnerable groups of communities.

Climate-related health impacts

Figure 13.1 illustrates the direct and indirect relationships between climate change and health.

Temperature-related illness

Human physiology can only tolerate a small range in core temperature (36 °C to 38 °C). Above 39 °C to 40 °C, dangerous health effects may occur, such as confusion, heat stroke, cardiac and renal impairment, organ failure, unconsciousness, and eventually death. The body's thermo-regulation mechanisms diminish in efficacy with advancing age, making the elderly particularly susceptible. The aged also have impaired thirst drives, predisposing them to dehydration, and cardiac and renal failure. Most deaths and hospitalisations during extreme heat waves are from cardiovascular events.

Another group at risk from heat are outdoor workers (Kjellstrom 2009). Continued exercise raises the core temperature, so occupational health strategies involving rest, fluids, and shade are required to protect worker health in a warming climate. Air conditioning is effective for indoor workers but relies on electricity, most of which is still fuelled by fossil or nuclear fuels. In many hot, low-income countries, where heat stress is most acute, air conditioning is unaffordable to the poor, and electricity, even if connected, is often unreliable.

Heat waves also test infrastructural capacity in rich nations. An extreme heatwave in 2009 brought temperatures approaching 50 °C (122 °F) across south-eastern Australia (Melbourne and Adelaide), with widespread power failures, buckled train lines, and interrupted telecommunications. Facilities for the aged lost air conditioning, commuters were stranded in the heat, and emergency services were overwhelmed and interrupted during the ensuing heat-related bushfires in Victoria that destroyed 2,000 homes and claimed 173 lives.

Extreme weather

The IPCC predicts increasing intensity of extreme weather events – a major source of injury and death, often followed by mental health problems, outbreaks of infectious diseases, and, in poor populations, food shortages. Intense storms damage property and infrastructure, and interrupt services, food, and water supply. In 2008, there were 41 Category 5 storms, defined as causing 'overall losses exceeding US\$ 500 million and more than 500 fatalities'. This is the highest number on record and is part of an upward trend (Munich Re 2009). Immediate health concerns of safety and treatment of injuries shift to the challenge of maintaining ongoing health needs in an environment struck by devastation. The aftermath of these events can overwhelm capacity of local infrastructure, public health, and external aid.

Sea-level rise

Sea-level rise (SLR) poses significant health risks and other concerns for the approximately 630 million people living in coastal zones at or below 10 metres above 2009 sea levels. Health consequences include heightened physical risks from storm surges, contamination of coastal

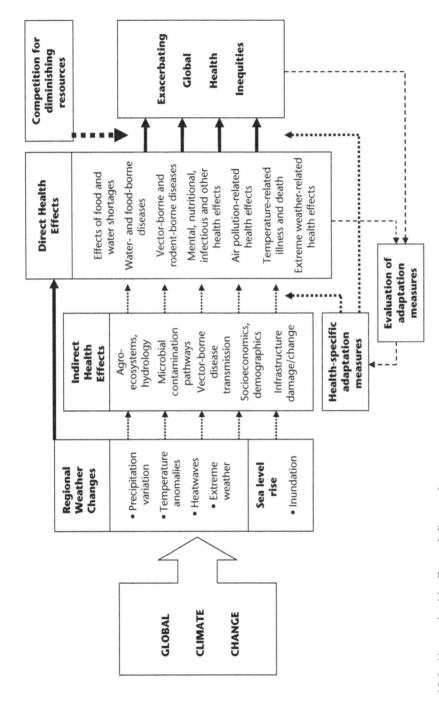

Figure 13.1 Human health effects of climate change
Source: Modified from McMichael *et al.* 2003.

freshwater supplies with encroaching sea water, the degradation of fishing and agricultural areas, and the many health effects of community disruption and displacement.

Recent estimates indicate at least a 1-metre rise by 2100; however, there is concern that melting of the ice caps covering Greenland and parts of Antarctica could raise this to several metres. A 1-metre rise would inundate many low-lying islands, such as the Maldives, many South Pacific islands, urban coastal strips, and various river deltas.

Air pollution

Heat waves exacerbate some aspects of air pollution, particularly the formation of ozone. Particulates from dust storms and bushfires diminish air quality and aggravate respiratory and cardiac conditions. One-third of the estimated 70,000 excess deaths resulting from the 2003 European heat wave were attributed to excessive ozone concentrations occurring on hot days in urban centres (Dear *et al.* 2005). Warmer and moister conditions, along with higher carbon dioxide concentrations, may increase the production of allergenic plant pollen and exacerbate asthma and hayfever symptoms (Johnston *et al.* 2009).

Water security

Changes in rainfall patterns will jeopardise water security and, hence, health in many regions. So too will the reduction in river flows from alpine glaciers. Beyond diarrhoeal disease, health risks also arise from chemical contamination of water supplies as people seek alternative sources. Melting ice can release trapped chemicals (Noyesa *et al.* 2009), and water wells can carry high arsenic loads presenting risks of skin pigmentation, hyperkeratosis, cardiovascular disease, neuropathy, and cancer (McMichael *et al.* 2008).

A shortage of safe water for drinking and sanitation is a major hazard to health, especially child mortality. The current rapid pace of population growth and urbanisation creates new water needs, while a rural backlog remains unserved. An estimated 1.6 million people die every year from diarrhoeal diseases attributable to lack of access to safe drinking water and basic sanitation, with 90 per cent of these children under five. During 1990 to 2004, the number of people without access to drinking water in sub-Saharan Africa increased by 23 per cent, and the number without sanitation increased by over 30 per cent[2] (WHO/UNICEF Joint Monitoring Programme for Water Supply and Sanitation 2006). Against that background, climate change looms as a serious threat to the quantity and quality of water supplies.

Diminished rainfall is predicted for the mid-latitude regions, as rainfall systems move poleward. The Organisation for Economic Co-operation and Development (OECD) calculates that by 2030, some 3.9 billion people – 47 per cent of the global population – will be living in areas with high water stress, mostly in developing countries. South and Southeast Asia, the new mega-cities, the Americas, and sub-Saharan Africa remain areas of great concern where a warming of +2.0 to +4.5 °C by 2100 is expected (Müller 2009). Drying is also affecting many wealthier countries. Brazil, the Mediterranean, Australia, and parts of the US have all suffered extreme droughts and more fires. These are forecast to continue, threatening agriculture and domestic water supplies.

Vector-borne infectious disease

Many infectious disease pathogens, vector organisms, and intermediate host species are sensitive to climate conditions. Climate change can affect the geographic range, seasonality, and transmissibility of infectious diseases. A particular concern is that vector habitat may increase, facilitating the entry of vector-borne infectious diseases (VBDs), such as malaria, dengue, West Nile virus, and Rift Valley fever, into previously disease-free areas with non-immune populations. The rate of parasite maturation, vector reproduction, and biting frequency all rise with increasing temperature. Several continents have reported expansion of vector range (FAO 2008), although the extent to which this is climate-related or due to other factors remains contested. More research is needed to differentiate causal relationships.

The precautionary principle dictates that public health must anticipate substantial increases in health risks. Models estimate that climate change could result in an additional 220 to 400 million people being exposed to malaria by 2080, and that 1.5 billion to 3.5 billion people could face the risk of being afflicted by dengue by 2080 (UNDP 2007).

Food security

Food security has been prominent in the rise and fall of past civilisations. The total numbers of food insecure persons has risen steadily during this decade, from around 900 million to 1 billion. Models consistently indicate that changes in temperature, rainfall, and soil moisture due to climate change are predicted to decrease the yields of many foods, on land and at sea, thus jeopardising nutritional status – and, in particular, maternal health and child growth and development (Homer et al. 2009).

Food security may become a so-called 'wicked [nigh insoluble] problem'. Food production must increase by 50 per cent to feed the projected population rise to 9 billion people. However, the United Nations Environment Programme (UNEP) warns that up to 25 per cent of the world's food production may become lost due to environmental breakdown by 2050 unless action is taken (UNEP/GRID-Arendal 2009).

Increased intensity and frequency of storms and droughts, and inundation by rising sea levels associated with storm surges, will place additional stresses on agricultural lands. The Global Food Crisis of 2008 may be a preview of the future. The compounded effects of speculation in food stocks, extreme weather events, including droughts in many of the food growing regions, growth in bio-fuels competing for cropland, and high oil prices led to a significant fall in global cereal stocks in 2008 (FAO 2009). The rapid 50–200 per cent increase in selected commodity prices pushed staples beyond the reach of many undernourished people, who were already spending 70–80 per cent of their daily income on food. This further reduction in caloric intake elevated infant and child mortality and increased susceptibility to disease. Prices curtailed the World Food Programme, pushed an additional 110 million people into poverty, and 44 million more to the undernourished (FSN Forum 2008), generating unrest and food riots in 22 countries.

Mental health

The prospect of facing an uncertain climatic future can affect mental health, as can the experience of extreme weather events and other climate-related social and personal disruptions (droughts, coastal displacement, etc.) (Berry et al. 2008, Fritze et al. 2008). Health outcomes will be determined by the nature and magnitude of exposure, loss, and life disruption – modulated by the degree of resilience. Most of the relevant literature comes from developed countries, whereas little research has examined mental health problems in developing countries (Patel 2008), or in children, who must be considered especially vulnerable. There is a relative dearth of research on climate change and mental health.

Social upheaval

Large-scale population displacement can follow extreme weather events that create natural disasters, environmental degradation, or sea-level rise. Droughts, food and water shortages, fires, failed infrastructure, and conflict may also force people to leave their homelands (Oxfam 2009). Worldwide, an estimated 26 million people have been displaced as a direct result of climate change, most of them within the borders of their country of origin (GHF 2009). However, further warming in conjunction with environmental degradation and water shortages may force 50–200 million people to relocate by mid-century (UNHCR 2009).

The many millions forcibly displaced by disasters, inundation, hunger, and slow-onset change will require substantial protection and humanitarian assistance. Receiving areas may be overcrowded and stressed. At the destination point, mass provision of food, water, shelter, sanitation, and basic health services, as well as information, communications, and governance must be arranged. Immediate public health concerns include the prevention of infectious diarrhoeal and sexually transmitted disease outbreaks among the overcrowded refugee camps. Durable solutions will be needed for those who cannot return to their homes in the aftermath of a disaster. Helping to establish self-sufficiency (e.g. employment options, food production) are, therefore, public health priorities.

Acquiring knowledge for health-protecting adaptive actions

Key determinants of climate change impacts are the magnitude of change in climatic conditions and short-term weather patterns, the rate of this change, and occurrence of low-frequency, high-impact events, such as extreme weather disasters. Thresholds will exist, below which changes can be absorbed with little observable deviation. Complex interactions can create tipping points, above which further pressure results in substantially greater sensitivity to additional stimuli, causing a cascade of change or indeed collapse (IPCC 2001).

Key factors in a nation's capacity to respond will be the resilience and technological and economic capacity to absorb the changes and adapt. The initial state of environmental systems and socio-economic conditions plays a pivotal role in determining a nation's vulnerability and capacity to adapt. These variables include population (density), economic trends (e.g. income levels, sectoral composition of GDP), and other socio-economic indicators (e.g. equity, culture, social cohesion, education levels, health, and nutritional status). Given the multisectoral, multi-regional, multidisciplinary, and multi-institutional nature of climatic change assessments of effects, impacts, and policy options, the IPCC recommends that integrated assessments be used to explore how diverse assumptions in relation to those several domains affect the modelled outcome (IPCC 2001).

Vulnerability

Vulnerability to climate change is a key consideration for policy and action. Vulnerability is defined as the degree to which a system (e.g. a defined community of persons) is exposed to a change in ambient climatic–environmental conditions and is susceptible (sensitive) to and unable to adapt to the external exposure. The system's adaptive capacity is defined as the ability to prepare for and accommodate changes and continue to function. In population health terms, adaptive capacity is a function of the local infrastructure and its capacity to respond sufficiently to protect those in need, and is analogous to public health (Ebi *et al.* 2008).

Lack of adaptive capacity exacerbates vulnerability. Stressed populations may have exhausted their reserve capacity, and, if struggling under present conditions, will find it difficult to cope with further deprivations from climate-induced environmental deterioration such as intensifying water shortages, more violent storms, deepening of food shortages, soil erosion, or inundation by rising seas. Loss of healthy life-years in low-income African countries due to climate change is predicted to be 500 times that in Europe (McMichael *et al.* 2008).

Role for public health

The primary task is to develop and implement a range of health-protecting 'adaptive' strategies. These should address both the existing effects of climate change on health, and the effects anticipated over the coming decades. Strategies should combine immediate heightened protection of communities and vulnerable groups (e.g. improved infectious disease surveillance, and effective early-warning systems for impending heat waves and storms) with strategies that render populations and habitats more climate-proof in the long run (e.g. enhanced water supplies and sanitation systems, and more 'sustainable' and temperature-tolerant urban and housing design).

Many mitigation strategies to reduce GHG emissions can enhance local population health. For example, a shift away from fossil fuel as an energy source delivers a series of 'co-benefits' via cleaner local air and alternative transport options. Cycling and walking bring benefits such as increased fitness, reduced obesity, social connectedness, and reductions in exposure to vehicle fumes. Vegetables grown in urban gardens reduce 'carbon footprints', while helping to secure (fresh) local food supplies.

An estimation of these potential health 'co-benefits' should be included in national health-risk assessments, and factored into cost estimates to provide more accurate analysis of costs. Delivering the positive message about the incidental social benefits of climate change mitigation also helps to highlight the central relevance of population health considerations in policymaking in general.

Meanwhile, many climate-adaptive strategies simply involve boosting public health capacity and action, which brings its own direct health rewards, and so constitute a 'no regrets' policy. Priority strategies may include taking action – often inter-sectoral action. Examples include:

1. Reducing local air pollution, especially the volatile organic compounds that are precursors for the temperature-sensitive formation of ozone
2. Reducing diarrhoeal disease by improving food safety, drinking water, and sanitation
3. Reducing the prevalence of cardiovascular and chronic respiratory diseases, major sources of heat-wave vulnerability
4. Improving housing design with insulation, mosquito-proofing, etc.
5. Improving the monitoring and control of vector species
6. Improving food availability and equity, thereby reducing food insecurity
7. Securing supplies of freshwater, to avert future shortage (health risks) and conflict.

Challenges for national government

Climate change will affect all countries. Under the United Nation's Framework Convention on Climate Change of 1992, nations are required to carry out formal assessments of the risk to their population's health posed by global climate change (WHO n.d.). This can only be achieved with support for (and collaboration in) research. Much of the research is needed at the local level, to identify climate-related risks and differential vulnerabilities, and will require collaboration from individuals and agencies within the health care system. International cooperation, financial assistance, and skills transfer are needed.

Public education and training of professionals and community leaders will assist reorientation to low-carbon economies and mainstreaming climate change adaptation. The major task globally is advocacy of rapid and substantial climate change mitigation. The fact that climate change poses risks to health is a potentially powerful message for inclusion in the wider policy discourse. Health professionals have the opportunity, and responsibility, to help ensure a fully informed and motivated community and polity.

Conclusion

Climate change impacts on physical and biotic systems have already been widely observed. The evidence for health impacts, studied against the much more complex and noisy background of human culture and behaviour, is as yet less definite – although suggestive evidence is now emerging, and the expectation of future, greater, health impacts is unarguable.

Climate science models predict that changing climate will deliver both health benefits and harms, but mostly harms, as global temperatures rise between 2 °C and 4.5 °C by 2100. Vulnerability to these changes will depend upon the nature of the local geography and new climate, and will be moderated by the underlying health and well-being of the population, existing infrastructure and governance, and adaptive capacity.

As a species, our adaptive capacity is evident in the extreme diversity in environments inhabited by humans: jungles, deserts, small islands, frozen lands, and mega-cities. Climate change portends challenges to human habitat on a scale not previously encountered. The long-term health and well-being of populations depends on the continued stability and functioning of the biosphere's ecological and physical systems. With good reason, these are referred to as 'life-support systems'. The world's climate system is an integral part of this complex of life-supporting processes, one of many large natural systems that are now coming under pressure from the increasing weight of human numbers and economic activities.

We need, today, a new solidarity around the concept of climate justice, and decisive action to reduce GHG emissions to secure our future.

The health sector should have engaged earlier and more vigorously in this crucial international and national topic. The public health sector must become educated about climate change and its local manifestations, likely health and social impacts of these, and identify vulnerabilities. Adaptation strategies should build public health capacity to boost resilience of populations, especially those who are most vulnerable. Wealthy countries, while attending to their own internal needs, must assist countries in need. Climate change is a call to action as challenging times are ahead for public health, a time for compassion and humanitarianism on personal, regional, and international scales.

Notes

1 Reinsurance underpins the global insurance system, by insuring insurance companies. The effect is to spread risk across all lines of reinsurance business and many geographical regions.
2 For further reading on this issue: World Health Organization and UNICEF (2006) *Meeting the MDG Drinking Water and Sanitation Target: The Urban and Rural Challenge of the Decade*, available at http://www.who.int/water_sanitation_health/monitoring/jmpfinal.pdf (accessed 19 April 2010).

References

Berry, H.L., Kelly, B.J., Hanigan, I.C., Coates, J.H., McMichael, A.J., Welsh, J.A., and Kjellstrom, T. (2008) *Garnaut Climate Change Review: Rural Mental Health Impacts of Climate Change*, Canberra: The Australian National University.

Butler, C.D. (2009) 'Food Security in the Asia-Pacific: Climate Change, Phosphorus, Ozone and Other Environmental Challenges', *Asia Pacific Journal of Clinical Nutrition*, 18: 590–7.

Dear, K., Ranmuthugala, G., Kjellstrom, T., Skinner, C., and Hanigan, I. (2005) 'Effects of Temperature and Ozone on Daily Mortality during the August 2003 Heat Wave in France', *Archives of Environmental & Occupational Health*, 60: 205–12.

Ebi, K.L., Balbus, J., Kinney, P.L., Lipp, E., Mills, D., O'Neill, M.S., and Wilson, M. (2008) 'Effects of Global Change on Human Health', in J.L. Gamble, K.L. Ebi, F.G. Sussman, and T.J. Wilbanks (eds) *Analyses of the Effects of Global Change on Human Health and Welfare and Human Systems: Synthesis and Assessment Product 4.6*, Washington, DC: US Environmental Protection Agency.

FAO (Food and Agriculture Organization of the United Nations) (2008) 'Climate-Related Transboundry Pests and Diseases', technical background document from the expert consultation in 'Climate Change, Energy and Food Conference', 3–5 June. Rome: FAO.

FAO (Food and Agriculture Organization of the United Nations) (2009) *Climate Change: Implications for Food Safety*, Rome: FAO.

Fritze, J.G., Blashki, G.A., Burke, S., and Wiseman, J. (2008) 'Hope, Despair and Transformation: Climate Change and the Promotion of Mental Health and Wellbeing', *International Journal of Mental Health Systems*, 2: 13.

FSN Forum (Food Security and Nutrition Forum) (2008) 'GLOBAL: Food Crisis could Worsen, Warns FAO' (media release), Johannesburg: Global Forum on Food Security and Nutrition, UN Food and Agriculture Organization (FAO).

GHF (Global Humanitarian Forum) (2009) *Human Impact Report: Climate Change – The Anatomy of a Silent Crisis*, Geneva: Global Humanitarian Forum.

Homer, C.S.E., Hanna, E.G., and McMichael, A.J. (2009) 'Climate Change Threatens the Achievement of the Millennium Development Goal for Maternal Health', *Midwifery*, 25: 606–12.

IPCC (Intergovernmental Panel on Climate Change) (2001) *Climate Change 2001: Impacts, Adaptation and Vulnerability*, report of Working Group II of the Intergovernmental Panel on Climate Change, ed. McCarthy J.J., Canziani, O.F., Leary, N.A., Dokken, D.J., and White, K.S., Cambridge, UK: IPCC.

IPCC (Intergovernmental Panel on Climate Change) (2007a) *Climate Change 2007: Impacts, Adaptation and Vulnerability*, contribution of Working Group II to the Fourth Assessment Report of the Intergovernmental Panel on Climate Change, ed. M.L. Parry, O.F. Canziaani, J.P. Palutikof, P.J. van der Linden, and C.E. Hanson, Cambridge: IPCC.

IPCC (Intergovernmental Panel on Climate Change) (2007b) *Climate Change 2007: Synthesis Report*, contribution of Working Groups I, II and III to the Fourth Assessment Report of the Intergovernmental Panel on Climate Change, ed. R.K. Pachauri and A.E. Reisinger, Geneva, Switzerland: IPCC.

Johnston, F.H., Hanigan, I.C., and Bowman, D.M.J.S (2009) 'Pollen Loads and Allergic Rhinitis in Darwin, Australia: A Potential Health Outcome of the Grass-Fire Cycle', *EcoHealth*, 6 (1): 99–108.

Kjellstrom, T. (2009) 'Climate Change, Direct Heat Exposure, Health and Well-Being in Low and Middle-Income Countries', *Global Health Action*, available at http://www.globalhealthaction.net/index.php/gha/article/viewArticle/1958/2183 (accessed 7 September 2010).

McMichael, A.J., Campbell-Lendrum, D.H., Corvalan, C.F., and Ebi, K.L. (eds) (2003) *Climate Change and Human Health – Risks and Responses*, Geneva: World Health Organization, World Meteorology Organisation, and United Nations Environment Programme.

McMichael, A.J., Friel, S., Nyong, A., and Corvalan, C. (2008) 'Global Environmental Change and Health: Impacts, Inequalities, and the Health Sector', *British Medical Journal*, 336: 191–4.

Müller, C. (2009) 'Climate Change Impact on Sub-Saharan Africa? An Overview and Analysis of Scenarios and Models', discussion paper, Bonn: Deutsches Institut für Entwicklungspolitik.

Munich Re (2009) *Topics Geo. Natural Catastrophes 2008: Analyses, Assessments, Positions*, Munich: Munich Re, available at http://www.munichre.com/publications/302-06081_en.pdf (accessed 7 September 2010).

Noyesa, P.D., Mcelweea, M.K., Millera, H.D., Clarka, B.W., Van Tiema, L.A., Walcotta, K.C., Erwina, K.N., and Levina, E.D. (2009) 'The Toxicology of Climate Change: Environmental Contaminants in a Warming World', *Environment International*, 35: 971–86.

OXFAM (2009) *Suffering the Science: Climate Change, People, and Poverty*, Copenhagen: Oxfam International.

Patel, V. (2008) *Mental Health in the Developing World: Time for Innovative Thinking*, London: London School of Hygiene & Tropical Medicine.

Rahmstorf, S. (2009) 'Sea Level Rise', United Nations Climate Change Conference, 10 March, Copenhagen.

Richardson, K., Steffen, W., Schellnhuber H.J., Alcamo, J., Barker, T., Kammen, D.M., Leemans, R., Liverman, D., Munasinghe, M., Osman-Elasha, B., Stern, N., and Wæver, O. (2009) *Synthesis Report from Climate Change: Global Risks, Challenges & Decisions*, Copenhagen: University of Copenhagen.

UNDP (United Nations Development Programme) (2007) *Human Development Report 2007/2008. Fighting Climate Change: Human Solidarity in a Divided World*, New York: United Nations Development Programme.

UNEP (United Nations Environment Programme) and GRID-Arendal (2009) *Environmental Food Crisis: Rapid Response Assessments*, Geneva: UNEP.

UNHCR (United Nations High Commissioner for Refugees) (2009) 'Forced Displacement in the Context of Climate Change: Challenges for States Under International Law', submission to the 6th session of the Ad Hoc Working Group on Long-Term Cooperative Action under the Convention Bonn: Office of the United Nations High Commissioner for Refugees, Norwegian Refugee Council, Secretary General on the Human Rights of Internally Displaced Persons, United Nations University.

Weart, S.R. (2003) *The Discovery of Global Warming*, Cambridge, MA: Harvard University Press.

WHO (World Health Organization) (2009) *National Assessments of Health Impacts of Climate Changes*, available at http://www.who.int/globalchange/climate/summary/en/index8.html (accessed 13 August 2009), Geneva: WHO.

WHO and UNICEF Joint Monitoring Programme for Water Supply and Sanitation (2006) *Meeting the MDG Drinking Water and Sanitation Target: The Urban and Rural Challenge of the Decade*, Geneva and New York: WHO and UNICEF.

14

Water and Health

Fragile Sources

Peter G. McCornick and John Pasch

Introduction

Water is a foundational resource for development and is essential for sustaining life. The world's population must have adequate supply to survive and thrive. The human body relies on a consistent supply of water to function; equally important is human beings' need for water to grow food and support adequate nutrition. Approximately 80 per cent of water use worldwide is for agriculture, and although there are opportunities to conserve water in this sector and transfer it for higher-value uses (such as drinking water), the absolute demand from agriculture is projected to increase, a fact of critical importance for the world's future food supply.

Renewable fresh water per capita is a basic measure of the relative water scarcity of a country or a basin (Falkenmark and Widstrand 1992). If a country has between 1,000 and 1,700 cubic metres (m^3) of water per capita per annum, it is considered to be *water-stressed*; if it has less than 1,000 m^3/capita/annum but more than 500 m^3/capita/annum, it is considered *water-scarce*, and thus presents a danger to human health and a threat to a country's economic development. A country with less than 500 m^3/capita/annum is considered *absolutely water-scarce*. The extent to which a country's capacity to meet the water needs of its population and economy depends on a number of factors, particularly its financial capacity to develop the available water resources and make water available where it is required. Many countries in sub-Saharan Africa and certain areas of South Asia do not have the financial means to meet the basic water needs of a large portion of their population, and thus are considered economically water-scarce (de Fraiture *et al.* 2007).

Millions of people die each year from diseases brought on by poor water quality, water shortages, or floods. The World Health Organization (WHO) estimates that one-tenth of the global disease burden could be prevented by improving water supply, sanitation, hygiene, and management of water resources (Pruss-Ustun *et al.* 2008). It is estimated that returns on investment in water supply, sanitation, and hygiene are fourfold, sevenfold, and ninefold, respectively (Hutton *et al.* 2007). For example, in rural parts of sub-Saharan Africa, the reduction of diarrhoeal diseases from the introduction of an improved water source, integrated with appropriate sanitation and hygiene practices, reduces the time lost from productive activities and the burden of caring for the sick, which often falls on the girls in the household. While significant progress has been made towards addressing the challenge of providing basic water access, there are still nearly 1 billion people who lack convenient access to safe water, most of them in sub-Saharan Africa and South and East Asia (WHO and UNICEF 2008a). Furthermore, other demands and pressures on water resources – including from agriculture, industry, increasing pollution loads, and the effects of climate change – and the inherent interconnectivity of the resource will further stress existing water supplies, and make finding new, clean sources increasingly challenging.

According to De Fraiture *et al.* (2007), around one-third of the world's population was already experiencing water scarcity by the year 2000, with the vast majority being in the drier basins of the developing world.

Even in relatively water-abundant regions, water availability changes seasonally, and unless communities have the capacity to store water, they can be faced with acute water shortages on an annual basis. For example, in the wetter parts of the highlands of Ethiopia, most of the rain falls in a three- to four-month period. While community-level rainwater harvesting systems can extend the period in which water is available for a few more months, this is often not sufficient for the full year.

Water supply and demand: implications for health

In water-rich areas, supply is greater than demand, with competition between different water uses low, and water allocation and management policy typically not well-developed as the communities rarely experience shortages. Freshwater resources are often adequate to meet all major demands (domestic, agricultural, and industrial), as illustrated in Figure 14.1. This limits the health-related risks faced by populations. In contrast, in regions that are approaching water scarcity, demand often exceeds supply, resulting in stiff competition for limited resources and sometimes yielding complex policy approaches and management schemes. Ultimately, however, as water supply becomes relatively more scarce (generally driven by increasing population and economic growth), competition increases, and the available supplies are transferred from lower- to higher-value uses, including those necessary to meet the immediate needs of the population. This can be planned for, but in many cases it happens in an unplanned manner as decisions regarding development do not account for the interconnectivity of the water resources. For instance, a decision to develop groundwater to improve water supply to a growing urban area does not account for the fact that the groundwater feeds springs downstream that are used for agriculture. The loss of freshwater for certain uses can mean that certain water-dependent systems, such as agricultural production, become unsustainable. In some such cases, tapping marginal water resources, such as wastewater or brackish groundwater, are viable alternative sources for agricultural or industrial uses and can be used to offset the freshwater

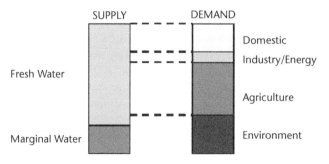

Figure 14.1   Balancing supply and demand in a water-rich region

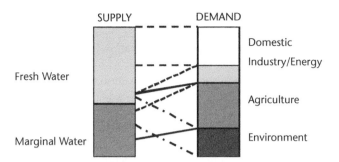

Figure 14.2   Balancing supply and demand in a water-scarce region

used elsewhere. Figure 14.2 illustrates a balance of water supply and demand in an area where available freshwater resources are less than the total demand. In this illustrative case, marginal resources are used to supplement freshwater resources and meet agricultural demand (thus sustaining the capacity of the agricultural sector to contribute to food security and nutritional needs, and the contribution of agriculture to the economy). Freshwater resources are prioritised for domestic and industrial applications in this example.

Across the globe, areas such the Middle East and North Africa, the southwestern United States, northern China, and southern India are trending toward greater water scarcity. The challenge faced by water resource managers to maintain the balance between supply and demand is thus increasing as pressures on resources mount within countries and river basins. These pressures are the result of:

- Demographic Growth – A continuously growing global population increases demand for water supply (potable and agricultural) in order to stay healthy. While population growth rates have been declining since their peak in the early 1960s, a population growth of greater than 1 per cent per year persists, placing a tremendous strain on limited water resources, especially in water-scarce regions.
- Water Quality Degradation – Competition for water resources results in decreasing quality of available water over time. As resources are withdrawn from the water cycle for domestic, industrial, agricultural, and other uses with greater frequency and volume, the loss of freshwater to the natural system can increase the concentration of natural contaminants, such as salt. Furthermore, increasing usage of the water supply results in greater volumes of wastewater, which in turn introduces more pollutants back into the environment.

While the portion of the overall water supply needed to meet basic domestic water demands (e.g. drinking, bathing, cleaning, washing) is relatively small, the requirement for an assured quantity and high quality of supply within the context of the above new water resource challenges is not a straightforward problem.

Compounding the situation, the present and potential future impacts of climate change are introducing new pressures and challenges for water resource managers and creating additional risks of negative health impacts from the increasingly limited and poor-quality global water supply (WHO 2009). These added pressures include:

- Increased Variability of Availability – Seasonal and geographic shifts (such as more intense rainstorms or more protracted droughts) introduce instability in water resource planning approaches. In the past, such approaches have relied on historical data to determine the future availability of water resources, but likely effects of climate change make this less predictable. Anticipated climate change scenarios include a greater frequency and magnitude of extreme climatic events (e.g. heavy precipitation and drought). With the majority of annual precipitation likely to be concentrated in several storm events, many areas will be vulnerable to seasonal oscillation between flood and drought conditions. These in turn will have potential impacts on population health as both conditions make accessing clean drinking water more challenging.

- Change in Water Requirements – Change in climatic conditions can have significant effects on crop water demand. Increased temperatures resulting from climate change will undoubtedly result in higher crop water requirements due to greater evapotranspiration.[1] Shortages of water for agriculture threaten food security, which has significant implications for the nutrition of local populations.

- Saltwater Intrusion – Rising sea levels, as a result of global climate change, will result in loss of freshwater resources (e.g. drinking water) due to saltwater intrusion in some areas. Regions such as the coastal areas of Bangladesh are at risk from such intrusion.

The impact of these water resource pressures on human health is potentially grave. A future where scarcity is common and demand is increased, without appropriate actions to improve management, will inevitably lead to severe health impacts due to poor water quality and poor nutrition. These impacts may be crippling to development in certain geographic areas such as sub-Saharan Africa and certain parts of South Asia unless responsive policy mechanisms and management approaches are introduced, along with prudent development of water-related infrastructure and focused investment in key technological advances (e.g. energy-efficient desalination of brackish water).

Case study: Jordan

In order to inform planning and prepare a water management framework that meets present needs, is responsive to the future requirements, considers the major changes that are likely to occur in water resources due to the interplay of other sectors, and is resilient to the uncertainty brought on by climate change, it is informative to look to lessons and experiences from regions that are presently water-scarce and that experience significant seasonal variability in precipitation amounts. The specific case of Jordan offers relevant climate, resource, and demand conditions, and important lessons learned that are informative for climate change adaptation. Such lessons are critical for those regions which must address such water-related realities in the coming years if they are to protect their population's health and well-being.

Jordan

At less than 150 m^3/capita of renewable freshwater per annum, the Hashemite Kingdom of Jordan is extremely water-scarce. It is projected to fall below 100 m^3/capita/annum before 2025. Approximately 80 per cent of the population lives in the Amman-Zarqa basin (see Figure 14.3). Water supplies for domestic and industrial use are sourced from the Yarmook River in the Jordan Valley (King Abdullah Canal), aquifers in the highlands of the Amman-Zarqa and Azraq basins, and recently developed brackish springs (Zara-Ma'in) near the Dead Sea. Presently the daily per capita water supply in the Amman-Zarqa urban area is less than 100 litres per day, which is around one-fourth of the average daily per capita domestic water supply in the US (USGS 2009).

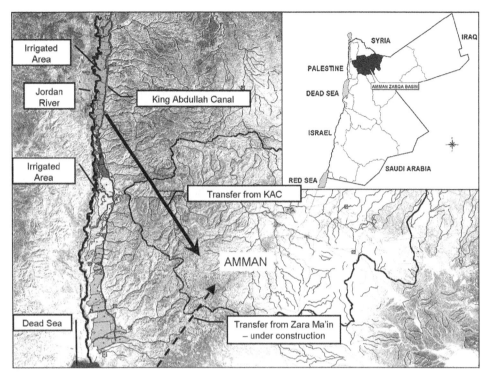

Figure 14.3 Sources of water supply for the Amman-Zarqa urban areas, and for the irrigated areas of the Jordan Valley

As the country has become more water-scarce, the portion of the available water supply going to meet the population's domestic and industrial demands has increased, while the quantity of freshwater used in agriculture has declined. Concurrently, the volume of domestic wastewater being generated from urban areas has increased, and the groundwater (which was freshwater) in the highlands, which is being over-pumped to meet the demands of the urban areas, has become increasingly brackish. As a result of these changes, the wastewater collected by the conventional sewer system and treated before being discharged into the Zarqa River, has gradually replaced fresh-water as the dominant source of water for irrigated agriculture in two-thirds of the Jordan Valley.

In spite of the scarcity of resources, Jordan has maintained a very high rate of access for its population to an improved drinking water supply. According to the Joint Monitoring Programme's (JMP) July 2008 Jordan country report (WHO and UNICEF 2008b), 99 per cent of Jordanians have access to an improved water source. Further, nearly 100 per cent of urban Jordanians and over 80 per cent of rural Jordanians have a piped water supply. Access to improved sanitation is also generally good in Jordan. The JMP's Jordan country report states that approximately 88 per cent of urban residents and 71 per cent of rural residents have access to improved sanitation. However, when the data are disaggregated, it reveals that approximately two-thirds of urban residents are connected to a sewer system, while less than 5 per cent of rural residents have sewer connections. The remainder use some form of household-level sanitation, such as systems based on septic tanks.

Infant mortality due to diarrhoeal diseases is 11 per cent (of all infant deaths), which is below the regional average of 15 per cent. Total deaths from diarrhoeal disease in Jordan in 2002 were less than 1,000. Clearly, Jordan has adapted to changes in water quality and availability in order to maintain a good supply of freshwater for domestic use under particularly challenging water supply conditions. That said, the country remains vulnerable to relatively moderate changes in the availability of water supply, whether it be due to competition from neighbouring countries, the effects of climate change, or other factors.

In urban areas, most water-related health issues are addressed with conventional treatment[2] of water supply. Because of over-abstraction, however, salinity levels in the groundwater from a number of wells in the Amman-Zarqa basin now exceed the 500 mg/litre level recommended by the WHO and must be blended with other sources of water to attain salinity levels low enough to meet this basic drinking water standard.

Given the acuteness of water scarcity in the Amman-Zarqa basin and the relative dominance of treated wastewater in the overall water balance, the wastewater management system is particularly important for population health, not only from the perspective of pollution control, but also for recognising wastewater as a resource. In the case of Amman-Zarqa, the wastewater management system has included expanding the number of households connected to the sewer system, enhancing the sewer system itself, developing rigorous systems to prevent industrial contaminants from entering the domestic wastewater system, and constructing new wastewater management facilities.

The absence of effective wastewater management systems also leads to health risks for the local population. The groundwater underlying the urban areas of the basin is generally contaminated by domestic and industrial wastewater, due in part to the households that are not connected to the sewer systems. These same sources, together with the smaller communities not connected to wastewater management facilities, are responsible for the elevated levels of faecal coliforms (a leading cause of diarrhoeal disease) in the Zarqa River. Fortunately, there are no diversions for domestic water supplies downstream (which protects the population from an unsafe domestic water supply). However, this contaminated water does pose health risks for the field workers exposed to the water and to those in the local population likely to consume raw vegetables which have been contaminated in the fields by the raw water. As with the water supply and wastewater management systems, Jordan has had the economic and technical capacity to evolve the management of treated wastewater in the agricultural sector.

After the development of a new national water strategy in 1997, Jordan developed a set of policies aimed at managing the country's scarce water resources. The resultant policies included improving groundwater management and managing wastewater as a resource, while simultaneously protecting the public's health and the environment. Since these policies were developed, Jordan has been progressively implementing and revising the initial policies. Opportunities for developing new freshwater resources are particularly limited, expensive to develop, and come with high operating costs, especially energy costs. This requires that the country makes careful decisions regarding the management of the resource.

General insights

While the case of Jordan is unique, there are a number of broader lessons that can be drawn from this situation and experience elsewhere in the world.

Quality is value

Given the increasing pressure on the resource and the interconnectivity among users, securing and maintaining the quality of water supply is paramount for maintaining a healthy population.

Setting aside particular national and local anomalies, including political realities, the highest-quality supplies of water are generally reserved for potable use. In most countries, national water policies assign domestic water supply as the highest priority. Industrial and agricultural water demands are then expected to be met with less, and in water-scarce areas, poorer-quality water, including marginal-quality supplies. Where marginal-quality resources are likely to be a viable source for sectors other than domestic water supply, care needs to be taken to consider the overall water system, including management of wastewater. Research, policy development, and strategic investments in infrastructure to support the use of marginal-quality water resources for a range of appropriate uses will expand the available supply and increase reliability of water within a country to maintain population health.

Storage is security

Increasing water storage can effectively reduce vulnerability to seasonal fluctuations in supply. Storage should be considered at all levels (household, community, river basin, and groundwater) and designed appropriately and consistently with anticipated changes in climate and hydrologic regime. In Jordan, the western US, and other water-scarce regions of the world, the careful balance maintained between supply and demand has fostered an appreciation for storage as security – much like we view a savings account in our personal financial dealings. In more water-rich regions, water storage has often been forgone out of consideration for the high environmental costs of storage facilities and management schemes. In regions of advancing water scarcity, the cost and benefits between storage schemes and environmental impacts should be reevaluated in terms of the changing conditions described above.

Wastewater as a resource

While much of the developing world does not have the same capacity to manage wastewater as Jordan, there is increasing emphasis on improving health conditions by expanding access to improved sanitation. There are interventions that are effective from a health perspective, such as latrines and septic systems, which do not require connections to a comprehensive wastewater management system. These approaches are usually significantly less expensive and easier to develop at the community level. However, the adoption of latrines and septic systems across a wide scale in urban areas and when combined with improved domestic water supply (i.e. increased volumes) does pose challenges in protecting groundwater and local surface water resources. This contamination of the water resources impacts the available local water supplies, especially where wastewater treatment is not available. Given this, especially where water resources are scarce, the strategic management of wastewater needs to be carefully considered. This might entail, for instance, planning for the future development of sewer systems or ensuring that industrial wastes remain separate from domestic wastewater.

Treatment is health

The degrading quality of water resources around the globe is rapidly becoming an issue of equal or greater importance than water scarcity. Potable raw water resources are extremely rare and the need for complex treatment processes in order to provide safe water is increasing. With continued global changes, we can expect a future where the need and responsibility for water treatment stretches from the government to the individual. To prevent disease, many regions will need to continue to require treatment of water at the household level. In water-scarce regions, improved technologies and efficiencies in desalination processes will make this financially viable where suitable resources are available, although their sustainability in developing countries will remain an obstacle to their adoption. There is a clear and immediate need to develop less costly and more accessible technology for drinking water treatment. Accompanying technology innovation, there will also be a need to change behaviour so that household water treatment is a standard practice.

Conclusions

Future changes in the socio-economic needs and climate conditions in regions around the world will undoubtedly have deep local, regional, and global impacts on the availability and quality of water supply. These in turn have the potential to severely and negatively affect human health. Increasing demands for food, compounded by changing precipitation patterns, and in some cases, increasing temperatures, will increase the demand for water in the agricultural sector. Over-pumping and rising sea levels will marginalise near-shore groundwater resources due to saltwater intrusion, impacting the availability of water for domestic use. In summary, water supplies will be scarcer and less reliable. These tenuous and unpredictable conditions are similar to those already faced by water-scarce countries such as Jordan. Jordan's successful policy and technology response to water resource management yields important insights that will be helpful to national and regional efforts to meet these challenges.

Notes

1 The loss of water to the atmosphere by the combination of transpiration from plants and evaporation from the soil surface.
2 Depending on the quality of the source water, this is some combination of filtration, flocculation (the process by which smaller particles are combined into large particles and thereby settle out), sedimentation, and disinfection.

References

Falkenmark, M. and Widstrand, C. (1992) 'Population and water resources: A delicate balance', *Population Bulletin*, 47(3): 1–36.
de Fraiture, C., Wichelns, D., Rockstrom, J., and Kemp-Benedict, E. (2007) 'Looking ahead to 2050: Scenarios of alternative investment approaches', in D. Molden (ed.), *Water for Food, Water for Life: A Comprehensive Assessment of Water Management in Agriculture*, London: Earthscan, and Colombo: International Water Management Institute.
Hutton, G., Haller, L., and Bartram, J. (2007) 'Economic and Health Effects of Increasing Coverage of Low Cost Household Drinking Water Supply and Sanitation Interventions to Countries Off-Track to Meet MDG Target 10', Geneva: World Health Organization, available at www.who.int/water_sanitation_health/economic/mdg10_offtrack.pdf (accessed 31 August 2010).
Pruss-Ustun, A., Bos, R., Gore, F., and Bartram, J. (2008) *Safer Water, Better Health: Cost, Benefits and Sustainability of Interventions to Protect and Promote Health*, Geneva: World Health Organization.
USGS (United States Geological Survey) (2009) *Estimated Use of Water in the United States in 2005: US Geological Survey Circular 1344*, Reston, VA: US Department of the Interior and USGS.
WHO (World Health Organization) (2009) *Vision 2030: The Resilience of Water Supply and Sanitation in the Face of Climate Change*, Geneva: WHO.
WHO (World Health Organization) and UNICEF (United Nations Children's Health Fund) (2008a) *World Health Organization and United Nations Children's Fund Joint Monitoring Programme for*

Water Supply and Sanitation (JMP). *Progress on Drinking Water and Sanitation: Special Focus on Sanitation*, New York: UNICEF, and Geneva: WHO.

WHO (World Health Organization) and UNICEF (United Nations Children's Health Fund) (2008b) *World Health Organization and United Nations Children's Fund Joint Monitoring Programme for Water Supply and Sanitation (JMP)*. *Coverage Estimates: Jordan, Improved Drinking Water and Improved Sanitation*, New York: UNICEF, and Geneva: WHO.

15

Double Jeopardy

Vulnerable Children and the Possible Global Lead Poisoning/Infectious Disease Syndemic

Merrill Singer

Introduction

Worldwide estimates suggest that 25 to 33 per cent of the global burden of disease is attributable to environmental factors, while infectious diseases are the actual leading cause of death (Clark 2001). Although these two sources of human morbidity and mortality have been studied extensively, far less attention has been paid to the ways in which they may interact, and thereby exacerbate their total adverse impact on human health. This chapter addresses this gap by examining a potential adverse interaction between lead poisoning and infectious disease.

In terms of environmental factors, lead is among the best-known threats to health. An indestructible metal that accumulates in the body, lead has been called 'the mother of all industrial poisons ... the paradigmatic toxin [linking] industrial and environmental disease' (Markowitz and Rosner 2002: 137). While not a xenobiotic, and in use in human communities for over 5,000 years, lead levels in inhabited areas began to mount dramatically during the Industrial Revolution (Davidson and Rabinowitz 1992).

Children are at greatest risk for lead poisoning because of dietary, behavioural, and developmental factors. First, children do not consume enough food to slow absorption of lead, and because of inadequate or imbalanced diets their bodies often do not receive enough iron and calcium. Consequently, 30 to 70 per cent of ingested lead reaches a child's digestive tract compared to only 11 per cent for adults. Secondly, children absorb as much as 50 per cent of inhaled lead (primarily from paint dust or, in some parts of the world, leaded gas exhaust), significantly more than adults, and tend to spend more time close to the ground where lead dust accumulates. Finally, young children (during the first three years of life) are especially vulnerable because their rapidly developing nervous systems are highly sensitive to the toxic effects of lead exposure (CDC 1991).

Although no lead level is considered safe – and the definition of childhood lead poisoning has been revised downward four times in recent years – an elevated blood lead level (BLL) in children is now defined by the Centers for Disease Control and Prevention (CDC) (1997) as ≥10 μg/dL (10 micrograms of lead per one-tenth litre of blood).

Globally, this primarily anthropogenic environmental threat is of special importance in developing nations, given the multiple sites of intensive lead exposure in children that have been identified, such as Tiangying, China, La Oroya, Peru, Dzerzhink, Russia, and Labwe, Zambia (Blacksmith Institute 2007). It is estimated that worldwide, 120 million people are currently being overexposed to lead, which, as Gottesfeld notes, is 'three times the number infected by HIV/AIDS. And this problem is going largely unnoticed under the radar screen' (quoted in Public Radio International 2009).

The health-related consequences of lead exposure include the disruption of three biological processes: (1) molecular interactions, (2) inter-cell signaling, and (3) cell functioning, which result in nervous system damage, decreased IQ, decreased growth, sterility, hyperactivity, impaired hearing, and seizures. In addition, as will be discussed in this chapter, there is growing, if incomplete, evidence of the adverse impact of lead on the immune system, and of a possible biological link between exposure to lead and heightened rates of infection, especially among children.

The nature and distribution of lead risk

Lead poisoning in children has been acknowledged as a significant public health issue in developed nations for only about 40 years. Exposure includes inhalation of contaminated air, breathing or ingesting contaminated dust and soil, drinking water delivered by lead and lead-soldered pipes, and eating food made in leaded containers. Despite decades of environmental release and build-up of lead, it is possible to take measures that lower blood lead in children. In the United States, for example, median BLLs in children under five years declined 89 per cent from 1976 to 2004, primarily because of the phase-out of leaded gasoline (EPA 2008). However, such efforts have not been adequate to eliminate lead exposure. Overall, the CDC estimates that one in 22 children in the United States have elevated BLLs (Meyer *et al.* 2003), and associated annual health care costs have been estimated to be over $40 billion, compared to less than $1 billion for childhood cancer (Landrigan *et al.* 2002).

Older housing stock that retains lead-based paint remains one of several significant sources of exposure. It is estimated that 75 per cent of homes built before 1978 contain lead-based paint and that 24 million US housing units, disproportionately in the north-east and midwest, are affected (Woolf *et al.* 2007). Despite warnings about the potential dangers of lead-based paint dating to the early twentieth century, companies continued to manufacture and sell this 'killer commodity' (Singer and Baer 2008) until well past 1940 (Rabin 1989). Older housing is disproportionately occupied by poor and socially marginalised populations. According to the US National Health and Nutrition Examination Survey (NHANES) Ill-Phase 2 study report, 8 per cent of impoverished children are lead poisoned, compared to 1 per cent of children from high-income families (CDC 1991).

In developing countries, lead poisoning remains one of the major environmental diseases found among children. The problem is more severe in developing nations because of limited attention historically to environmental health risks in light of infectious, nutritional, and other disease-related health burdens; inadequately controlled industrial emissions; incomplete enforcement of health safety protections; sale of lead-based commercial products; unregulated cottage industries; traditional cultural practices (e.g. leaded folk medicines, cosmetics, and ceramic glazes); the synergistic effects of dietary deficiencies; and inadequate prevention and treatment capacity.

The United Nations Children's Fund (UNICEF) (1997) estimates that 15–18 million children in developing countries suffer from permanent brain damage due to lead poisoning, and millions more are regularly exposed to environmental lead. Exemplary of contaminated areas is the shantytown known as Flammable (actual name) on the southeastern border of

Buenos Aires, Argentina; an urban slum comprised of 5,000 people. Residents are exposed to toxins from the surrounding petrochemical compound. Once used as a free dumping zone for industrial waste, the ground beneath the community is believed to be heavily polluted. Illegal dumping continues into the present and contributes to the 'nauseating stench' (Auyero and Swistun 2007: 133) that permeates the air locally. Tests show that the children in Flammable are routinely exposed to various industrial chemicals. As Auyero and Swistun point out, however, it is the lead in their bodies that most distinguishes the children of Flammable from those in other poor neighbourhoods:

> Fifty percent of the children tested in this neighborhood had higher-than-normal blood levels of lead (against 17% in the control population) …. [T]he study [also] found lower-than-average IQ among Flammable children and a higher percentage of neurobehavioural problems … Flammable children also reported more dermatological problems (eye irritation, skin infections, eruptions, and allergies), respiratory problems (coughs and broncospasms), neurological problems (hyperactivity) and sore throats and headaches.
>
> (2007: 134)

Several studies of urban children in Nigeria also have found significant BLLs. A study of children in three Nigerian cities by Nriagu *et al.* (2008), which found high BLLs, linked lead exposure to several sources including 'homegrown' food, a needed practice in light of food insecurity. Because lead is deposited in urban soils from multiple sources, as well as from manure and fertiliser used by urban farmers, food plants grown in Nigerian cities accumulate high concentrations of lead (Eriyamremu *et al.* 2005).

Elsewhere, the source of lead pollution is more concentrated at local occupation sites. In August 1987, for example, public health officials in Jamaica learned that 19 of 22 (86 per cent) recently hospitalised children with lead poisoning in the capital city of Kingston lived near cottage factories in residential areas that were involved in automobile battery repair (CDC 1989). In response, the Jamaican Ministry of Health sponsored an assessment of the prevalence and causes of lead absorption, which found that repair shops commonly employ a few workers but share a yard with several households, many with children (Matte *et al.* 1989). Most are not subject to environmental monitoring, nor are workers informed about risks. Comparison of households exposed to lead in battery repair shops to control households found elevated BLLs in repair shop-exposed children less than 12 years of age, 43 per cent of whom had levels higher than 70 μg/dl. By contrast, in the control households, BLLs were significantly lower, with less than 10 per cent of subjects exhibiting elevated lead levels. Examples like this suggest the growing role of globalisation, and the flow of materials and people in exposure to lead (Fassin and Naudé 2004; Handley *et al.* 2007).

While international efforts have focused on removing lead from gasoline, this commodity continues to be a source of exposure among children in many developing countries (Sharma and Pervez 2003). As Kitman (2000) explains, blocked by laws in developed countries, the sellers of lead additives focused on markets in the developing world. Internal conflict in developing nations and the relocating of displaced refugees in environmentally risky sites for temporary shelter is another source of exposure. This problem is exemplified by the case of the Roma in Kosovo, in the former nation of Yugoslavia. Before the Balkan conflict (1990–99), the Roma primarily lived in a neighbourhood known as Roma Mahala. This neighbourhood was destroyed during the conflict and the United Nations (UN) constructed two internal displacement camps for homeless Roma families. The camps were located in highly lead-contaminated areas near the

Trepca smelter. Testing found that BLLs were dangerously high (>45 µg/dL) among Roma children under 14 years of age (Brown and Brooks 2007).

As this review suggests, children and some adults in developed and especially developing nations are at risk for lead exposure from multiple sources. Additionally, because of the specific effects of lead on the body, they may be placed at heightened risk for infection.

The environmental role in syndemics

Recently, King *et al.* (2009: 145), in discussing AIDS patients, noted that 'Treating [disadvantaged] persons with multiple diagnoses … is complicated – not only because of [both] independent and synergistic disease processes but also because of disparate access to care, limited or no insurance, and unmet subsistence needs…'. Disease interactions, and the interaction of diseases with social and physical environments, are the two defining features of *syndemics*, which entail the concentration within a population and deleterious interface of two or more diseases or other health conditions, especially as a consequence of social inequity and the unjust exercise of power (Singer 2009). Syndemic research focuses on disease synergies (i.e. impacts of one disease that facilitate the activation, spread, progression, treatment resistance, or damage caused by another) that increase the overall health burden of a population.

Many syndemics are mediated by anthropogenic environmental factors. In the case of the suggested *lead poisoning/infectious disease syndemic*, the likely causal chain involves:

(1) human activities that significantly increase environmental lead in residential, occupational, and other behavioural settings, resulting in
(2) increased exposure and bodily lead levels, especially among children;
(3) consequent symptoms of lead poisoning, including immunosuppression; and
(4) subsequent increase in vulnerability to infection.

The evidence, both animal and human, for syndemic development is described below.

Exploring the lead poisoning/infectious disease syndemic: animal studies

The possibility that lead might damage components of the immune system is not surprising in light of the observation that 'There is probably no biological function and no enzyme activity that is not affected by lead in sufficiently high concentrations' (Hernberg 2000: 252). Yet, as Dietert and Piepenbrink (2006) point out, it is only in recent years that lead has been recognised as belonging among a newly identified category of immunotoxicants. These chemicals and other substances do not directly kill immune cells but rather consequentially shift immune function biochemistry. In particular, lead affects a component of the immune system known as the helper T cell, which comes in two varieties: Th1 and Th2. Each of these produces its own type of cytokine, a hormonal messenger that controls the activity of other immune cells, especially those involved in immune inflammation reactions. As Playfair (2004: 126) explains, each of the 30 or so varieties of cytokine produced by the body has a specific function, such as stimulating immune cells 'to enlarge, to divide, to release antibody, to switch from making IgM to IgG, [immunoglobulin M and G] etc.'. Th1 cytokine triggers a pro-inflammatory response that aids the body in fighting infection by both activating immune defenses and by slowing the flow of blood that would otherwise carry pathogens away from the infected site to new locations. Excessive inflammation, however, is dangerous, as it can harm body tissues. This is where Th2 production is critical, as it triggers an anti-inflammatory response, although excessive production of Th2 weakens the protective functions of inflammation. Consequently, in a healthy body there is a natural balance between Th1 and Th2, allowing sufficient inflammation to effectively fight infection without going overboard and causing injury.

Lead has been found to impact the immune capacity in three ways: (1) elevation of the level of production of the antibody immunoglobulin E (IgE), as well as the creation of Th2 cytokines (such as IL-4), a shift associated with the development of asthma and allergy (Wu *et al.* 2004); (2) suppression of Th1 immune response and the production of Th1 cytokines; and (3) impairment in the functioning of macrophages (an important immune system component), causing a jump in pro-inflammatory cytokine production (e.g. IL-6), which, in turn, heightens the risk of inflammation-related tissue damage while reducing the macrophage's ability to kill bacteria. The extent of these various types of immune system damage is affected by the dose and duration of lead exposure, as well as the life stage and possibly the gender of the affected individual.

Studies with animal populations strongly suggest the potential of a lead poisoning syndemic. In an early study, Gainer (1974) administered lead in the drinking water of male mice beginning at four weeks of age. He found that lead increased the adverse response of the mice to all classes of viruses against which they were tested. He suggested that lead may aggravate viral infection because it represses components of the natural immune response, such as the synthesis of mouse interferon (a type of protein that helps to activate the immune system's protective defenses). In subsequent animal studies, the relationship between BLL and IgE level was established, which, as noted, has relevance to understanding increasing levels of asthma and other allergic reactions.

Animal studies demonstrate that exposure to lead increases susceptibility to viral and bacterial infections (Gupta *et al.* 2002), and suggests there may be decreased resistance to parasites, as well. Based on their research with mice, Listeria, Dyatov, and Lawrence (2002: 477) suggested that 'children with blood Pb [lead] during bacterial infection may exhibit enhanced and prolonged sickness behaviour …'.

Exploring the lead poisioning/infectious disease syndemic: human studies

As with animals, studies with humans affirm that the 'immune system appears to be one of the more sensitive systems to the toxic effects of lead' (Dietert and Piepenbrink 2006: 379). In assessing the immune impact of lead, Anetor and Adeniyi (1998) compared a sample of Nigerian lead industry workers with a matched sample of controls. They found that these workers had significantly higher blood lead levels and were more likely to have a depressed immune status. Similar findings were reported by Heo *et al.* (2004) based on a study of workers in a Korean battery factory. Among children, Li *et al.* (2005) compared age- and gender-matched preschool children from a rural area in Zhejiang Province, China, with high and low blood lead levels, and found a significant reduction in the percentage of CD4+ cells and a significant increase of CD8+ cells in the high-lead group. Both of these specialised white blood cells have immune system functions; while CD4+ cells are helper cells involved in directing the activities of other immune components, including maximising the bactericidal capacity of macrophages, CD8+ cells are directly involved in the killing of body cells that are damaged or infected with pathogens. These differences in cell counts suggest an important alteration in the immune function of lead-exposed young children. Similar findings among adult women exposed to lead in an occupational setting have been reported by Qiao *et al.* (2001).

Overall, recent human studies confirm the findings of earlier animal studies, namely that in humans, lead impacts both T-cell-dependent and macrophage immune functions (Maezawa *et al.*

2004; Sun *et al.* 2003). Furthermore, the findings from human studies parallel those from animal research, with data suggesting that exposure to lead alters the production of cytokines, which in turn shifts the immune system towards a Th2 immune response that 'might contribute to increased susceptibility to pathogenic agents' (Hemdam *et al.* 2005: 75). Finally, existing human research suggests that sufficient exposure to lead impairs macrophage functionality (Dietert and Piepenbrink 2006), further impacting the immune system. Missing from this body of research are actual studies of rates and consequences of infection in children or adults with high BLLs.

Conclusions

Despite considerable evidence from both animal and human studies indicating the immuno-toxicity of lead, and of resulting impairment in immune response to infection – suggesting the possibility of a *lead poisoning/infectious disease syndemic* – there is a paucity of focused clinical and epidemiological studies of the kinds, frequencies, and health outcomes of infection among both children and adults with high blood lead levels. Based on their review of the available evidence on the maternal and child health role of environmental contaminants like lead, Wigle *et al.* (2009: 373–4) emphasise, 'There is a great need for population-based, multidisciplinary and collaborative research on the many relationships supported by inadequate evidence, as these represent major knowledge gaps …'. Additionally, because of the difficulties of extrapolating immune system findings from animals to humans, 'many more data on humans and non-human primates … are necessary and should be on the main line of research' (Neubert *et al.* 2002: 564). Also needed are ethnographic studies that help clarify the social conditions and social structural relations that increase the likelihood of lead exposure, and create, as a result, the potential for syndemic interaction with infection.

References

Anetor, J. and Adeniyi, F. (1998) 'Decreased Immune Status in Nigerian Workers Occupationally Exposed to Lead', *African Journal of Medicine and Medical Science*, 27(3–4): 169–72.

Auyero, J. and Swistun, D. (2007) 'Confused because Exposed: Towards an Ethnography of Environmental Suffering', *Ethnography*, 8(2): 123–44.

Blacksmith Institute (2007) *The World's Ten Most Polluted Places*, New York: Blacksmith Institute.

Brown, M.J., and Brooks, B. (2007) *Recommendations for Preventing Lead Poisoning Among the Internally Displaced Roma Population in Kosovo*, Atlanta, GA: Lead Poisoning Prevention Branch, Centers for Disease Control and Prevention.

CDC (Centers for Disease Control and Prevention) (1989) 'Occupational and Environmental Lead Poisoning Associated with Battery Repair Shops – Jamaica', *MMWR Morbidity and Mortality Weekly Report*, 38(27): 479–81.

CDC (Centers for Disease Control and Prevention) (1991) *Preventing Lead Poisoning in Young Children: A Statement by the Centers for Disease Control*, Atlanta, GA: US Department of Health and Human Services, Public Health Service.

Clark, C. (2001) 'Environmental Wellness', in C. Clark (ed.) *Health Promotion in Communities*, New York: Springer Publishing Company.

Davidson, C. and Rabinowitz, M. (1992) 'Lead in the Environment: From Sources to Human Receptors', in H. Needleman (ed.) *Human Lead Exposure*, Boca Raton, FL: CRC Press.

Dietert, R., Lee, J., Hussain, I. and Piepenbrink, M. (2006) 'Developmental Immunotoxicology of Lead', *Toxicology and Applied Pharmacology*, 198(2): 86–94.

Dietert, R. and Piepenbrink, M. (2006) 'Lead and Immune Function', *Critical Reviews in Toxicology*, 36(4): 359–85.

EPA (Environmental Protection Agency) (2008) *America's Children and the Environment. Measure B1: Lead in the Blood of Children*, available at http://www.epa.gov/envirohealth/children/body_burdens/b1-graph.htm (accessed 2 March 2009).

Eriyamremu, G., Asagba, S., Akpoborie, I., and Ojeaburu, S. (2005) 'Evaluation of Lead and Cadmium Levels in some Commonly Consumed Vegetables in the Niger-Delta Oil Area of Nigeria', *Bulletin of Environmental Contamination and Toxicology*, 75: 278–83.

Fassin, D. and Naudé, A.-J. (2004) 'Plumbism Reinvented: Childhood Lead Poisoning in France, 1985–1990', *American Journal of Public Health*, 94(11): 1,854–63.

Gainer, J. (1974) 'Lead Aggravates Viral Disease and Represses the Antiviral Activity of Interferon Inducers', *Environmental Health Perspectives*, 7: 113–19.

Gupta, P., Husain, M., Shankar, R., Seth, P. and Maheshwari, R. (2002) 'Lead Exposure Enhances Virus Multiplication and Pathogenesis in Mice', *Veterinary and Human Toxicology*, 44(4): 205–10.

Handley, M., Hall, C., Sanford, E., Diaz, E., Gonzalez-Mendez, E., Drace, K., Wilson, R., Villalobos, M., and Croughan, M. (2007) 'Globalization, Binational Communities, and Imported Food Risks: Results of an Outbreak Investigation of Lead Poisoning in Monterey County, California', *American Journal of Public Health*, 97: 900–06.

Hemdan, N., Emmrich, F., Adham, K., Wichmann, G., Lehmann, I., El-Massry, A., Ghoneim, H., Lehmann, J., and Sack, U. (2005) 'Dose-dependent Modulation of the In Vitro Cytokine Production of Human Immune Competent Cells by Lead Salts', *Toxicological Sciences*, 86(1): 75–83.

Heo, Y., Lee, B.-K., Ahn, K.-D., and Lawrence, D. (2004) 'Serum IgE Elevation Correlates with Blood Lead Levels in Battery Manufacturing Workers', *Human and Experimental Toxicology*, 23: 209–13.

Hernberg, S. (2000) 'Lead Poisoning in Historical Perspective', *American Journal of Industrial Medicine*, 38(3): 244–54.

King, W., Larkins, S., Hucks-Ortiz, C., Wang, J., Gorbach, P., Veniegas, R., and Shoptaw, S. (2009) 'Factors Associated with HIV Viral Load in a Respondent Driven Sample in Los Angeles', *AIDS and Behavior*, 13(1): 145–53.

Kitman, J. (2000) 'The Secret History of Lead', *The Nation*, available at http://www.thenation.com/doc/20000320/kitman (accessed 13 April 2009).

Landrigan, P., Schechter, C., Lipton, J., Fahs, M., and Schwartz, J. (2002) 'Environmental Pollutants and Disease in American Children: Estimates of Morbidity, Mortality, and Costs for Lead Poisoning, Asthma, Cancer, and Developmental Disabilities', *Environmental Health Perspectives*, 110(7): 721–8.

Li, S., Zhengyan, Z., Rong, L. and Hanyun, C. (2005) 'Decrease of CD4+ T-Lymphocytes in Children Exposed to Environmental Lead', *Biological Trace Element Research*, 105(1–3): 19–25.

Maezawa, Y., Nakajima, H., Seto, Y., Suto, A., Kumana, K., Kubo, S., Karasuyama, H., Saito, Y., and Iwamoto, I. (2004) 'IgE-dependent Enhancement of Th2 Cell-mediated Allergic Inflammation in the Airways', *Clinical and Experimental Immunology*, 135(1): 12–18.

Markowitz, G. and Rosner, D. (2002) *Deceit and Denial: The Deadly Politics of Industrial Pollution*, Berkeley, CA: University of California Press.

Matte, T., Figueroa, J.P., Ostrowski, S., Burr, G., Jackson-Hunt, L., Keenlyside, R., and Baker, E. (1989) 'Lead Poisoning among Household Members Exposed to Lead-Acid Battery Repair Shops in Kingston, Jamaica', *International Journal of Epidemiology*, 18(4): 874–81.

Meyer, P., Pivetz, T., Dignam, T., Homa, D., Schoonover, J., and Brody, D. (2003) 'Surveillance for Elevated Blood Lead Levels among Children: United States, 1997–2001', *Morbidity and Mortality Week Report*, 52 (Surveillance Summary 10): 1–21.

Neubert, R., Webb, J., and Neubert, D. (2002) 'Feasibility of Human Trials to Assess Developmental Immunotoxicity, and some Comparison with Data on New World Monkeys', *Human and Experimental Toxicology*, 21(9–10): 543–67.

Nriagu, J., Afeichea, M., Lindera, A., Arowolob, T., Anac, G., Sridharc, M., Oloruntobac, E., Obid, E., Ebenebed, J., Orisakwed, O., and Adesina, A. (2008) 'Lead Poisoning Associated with Malaria in Children of Urban Areas of Nigeria', *International Journal of Hygiene and Environmental Health*, 211(20): 591–605.

Playfair, J. (2004) *Living with Germs in Health and Disease*, New York: Oxford University Press.

Public Radio International (2009) *Lead Poisoning in Developing Countries*, available at http://www.pri.org/health/Global-Health/lead-battery-poisoning.html (accessed 29 March 2009).

Qiao, N., Di Giaocchino, M., Shuchang, H., Youxin, L., Paganelli, R., and Boscolo, P. (2001) 'Effects of Lead Exposure in Printing Houses on Immune and Neurobehavioural Functions in Women', *Journal of Occupational Health*, 43: 271–7.

Rabin, R. (1989) 'Warnings Unheeded: A History of Child Lead Poisoning', *American Journal of Public Health*, 79(12): 1,668–74.

Sharma, R. and Pervez, S. (2003) 'Enrichment and Exposure of Particulate Lead in a Traffic Environment in India', *Environmental Geochemistry and Health*, 25: 297–306.

Singer, M. (2009) *Introduction to Syndemics: A Systems Approach to Public and Community Health*, San Francisco, CA: Jossey-Bass.

Singer, M. and Baer, H. (eds) (2008) *Killer Commodities: Public Health and the Corporate Production of Harm*, Lanham, MD: AltaMira/Roman Littlefield Publishers, Inc.

Sun, L., Hu, J., Zhao, Z., Li, L. and Cheng, H. (2003) 'Influence of Exposure to Environmental Lead on Serum Immunoglobulin in Preschool Children', *Environmental Research*, 92: 124–8.

Wigle, D., Arbuckle, T., Turner, M., Bérub, A., Yang, Q., Liu, S., and Krewski, D. (2008) 'Epidemiologic Evidence of Relationships Between Reproductive and Child Health Outcomes and Environmental Chemical Contaminants', *Journal of Toxicology and Environmental Health*, 11(5–6): 373–517.

Woolf, A., Goldman, R., and Bellinger, D. (2007) 'Update on the Clinical Management Childhood Lead Poisoning', *Pediatric Clinics of North America*, 54: 271–94.

Wu, W., Rinaldi, L., Fortner, K.A., Russell, J.Q., Tschoop, J., Irvin, C., and Budd, R.C. (2004) 'Cellular FLIP Long-transgenic Mice Manifest a Th2 Cytokine Bias and Enhanced Allergic Airway Inflammation', *Journal of Immunology*, 172(8): 4,724–32.

16

Air Pollution and Global Public Health

Christopher J. Paul and Marie Lynn Miranda

Introduction

Air is a primary component of the environment. A healthy adult respirates between 10 and 20 cubic metres of air each day, and this air is exchanged across lung tissue with a surface area between 50 and 100 square metres (Colls 2002). Significant public health concerns exist due to the pervasive nature of air pollution and its associated negative health impacts. The World Health Organization (WHO) estimates that air pollution results in more than 2 million premature deaths globally each year (WHO 2005).

This chapter describes the key sources and effects of air pollution exposures around the world. Air pollution can broadly be considered in terms of the indoor and outdoor environments. Most air pollution originates through combustion, which includes mobile and stationary sources such as land clearing, forest fires, fossil fuel-fired coal-burning power plants, and automobiles. Around half of the world's population uses solid fuels for their cooking and heating, which constitutes a significant source of indoor air pollution (Bruce *et al.* 2000). The largest source of outdoor air pollution comes from the burning of coal, oil, and natural gas (and their derivatives like gasoline), with vehicular emissions contributing the most substantial proportion (Holman 1999).

The negative health effects of air pollution include asthma, airway hyper-reactivity (airway narrowing due to stimuli), chronic obstructive pulmonary disease and exacerbation of other cardio-pulmonary diseases, lung cancer, respiratory infections, conjunctivitis, and negative reproductive health outcomes. In many cases, air pollution may exacerbate existing disease rather than cause disease (Lipfert 1994). For example, sulphate air pollution from the burning of coal exacerbates symptoms of shortness of breath in asthmatics (Ostro *et al.* 1999). Specific at-risk populations include infants, youth, and the elderly. The very young and the very old spend the majority of their time indoors, making the quality of the indoor environment a critical contributor to their health. In regions of the world where solid fuels are used for cooking, women and their young children are particularly likely to be heavily exposed to smoke (Bruce *et al.* 2000). Acute respiratory infections (ARIs) are the primary cause of infant and child mortality in sub-Saharan Africa and Asia (Krzyzanowski and Schwela 1999). Reducing pollution from solid fuel fires indoors could reduce the incidence of ARIs by as much as 8 per cent (Krzyzanowski and Schwela 1999).

While there have been significant improvements in air quality in high-income countries, many sources of air pollution in low- and middle-income countries (LMIC) are increasing (with air quality degrading) as industrial output and car ownership grow. The concentration of populations in urban environments often creates poor background air quality. Many countries have legislation regulating sources of air pollution to improve air quality. However, the reach (and enforcement) of these guidelines and regulations may be limited.

Even in high-income countries, poor air quality in urban and industrial areas remains a concern. Drastic improvements have occurred after the implementation of clean air laws and technological advances, such as laws encouraging the use of cleaner fuels (such as gas) or abatement technologies (such as 'sulphur scrubbers'). Despite these gains, evidence suggests that current levels of air pollution, specifically particulate matter (particles suspended in the air), are associated with shorter life expectancies. Exposure to fine particulate matter has been estimated in a number of studies to result in shortening lives by one year, a consequential amount of time (Brunekreef and Holgate 2002). Exposure to air pollution may result in upwards of 2 million excess deaths in LMIC, and 4 per cent of the global disease burden (Bruce et al. 2000). Levels of outdoor pollutants are frequently much higher in LMIC (Krzyzanowski and Schwela 1999). Open fires, such as those used to clear land or burn rubbish, are common in most low-income countries, as are cars and motor bikes with highly polluting engines (Krzyzanowski and Schwela 1999).

Research in LMIC highlights pollution within the context of local settings (Murray and McGranahan 2003). For example, Malaysia experienced rapid economic growth (and consequently a growth in car ownership), but air pollution regulations lagged. Overall, the air quality in Malaysia is much better than that in nearby lower-income countries, such as Indonesia or Thailand, but concern over increasing pollution has driven Malaysia to adopt comprehensive air quality regulations (Afroz et al. 2003). In African countries such as Kenya, research is focusing on air pollution concerns relevant to changing urbanisation and car ownership patterns (Tanimowo 2000).

Chronic versus acute exposures

Even at lower levels, extended (or chronic) exposure to pollutants over time is cause for concern to population health. Along with exposure to smoke from cook fires, additional indoor air pollution risks exist such as allergens (e.g. mould, animal dander) or the toxic gaseous element, radon, which may have chronic effects on health at low levels of exposure. While residents of highly developed countries (and the rich across most countries) are much less likely to be exposed to harmful indoor smoke, they are more likely to spend much of their time indoors, with subsequent increased risks of exposure to the above-mentioned pollutants. In the United States, the average individual spends approximately 22 hours indoors every day (Bernstein et al. 2008). In poorer countries with colder climates, a majority of the population may be confined for extended periods of time inside structures with high concentrations of pollutants.

Events of extreme smog and industrial accidents (or acute exposures) have occurred throughout history and resulted in significant excess death (Lipfert 1994). The 1952 four-day smog event in London resulted in over 4,000 excess deaths, with some research suggesting the ultimate excess death toll was 12,000 people (Brunekreef and Holgate 2002). Acute exposures can also occur in industrial accidents, one of the most infamous being the Bhopal disaster of 1984 in India, where a toxic gas release killed thousands in one day, with additional longer-term effects continuing to harm the exposed population in subsequent years (Lipfert 1994).

Air pollution sources and exposure

Pollutants that are emitted into the atmosphere such as by combustion (burning) of fuels (e.g. carbon monoxide, sulphur dioxide) are termed *primary pollutants*. Pollutants that are formed or modified in the atmosphere, such as ozone (which is formed when nitrogen oxides and volatile organic compounds react in the atmosphere in the presence of sunlight), are called *secondary pollutants*. Secondary pollutants largely occur from reactions with pollutants from combustion, usually from car engines and power plants. Some pollutants fall into both categories, including particulate matter, which is released directly into the environment by the burning of fuels and can be formed by the recombination and interaction of aerosolised pollutants (such as sulphur oxides reacting to become droplets of sulphuric acid). While legislation aimed at controlling exhaust fumes may directly reduce primary pollutants, by requiring technological fixes such as catalytic converters, secondary pollutants may not decrease proportionally or may even increase (Holman 1999).

Indoor environment

Outdoor air pollution may contaminate indoor environments, but inside environments are also sites of high concentrations of certain pollutants. Key indoor pollutants include: smoke from heating, cooking, kerosene lights, and tobacco use; allergens from animals, moulds, and other organisms; and various other sources such as building materials and geologic sources. If building envelopes are tightly sealed, as would be the case in settings where energy conservation or insulation against extreme climate is prioritised, indoor pollution may concentrate and persist over long time periods. In high-income countries, most indoor pollution arises from non-combustion sources such as volatile compounds (substances that enter the air at normal temperature) from building materials (e.g. paint or carpets), or is circulated from outdoor sources, such as from nearby roadways. In low-income countries, indoor air pollution is dominated by fuel being burned for heating and cooking.

Cooking and heating smoke

Smoke from open combustion indoors can be one of the most pernicious pollutants for population health. It can include particulate matter, carbon monoxide, nitrogen and sulphur dioxides, and other carcinogenic and toxic compounds. The potential negative health effects include lung cancer, ARIs, carbon monoxide poisoning, and other health effects such as decreased immune ability. In a progression of what is described as an energy ladder from the dirtiest to cleanest methods, people may use animal dung, plant material, wood, charcoal, kerosene, gas, and electric energy to cook, depending on the local context, environment, and available resources. For the world's poor, open fires and other unventilated solid or dirty fuel stoves for heating and cooking are used nearly universally (both in rural and urban areas). In China alone, meta-analysis suggests that 420,000 premature deaths occur annually due to indoor solid fuel use (Zhang and Smith 2007). Cleaner fuel options, such as liquid propane, which can be used for cooking, are significantly more expensive and unavailable in much of the world. Even when it is available, many households will continue to use solid fuels, primarily due to cost concerns (Bruce *et al.* 2000).

Environmental tobacco smoke

In all countries, exposure to tobacco smoke through direct consumption is a significant health concern, with an estimated 1.3 billion adult smokers worldwide (Thun and da Costa e Silva 2003).

Exposure to tobacco smoke may begin *in utero* and continue throughout life. Smoking patterns have shifted globally, with the majority of smokers now in LMIC, where rates of tobacco use continue to increase and public health policymaking is limited (Thun and da Costa e Silva 2003). In addition, even non-smokers worldwide, especially women and children, experience significant environmental tobacco smoke (ETS) exposure. For example, while men in China smoke at roughly nine times the rate of women (~60 per cent versus ~7 per cent), 51.3 per cent of women report ETS exposure at home and 26.2 per cent report ETS exposure in the workplace (Gu *et al.* 2004). Around half of students in a global survey of 131 countries aged 13 to 15 years reported exposure to ETS in public places (Warren *et al.* 2006). ETS from other smokers (also known as 'second-hand smoke') has numerous documented negative health effects that are comparable to the harm caused by first-hand exposure to smoking tobacco. There can be a synergistic effect between tobacco smoke and other indoor pollutants, although tobacco smoke alone is sufficiently harmful and can contain upwards of 4,000 different chemicals including known pollutant health risks such as cadmium and particulate matter (Jeffrey 1999).

Other sources of air pollution

Due to the extensive time individuals spend in confined indoor environments, many other air pollution exposures may occur. For example, radon is a radioactive air pollutant generally arising from naturally occurring decaying uranium in the Earth's crust, and can be a source of indoor air pollution as a lung carcinogen. Radon is often concentrated in small buildings or homes in certain geological areas. Other indoor air-borne allergens arise from animals and other organisms including mice, cockroaches, and fungi. Building materials may include toxic materials, such as the carcinogenic substance asbestos (a silicate crystal used in insulation). Other factors augmenting the indoor air pollution challenge in low-income countries in particular are the lack of adequate regulations of building materials, and the challenge of housing which often has minimal filtering (such as air conditioning and sealable windows) or proper ventilation, particularly for cooking and heating smoke.

Outdoor environment

Outdoor air pollution is generally worse in urban areas in both low- and high-income countries, due to the concentration of vehicles, factories, and domestic sources of pollution. In addition, low-vegetation urban built environments may concentrate pollutants or limit their dispersion. Air pollution can also be trapped near the surface by temperature inversions, when warmer air stalls above cooler air, limiting circulation. This effect can be exacerbated by topographical features such as when urban areas are situated in valleys. Concentrated air pollution resulting from topography is a particular problem in cities like Mexico City, Mexico, and Kathmandu, Nepal (Edgerton *et al.* 1999; Regmi *et al.* 2003). The 20 million residents located in Mexico City experience increased exposure during the day to concentrated pollutants from the large amount of industry and 3 million cars, with concentrations of particulate matter in certain areas far exceeding Mexican and international standards. Despite improvements in most countries, including Mexico, such as the requirement of catalytic converters for cars and the introduction of modern, cleaner buses, air pollution remains a major problem, resulting in asthma and respiratory illnesses (Edgerton *et al.*1999; Escamilla-Nunez *et al.* 2008).

Particulate matter

Much particulate matter (PM) is produced by the burning of fossil fuels, but open fires, biogenic sources, erosion of cleared land, and dust are all additional significant sources that affect population health. PM varies in size and health effects, and is often classified as either ultrafine (particles with a diameter less than 0.1 µm: $PM_{0.1}$), fine (particles with a diameter less than 2.5 µm: $PM_{2.5}$), or coarse (particles with a diameter less than 10 µm: PM_{10}). A significant proportion of PM_{10} is dust from wind or roads, though the actual contribution of dust to PM levels is difficult to quantify (Holman 1999). Fine PM comes from the combustion of fossil fuels, open fires, and industrial processes such as smelting. Ultrafine PM particles are primarily generated by vehicles. Finer particles are of particular concern for population health because they can penetrate further into the respiratory system, may have other toxic substances (lead, sulphates, and various chemicals) absorbed onto their surface, and are transported to sites where they are more easily absorbed by the body (Brunekreef and Holgate 2002). Current research suggests that PM is harmful at all levels, with no discernible threshold of safety (Pope III and Dockery 2006).

Ozone

Ozone (O_3) is a highly oxidative and polluting substance. In the troposphere (the surface layer of the atmosphere), ozone is formed through the reactions of other pollutants (i.e. nitrogen oxides and volatile organic compounds) that are catalysed by sunlight. In the stratosphere ('the ozone layer'), ozone protects the earth from solar radiation. However at ground level, ozone is a harmful pollutant for human health, particularly for the lungs. Due to its reactive nature and production in sunlight, ozone levels vary throughout the day and year, peaking seasonally in the summer and daily in the afternoon. Ozone is very reactive, and the oxidative stress it creates in the lungs can cause inflammation and cellular damage (Jeffrey 1999). Exposure to ozone may reduce the body's ability to remove other toxins, such as asbestos (Jeffrey 1999). Asthmatics in particular are considered to be at greater risk for ozone-induced airway inflammation (Jeffrey 1999).

Nitrogen oxides, sulphur dioxide, carbon monoxide, and other by-products of combustion

Pollutants such as nitrogen oxides, sulphur dioxide, and carbon monoxide are all by-products of combustion. Nitrogen oxides are produced in high temperature combustion, so that in addition to anthropogenic sources of fuel engines, they are produced by lightning and forest fires (Holman 1999). Nitrogen oxides are important because they are a catalyst for ozone production, with the above-mentioned associated health effects. Nitrogen dioxide is a strong oxidant and can cause significant oxidative stress to the respiratory system, which can lead to cellular damage and subsequent susceptibility to other diseases (Jeffrey 1999).

Sulphur dioxide is produced by the burning of certain types of fossil fuels, particularly certain coals and fuel oils in power and heat generation (Holman 1999). Sulphur dioxide can react to produce sulphuric acid, a pollutant of particular concern in heavy smog. Due to technological and regulatory controls, its presence and effects are decreasing in higher-income countries, but the use and pollution of coal is high and increasing in some rapidly industrialising countries, such as China and India. Sulphur dioxide can cause an aggravation of symptoms in asthma sufferers and has been associated with increased mortality, though the direct health effects are uncertain (WHO 2005).

Carbon monoxide is produced through combustion, primarily from vehicles. Carbon monoxide reduces the oxygen-carrying capacity in blood, and can cause death. Lastly, the combustion of compounds containing chlorine, particularly from waste incineration, can produce dioxins and furans which are considered carcinogenic toxics.

Air toxics and other air pollutants

The combustion of fossil fuels and the use of other chemicals in vehicles (e.g. buses, cars, trucks) are an important source of thousands of toxic substances that may be present in air pollution. More generally, these other air contaminants are termed 'air toxics'. Air toxics include benzene compounds, toxic metals, and volatile organic compounds (VOCs). VOCs are primarily a concern for their contribution to ozone production and photochemical smog, though some are known toxics, including benzene (Holman 1999). VOCs originate from solvents, fuels, and other industrial processes, such as coating materials, and often enter the environment from materials used in buildings, including carpet, paint, and furniture.

Many heavy metals are a concern as a component of air pollution. They can also easily be transferred to other forms of contamination and exposure within the environment, affecting population health. One example is lead, which is of particular concern because of its history as a fuel additive in many countries. Lead contamination remains high near roadways in both high- and low-income countries, and can be remobilised when the soil surrounding roadways is disrupted. Remobilisation of lead into dust and the air is also a serious risk when renovating or demolishing old houses which may contain lead-based paint. Lead causes a wide variety of health problems, most notably impaired cognitive development in infants and young children, even with low levels of exposure. Other heavy metals are also present in fossil fuels and industrial processes. Such metals include antimony, arsenic, cadmium, chromium, manganese, mercury, and nickel. These act in a variety of ways to adversely affect health, including as neurotoxic substances and carcinogens. In addition to industrial, combustion, and natural sources, the heavy metals chromium and cadmium are also present in tobacco smoke.

Nanoparticles, which are increasingly being manufactured in higher-tech settings, are an emergent concern in air pollution as they are similar in size and composition to many existing known detrimental pollutants (Stone *et al.* 2007). Lastly, mould and plants can also be significant sources of allergens in the outdoor environment in regions around the world. Such allergens are frequently a trigger for respiratory morbidities, particularly asthma.

Regulations and interventions

In many countries, particularly in high-income countries, regulations have reduced air pollution levels and exposures. In the United States, for example, the Clean Air Act of 1970, and its several subsequent amendments, form the regulatory basis upon which significant air quality improvements have been achieved. The European Union has harmonised air pollution policies among its member and affiliated states with a series of guidelines on ambient air pollutants, including particulate matter and nitrogen dioxide. Individual countries enforce the targets, though the European courts may be used to pursue action on air pollution. The WHO issued guidelines on air pollution for policymakers around the world, originally in 1987 and updated in 2005, based upon evaluation of the scientific evidence (WHO 2005).

Recent research increasingly recognises that known pollutants have health impacts at much lower levels than previously understood, and that there are additional previously unknown pollutants of significant concern for population health (Murray and McGranahan 2003). Given that no safe threshold for health impact seems to exist for many known pollutants, the WHO guidelines must be considered in relation to the realistic level of regulatory stringency that can be enacted within local and national contexts (Murray and McGranahan 2003). Guidelines are most commonly adapted (if adopted at all) to be economically and socially feasible within local conditions. Problematically, even in the most stringent regulatory settings, regulations rarely reach the indoor residential environment, instead focusing on industrial sources, power generation, and vehicles.

Murray and McGranahan suggest six important elements of air pollution management for national policymakers: (1) local air pollution monitoring; (2) public awareness; (3) land use planning; (4) transport policy; (5) industrial pollution control; and (6) energy policy (Murray and McGranahan 2003). All six of these areas represent active areas of public debate and policy reform in high-income countries – less so in LMIC. Lower-income countries engage in patchwork air quality policymaking and enforcement, but there is huge variation in efficacy. For example, most power plants in China have controls for particulate matter, but only the newest plants control for nitrogen oxides and sulphur oxides (Lovely and Popp 2008). In Turkey, the municipal government of Istanbul implemented rules requiring the treatment of coal entering the city in order to reduce the amount of sulphur, decreasing the air pollution locally (Tayanc 2000).

Technology has been an important means for pollution reduction, notably in vehicles and power generation (Holman 1999). For example, in the United States, current emissions are 1 per cent of the pre-1970s levels (Holman 1999). Future technological advances, both with existing fuels and new fuels, can have a significant impact on air pollution and air quality. However, poorer countries may have minimal access to new technology, both through a lack of purchasing power and a lack of advanced industry. In many countries, including Kenya and China, the introduction of simple improved solid fuel stoves (with improved fuel efficiency and reduced air pollution) has the potential to significantly reduce ARIs due to reduced pollution (Ezzati and Kammen 2001; Saksena and Smith 2010).

Countries of different income levels have different means and different incentives for regulating polluting industries. The cost of controlling pollution comprises local research, law-making, monitoring, enforcement, and the adaptation of technologies or processes to reduce pollution. Certain circumstances may bring popular support (and thus pressure on the government or polluters) for pollution control, but this may focus on prominent sources even if other sources (such as indoor stoves) are more detrimental (Pargal and Wheeler 1996). Governments of LMIC may also be hesitant to introduce pollution controls that might impede economic growth.

Conclusions

Air pollution is pervasive in the environment. Thus, communities locally, regionally, and globally can suffer the effects of another's pollution. The effects of air pollution are pernicious – and variable across time, geographies, and populations. In high-income countries, emissions from power plants and industrial sources are regulated, and estimates can be made of the contribution to air pollution (Holman 1999), enabling the tracking of pollution's impacts on population health. Vehicles and other small sources (such as generators and cook fires) are much more difficult to evaluate. This is particularly important as the number of vehicles worldwide increases, especially in lower-income countries. South America is producing more than 2 million vehicles per year, and China is producing more than 10 million motorcycles per year, most of which are aimed at markets in Southeast Asia – markets that are mostly unregulated and unmonitored.

Improvements in air pollution will affect the entire global population, but will have the largest effect on at-risk populations. Even low-level exposures can have significant health effects, especially for vulnerable sub-populations. The growth and development of economies in LMIC will likely bring increased emissions, but these countries can take advantage of advanced control technologies (Lovely and Popp 2008). Ensuring clean air for everyone – which will take careful study, effort and investment, and cooperation – will have significant implications for public health throughout the world.

References

Afroz, R., Hassan, M.N., and Ibrahim, N.A. (2003) 'Review of Air Pollution and Health Impacts in Malaysia', *Environmental Research*, 92(2): 71–7.

Bernstein, J.A., Alexis, N., Bacchus, H., Bernstein, I.L., Fritz, P., Horner, E., Li, N., Mason, S., Nel, A., Oullette, J., Reijula, K., Reponen, T., Seltzer, J., Smith, A., and Tarlo, S.M. (2008) 'The Health Effects of Nonindustrial Indoor Air Pollution', *Journal of Allergy and Clinical Immunology*, 121(3): 585–91.

Bruce, N., Perez-Padilla, R., and Albalak, R. (2000) 'Indoor Air Pollution in Developing Countries: A Major Environmental and Public Health Challenge', *Bulletin of the World Health Organization*, 78(9): 1,078–92.

Brunekreef, B. and Holgate, S.T. (2002) 'Air Pollution and Health', *The Lancet*, 360: 1,233–42.

Colls, J. (2002) *Air Pollution*, 2nd edn, New York: Spon Press.

Edgerton, S.A., Bian, X., Doran, J.C., Fast, J.D., Hubbe, J.M., Malone, E.L., Shaw, W.J., Whiteman, C.D., Zhong, S., Arriaga, J.L., Ortiz, E., Ruiz, M., Sosa, G., Vega, E., Limon, T., Guzman, F., Archuleta, J., Bossert, J.E., Elliot, S.M., Lee, J.T., Mcnair, L.A., Chow, J.C., Watson, J.G., Coulter, R.L., Doskey, P.V., Gaffney, J.S., Marley, N.A., Neff, W., and Petty, R. (1999) 'Particulate Air Pollution in Mexico City: A Collaborative Research Project', *Journal of the Air & Waste Management Association*, 49(10): 1,221–29.

Escamilla-Nunez, M.C., Barraza-Villarreal, A., Hernandez-Cadena, L., Moreno-Macias, H., Ramirez-Aguilar, M., Sienra-Monge, J.J., Cortez-Lugo, M., Texcalac, J.L., del Rio-Navarro, B., and Romieu, I. (2008) 'Traffic-related Air Pollution and Respiratory Symptoms among Asthmatic Children, Resident in Mexico City: The EVA Cohort Study', *Respiratory Research*, 9: 74.

Ezzati, M. and Kammen, D. (2001) 'Indoor Air Pollution from Biomass Combustion and Acute Respiratory Infections in Kenya: An Exposure-Response Study', *The Lancet*, 358 (9,282): 619–24.

Gu, D., Wu, X., Reynolds, K., Duan, X., Xin, X., Reynolds, R.F., Whelton, P.K., and He, J. (2004) 'Cigarette Smoking and Exposure to Environmental Tobacco Smoke in China: The International Collaborative Study of Cardiovascular Disease in Asia', *American Journal of Public Health*, 94(11): 1,972–6.

Holman, C. (1999) 'Sources of Air Pollution', in S.T. Holgate, H.S. Koren, J.M. Samet, and R.L. Maynard (eds) *Air Pollution and Health*, New York: Academic Press: 115–148.

Jeffrey, P. (1999) 'Effects of Cigarette Smoke and Air Pollutants on the Lower Respiratory Tract', in S.T. Holgate, H.S. Koren, J.M. Samet, and R.L. Maynard (eds) *Air Pollution and Health*, New York: Academic Press: 219–68.

Krzyzanowski, M. and Schwela, D. (1999) 'Patterns of Air Pollution in Developing Countries', in S.T. Holgate, H.S. Koren, J.M. Samet, and R.L. Maynard (eds) *Air Pollution and Health*, New York: Academic Press: 105–14.

Lipfert, F.W. (1994) *Air Pollution and Community Health: A Critical Review and Data Sourcebook*, New York: Van Nostrand Reinhold.

Lovely, M. and Popp, D. (2008) 'Trade, Technology and the Environment: Why Do Poorer Countries Regulate Sooner', National Bureau of Economic Research (NBER), working paper no. 14286, Cambridge, MA: NBER.

Murray, F. and McGranahan, G. (2003) 'Air Pollution and Health in Developing Countries: The Context,' in G. McGranahan and F. Murray (eds) *Air Pollution and Health in Rapidly Developing Countries*, Sterling, VA: Earthscan Publications: 1–20.

Ostro, B.D., Chestnut, L.G., Mills, D.M., and Watkins, A.M. (1999) 'Estimating the Effects of Air Pollutants on the Population: Human Health Benefits of Sulfate Aerosol Reductions Under Title IV of the 1990 Clean Air Act Amendment', in S.T. Holgate, H.S. Koren, J.M. Samet, and R.L. Maynard (eds) *Air Pollution and Health*, New York: Academic Press: 899–916.

Pargal, S. and Wheeler, D. (1996) 'Informal Regulation of Industrial Pollution in Developing Countries: Evidence from Indonesia', *Journal of Political Economy*, 104(6): 1,314–27.

Pope III, C.A. and Dockery, D.W. (2006) 'Health Effects of Fine Particulate Air Pollution: Lines that Connect', *Journal of Air and Waste Management Association*, 56: 709–42.

Regmi, R.P., Kitada, T., and Kurata, G. (2003) 'Numerical Simulation of Late Wintertime Local Flows in Kathmandu Valley, Nepal: Implication for Air Pollution Transport', *Journal of Applied Meteorology*, 42(3): 389–403.

Saksena, S. and Smith, K.R. (2010) 'Indoor Air Pollution', in G. McGranahan and F. Murray (eds) *Air Pollution and Health in Rapidly Developing Countries*, Sterling, VA: Earthscan Publications: 129–45.

Stone, V., Johnston, H., and Clift, M.J. (2007) 'Air Pollution, Ultrafine and Nanoparticle Toxicology: Cellular and Molecular Interactions', *Institute of Electrical and Electronics Engineers Transactions on Nanobioscience*, 6(4): 331–40.

Tanimowo, M.O. (2000) 'Air Pollution and Respiratory Health in Africa: A Review', *East African Medical Journal*, 77(2): 71–5.

Tayanc, M. (2000) 'An Assessment of Spatial and Temporal Variation of Sulfur Dioxide Levels over Istanbul, Turkey', *Environmental Pollution*, 107(1): 61–9.

Thun, M.J. and da Costa e Silva, V.L. (2003) 'Introduction and Overview of Global Tobacco Surveillance', in O. Shafey, S. Dolwick, and G.E. Guindon (eds) *Tobacco Control Country Profiles*, 2nd edn, Atlanta: American Cancer Society: 7–12.

Warren, C.W., Jones, N.R., Eriksen, M.P., and Asma, S. (2006) 'Patterns of Global Tobacco Use in Young People and Implications for Future Chronic Disease Burden in Adults', *The Lancet*, 367(9,512): 749–53.

WHO (World Health Organization) (2005) *WHO Air quality guidelines for particulate matter, ozone, nitrogen dioxide and sulfur dioxide: Global update 2005*, Geneva: WHO.

Zhang, J.J., and Smith, K.R. (2007) 'Household Air Pollution from Coal and Biomass Fuels in China: Measurements, Health Impacts, and Interventions', *Environmental Health Perspectives*, 115(6): 848–55.

Part IV

Population and Reproductive Health

17

The Evolution of Reproductive Health and Rights

Susan Purdin, Anne Langston, and Ashley Wolfington

Introduction

This chapter provides an overview of how our understanding of human rights has evolved to inform our understanding of reproductive health and rights, and how this has in turn changed humanitarian practice to better fulfil those rights. It offers a definition of commonly used terms, an historical perspective on selected international legal instruments, a review of key reproductive rights, a glimpse at reproductive health for persons affected by man-made and natural disasters, and a listing of essential reproductive health services.[1]

Tracing the evolution of *reproductive health and rights* calls for a broad historical perspective. Many topics come together under this rubric – the study of human reproduction, the legal underpinnings of human rights, and the feminist movement to overturn gender inequality and historic cultural teachings. While reproductive rights are understood as rights of both men and women, and both men and women are participants in human reproduction, in recent decades the evolution of reproductive rights has become entangled with efforts to promote women's rights as human rights.

Reproductive health is a vitally important health issue – a leading area of morbidity and mortality globally – and a too-often neglected area of health care. In October 2006, recognising the critical role that sexual and reproductive health plays in achieving the Millennium Development Goals (MDG), universal access to reproductive health was incorporated into the MDG framework. The global data underpinning this decision illustrates the magnitude of morbidity and mortality related to reproductive health. The disparities noted across countries demonstrate a lack of equity in access to health services that is a major deficit in the realisation of reproductive rights. According to the World Health Organization (WHO) (2009), each year:

- 536,000 women die from causes related to pregnancy and childbirth. Ninety-nine per cent of these deaths occur in developing countries.
- 700,000 infants are born with congenital syphilis.
- 120 million couples have an unmet need for safe and effective contraception.
- 340 million people acquire a new curable sexually transmitted infection (STI).
- 80 million unwanted pregnancies are conceived.

- 68,000 deaths occur as the result of unsafe abortion.
- 2,800,000 deaths result from AIDS. Sixty-five per cent of these occur in Africa.
- 500,000 infants become infected with HIV.
- 3 million girls are subjected to female genital mutilation.

Definitions

The term *reproductive health* was first defined in an international policy statement, and agreed to by 179 member states at the 1994 International Conference on Population and Development (ICPD) in Cairo.

> Reproductive health is a state of complete physical, mental and social well-being and not merely the absence of disease or infirmity, in all matters relating to the reproductive system and to its functions and processes. Reproductive health therefore implies that people are able to have a satisfying and safe sex life and that they have the capability to reproduce and the freedom to decide if, when and how often to do so. Implicit in this last condition are the right of men and women to be informed and to have access to safe, effective, affordable and acceptable methods of family planning of their choice, as well as other methods of their choice for regulation of fertility which are not against the law, and the right of access to appropriate health-care services that will enable women to go safely through pregnancy and childbirth and provide couples with the best chance of having a healthy infant. In line with the above definition of reproductive health, reproductive health care is defined as the constellation of methods, techniques and services that contribute to reproductive health and well-being through preventing and solving reproductive health problems. It also includes sexual health, the purpose of which is the enhancement of life and personal relations, and not merely counselling and care related to reproduction and STIs.
>
> (United Nations 1994: para. 7.2)

Clearly, the concept of *reproductive rights* is embedded in the definition of *reproductive health*. In the subsequent paragraph, the Programme of Action described reproductive rights as:

> embrac[ing] certain human rights that are already recognised in national laws, international human rights documents and other relevant UN consensus documents. These rights rest on the recognition of the basic right of all couples and individuals to decide freely and responsibly the number, spacing and timing of their children and to have the information and means to do so, and the right to attain the highest standard of sexual and reproductive health. They also include the right of all to make decisions concerning reproduction free of discrimination, coercion and violence. Full attention should be given to promoting mutually respectful and equitable gender relations and particularly to meeting the educational and service needs of adolescents to enable them to deal in a positive and responsible way with their sexuality.
>
> (United Nations 1994: para. 7.3)

An historical perspective

Starting with the earliest known legal systems such as Urukagina's Code in Mesopotamia, which declared in 2350 bc that adulteresses be punished with death by stoning with stones inscribed with the name of their crime (Duhaime 2006), women's rights were articulated separately from men's rights. Descriptions of women's rights often centred on their reproductive capacity, and uncovered society's greater interest in a woman's sexuality versus a man's. Women and girls were often described as possessions of husbands and fathers. However, some early legal systems upheld access to reproductive rights that are currently contested in modern discourse. For example, in the Middle Ages, Islamic writings codified conditions for legal abortions, for example, 'not after ensoulment, [said to take place between 40 and 120 days after conception]' or 'to save the life of the mother' (Sachedina 2009). More recently, there were no laws limiting abortion in the United States prior to the 1820s.

The movement towards international human rights which emerged following World War II gave rise to broad human rights language first in the 1945 UN Charter, and three years later in the Universal Declaration of Human Rights. In 1968, reproductive rights emerged as a subset of human rights in the Proclamation of Tehran, which averred that 'Parents have a basic right to decide freely and responsibly on the number and spacing of their children and a right to adequate education and information in this respect' (United Nations 1968). As explained above, the 1994 Cairo ICPD Programme of Action articulated an internationally agreed upon definition of reproductive health, which has been the underpinning of efforts to assure access to a range of reproductive health services for women, men, and adolescents globally since the Cairo meeting. The 1995 Fourth World Conference on Women in Beijing Platform for Action reinforced the Cairo definition of reproductive health, and further established interrelated areas of 'indivisible, universal and inalienable reproductive rights' described in the following section (United Nations 1995).

The term 'reproductive rights' is variously used to include some or all of the following rights: the right to legal or safe abortion, the right to control one's reproductive functions, the right to access quality reproductive health care, and the right to education and access to health services in order to make reproductive choices free from coercion, discrimination, and violence (Amnesty International 2007). Reproductive rights may also be understood to include education about contraception and STIs, freedom from coerced sterilisation and contraception, and protection from gender-based practices such as genital cutting. In 2000, reproductive rights were incorporated into the UN MDGs, with governments agreeing that addressing reproductive health is key to promoting development.

Time has shown that national and global swings between liberal and conservative political directions play out in legal challenges to previously secured reproductive rights, even as science advances to provide new technologies which change the underlying issues. This has been seen in areas such as treatment of HIV, prevention of post-partum haemorrhage, methods of contraception, and medical abortion. For example, on his second day in office in 2001, President Bush reinstated the Mexico City Policy that denied US government assistance to non-US-based agencies which offered abortion counselling or services. This presidential directive originated during Ronald Reagan's presidency and is named after the 1984 International Conference on Population, which was held in Mexico City, where the US delegation first announced the policy (Willson 1984). The policy has been operative when Republican presidents were in office (Ronald Reagan, George H. W. Bush, George W. Bush), and overturned during the terms of Democrat presidents (Bill Clinton and Barack Obama).

Key rights

The Center for Reproductive Rights, a global legal advocacy organisation (http://reproductiverights. org/), outlines specific human rights as key elements of a reproductive rights framework (Center for Reproductive Rights 2009). The rights to sexual and reproductive health are articulated in international treaties and conventions, including the Convention on the Rights of the Child, and the Convention on the Elimination of All Forms of Discrimination against Women (CEDAW). Governments that have ratified these documents are obligated to ensure equitable access to reproductive health services, and uphold the rights described below. Regional conventions and international conference declarations have further established the human rights principles that are used to shape programmes and guide health workers in countries around the globe (Freedman 2001).

The *right to life* was established with the Universal Declaration of Human Rights and is upheld in a range of international human rights instruments. This right is fundamental to the arguments in support of access to reproductive health care (Center for Reproductive Rights 2009).

The *right to liberty and security of person* is the basis for ensuring that people are able to make reproductive decisions free of discrimination, coercion, and violence; and that reproductive health services ensure voluntary, informed consent for all procedures.

The *right to health, including sexual and reproductive health*, supports protection to mothers before and after childbirth, access for everyone to family planning, medical attention, and social services, non-discrimination for persons with disabilities, the provision of sexual and reproductive health education, ethical research standards, and access to safe abortion in cases of sexual assault.

The *right to decide the number and spacing of children* ensures men and women have access to information, education, and the means to exercise this right, including a full range of safe and effective methods of fertility control.

The *right to consent to marriage and to equality in marriage* assures that men and women, of full adult age, without any limitation due to race, nationality, disability, or religion, have the right to marry and found a family, that each individual may consent only for him/herself, and that each has equal rights with regard to decisions within the marriage, property ownership, and the dissolution of marriage.

The *right to privacy* prevents arbitrary interference with privacy or family, prevents attacks on honour, supports the confidentiality of health information, and supports the right of young people to privately and confidentially access sexual and reproductive health information and services.

The *right to equality and non-discrimination* prevents discrimination on the basis of race, colour, sex, language, religion, political or other opinion, national extraction or social origin, health, minority status, or maternity; and assures that adolescents, in a manner consistent with their evolving capacities, may access appropriate direction and guidance in sexual and reproductive matters.

The *right to be free from practices that harm women and girls* prohibits practices based on ideas of inferiority or superiority of either sex, prohibits harmful cultural and traditional practices, specifically child marriages and female genital mutilation, and mandates provision of support to victims of harmful practices.

The *right not to be subjected to torture or other cruel, inhuman, or degrading treatment or punishment* requires that no one shall be subjected to scientific experiment without consent, and requires full assistance for survivors of rape in war.

The *right to be free from sexual and gender-based violence* prevents human trafficking, child sexual abuse or exploitation, violence against women, sexual harassment, rape, sexual slavery, enforced prostitution, forced pregnancy, and enforced sterilisation or any other form of sexual violence of comparable gravity.

The *right to access sexual and reproductive health education and family planning information* ensures access to equal education opportunities for men and women, the elimination of gender stereotypes in educational content, information on family well-being, including family planning, information and services to protect against STIs, and information on health status.

The *right to enjoy scientific progress* assures that all persons may benefit from scientific advancement but cautions that the dignity and rights of individuals must be respected (Center for Reproductive Rights 2009).

While these rights have been accepted by international bodies and embedded in international conventions, their meanings continue to be contested. In particular, the right to safe abortion services continues to be debated, in both high- and low-income countries around the globe. However, focusing primarily on areas of agreement (such as access to essential obstetric care) has allowed the international community to make progress towards a broad consensus on what reproductive health services are needed to allow individuals and couples to realise their right to reproductive health.

Reproductive health among forced migrants

One new reproductive health and rights-related movement – that of assuring access to reproductive health care for refugees and others displaced by conflict and disaster – was initiated following the 1994 ICPD Conference in Cairo. This was also the year of the Rwanda genocide, and Rwandan women refugees spoke out at the Cairo meeting to demand their own right to reproductive health care – care they had had access to in their home country, but which was absent from the services provided by humanitarian relief agencies aiding Rwandan refugees in camps outside Rwanda's borders. In the ensuing years, significant progress has been made, from mobilising a coalition of UN agencies, academics, field practitioners, and donors to raise awareness of the unique needs of refugees and displaced persons for reproductive health care and access, to developing guidelines for reproductive health service delivery in emergency settings, and publishing in the scientific literature. An interagency evaluation published in 2004 reviewed ten years of work to improve access to reproductive health care for refugees and internally displaced persons. The evaluation identified areas of clear progress, such as increased access to obstetric and contraceptive services for refugees, as well as areas of persistent deficiencies, including a lack of services for survivors of sexual assault, inadequate care for persons living with HIV, and very little attention paid to the reproductive health needs of people who had been internally displaced by conflict. The evaluation also showed that funding for reproductive health declined after 2000, reflecting a weakening of political support for reproductive health programmes (UNHCR 2004).

Attention on rape as a weapon of war has led to watershed decisions of criminal tribunals affirming rape as a war crime, and declaring sexual offences could constitute genocide and crimes against humanity. In 1996, the International Criminal Tribunal for the Former Yugoslavia stated that organised rape and other sexual offences could constitute crimes against humanity, and in 1998, the Rwanda Tribunal found that rapes and sexual assaults committed during the conflict could constitute genocide if they were committed as part of an intentional desire to destroy a protected group (Purdin *et al.* 2004).

In September 2009, a convocation of practitioners directly involved in the provision of services in conflict-affected countries, representatives from UN organisations, academic experts, and donors produced the 'Granada Consensus on Sexual and Reproductive Health in Protracted Crises and Recovery', which identified four priorities for action in these settings: mainstreaming sexual and reproductive health in policies and strategies, sustaining sexual and reproductive health services, bridging gaps in funding and services, and supporting local leadership (Excuela Andaluza de Salud Pública et al. 2009).

Components of reproductive health services

In 1972, the WHO, co-sponsored by the United Nations Development Programme (UNDP), the United Nations Population Fund (UNFPA), and the World Bank, established a Special Programme of Research, Development, and Research Training in Human Reproduction (www. who.int/hrp/en/). This programme has provided a foundation for evidence-based programming in support of sexual and reproductive health globally.

Within the ICPD, definition of reproductive health is a reflection of the package of services to be offered that will enable men, women and adolescents to realise their reproductive rights. In adhering to this guidance, UNFPA suggests that, for the convenience of users and to avoid duplication of management structures, sexual and reproductive health services should be integrated within a primary health care system rather than offered as separate 'vertical' programme activities (UNFPA 2009). The debate about selective, or vertical, programmes versus comprehensive, or integrated, primary health care services has been underway since 1979, a year after the concept of 'health for all' was introduced at Alma-Ata (Magnussen et al. 2004). This chapter will not explore the debate, but suggests that whether or not a vertical sexual and reproductive health programming strategy is employed, focused attention is necessary in order to assure that men, women, and adolescents have equitable access to good quality, comprehensive services.

As outlined by UNFPA (2009), a full sexual and reproductive health package includes:

Age-appropriate sexual and reproductive health information for men, women, and adolescents

Correct information made available in a manner that is accessible and respectful of the individual enhances one's ability to develop and maintain his or her reproductive health. Relevant activities include health education programmes for in- and out-of-school youth, life skills education to build critical decision-making proficiency, behaviour change communication on how to protect oneself from STIs or unintended pregnancy, and community awareness-raising on the availability of reproductive health services.

Care during pregnancy, at the time of delivery, including emergency obstetric care, and after delivery for the mother and baby

For pregnant women, the WHO advises that a 12-step process be followed over four routine antenatal visits. Emergency obstetric services should be accessible to all pregnant women, as well as safe abortion and post-abortion care. Postpartum care requires on-site surveillance during the first two hours after delivery, followed by additional check-ups on the first two days after delivery, as well as at one week and six weeks. Postpartum care includes identification and treatment of complications, along with promotion of healthy behaviours such as breastfeeding, family planning, and infant immunisations (WHO 2003).

Family planning/birth spacing services

If women are able to avoid unwanted pregnancy, up to one-third of maternal deaths and one-quarter of child deaths can be prevented. Shorter birth intervals put the mother's life at

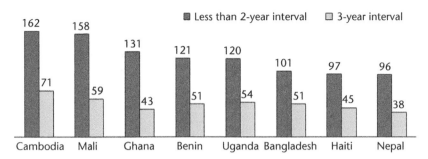

Figure 17.1   Deaths per 1,000 infants under age 1 year
Source: Adapted from Smith *et al.* (2009).

risk and contribute to poor health outcomes for infants. Figure 17.1 illustrates the reduction in infant mortality which would occur in developing countries if women spaced their births two or more years apart. A good quality family planning service includes clear information and respectful treatment for clients, technically competent staff, a range of methods, and a plan for user follow-up (Bruce 1990).

Prevention and treatment of reproductive tract infections and STIs, including HIV/AIDS

Men, women, and young people need basic information, access to free condoms, and well-stocked services in order to minimise their risk of morbidity and mortality associated with STIs. Currently, it is estimated that only about 31 per cent of people living with HIV who are medically eligible for antiretroviral medications have access to these life-saving drugs (Global AIDS Alliance 2009).

Early diagnosis and treatment for breast and cervical cancer

In 2000, cancer of the breast was, for the first time, the most commonly diagnosed tumour among women in low-income regions of the world, with 470,000 new cases per year (International Agency for Research on Cancer 2002). Cervical cancer is the second most common type of cancer in women and was responsible for over 250,000 deaths in 2005 – approximately 80 per cent of which occurred in developing countries (WHO 2006).

Prevention and management of gender-based violence

Gender-based violence (GBV) has been recognised as an epidemic in settings of armed conflict, but, in fact, the practice of violence against women is endemic in human society. Addressing GBV in conflict settings has proven to be the thin edge of a wedge that can open community dialogue on a traditionally taboo subject. Effective programmes to address GBV are multi-faceted, encompassing the health, social, security, and justice sectors, and build from a singular focus such as rape in war to a broader platform of women's rights that eventually enables communities to tackle intimate partner violence and female genital cutting. Men, as community members who perpetrate violence and may be subjected to it themselves, must be constructively engaged (Marsh *et al.* 2006).

Adolescent sexual and reproductive health

Adolescents transit a challenging passage from child to adult which involves not only physical changes resulting in sexual maturation, but also a social transition characterised by movement towards decision-making autonomy and economic self-reliance. All the components of reproductive health programming described above need to include attention to the unique needs of adolescents (Save the Children and United Nations Population Fund 2009).

Prevention and appropriate treatment of sub-fertility and infertility

Infertility remains an unrecognised reproductive rights issue that carries a high social cost for individuals, especially women, and couples who are unable to bear children. Services can range from counselling to the application of reproductive technologies depending on available resources in a particular setting.

Conclusion

International treaties and consensus documents provide a clear mandate for governments to meet the reproductive rights of their citizens. However, the full range of required services is rarely available to the poor, whether they reside in a high- or low-income country. The crucial issue remains that men, women, and adolescents need unobstructed access to high-quality, comprehensive sexual and reproductive health services in order to realise their basic right to reproductive health.

Note

1 For more in-depth reading, please see: *Reproductive Health and Human Rights: The Way Forward*, edited by Laura Reichenback and Mindy Jane Roseman (Philadelphia: University of Pennsylvania Press, 2009).

References

Amnesty International (2007) 'Reproductive Rights', available at http://www.amnestyusa.org/violence-against-women/stop-violence-against-women-svaw/reproductive-rights/page.do?id=1108242 (accessed 15 December 2009).

Bruce, J. (1990) 'Fundamental Elements of the Quality of Care: A Simple Framework', *Studies in Family Planning*, 21: 61–91.

Center for Reproductive Rights (2009) 'Twelve Human Rights Key to Reproductive Rights', available at http://reproductiverights.org/en/document/twelve-human-rights-key-to-reproductive-rights (accessed 14 December 2009).

Duhaime, L. (2006) 'The Timetable of World Legal History', available at http://duhaime.org/LawMuseum/LawArticle-44/Duhaimes-Timetable-of-World-Legal-History.aspx?lk=mm (accessed 12 January 2010).

Excuela Andaluza de Salud Pública, United Nations Population Fund, World Health Organization (2009) 'Granada Consensus on Sexual and Reproductive Health in Protracted Crises and Recovery', available at http://www.who.int/hac/techguidance/pht/reproductive_health_protracted_crises_and_recovery.pdf (accessed 12 January 2010).

Freedman, L.P. (2001) 'Using Human Right in Maternal Mortality Programmes: From Analysis to Strategy', *International Journal of Gynecology and Obstetrics*, 75: 51–60.

Global AIDS Alliance (2009) *Treat the People*, available at http://www.globalaidsalliance.org/issues/treat_the_people/ (accessed 14 December 2009).

IARC (International Agency for Research on Cancer) (2002) *IARC Handbooks of Cancer Prevention Programme*, Vol. 7: *Breast Cancer Screening*, ed. H. Vainio and F. Bianchini, Lyon: IARC Press.

Magnussen, L., Ehiri, J., and Jolly, P. (2004) 'Comprehensive Versus Selective Primary Health care: Lessons For Global Health Policy', *Health Affairs*, 23: 167–76.

Marsh, M., Purdin, S., and Navani, S. (2006) 'Addressing Sexual Violence in Humanitarian Emergencies', *Global Public Health*, 1 (2): 133–46.

Purdin, S., McGinn T., and Miller, A. (2004) Reproductive Health among Forced Migrants – An Issue of Human Rights', *The Lancet*, available at http://image.thelancet.com/extras/03art4174webappendix.pdf (accessed 10 October 2009).

Sachedina, A.A. (2009) *Islamic Biomedical Ethics: Principles and Application*, New York: Oxford University Press.

Save the Children and United Nations Population Fund (UNFPA) (2009) *Adolescent Sexual and Reproductive Health Toolkit for Humanitarian Settings*, Westport, CT and New York: Save the Children and UNFPA.

Smith, R., Ashford L., Gribble, J., and Clifton, D. (2009) *Family Planning Saves Lives*, Washington, DC: Population Reference Bureau.

UN (United Nations) (1968) *Proclamation of Teheran*, International Conference on Human Rights, Teheran, Iran, 13 May.

UN (United Nations) (1994) *Report of the United Nations International Conference on Population and Development (ICPD)*, Cairo, Egypt, 5–13 September. New York: UN.

UN (United Nations) (1995) *Beijing Declaration and Platform for Action*, United Nations World Conference on Women, Beijing, China, 4–15 September. New York: UN.

UNHCR (United Nations High Commissioner for Refugees) (2004) *Reproductive Health Services for Refugees and Internally Displaced Persons: Report of an Inter-agency Global Evaluation*, Geneva: UNHCR.

UNFPA (United Nations Population Fund) (2009) 'Improving Reproductive Health Services', available at http://www.unfpa.org/rh/services.htm (accessed 14 December 2009).

Willson, P. (1984) 'The 1984 International Conference on Population: What Will Be the Issues?' *International Family Planning Perspectives*, 10: 43–8.

WHO (World Health Organization) (2003) *Pregnancy, Childbirth, Postpartum and Newborn Care: A Guide for Essential Practice*, Geneva: WHO.

WHO (World Health Organization) (2006) *Comprehensive Cervical Cancer Control: A Guide to Essential Practice*, Geneva: WHO.

WHO (World Health Organization) (2009) 'Partner Brief', Department of Reproductive Health and Research, available at http://whqlibdoc.who.int/hq/2009/WHO_RHR_09.02_eng.pdf (accessed 12 January 2010).

18

A Generation at Risk
Prioritising Child and Youth Health

Caroline W. Kabiru, Chi-Chi Undie, and Alex C. Ezeh

The health and social needs of vulnerable and disenfranchised young people serve as an early warning system of threats that will ultimately engulf larger populations.
(Michael Resnick and Glenn Bowes (2007), drawing from the words of Marian Wright Edelman)

Introduction

In this chapter, we draw attention to the health and well-being of children and youth, paying particular attention to the sub-Saharan African (SSA) region. We draw on existing literature and our experiences working in Nairobi's urban slums, highlighting the opportunities and challenges faced by young people as they grow up in a changing world. We underscore implications for policy and programmatic efforts aimed at prioritising child and youth health in national agendas.

Why focus on young people?

Young people under the age of 25 years represent just under one half (44 per cent) of the world's population (US Census Bureau 2009). Ninety per cent of these young people live in the developing world. It is estimated that while countries in Europe will experience a decline in the number of young people (from 140 million in Europe in 2006 to about 111 million in 2025), Africa will experience an increase from 305 million to 424 million (Blum 2009). While young people comprise a significant proportion of the world's population, their health and developmental needs are often obscured in the health and development agendas of many countries. Yet the primary causes of poor health and social outcomes in this group are largely preventable. Further, as noted by the Panel on Transitions to Adulthood in Developing Countries (National Research Council and Institute of Medicine 2005), 'the successful achievement by 2015 or beyond of many of these [UN Millenium Development Goals] will require that policy makers center their attention on young people' (575).

The health profile of children and youth

Leading causes of death among the youth

A recent study by Patton and colleagues (2009) reported 2.6 million deaths among children and youth aged 10–24 years, with the majority of these deaths occurring in the least developed countries. While more deaths occurred in Southeast Asia, the relative risk for death was highest in Africa. Unlike other regions, females aged 10–24 years in Africa and Southeast Asia had a greater risk of death than males. Cause of death data show that the leading causes of death among females could be grouped as either maternal-related causes (e.g. haemorrhage, abortions, etc.), or as communicable, perinatal, and nutritional-related causes, which together account for 48 per cent of all females deaths globally. In Africa, maternal mortality accounts for 26 per cent of all female deaths, while HIV/AIDS and TB account for more than 20 per cent of all deaths among Africans aged 10–24 years. With increasing age, non-communicable causes and injuries gain prominence, with injuries accounting for 51 per cent of all male mortality among 20–24 year olds globally. Road traffic-related fatal injuries are the most common cause of death, and although the number of deaths per registered vehicle is higher in poorer countries, the death rates are higher in upper-middle-income countries (National Research Council and Institute of Medicine 2005). With the growth of motorised transportation globally, road-traffic-related morbidity and mortality is expected to increase, especially where there are no improvements in preventive and safety measures, such as enforcement of policies on seatbelt and helmet use, as well as improvements in road infrastructure, including pedestrian walkways.

The maternal-related causes described above represent the largest gap between Africa and the rest of the world with regard to deaths among young people aged 15–24 years. In Africa, maternal deaths dwarf other causes of death among older adolescent women aged 15–19 years and account for nearly three-quarters of all maternal, communicable, perinatal, and nutritional causes of death. The high levels of mortality in young adult women continue into early adulthood (20–24 years) (Patton *et al.* 2009).

For many young women in the developing world, early childbearing, particularly in impoverished areas such as urban slums, contributes to high rates of maternal mortality. In these settings, where access to obstetric services is hindered by the lack of basic health facilities and the high cost of care (Izugbara *et al.* 2009), early childbearing becomes a dangerous process for the health of not only the young women, but also for their children. Other negative impacts of early childbearing, including school dropout and reduced opportunities for future employment (National Research Council and Institute of Medicine 2005), further expose young mothers and their children to other adverse health and social outcomes (Koniak-Griffin and Turner-Pluta 2001). These risks are heightened in the slum settlement context of relatively high HIV/AIDS prevalence (APHRC 2008b). Thus, there is an urgent need to ensure that young people have access to sexual and reproductive health (SRH) services, and that early (unwanted) childbearing is prevented.

Emerging trends impacting on child and youth health

Globalisation

Children and youth are growing up in a context characterised by rapid changes in technology, increased intranational and international travel, and the expansion of global markets. Globalisation has had both positive and negative impacts on the health of young people around the world. For example, global communication and the expansion of inter- and intra-continental travel has increased access to information, and widened access to job and educational opportunities. However, global forces have also led to widespread negative social disruptions, such as increased access to illicit drugs, which are easily transported across national boundaries, and the breakdown of social structures and community cohesion. The benefits of globalisation are not uniformly spread, and the effects are often concentrated in cities, resulting in large inequalities (National Research Council and Institute of Medicine 2005). Industrialisation, technological advances, and other market changes mean that education has become an important prerequisite for future careers. In many developing countries, especially in sub-Saharan Africa, where the expansion of educational opportunities has not kept pace with the growth in child and youth populations, competition for access to formal education has stiffened, with many unintended consequences for the emotional and social development of young people (such as increased stress and frustrations, particularly for average learners), as well as for their potential to meaningfully engage in an economy that is heavily dependent on an educated labour force.

Urbanisation

> Cities are the materialization of humanity's noblest ideas, ambitions and aspirations, but when not planned or governed properly, can be the repository of society's ills. Cities drive national economies by creating wealth, enhancing social development and providing employment but they can also be the breeding grounds for poverty, exclusion and environmental degradation.
>
> (United Nations Human Settlements Programme
> [UN-HABITAT] 2008b)

Half of the world's population live in urban areas. However, the proportion that is urban varies from region to region. Over 70 per cent of the population in Europe, North America, and Latin America live in urban areas. While the majority of Asian and African populations are rural dwellers, it is estimated that by 2050 more than half of Africa's population will be urban. In Asia, the transition will occur much earlier, fuelled largely by rapid urbanisation in China (UN-HABITAT 2008b). Unfortunately, rapid urbanisation in many developing countries occurs amid floundering economies and poor governance. Thus, many low-income countries have been unable to provide basic services to meet the demands of urban populations, in turn leading to the growth of informal settlements that are characterised by a youthful population. For example, slums in Nairobi (Kenya) house over 2 million people, about 50 per cent of whom are 24 years or younger (APHRC 2002; UN-HABITAT 2008a). These slums are characterised by poor housing, sanitation, and infrastructure, high unemployment rates, and high rates of violence. Limited access to formal education (APHRC 2008a) and the lack of employment opportunities (World Bank 2008) means that young people in these settings are prone to involvement in crime, violence, and risky behaviours that place them at heightened risk for poor health and social outcomes.

Studies conducted in Nairobi's slums indicate that slum dwellers fare much worse in terms of risky sexual behaviour than their peers living outside slums (Dodoo et al. 2003, 2007; Zulu et al. 2002, 2003). Yet slum dwellers do not necessarily fare worse in terms of the presence or absence of protective and risk factors, such as models for pro-social behaviour or parental monitoring (Kabiru et al. 2010). Other attributes of the social context in urban slums may, therefore, mute the effects of these factors and contribute to health disparities between young people living within and outside slum settings. Thus, governments and other agencies aiming to improve sexual and reproductive health outcomes among young people should target the youth in especially vulnerable contexts, such as urban informal settlements.

The HIV/AIDS pandemic

Young people's sexual behaviours and their socio-economic and cultural contexts place them at a high risk of acquiring HIV and other sexually transmitted infections. Indeed, young people are disproportionately affected by the HIV/AIDS pandemic. In 2007, more than 90 per cent of new HIV infections were in low- and middle-income countries, with about 45 per cent of infections occurring among young people aged 15 to 24 years (UNAIDS 2008). The HIV/AIDS pandemic has heightened the need to understand the drivers of HIV infections among young people. An unpublished manuscript by Ndugwa and colleagues, based on data collected from adolescents living in two slums in Nairobi, Kenya, highlights potential contributing factors (Ndugwa *et al.* ms). For example, although over 95 per cent of these adolescents are able to correctly answer questions on modes of HIV transmission, several HIV/AIDS knowledge misconceptions among slum adolescents remain with regard to identifying asymptomatic carriers, mother-to-child transmission, and having sexual relations with people who are actively involved in injecting drugs. In line with other studies, sexual risk behaviour is high among these communities, and is mostly driven by key socio-demographic and economic factors such as age, ethnicity, and poverty status (Bankole *et al.* 2007; Zulu *et al.* 2002). Ndugwa and colleagues (ms) also note that sexual debut occurs much earlier among girls living in the slums compared to their male peers, although boys are three times more likely than girls to have more than one sexual partner. The finding of gender differences in sexual behaviour, but not for knowledge of HIV, highlights a key area for designing gender-based interventions for adolescent slum residents. On the one hand, this finding may suggest a much higher pressure on girls to have sex in the communities than on boys. For example, Dodoo and colleagues (2007), in their examination of qualitative reports from the Sexual Networking and Associated Reproductive and Social Health Concerns study (conducted in four slum settlements in Nairobi), noted that some young girls are forced into transactional sexual partnerships so that they can contribute to household income. Strengthening the pace of sexual and reproductive health interventions is key, while further studies are needed to clarify the observed gender-related differences in sexual behaviour. Finally, to promote healthy sexuality among young people in slums, programmes that incorporate local knowledge and cultural norms may be required.

HIV testing-related data from a study by Kabiru and colleagues (ms) highlight four key lessons for policies and programmes that aim to address the high HIV prevalence among youth, and in particular, to increase HIV testing among this population. First, study findings suggest that young people are unable (or unwilling) to assess their risk of infection based on behaviour. Thus, programmatic efforts to enable young people to accurately assess their levels of risk based on prior behaviour may lead to an increase in use of appropriate health services. Second, encouragement from referent others (e.g. peer educators, counsellors, peers, partners, and parents) plays an important role in encouraging young people to get tested. Third, adolescents who report a history of pregnancy are more likely to be tested. There is widespread promotion of interventions to prevent mother-to-child transmission (PMTCT) of HIV in the region (PEPFAR 2004). Targeting pregnant adolescents is important in preventing paediatric HIV/AIDS; nevertheless, it is important that HIV testing interventions target both males and females who may not be reached through PMTCT initiatives (Arrington-Sanders and Ellen 2008). Finally, although the HIV testing guidelines issued by the Kenyan Ministry of Health recommend that appropriate counselling precede and follow all testing (National AIDS and STD Control Programme 2006), the data show that counselling is less than universal. Study findings show that those who receive counselling are more likely to receive their test results, hence it may be important for governments to take steps to ensure compliance with policies and guidelines on HIV testing.

The HIV/AIDS pandemic has brought youth sexual behaviour to the forefront of research, as well as programmatic efforts targeting young people aged between ten to 24. The validity and reliability of sexual behaviour data are critical in addressing sexual and reproductive health concerns of young people, and in informing successful targeting and evaluation of sexual and reproductive health interventions. However, measuring sexual behaviour is subject to numerous biases. Indeed, several studies document the challenges of measuring sexual behaviour among young people (Beguy et al. 2009; Mensch et al. 2003; Palen et al. 2008; Plummer et al. 2004) and highlight several important lessons for researchers and users of sexual behaviour data based on studies conducted among youth. For example, Beguy et al. (2009) found that a relatively high proportion of adolescents provided inconsistent information on their sexual behaviour, and observed that males, slum residents, and in-school adolescents were more likely to give inconsistent sexual information. Given widespread disapproval of adolescent sexual behaviour among local societies and communities, contradictory information on the timing of first sex may reflect possible discomfort by young people in disclosing sexual activity (especially among females), or external pressures to be perceived to be sexually active (particularly among males for whom sexual prowess is widely accepted, if not glorified). Further research on methodologies to improve the quality of data collected is warranted. These findings also have implications for sexual and reproductive health programmes targeted towards youth. In particular, these programmes should endeavour to provide confidential settings where young people feel comfortable enough to disclose information about sensitive matters that may ultimately impact on their health and well-being.

Education

Changes in the global economy have increased the demand for formal education, and earnings are substantially higher for more educated persons. With increasing school enrolment rates across the world, large proportions of young people are spending substantial amounts of time in school. Thus, schooling not only enhances so-called 'book knowledge' but, in addition, also provides an important context for shaping youth socialisation and development. Data collected by the Panel on Transitions to Adulthood in Developing Countries (National Research Council and Institute of Medicine 2005) indicate that three-quarters of young people aged 10–14 are enrolled in school, with fewer girls than boys in school. Across the developing world, enrolment rates drop significantly among 15–19 year olds. Within countries, there is strong evidence that young people in the wealthiest social class are more likely to be enrolled in school, while school attendance is higher among urban dwellers compared to their rural counterparts (National Research Council and Institute of Medicine 2005). The changing family, social, and economic context has contributed to shifts in educational participation. For example, decreasing family size has been linked to greater enrolment and lower gender disparities in enrolment rates, greater parental schooling translates to greater child enrolment, and increasing urbanisation means that young people have greater access to educational opportunities (National Research Council and Institute of Medicine 2005). In addition to increased job opportunities and greater potential for higher earnings, school attendance delays entry into marriage and childbearing. Studies show that education has been linked to lower rates of sexually transmitted infections, including HIV, lower substance use, and better health (Blum 2007). Our studies of Nairobi slums also suggest that school attendance is a protective factor for girls (Kabiru et al.

2010). We postulate that schools may provide an environment that protects girls from exposure to high-risk activities because the level of supervision, and schooling may empower women by providing them with knowledge about the health and social consequences of precocious sexual activities, and may arm them with the necessary psychological tools to refuse unwanted sexual advances. The finding that schools appear to be protective of girls raises a need for more in-depth analysis and research to understand why and how this is so, and also particularly how boys can be helped to enjoy the benefits of the school-setting.

Marriage

Marriage trends indicate that young people around the globe are marrying later in life. Similar trends have been observed in Africa. Mensch and colleagues (2006), in a review of Demographic and Health Survey (DHS) data from 27 sub-Saharan African countries, observed a significant decline in the proportion of African females getting married in their teens. However, many young women still get married in their teens across Africa. For example, in counties such as Chad and Niger, more than 70 per cent of 20–24 years old reported being married before age 18. Clark and colleagues (2006), in their analyses of data from 22 African countries and seven Latin American and Caribbean countries, also found high rates of early marriage in all sub-Saharan African countries, with the exception of South Africa. Specifically, about 40 per cent of women in the sub-Saharan African countries were married by age 20 compared to about 25 to 30 per cent among women in Latin America and the Caribbean.

Drawing on the existing literature, Mensch and colleagues (2006) postulate that the decline in female teen marriages stems in part from increased mobility of young men; the changing dynamics of the marriage process, including cash-based dowry payment and individual spouse selection; and increased opportunities for employment. Other reasons include changes in the legal age at marriage, increased access to formal education, and increased women's labour force participation (National Research Council and Institute of Medicine 2005).

While there is a decrease in both marriage and sexual initiation before age 18, the increase in age at first marriage has occurred more rapidly than the increase in age at first sex. Thus, while marriage may have been a more common context for sexual initiation, pre-marital sexual initiation is increasingly common. Although pre-marital sex is often cited as problem behaviour, recent evidence suggests that young married women are often at higher risk of pregnancy and STIs, including HIV/AIDS (Glynn et al. 2001). Clark and colleagues (2006) report higher HIV prevalence rates among married females compared to their unmarried, sexually active counterparts. Limited condom use within marriage, due in part to the unfounded assumption of marriage as a protective factor, may explain the greater vulnerability to poor sexual and reproductive health outcomes among young married women. Clark et al. (2006) also postulate that the large age differences between spouses compared to age differences between non-spousal partners may contribute to differences in the risk for HIV infection. However, further research is needed to fully clarify the pathways through which marriage increases the vulnerability of young women to poor sexual and reproductive health outcomes. Some questions worth further investigation include: to what extent are these outcomes due to gender and power relations between these adolescent girls and their often much older husbands? Or to young women's limited access to information and SRH services? Given the fact that a considerable proportion of sexually active young people in SSA are married, it is important to clarify the extent to which marriage is a protective or risk factor for sexual and reproductive health outcomes.

The labour market

> The energy, skills and aspirations of young people are invaluable assets that no country can afford to squander, and helping them to realise their full potential by gaining access to employment is a precondition for poverty eradication, sustainable development, and lasting peace.
>
> (World Bank 2009)

The large number of young people, coupled with relatively high fertility rates in many parts of the developing world, means that most countries have to grapple with the provision of job opportunities to meet the growing demands. However, due to limited economic growth, many young people are shut out from the labour market. Thus, youth comprise a significant proportion of the unemployed: 43.7 per cent globally and 60 per cent in sub-Saharan Africa (World Bank 2009). Limited employment opportunities also trigger widespread migration among youth, with data from around the world showing that young people aged 15–30 years are the most mobile segment of the population, moving primarily in search of employment opportunities (National Research Council and Institute of Medicine 2005). For many young people, entry into the labour force is prompted by a need to be able to support themselves and others. For some young people, however, entry into the labour market comes too early in life, which may bring short-term benefits of increased family earnings, but at high long-term costs in relation to lost educational opportunities (World Bank 2009). Studies are needed to fully clarify the short- and long-term implications of early entry into the labour force.

Conclusions

Young people today are growing up in a rapidly changing world where improvements in health mean heightened chances of survival to old age; where widespread educational opportunities enhance livelihood prospects; and where globalisation and technological advances increase access to vital information, provide opportunities for civic participation, and enable interactions with diverse groups of people. While many of the changes have beneficial outcomes, the reality is that they also expose young people to numerous risks that threaten their well-being. In sub-Saharan Africa in particular, young people are growing up in a context characterised by the HIV/AIDS pandemic, rapid urbanisation amid floundering economies, increased competition for educational opportunities, rising unemployment, and widespread social disruption. Yet the complex health and social needs of young people, who represent a significant proportion of the population, are often ignored in the health agendas of many countries, especially those in the developing world. Failure to address these needs represents a lost opportunity to meet health and development goals.

References

APHRC (African Population and Health Research Center) (2002) *Population and Health Dynamics in Nairobi's Informal Settlements: Report of the Nairobi Cross-sectional Slums Survey (NCSS) 2000*, Nairobi: African Population and Health Research Center.

APHRC (African Population and Health Research Center) (2008a) *Policy and program issues emerging from APHRC's education research in urban informal settlements of Nairobi, Kenya (Occasional Report No. 2)*, Nairobi: African Population and Health Research Center.

APHRC (African Population and Health Research Center) (2008b) *The Social, Health, and Economic Context of HIV/AIDS in Informal Urban Settlements of Africa*, Nairobi: African Population and Health Research Center.

Arrington-Sanders, R. and Ellen, J. (2008) 'Prevalence of self-reported HIV testing among a population-based sample of urban African American adolescents', *Journal of Adolescent Health*, 43(3): 306–308.

Bankole, A., Biddlecom, A., Guiella, G., Singh, S., and Zulu, E. (2007) 'Sexual behavior, knowledge and information sources of very young adolescents in four sub-Saharan African countries', *African Journal of Reproductive Health*, 11(3): 28–43.

Beguy, D., Kabiru, C.W., Nderu, E.N., and Ngware, M.W. (2009) 'Inconsistencies in self-reporting of sexual activity among the young people in Nairobi (Kenya)', *Journal of Adolescent Health*, 45: 595–601.

Blum, R.W. (2007) 'Youth in sub-Saharan Africa', *Journal of Adolescent Health*, 41: 230–38.

Blum, R.W. (2009) 'Young people: Not as healthy as they seem (Comment)', *The Lancet*, 374: 853–84.

Clark, S., Bruce, J., and Dude, A. (2006) 'Protecting young women from HIV/AIDS: The case against child and adolescent marriage', *International Family Planning Perspectives*, 32(2): 79–88.

Dodoo, F.N., Zulu, E.M., and Ezeh, A.C. (2007) 'Urban-rural differences in the socioeconomic deprivation-sexual behavior link in Kenya', *Social Science & Medicine*, 64: 1,019–31.

Glynn, J.R., Caraël, M., Auvert, B., Kahindo, M., Chege, J., Musonda, R., Kanoa, F., Buvé, F., and Study Group on the Heterogeneity of HIV Epidemics in African Cities (2001) 'Why do young women have a much higher prevalence of HIV than young men? A study in Kisumu, Kenya and Ndola, Zambia', *AIDS*, 15(Supplement 4): S51–S60.

Izugbara, C.O., Kabiru, C.W., and Zulu, E.M. (2009) 'Urban poor Kenyan women and hospital-based delivery', *Public Health Reports*, 124: 585–9.

Joint United Nations Programme on HIV/AIDS (UNAIDS) (2008) *Report on the Global HIV/AIDS Epidemic 2008*, available at http://www.unaids.org/en/HIV_data/2006GlobalReport/default.asp (accessed 29 December 2009).

Kabiru, C.W., Beguy, D., Crichton, J., and Zulu, E. (ms) 'HIV/AIDS among adolescents in urban informal settlements in Kenya: What predicts the likelihood of HIV testing?'.

Kabiru, C., Beguy, D., Undie, C., Zulu, E., and Ezeh, A.C. (2010) 'Transition into first sex among adolescents in slum and non-slum communities in Nairobi, Kenya', *Journal of Youth Studies*, 13(4): 453–71.

Koniak-Griffin, D. and Turner-Pluta, C. (2001) 'Health risks and psychosocial outcomes of early childbearing: a review of the literature', *Journal of Perinatal & Neonatal Nursing*, 15(2): 1–17.

Mensch, B.S., Hewett, P.C., and Erulkar, A.S. (2003) 'The reporting of sensitive behavior by adolescents: A methodological experiment in Kenya', *Demography*, 40(2): 247–68.

Mensch, B.S., Grant, M.J., and Blanc, A.K. (2006) 'The changing context of sexual initiation in sub-Saharan Africa', *Population and Development Review*, 32(4): 699–727.

National AIDS and STD Control Programme (2006) *Guidelines for HIV testing in clinical settings*, 3rd edn, Nairobi, Kenya: Ministry of Health.

National Research Council and Institute of Medicine (2005) *Growing Up Global: The Changing Transitions to Adulthood in Developing Countries. Panel on Transitions to Adulthood in Developing Countries*, Washington, DC: The National Academies Press.

Ndugwa, R., Cleland, J., Kabiru, C., and Zulu, E. (ms) 'Adolescents Sexual experiences and HIV/AIDS knowledge in Nairobi Urban informal settlements'.

Palen, L.-A., Smith, E.A., Caldwell, L.L., Flisher, A.J., Wegner, L., and Vergnani, T. (2008) 'Inconsistent reports of sexual intercourse among South African high school students', *Journal of Adolescent Health*, 42: 221–7.

Patton, G.C., Coffey, C., Sawyer, S.M., Viner, R.M., Haller, D.M., Bose, K., Vos, T., Ferguson, J., and Mathers, C.D.(2009) 'Global patterns of mortality in young people: a systematic analysis of population health data', *The Lancet*, 374(9,693): 881–92.

Plummer, M.L., Ross, D.A., Wight, D., Changalucha, J., Mshana, G., Wamoyi, J., Todd, J., Anemona, A., Mosha, F.F., Obasi, A.I., and Hayes, R.J. (2004) ' "A bit more truthful": the validity of adolescent sexual behaviour data collected in rural northern Tanzania using five methods', *Sexually Transmitted Infections*, 80 Supplement 2: ii49–56.

President's Emergency Plan for AIDS Relief (PEPFAR) (2004) *Annual Report on Prevention of Mother-To-Child Transmission of the HIV Infection*, available at http://www.state.gov/documents/organization/34001.pdf (accessed 14 October 2008).

Resnick, M.D., and Bowes, G. (2007) 'Us and them: worldwide health issues for adolescents', *The Lancet*, 369: 1,058–60.

UN-HABITAT (United Nations Human Settlements Programme) (2008a) *The State of African Cities 2008: A Framework for Addressing Urban Challenges in Africa*, Nairobi: UN-HABITAT.

UN-HABITAT (United Nations Human Settlements Programme) (2008b), *State of the World's Cities 2008/2009: Harmonious Cities*, Nairobi: UN-HABITAT.

US Census Bureau (2009) *International Data Base (IDB): World Population by Age and Sex*, available at http://www.census.gov (accessed 31 December 2009).

World Bank (2008) *Kenya Poverty and Inequality Assessment (Volume 1: Synthesis Report) – Draft Report (44190-KE)*, available at www.hackenya.org/ (accessed 13 April 2010).

World Bank (2009) *Youth and Employment in Africa: The Potential, the Problem, the Promise*, Washington, DC: World Bank.

Zulu, E.M., Dodoo, F.N., and Ezeh, A.C. (2002) 'Sexual risk-taking in the slums of Nairobi, Kenya, 1993–98', *Population Studies*, 56(3): 311–23.

19

Reducing Death and Disability from Unsafe Abortion

Therese McGinn

In this chapter, we will examine the global scope of abortion and the challenges faced by public health professionals in reducing death and disability from unsafe abortion. The challenges are programmatic and political, some linked to the larger issues of weak health systems in the developing world generally and some specific to the issue of abortion.

The global scope of abortion

Abortion is the death and expulsion of the foetus from the uterus either spontaneously or by induction before the 22nd week of pregnancy, though the specific number of weeks may vary from one country to another depending on local legislation (WHO 2003). The World Health Organization (WHO) estimates that 80 million women per year have an unplanned pregnancy and that 42 million pregnancies were voluntarily terminated throughout the world in 2003, or 32 abortions for every 100 live births (WHO 2007). When abortion is induced by qualified staff using correct techniques in sanitary conditions, it is a very safe procedure. In the US, for example, the death rate from induced abortion is 0.6 per 100,000 procedures, making it as safe as an injection of penicillin (WHO 2007). However, approximately half (48 per cent) of the 42 million annual induced abortions are unsafe, and virtually all (98 per cent) of the unsafe abortions are in the developing world (WHO 2007).

Unsafe abortion is a major direct cause of maternal mortality, accounting for an estimated 13 per cent or 65,000–70,000 maternal deaths per year (WHO 2007). Additionally, unsafe abortion leads to 5 million women suffering temporary or permanent disability annually (WHO 2007).[1] Reducing abortion-related maternal deaths would contribute substantially to the attainment of Millennium Development Goal No. 5, 'Reduce by three-quarters the maternal mortality ratio', which the United Nations (UN) reports requires accelerated progress (UN 2009).

Challenges to reducing death and disability from unsafe abortion

Few women die from unsafe abortion in some countries; what prevents women in other countries from attaining the same level of safety? We will review the challenges women face in obtaining safe abortion services, which include real and perceived national policy constraints, limited availability and quality of safe abortion services, and the influence of donors, specifically the US government.

The challenge of national policy

Only five countries in the world ban abortion entirely: Chile, El Salvador, the Holy See, Malta, and Nicaragua. The remaining countries, covering 99 per cent of the world's population, permit abortion under at least some circumstances.

As Table 19.1 shows, most countries permit abortion for a range of reasons. Of the 194 countries included in the UN's 2007 review of abortion policies, 55 countries covering 40 per cent of the world's population permit abortion 'on request'. This is the least restrictive policy category: most of these countries impose limits on the period during which women may access abortion but, within those limits, women need not give a reason for requesting an abortion. Most of the countries with such policies are in the developed world. A greater number, 66 countries covering 61 per cent of the world's people, permit abortion for women who can demonstrate economic or social need. Additional countries allow abortion when the foetus is impaired, and 94 countries, with 72 per cent of the world's population, specifically allow abortion in cases of rape or incest. The majority of countries permits abortion to preserve women's mental or physical health – 125 and 130 countries respectively, covering over three-fourths of the world's people. The mental or physical health provision may be used to approve abortion for rape or incest survivors in countries without specific allowance for those conditions. As noted, almost all countries – 189 of the 194 included in the UN's 2007 review, covering 99 per cent of the world's population – permit abortion to save the life of a woman (UN Population Division 2007). Typically, health, mental health, or other professionals must approve the abortion procedure under the economic or social need, mental health, physical health, or life of the women allowances, and interpretation may vary among these professionals across and within countries.

Changes in abortion policies have been linked to changes in maternal death. Legalising abortion has been shown to reduce maternal mortality while restricting abortion has been

Table 19.1 Grounds on which abortion is legally permitted in 194 countries, 2007

	To save the woman's life	To preserve physical health	To preserve mental health	Rape or incest	Foetal impairment	Economic or social reasons	On request
All countries (n = 194)							
• Permitted	189	130	125	94	88	66	55
• Not permitted	5	64	69	100	106	128	139
Proportion of world's population covered							
• Permitted	99	78	75	72	64	61	40
• Not permitted	1	22	25	28	36	39	60

Source: United Nations Population Division 2007.

shown to increase maternal death. The case of Romania is often cited to illustrate the link. In 1966, Romania reversed the legal status of abortion and then, in 1985, introduced further restrictions. Data show that maternal mortality in Romania from 1979 to 1989 was ten times higher than in any other European country. In 1989, the new government overturned the restrictions and again permitted abortions. From 1989 to 1992, the maternal mortality ratio declined from 170 to 60 deaths per 100,000 live births, a decline reported to be due entirely to the reduction in abortion-related deaths (Serbanescu et al. 1995). In South Africa, the 1996 Choice of Termination of Pregnancy Act legalised abortion and resulted in a 91 per cent reduction in deaths due to unsafe abortion between 1994 and 1998 to 2001 (Jewkes and Rees 2005). Policy restrictions also affect mortality: Nicaragua introduced a total ban on abortion in July 2008, a change from the 1983 law which permitted abortion to save a woman's life. Government data show that maternal deaths increased by 65 per cent from January to August 2009 compared to the same period in 2008; these figures are thought by health and human rights to be underestimates (Moloney 2009).

Thus, while national policies may restrict abortion in many countries of the world, it is nevertheless true that almost all women live in countries where abortion is permitted at least under some conditions. Most live in countries in which abortion is allowed for a range of health and social reasons. Having a policy that permits abortion is an important foundation for saving women's lives. The challenge of applying policy by ensuring that safe abortion is available is also critical, and is addressed below.

The challenge of limited availability and quality of safe abortion

Safe abortion procedures

Most abortions are carried out in the first trimester (the first 12 weeks of pregnancy). Even where laws permit later abortions, such as in France, the United States, and the United Kingdom, the proportions of abortions carried out after 12 weeks were 6, 11, and 12 per cent, respectively, in 2002, 2004, and 2006 (Singh et al. 2009).

Protocols for safe abortion are well-established and consistent throughout the world (WHO 2003). First trimester abortion may be done by manual or electric vacuum aspiration or newer medication methods.

Manual vacuum aspiration (MVA) – better suited to low-resource settings than electric vacuum aspiration – is a procedure in which the provider uses a hand-held, hand-activated plastic aspirator or syringe attached to a vacuum source. A thin plastic cannula is attached to the syringe, inserted through the cervix to the uterus, and the products of conception are suctioned out. Dilatation of the cervix before cannula insertion is usually but not always required, and clients may be given analgesics or local anaesthesia for pain. The procedure takes 3–10 minutes, and most clients are ready to leave the recovery room within 30 minutes (WHO 2003).

Abortion using orally administered drugs, called medical or medication abortion, has become more widely used in the last decade. The most common regimen requires taking two sets of oral pills within 48 hours. The first dose is mifepristone, an antiprogestogen which interferes with the continuation of the pregnancy. The second dose is a prostaglandin, such as misoprostol, which enhances uterine contractions. The result is the expulsion of the foetus, with effects similar to those associated with a spontaneous abortion. Bleeding occurs for an average of nine days, and women may experience cramping. Medication abortion fails for 2 to 5 per cent of clients, who then require vacuum aspiration to complete the abortion (WHO 2003). This regimen is proven effective for up to nine weeks' gestation, and studies testing its use at 10 to 12 weeks are likely to show its effectiveness for this gestational period (Singh *et al.* 2009). Using oral or vaginal misoprostol alone up to nine weeks' gestation is also a safe option, though not as effective as the mifepristone-misoprostol combination (Singh *et al.* 2009).

Medication abortion is increasingly chosen where it is offered as an option. For example, medication abortion accounted for 40 per cent of abortions in England and Wales in 2009 (UK Department of Health 2010), 70 per cent in Scotland in 2009 (ISD Scotland 2010), and 46 per cent in France in 2006 (Vilain 2008). In Sweden, 86 per cent of all abortions performed before the ninth week of pregnancy were done with medication in 2009 (National Board of Health and Welfare, Sweden, 2010).

Safe abortion providers

Protocols for safe abortion also determine which cadres of health workers are permitted to provide the procedures. While some countries specify that only physicians may perform MVA or medication abortion, studies have consistently shown that mid-level providers – such as midwives and nurses – can provide care as well as physicians. For example, randomised controlled equivalence trials in South Africa and Vietnam compared complication rates for MVA procedures done by physicians and by mid-level providers, most of whom were midwives, and found the rates equivalent (Warriner *et al.* 2006). Non-physician clinicians in Mozambique (Pereira *et al.* 1996), Malawi (Chilopera *et al.* 2007), and Tanzania (McCord *et al.* 2009) provide MVA as well as more complex obstetric procedures such as Caesarean section, also with outcomes comparable to physicians. Where medication abortion is widely available, mid-level providers routinely manage the service (Yarnall *et al.* 2009). With appropriate pre-service and in-service training and regular clinical support, the evidence demonstrates that mid-level staff can provide safe abortion services, using both MVA and medication.

Delivering safe abortion

Performing abortion safely is neither a complex nor dangerous procedure. It does not require running water, electricity, sophisticated equipment, or high level staff. It can be done in rural health centres by trained mid-level providers. Why then do 65,000 to 70,000 women die and another 5 million women become disabled each year from unsafe abortion? (WHO 2007).

Fundamentally, abortion-related deaths and disability occur because good quality safe abortion services – even when permitted by national policy – are not available to women who want and need them. Post-abortion care, the set of services needed to treat women with complications of unsafe abortion and to provide family planning to prevent further unplanned pregnancies, is also often unavailable. These services are not available because overall health systems are often weak and because, within these weak systems, women's health care, and abortion specifically, may receive low priority.

For any health service to be delivered well – whether safe abortion, family planning, delivery, immunisation, HIV/AIDS care and treatment, or the many other services people need – all components of the health system must function and they must function well together. Hospital and health centre infrastructure, including water and sanitation systems, must be developed and maintained. Equipment and supplies must be ordered, installed, maintained, tracked, and reordered. Staff must be trained, hired, posted, supervised, and retrained for their clinical responsibilities. The public must be engaged in ways that enhance their knowledge and their power to make decisions as individuals and as communities. Outreach, referral links, and feedback loops must be established across communities, health centres, and hospitals. Systems to manage the human resources, logistics, supervision, quality of care, referral, and data needs must be established, and managers trained in their use at province, district, and facility levels.

When any of these health system components is missing or functioning badly – for example, when there are staff but no supplies, supplies but no working equipment, poor infection prevention procedures, health facilities that do not earn the trust and confidence of the communities they serve – then all health services, not only safe abortion, are weak. Gaps such as these are common in developing countries and it is the responsibility of Ministries of Health to address them, often with the involvement and support of foreign government and private donors, and local and international technical organisations.

Making safe abortion a priority

Determining priorities when the needs are many and resources few is a major challenge. It is in the choice of priorities that women's health, and especially safe abortion services, are often disadvantaged. Many services, such as child survival and malaria prevention, are not only critically important but virtually controversy-free; improving such care is often determined a priority. Some needs, notably HIV prevention and HIV/AIDS care and treatment, are also critically important and have substantial, dedicated funding available from sources such as the Global Fund to Fight AIDS, Tuberculosis and Malaria and the US President's Emergency Plan for AIDS Relief (PEPFAR). The true need for greater HIV/AIDS programmes combined with the availability of resources also influences the selection of priorities.

In addition to the factors that support other health needs as priorities, several factors work against choosing women's health and abortion specifically as a priority. Abortion is controversial in many societies and carries stigma for women who seek abortion and the workers who provide it. Even in a largely unrestricted policy environment, individual providers may prefer not to be involved in safe abortion care. The controversy or fear of controversy can stifle discussion. Neither the public nor health providers may understand the actual status of abortion policy in their countries but fear voicing their questions, and so continue to act under the assumption that it is illegal in all cases. Donors and assistance agencies too often collude in this silence, being unwilling to raise what is assumed to be a sensitive topic for fear of offending local sensibilities, government donors, or their public. Many programme managers and health care providers are simply confused, unsure of what they are allowed to say or not say, do or not do.

The challenge of US government influence

In fact, their fear and confusion are justified with respect to the US government, a large and influential donor.[1] The US government has periodically instituted and rescinded abortion-related policies associated with its foreign aid. Most attention has been paid to the 'Mexico City Policy', named because it was articulated by the US government under President Ronald Reagan at the 1984 International Conference on Population and Development in Mexico City (Anon. 1984). The Mexico City Policy prohibited overseas non-governmental organisations from receiving US family planning assistance if they provided abortion-related information, counselling, or services, or carried out any abortion rights activity, even though such work would be covered by non-US funds (the Helms Amendment, discussed below, already prohibited US funds from being used for abortion). The Mexico City Policy was rescinded by President Bill Clinton in 1993, reinstated by President George W. Bush in 2001, and again rescinded by President Barack Obama in 2009, all in the first days of their administrations (PAI 2006). Ironically, the Mexico City regulations may have been interpreted far more broadly than their provisions actually required. For example, the restrictions applied only to foreign non-governmental agencies, not to foreign governments, multilateral agencies, or US agencies; they applied only to US family planning funding, not to other US funding, including that for HIV/AIDS; and they made allowances for abortion to save the life of a woman and in cases of rape and incest (PAI 2006). However, the fear of running foul of this highly politicised and confusing set of regulations and the impracticalities of determining when the restrictions applied and when they did not – especially within highly integrated field programmes – led many organisations to instruct their staff to simply never discuss abortion. This chilling effect led to the policy becoming known as the 'global gag rule'.

The substantial political attention to the Mexico City Policy distracts from a more encompassing and longstanding US government restriction. The 1973 Helms Amendment to the 1961 Foreign Assistance Act, named for its sponsor, Senator Jesse Helms of North Carolina, prohibits the use of US government funds to support abortion as a method of family planning or to motivate or coerce any person to practice abortion (USAID 2009). This has been interpreted in US foreign aid implementation as prohibiting abortion information, education, and services even when a woman's life is in danger or in cases of rape or incest, regardless of countries' own policies; the subsequent Siljander Amendment extended the restrictions to speech for or against national abortion law reform (Ipas 2009). The Helms Amendment applies to any entity that receives US funding, including US organisations, foreign agencies, national governments, and multilateral agencies. Unlike the Mexico City Policy, which was issued and can be changed by executive order, the Helms Amendment was enacted and would have to be changed by Congress.

Few developing country governments or non-governmental organisations will risk losing US government funding – a substantial amount and proportion of total budgets for many – over the issue of abortion.

The case for safe abortion for women who are raped, including in war

The need for safe abortion in the developing world is neglected because it is highly politicised globally and because many assume, wrongly, that national abortion laws make abortion illegal in all instances. As we have seen, that is not the case. It is a public health imperative to advance the conversation about safe abortion.

Safe abortion for women who are raped, including during conflict, may provide common ground for discussion. Sexual assault, especially by strangers or by combatants during war, is commonly agreed to be a social wrong and is a crime in most countries. Almost three-quarters of the world's population (72 per cent) live in countries which recognise rape or incest as special circumstances and so permit abortion. International human rights laws and treaties include the right to safe abortion, at least in some circumstances (Shaw 2010). When committed as part of systematic attacks directed at civilians, sexual slavery, rape, and forced pregnancy are defined by the International Criminal Court as crimes against humanity (United Nations General Assembly 2002).

Humanitarian organisations provide a range of services to respond to the needs of refugees and internally displaced persons during and in the period following conflicts and natural disasters. In addition to food, water, sanitation, and shelter, standards-based health services are offered (Sphere 2010). To prevent and respond to sexual violence, programmes may be implemented to enhance security, offer social support to survivors, and train women to generate income. Health services may include emergency contraception, treatment for sexually transmitted infections, and prophylaxis to prevent HIV transmission, if survivors come early enough to clinics and if the clinics have what they need to provide those services. Legal assistance may be available for women to seek justice through the courts.

However, a service rarely available to women who become pregnant as a result of rape is safe abortion, even though international laws authorise it and even where national policy allows it (Lehmann 2002). Organisations receiving US funding are caught between their obligation to apply humanitarian standards, which require that they act to prevent forced pregnancy and carry out other rape-related prevention and response activities, and the Helms Amendment, which bars them from providing abortion information, education, or services with their US funds (Centre for Global Justice 2010). Women are the losers in this stand-off.

Providing safe abortion information, education, and services to women who become pregnant through rape, including in conflict, may be a useful starting point for discussion. Such activities may be done currently with non-US funds, though challenges to the Helms Amendment on grounds that it violates international humanitarian law may result in changes to US policy and practice (Centre for Global Justice 2010).

Note

1 The US provides the highest dollar amount of official development assistance (ODA) of any country, $28.7 billion in 2009 or 24 per cent of the ODA provided by 23 donor governments (OECD 2010).

References

Anon. (1984) 'US Policy Statement for the International Conference on Population', *Population and Development Review*, 10(3): 574–9.

Centre for Global Justice (2010) *United States of America, Submission to the UN Universal Periodic Review, Ninth Session of the UPR Working Group of the Human Rights Council*, New York: Centre for Global Justice.

Chilopora, G., Pereira, C., Kamwendo, F., Chimbiri, A., Malunga, E. and Bergström, S. (2007) 'Postoperative Outcome of Caesarean Sections and Other Major Emergency Obstetric Surgery by Clinical Officers and Medical Officers in Malawi', *Human Resources for Health*, 5: 17.

ISD (Information Services Division), Scotland (2010) *Sexual Health: Abortions Data*, available at http://www.isdscotland.org/isd/1918.html (accessed 6 June 2010).

Ipas (2009) *The Abortion Ban in US Foreign Assistance: How U.S. Policy Obstructs Efforts to Save Women's Lives*, Chapel Hill, NC: Ipas.

Jewkes, R. and Rees, H. (2005) 'Dramatic Decline in Abortion Mortality due to the Choice on Termination of Pregnancy Act', *South African Medical Journal*, 95: 4.

Lehmann, A. (2002) 'Safe Abortion: A Right for Refugees?', *Reproductive Health Matters*, 10(19): 151–5.

McCord, C., Mbaruku, G., Pereira, C., Nzabuhakwa, C., and Bergstrom, S. (2009) 'The Quality of Emergency Obstetrical Surgery by Assistant Medical Officers in Tanzanian District Hospitals', *Health Affairs*, 28(5): w876–w885.

Moloney, A. (2009) 'Abortion Ban Leads to More Maternal Deaths in Nicaragua', *The Lancet*, 374: 677.

National Board of Health and Welfare, Sweden (2010) *Induced Abortions 2009*, Sweden: National Board of Health and Welfare, available at http://www.socialstyrelsen.se/Lists/Artikelkatalog/Attachments/18031/2010-5-12.pdf (accessed 6 June 2010).

OECD (Organisation for Economic Cooperation and Development) (2010) *Table 1: Net Official Development Assistance in 2009 (Preliminary data for 2009)*, available at http://www.oecd.org/dataoecd/17/9/44981892.pdf (accessed 6 June 2010).

Pereira, C., Bugalho, A. and Bergstrom, S. (1996) 'A Comparative Study of Caesarean Deliveries by Assistant Medical Officers and Obstetricians in Mozambique', *British Journal of Obstetrics and Gynaecology*, 103: 508–12.

PAI (Population Action International) (2006) *What You Need to Know about the Mexico City Policy Restrictions on US Family Planning Assistance: An Unofficial Guide*, April, Washington, DC: PAI.

Serbanescu, F., Morris, L., Stupp, P. and Stanescu, A. (1995) 'The Impact of Recent Policy Changes on Fertility, Abortion, and Contraceptive Use in Romania', *Studies in Family Planning*, 26(2): 76–87.

Shaw, D. (2010) 'Abortion and Human Rights', *Best Practice and Research Clinical Obstetrics and Gynecology*, 24(5): 633–46.

Singh, S., Wulf, D., Hussain, R., Bankole, A., and Sedgh, G. (2009) *Abortion Worldwide: A Decade of Uneven Progress*, New York: Guttmacher Institute.

Sphere Project (2010) *Humanitarian Charter and Minimum Standards in Disaster Response*, Geneva: The Sphere Project.

United Kingdom Department of Health (2010) *Abortion Statistics, England and Wales: 2009*, available at http://www.dh.gov.uk/en/Publicationsandstatistics/Publications/PublicationsStatistics/DH_116039 (accessed 6 June 2010).

UN (United Nations) (2009) *Millennium Development Goals Report*, New York: United Nations.

United Nations General Assembly (2002) *Rome Statute of the International Criminal Court (last amended January 2002)*, Article 7: 'Crimes against Humanity', A/CONF. 183/9.

UN (United Nations) Population Division, Department of Economic and Social Affairs (2007) 'World Abortion Policies 2007 (Wallchart)', New York: United Nations Population Division.

USAID (US Agency for International Development) (2009) *Family Planning Guiding Principles and U.S. Legislative and Policy Requirements: Restrictions on Support for Abortions*, Washington, DC: USAID, available at http://www.usaid.gov/our_work/global_health/pop/restrictions.html (accessed 6 June 2010).

Vilain, A. (2008) *Les Interruptions Volontaires de Grossesse en 2006: Etudes et Résultats No. 659*, Paris: Ministry of Health, available at http://www.sante.gouv.fr/drees/etude-resultat/er-pdf/er659.pdf (accessed 6 June 2010).

Warriner, I.K., Meirik, O., Hoffman, M., Morroni, C., Harries, J., My Huong, N.T., Vy, N.D., and Seuc, A.H. (2006) 'Rates of Complication in First-trimester Manual Vacuum Aspiration Abortion done by Doctors and Mid-level Providers in South Africa and Vietnam: A Randomized Controlled Equivalence Trial', *The Lancet*, 368: 1,965–72.

WHO (World Health Organization) (2003) *Safe Abortion: Technical and Policy Guidance for Health Systems*, Geneva: WHO.

WHO (World Health Organization) (2007) *Unsafe Abortion: Global and Regional Estimates of the Incidence of Unsafe Abortion and Associated Mortality in 2003*, 5th edn, Geneva: WHO.

Yarnall, J., Swica, Y., and Winikoff, B. (2009) 'Non-physician Clinicians Can Safely Provide First Trimester Medical Abortion', *Reproductive Health Matters*, 17(331): 61–9.

20

Masculinity and Its Public Health Implications for Sexual and Reproductive Health and HIV Prevention

Margaret E. Greene and Gary Barker

Introduction

This chapter describes some of the main findings emerging from research on men, masculinities, and programmes that seek to change social norms related to violent or gender inequitable views of manhood in ways that improve health. Sexual and reproductive health (SRH), and to some extent prevailing HIV prevention paradigms, have used a gender lens to focus on the vulnerabilities and disempowerment of women and girls. Research in the reproductive health field often collects data on sexual and reproductive health only from women (Greene and Biddlecom 2000), and, in a mutually reinforcing cycle, it often uses a gender lens to focus on women's disadvantaged position without addressing the role of masculinity in both contributing to gender inequities and putting men and their partners at risk. In this chapter, we seek to bring in this perspective, highlighting how applying a gender perspective to men and masculinities provides a more nuanced view of the health needs and rights of both men and women.

Underlying this approach has been the assumption that women were in monogamous heterosexual marital relationships, and that they are primarily responsible for any fertility regulation. Sexuality really has not figured in this vision. In contrast, HIV prevention efforts have reflected greater attention to sexuality and the diversity of sexual relationships from the outset.

Programme interventions and policy responses in the public health arena have therefore tended to follow the research by emphasising women's and girls' vulnerabilities and disempowerment, while applying stereotypes to men and boys as either disinterested, risk-taking, sexually predatory, or always in control of heterosexual relations.

The case has now been made quite effectively that reducing gender inequality is key to improving sexual and reproductive health and reducing HIV. Where cultural and economic conditions privilege men's control over resources, men indeed exert considerable control over the timing and nature of sexual relations, the number of children a couple has, whether or not they protect themselves from disease, and often women's access to health care. Feminist advocates fought for the recognition of women's human rights, including the rights to decide freely whether, when, and with whom to have children, and the rights to determine whether, with whom, and under what circumstances to engage in sexual relations. The 1994 Cairo ICPD

Programme of Action was informed by extensive research on and activism related to women's subordinate status in most societies (UNFPA 1994).

The ongoing challenge is how to translate the rhetorical support for gender equity into a more holistic approach to sexual and reproductive health and rights. A growing number and range of programmes have attempted in recent years to incorporate men (and to some extent, young men and boys) into public health interventions that address sexuality, reproductive health, and HIV prevention. These programmes are diverse in their reach, approaches, and effectiveness. Yet, women- (and more recently, girl-) focused services – and women-focused or girl-focused 'social change' interventions – are still largely the norm.

This limited take on 'gender' negates the ways gender roles harm men's health, sidesteps widespread male control over sexuality and reproduction, and misses opportunities to catalyse social change and improve women's *and* men's health by involving both sexes. We assert that men are essential to 'gender', that changing the harmful gender norms that undermine health requires everyone's participation, and that efforts to engage men and empower women benefit both sexes.

What a unilaterally 'gendered' approach to SRH and HIV prevention has meant for health programmes

The way gender equity has been defined in the context of health programmes has had three negative consequences for health and development.

Advances for girls and women continue to encounter gender-related obstacles

First, girls and women who have benefitted from advances in other areas are still finding themselves held back by limited notions of what it means to be female. Global discourse on empowering girls and women has generally centred on increasing girls' enrolment in public education, reducing early marriage, and empowering women economically. But even where we see progress in achieving these goals, girls and women still struggle (Barker 2007). In Latin America and the Caribbean, for example, where almost all girls are enrolled in primary school, and girls' enrolment often exceeds that of boys in secondary school (UNESCO 2008), girls still experience harassment and unwanted sexual advances that affect their health and their success in school. Research from Kenya shows that school environments in which female students reported that girls and boys were not treated equally by the teachers and school administration – reinforcing societal discrimination – greatly increased girls' chances of dropping out (Mensch *et al.* 2001). In parts of sub-Saharan Africa and much of South Asia, girls studying in coeducational schools similarly report harassment and sexual violence at the hands of male students and teachers (Dunne *et al.* 2003; Jeejheebhoy *et al.* 2005). Thus, even as girls and women are empowered and encouraged to study or work, little is being done to engage men and boys to create environments free of harassment and abuse.

Unfavourable stereotypes of men abound in sexual and reproductive health programmes

The negative stereotypes of men that influence their exclusion from many programmes include the sense that they are disinterested, do not care about sexual and reproductive health, which they view as women's domain, and do not see what is in it for them. Second is the notion that men are invariably predatory in their sexual relationships and relations and unable to see their relationships with women as places for give and take and mutual respect and pleasure. Third, men are also viewed as being entirely in control of sexual relations, and reluctant to give up any of that control. Fourth, the recognition that men engage in risk-taking gives rise to the perspective that they are reckless to the point of not being interested in caring for their health or that of others. Finally, sceptics are suspicious that including men and boys may undermine gender equality, for example, men can appear 'politically correct' without actually ceding power and privilege.

If men were consistently like these negative stereotypes, there might be little point in engaging them. Fortunately, they are not. A growing body of qualitative and quantitative research on men's behaviours, attitudes, and lived experiences related to their sexual lives finds tremendous diversity among men in their attitudes, lives, and responses to their cultural contexts. Given the opportunity, many seem willing to question rigid gender norms. Still, if there is evidence that men and masculinities change, there also remains significant scepticism about whether they can change quickly and significantly enough to matter for this generation of women and girls (Barker 2007).

Working with men versus working with women is viewed as a 'zero sum game'

Men and boys can – and many do already – see that gender equality is not always a losing proposition. The tendency in the field, however, is to view women's and men's interests as competing directly with one another. Relationships based on greater equality and cooperation, a more equal division of household, and work activities outside the household, and equal pay to go with that equal division, are good for all of us – men and women (Barker 2007). Men in diverse contexts are coming to see the benefits of viewing their sexual and intimate relations in more equitable ways (Barker 2005). While giving up power and privilege is never easy, men in these studies voluntarily relinquished some of their power once they really understood the extraordinarily high costs of unequal power relations.

Given the risks, as well as benefits, male involvement poses to women's autonomy, privacy, and health, *how* men are included in reproductive health programmes is extremely important. The sexual and reproductive health field must address legitimate concerns as to whether engaging men and boys in gender equality will take away the already scarce resources for women's and girls' empowerment. Family planning, an important source of empowerment for women and for physiological and social reasons, must continue to address women's needs (Schuler *et al.* 1995, 1998). Though some worry that including men in service delivery may dissuade women from accessing services, strain existing services by increasing workloads, and channel scarce resources away from women to men, programmes and policies that integrate a holistic gender perspective have the potential to multiply the value of every dollar spent.

How to recognise women's greater sexual and reproductive vulnerabilities while acknowledging that men also face vulnerabilites?

The prevailing gender discourse in diverse fora has often ignored men's sexual and reproductive vulnerabilities, viewing them as secondary or as competing with women's needs and vulner-abilities. A 'relational' starting point on sexual and reproductive health is to acknowledge women's greater vulnerabilities on aggregate *and* to understand men as subjects of rights who can and sometimes are made vulnerable by prevailing gender norms. Problematic norms may suggest men are invincible, cause them to delay seeking health care, and persuade them that unprotected, unplanned sex is more exciting than safer sex, or that they require multiple sexual partners to fulfil physical and social expectations.

Indeed, while men face health vulnerabilities in the sexual and reproductive health arenas, the fact remains that women bear the greatest costs of problematic sexual and reproductive practices and poor reproductive health. Research has consistently shown that men largely drive the spread of sexually transmitted disease, and that women bear greater health hazards associated with sexual activity and reproduction than men (Foreman 1999).

A few key statistics show how far we have to go in engaging men more fully in sexual and reproductive health, and also suggest the potential positive health impacts of shifting gender norms. Despite advances in encouraging men to use male contraceptive methods, women continue to bear the responsibility for family planning worldwide (over 74 per cent of all contraceptive use) (Barker and Olukoya 2009). The recent WHO-sponsored multi-country study showed some 30–50 per cent of women worldwide have suffered physical violence at least once from a male partner (WHO 2002). Approximately 600,000 women die of maternal-health related causes each year, the majority of these deaths preventable (WHO 2007). Girls and women are especially vulnerable to HIV and recent data show that young women account for 75 per cent of 15- to 24-year-olds living with HIV in Africa (Global Coalition on Women and AIDS 2006), over 70 per cent in the Caribbean, and nearly 70 per cent of the infected young people in the Middle East and North Africa (Levine *et al.* 2007).

While there is some evidence of encouraging men and boys to question rigid forms of socialisation and power, harmful gender norms continue to pose major public health challenges. Much more could be done to engage men in the support and care of the women in their lives.

The neglect of men's vulnerabilites

Both men and women are made vulnerable by men's gendered attitudes and behaviours. In some settings, for example, being a man means being tough, brave, risk-taking, aggressive, and not caring for one's body. Men's and boys' engagement in some risk-taking behaviours, including substance use, unsafe sex, and unsafe driving, may be seen as ways to affirm their manhood. The need to appear invulnerable also reduces men's willingness to seek help or treatment for physical or mental health problems.

In some settings, men have more chronic health conditions than women, die earlier on average, and face greater rates of injuries and morbidities related to occupational illnesses, traffic accidents, and violence-related injuries. Men in some predominantly male institutions, such as police forces, the military, or in prisons, also face specific risks due to institutional cultures that may encourage domination and violence. If prevailing notions of manhood often increase men's own vulnerability to injuries and other health risks, they also create considerable risk for women and girls.

These health-related vulnerabilities for men are exacerbated by class differences – lower-income men, and men of socially excluded groups are even more likely to suffer from illnesses and injuries, and these same issues play out in the realm of sexual and reproductive health. Low-income men, men who migrate for work, and men with limited access to health services (generally low-income men) are more likely to have STIs, less likely to seek treatment for those STIs, and more likely have higher rates of HIV (Saggurti *et al.* 2009). Young and adult men in violent, low-income, or conflict-affected settings may suffer from a sense of helplessness and fatalism that contributes to lower rates of safer sex and health-seeking behaviour (Barker 2005).

In short, men suffer from poor health as a consequence of the same risk-taking and other behaviours that can harm their sexual partners, male and female. The vulnerabilities of masculinity are changeable and not simply determined by biology. Poverty and the economic and social marginalisation of men intensify these effects. Programmes miss out by not addressing masculinity and men's vulnerabilities as part of a comprehensive approach to health.

Programmes engaging men and boys in the struggle against gender inequality

The world has made the most progress in addressing gender inequality as it affects health in the sexual and reproductive health and HIV prevention arenas. The surge over the past 15 years in programmes that engage men has been lagged by an 'echo boom' of evaluations. These are providing the basis for a growing body of evidence that engaging men and boys in gender-specific, relevant programmes leads to improved health and other benefits. Emerging studies of programme models being implemented by a diverse range of institutions are showing that engaging men and boys can result in higher condom use, reduced rates of sexually transmitted infections, greater take-up by men of voluntary counselling and testing (VCT), and increased collaboration between couples on matters of sexual and reproductive health.

WHO and Promundo[1] recently reviewed 59 evaluation studies of programmes working to engage men and boys in health interventions in the areas of sexual and reproductive health, HIV/AIDS prevention, gender-based violence, fatherhood, and maternal and child health (Barker et al. 2007). The review classified the programmes by the extent to which they challenged harmful gender norms, and also ranked them with regard to their overall effectiveness, assessing whether the impact was on behaviours, attitudes, or knowledge, and combining this with the rigour of the evaluation design.

Few programmes engaging men and boys last for more than two to three years or get scaled up beyond the pilot stage. Yet the evidence we have from these indicates that carefully conceived programmes with men and boys can lead to positive changes in men's and boys' attitudes and behaviours related to sexual and reproductive health and HIV, maternal and child health, engagement with their children, their use of violence, and whether they seek out health care.

Programmes that seek to promote more gender-equitable relationships between men and women are more effective in producing behaviour change, as are programmes that address social context and not just the individual men. Programmes that include deliberate discussions of gender and masculinities and the benefits of transforming such gender norms appear to be more effective than programmes that merely acknowledge or mention gender norms and roles.

Integrated programmes that provide both individual engagement with men and community mobilisation or media-based messages were the most effective (Barker et al. 2007). Given that the ultimate goal of this work is to help men understand their choices and behaviours in a broader social context, the powerful effects of programmes that reach beyond the individual level, to men and boys' social contexts, including relationships, social institutions, gatekeepers, community leaders, and so on, make perfect sense.

Promundo's experience in applying their Programme H approach finds lower rates of STIs, higher rates of condom use, and more concern with their own health and their partners' health as a result of well-designed and consistently applied group education and community campaigns (Pulerwitz *et al.* 2006).

Programmes can respect and affirm the caring and responsible roles men may play already in their families. In Turkey, where withdrawal is widespread, the failure to support withdrawal in favour of 'modern' and 'effective' methods of birth control used by women actively discouraged male involvement where it was already high (Rogow and Horowitz 1995). By helping men learn parenting and negotiating skills, for example, programmes can assist men in questioning their limited notions of masculinity, and can transform the basis of male–female relationships. Men who are more involved in the health of their families themselves enjoy better health and closer relationships with their family members (Miedzian 1991). Young men who want to see their children grow up seem less likely to take serious risks (Cohen 1998).

By increasing men's security about their own masculinity (Segal 1990), programmes can contribute to a greater capacity to understand and communicate openly with women. Supporting men who are the exceptions to dominant masculinity can be difficult, but offers substantial payoffs (Montoya 1999). The Society for the Integrated Development of the Himalayas in India, for example, identifies men who are the *exceptions* to the disengaged norm, and supports them in spreading their more positive views of women and more active roles in fatherhood (Barker 1997: 26). When provided with positive alternatives and the possibility of questioning the limited roles with which they were raised, men are often glad to adapt their behaviour in ways that challenge traditional rules of masculinity.

Public policy addressing masculinities and health

Most of the innovative work in recent years to involve men in questioning harmful gender norms that undermine health has occurred in the context of programmes. It is time now to be more ambitious and to expand this work to the policy level. There is a great need for increased implementation of policies, legal structures, or laws, especially in developing country settings, to engage men in achieving gender equality.

Policies and national guidelines ensure that good ideas for engaging men and boys are taken to scale. They define approaches and increase programme consistency around objectives and strategies for working with men. The formulation and implementation process can facilitate coordination across sectors. This helps to prevent male engagement from being interpreted as a strictly clinical mandate for treating men as reproductive health clients.

The general tendency is for governments to endorse gender equity internationally, but to have little to say in *national* development policies about men and their potential roles in achieving it. A few notable exceptions stand out, however; a few governments are beginning to include discussions of men's vulnerabilities, as well as the need to engage men in specific ways in achieving gender equality and ending violence against women. In South Africa, for example, engaging men has been made part of the gender equality agenda, even if implementation lags behind policy pronouncements (Redpath *et al.* 2008).

Paternity leave policies in some European countries show evidence of increased participation by men in child-rearing and an increased use of paid paternity leave, which men previously often failed to use. An example from a middle-income country is Costa Rica's Responsible Paternity Law, which includes awareness-raising campaigns and public support for mothers to request DNA testing from men. Nearly a third of Costa Rican children had been unrecognised by their fathers, with all of the implications for name, support, and inheritance that this implied. In 2001, the government took action and adopted the innovative Law of Responsible Fatherhood, whose intention is to expand men's roles beyond biological paternity to social and cultural fatherhood. The law led to a dramatic decline in the number of children with unrecognised paternity – from 29.3 per cent in 1999 to 7.8 per cent in 2003 (Centro de Análisis Sociocultural – Universidad Centroamericana *et al.* 2005).

A consortium of Cambodian non-governmental organisations (NGOs) identified multiple male partnerships, the lack of reproductive health and HIV information among men, and poor couple communication as a major reason behind the spread of HIV and high maternal mortality in the country. The NGOs worked together for over two years to develop Male Involvement Guidelines and to advocate with the Ministry of Health to see they were integrated into the Strategic Plan for Reproductive Health in Cambodia for 2006–2010 (Greene *et al.* 2006).

The armed forces of most countries are groups with a heightened sense of masculinity, high levels of risk-taking, and an enormously influential role – for good or for ill – to play in the communities where they are deployed. The United Nations Population Fund (UNFPA) worked with the governments of nine countries to improve sexual and reproductive health and reduce the spread of HIV (UNFPA 2003). Their findings from settings as diverse as Benin and Botswana in Africa, Ecuador in Latin America, and Mongolia in Asia suggest the enormous promise of working with this captive audience of a huge fraction of a country's young men. In reporting on the initiative, UNFPA focused on changes in government institutions that would likely sustain the efforts to work with men.

As we seek to reduce gender inequities at a society-wide level, understanding the impact of policy change must be a priority for future innovation and research.

Conclusions

Social expectations of appropriate roles and behaviours for men and women, and the reproduction and reinforcement of these norms in institutions and cultural practices, are directly related to people's experience of health. In no area is this truer than in sexual and reproductive health and HIV. Programme planners have understood this and have made huge strides in addressing gendered social constraints to health in their work with both men and women.

NGOs have taken the lead in engaging men and boys in many settings, but the scale of their operations is limited. One solution is to form a network of NGOs to assemble the larger body of groups engaged in this work. MenEngage – a global alliance to engage boys and men in gender equality – is currently facilitating the sharing of disparate experiences and building the capacity of organisations of all shapes and sizes. Regional MenEngage consultations have brought together 75 like-minded NGOs in eastern and southern Africa, 65 in South Asia, and 80 in India alone. Additional consultations are planned for Southeast Asia and Latin America, and the network is building its membership in the Middle East and North Africa.[2] There are likely hundreds more NGOs keen to work with men and boys, whose experiences could provide platforms for taking gender equitable interventions with men and boys to scale. Many of these NGOs are also working with women and girls or are partnering with other groups that do.

The emerging conclusion from these programmatic efforts is that problematic gender norms are at the heart of poor sexual and reproductive health and the spread of HIV. These norms also represent a golden opportunity to improve health and well-being. The next revolution – already underway in a few places – will be to expand this understanding to the policy level. Both men and women stand to gain enormously from the processes of social transformation described here.

Notes

1 Promundo is a Brazilian NGO that has worked to engage men and boys in gender equality in Brazil and internationally. With partner NGOs, Promundo developed the Programme H group education and community campaign approach to engaging young men in achieving gender equality. For more information, see www.promundo.org.br.
2 For more information about the MenEngage Alliance, see www.menengage.org.

References

Barker, G. (2005) *Dying to be Men: Youth and Masculinity and Social Exclusion*, London: Routledge.

Barker, G. (2007) 'The Role of Men and Boys in Achieving Gender Equality', written statement submitted to the United Nations Commission on the Status of Women Fifty-first Session, New York, 26 February–9 March.

Barker, G. and Olukoya, P. (2007) 'Bringing Men into the Story', *Entre Nous: The European Magazine for Sexual and Reproductive Health*, 66: 8–9.

Barker, G., Ricardo, C., and Nascimento, M. (2007) *Engaging Men and Boys in Changing Gender-based Inequity in Health: Evidence from Programme Interventions*, Geneva: World Health Organization.

Centro de Análisis Sociocultural – Universidad Centroamericana, CEPAL, and United Nations Populations Fund (UNFPA) (2005) *Masculinidad y Factores Socioculturales Asociados al Compor-tamiento de los Hombres Frente a la Paternidad en Centroamérica*, Draft Summary, and *Estudio Masculinidad y Factores Socioculturales Asociados al Comportamiento de los Hombres Frente a la Paternidad en Centroamerica: Caso Nicaragua*, Draft, Managua: United Nations Population Fund and CEPAL.

Cohen, P. (1998) 'Daddy Dearest: Do You Really Matter?', *Washington Post*, 11 July: B7.

Dunne, M., Humphreys, S., and Leach, F. (2003) 'Gender and Violence in Schools', background paper prepared for All Global Monitoring Report 2003/4, 'Gender and Education for All: The Leap to Equality', New York: UNESCO.

Foreman, M. (ed.) (1999) *AIDS and Men: Taking Risks or Taking Responsibility?* London: PANOS/Zed Books.

Global Coalition on Women and AIDS (2006) *Keeping the Promise: An Agenda for Action on Women and AIDS*, Geneva: Joint United Nations Programme on HIV/AIDS.

Greene, M.E. and Biddlecom, A.E. (2000) 'Absent and Problematic Men: Demographic Accounts of Male Reproductive Roles', *Population and Development Review*, 26(1): 81–115.

Greene, M.E., Walston, N., Jorgensen, A., Reatanak Sambath, M, and Hardee, K. (2006) *From Adding to The Burden to Sharing The Load: Guidelines for Male Involvement in Reproductive Health in Cambodia*, Washington, DC: POLICY Project, available at http://www.policyproject.com/pubs/countryreports/Cambodia%20MI%20casestudy%20final%201%2024%2006.doc (accessed 1 November 2009).

Jejeebhoy, S., Shah, I., and Thapa, S. (2005) *Sex without Consent: Young People in Developing Countries*, London: Zed Books.

Levine, R., Lloyd, C., Greene, M., and Grown, C. (2008) *Girls Count: A Global Investment and Action Agenda*, Washington, DC: Center for Global Development.

Mensch, B.S., Clark, W.H., Lloyd, C.B., and Erulkar, A.S. (2001) 'Premarital Sex, Schoolgirl Pregnancy, and School Quality in Rural Kenya', *Studies in Family Planning*, 32(4): 285–301.

Miedzian, M. (1991) *Boys Will Be Boys: Breaking the Link Between Masculinity and Violence*, New York: Doubleday.

Montoya, O.T. (1999) *Swimming Upstream: Looking for Clues to Prevent Male Violence in Couple Relationships*, Nicaragua: Puntos de Encuentro.

Pulerwitz, J., Barker, G., Segundo, M., and Nascimento, M. (2006) *Promoting More Gender-equitable Norms and Behaviors among Young Men as an HIV/AIDS Prevention Strategy*, Washington, DC: Population Council/Horizons.

Redpath, J., Morrell, R., Jewkes, R., and Peacock, D. (2008) *Masculinities and Public Policy in South Africa: Changing Masculinities and Working Toward Gender Equality*, Johannesburg: Sonke Gender Justice Network.

Rogow, D. and Horowitz, S. (1995) 'Withdrawal: A Review of the Literature and an Agenda for Research', *Studies in Family Planning*, 26(3): 140–53.

Saggurti, Niranjan, Stephen L. Schensul and Ravi K. Verma (2009) Migration, Mobility and Sexual Risk Behavior in Mumbai, India: Mobile Men with Non-Residential Wife Show Increased Risk, *AIDS and Behavior*, 13(5): 921–27.

Schuler, S.R., Hashemi, S.M., and Jenkins, A.H. (1995) 'Bangladesh's Family Planning Success Story: A Gender Perspective', *International Family Planning Perspectives*, 21(4): 132–7, 166.

Schuler, S.R., Hashemi, S.M., and Shamsul, H.B. (1998) 'Men's Violence against Women in Rural Bangladesh: Undermined or Exacerbated by Microcredit Programmes?' *Development in Practice*, 8(2): 148–57.

Segal, L. (1990) *Slow Motion: Changing Masculinities, Changing Men*, Piscataway: Rutgers University Press.

UNESCO (United Nations Educational, Scientific and Cultural Organization) (2008) *Global Education Digest 2008: Comparing Education Statistics across the World and International Levels*, Montreal: UNESCO Institute for Statistics.

UNFPA (United Nations Population Fund) (1994) *Programme of Action of the International Conference on Population and Development*, New York: UNFPA.

UNFPA (United Nations Population Fund) (2003) *Enlisting The Armed Forces To Protect Reproductive Health And Rights: Lessons Learned From Nine Countries*, New York: UNFPA.

WHO (World Health Organization) (2002) *Multi-Country Study on Women's Health and Domestic Violence*, Geneva: WHO.

WHO (World Health Organization) (2007) *Maternal Mortality in 2005: Estimates developed by WHO, UNICEF, UNFPA and The World Bank*, Geneva: WHO.

21

Longevity and Ageing
The Success of Global Public Health

Linda P. Fried

We recognize that concerted action is required to transform the opportunities and the quality of life of men and women as they age and to ensure the sustainability of their support systems, thus building the foundation for a society for all ages. When ageing is embraced as an achievement, the reliance on human skills, experiences and resources of the higher age groups is naturally recognized as an asset in the growth of mature, fully integrated, humane societies. [We also recognize that we] must include ageing in development agendas. [Further,] We recognize that the growing needs of an ageing population require additional policies, in particular care and treatment, the promotion of healthy lifestyles and supportive environments. We shall promote independence, accessibility and the empowerment of older persons to participate fully in all aspects of society.

(UN Second World Assembly on Ageing, Madrid Declaration, 2002)

Success of public health globally is seen in increasing longevity

The world's population has been undergoing a dramatic demographic shift: people are living longer and, increasingly, having fewer children. As a result, the population profiles of countries around the world are changing radically. The United Nations (UN) estimates that, currently, 11 per cent of the world's population is aged 60 and over while 26.9 per cent is 14 or under (UN Population Division 2009). By 2030, only 22.7 per cent of the world's population will be aged 14 or under, while 16.5 per cent will be 60 and older – and more than 2 per cent will be aged 80 and over (UN Population Division 2009). By the year 2050, the world will reach a major demographic milestone: in that year, the percentage of the population aged 60 or over will surpass that of the population aged 14 and under (21.9 per cent and 19.6 per cent, respectively) (UN Population Division 2009).

Many of the most developed countries have already reached a point of equity in the proportion of children and older adults in society: this includes Germany, Austria, Belgium, Denmark, Luxembourg, Norway, and the United Kingdom, all of which reached the point of equity before 1990; as well as countries such as Belarus, Estonia, Ukraine, Poland, Canada, and Australia, which reached equity during the twenty-first century (UN Population Division

2009). Many other countries, including the United States (US), will reach this point of proportional equality in the population long before 2050. This is a population distribution never seen before in human history, and it has profound social and health implications.

The proportion of the population that is older is one marker of the world's ageing. However, for many countries where the proportion of the population will not be markedly older for another 10–20 years, the absolute numbers of older adults are now increasing rapidly and significantly. For example, the two countries with the largest number of people 65 and older, or 80 and older, are China and India. In China, there are currently 111 million adults aged 65 or older and 19 million aged 80 and older; in India, there are currently 60 million adults aged 65 and older, including 12 million aged 80 and older (UN Population Division 2009). In the next 20 years, the increase in older adults will lead China, for example, to have more older adults (aged 65+) than the total population of any other country, except India and the US (UN Population Division 2009).

A dominant reason for population ageing has been the change in fertility rates. Fertility rates worldwide have undergone a major decline over the last 60 years. Between 1950 and 2010, the average number of children born to each woman worldwide fell from 4.92 children per woman to 2.49 children per woman, and this total fertility rate is expected to fall further, to 2.15 children per woman, in 2030. By 2040, the global total fertility rate (2.04 children per woman) (UN Population Division 2009) will be below the replacement rate of 2.08 children per woman, the fertility level needed to maintain the global population at the same size (Castles 2003).

At the same time that the number of children born per woman has declined, life expectancy has increased dramatically since the middle of the twentieth century. In 1950, women world-wide had an average life expectancy of 48 years and men a life expectancy of only 45.2 years. By 2010, the average life expectancy worldwide for women will be 71.1, an increase of 23.1 years; for men it will be 66.7 years, an increase of 21.5 years (UN Population Division 2009). Improvements in life expectancy have occurred in all regions during this time (Figure 21.1) and been greatest in the least developed countries where life expectancies have historically been lowest. For example, life expectancy for women in Bangladesh has already increased by 32.3 years, from 37.1 years in 1950 to 69.0 years in 2010, and is projected to increase a further 6.3 years between 2010 and 2030 to 75.3 years. In comparison, life expectancy for women in the US increased by only 10.1 years between 1950 and 2010, and is projected to further increase by only 2.2 years by 2030, when women will have a life expectancy of 84.3 years. Increases in life expectancy lead to shifting population distributions, and are, significantly, a result of improved foundational public health: safer food and water, improved nutrition, decreased maternal and infant mortality, and decreases in infectious diseases (Figure 21.2).

There is some variation between nations in reasons for population ageing, although life expectancy has increased in all countries. In China, the one-child policy has radically shifted the ratio of children to older adults at the same time that life expectancy has increased dramatically. In the US, the baby boom after Second World War was a dominant driver, but increasing life expectancy with decreased fertility will sustain population ageing into the future. In Europe, the post-Second World War baby boom briefly compensated for birth rates which had been declining since the early 1900s (Grant *et al.* 2004). Currently, below-replacement birth rates, coupled with low immigration, are the dominant drivers of population ageing in Europe (Grant *et al.* 2004). In contrast, in countries where the parental-age population has been deeply affected by the HIV/AIDS epidemic, improvements in overall life expectancy have been much lower than expected. For example, in Swaziland, where the adult prevalence rate for HIV/AIDS is 26.1 per cent (CIA 2009), life expectancy increased by only 4.2 years for women between 1950 and 2010 – from 43.4 years to 47.6 years, and by only 10.3 years for men, from 39.4 years to

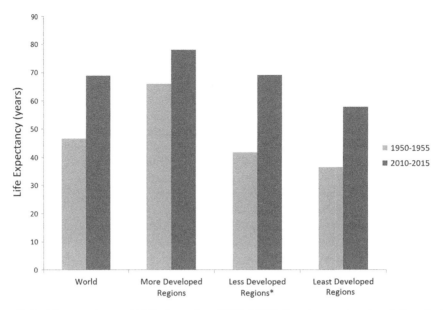

Figure 21.1   Life expectancy at birth, by region, 1950–2015. Development regions follow the UN Population Database regions. *Less developed regions excludes countries included in least developed countries
Source: http://esa.un.org/unpp/.

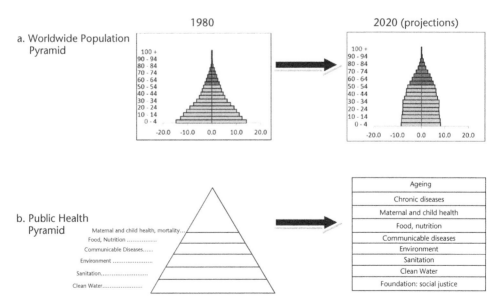

Figure 21.2   Transforming Public Health in accord with the 'rectangularisation' of society. Vertical axis: age group in years; horizontal axis: percentage of population in age group, by sex – negative values are percent of male population, positive values are percent of female population
Source: US Census Bureau – International Data Base; available at www.census.gov/ipc/www/idb/.

49.7 years (UN Population Division 2009). However, notably, life expectancy for those without HIV is increasing.

Economically developed countries have been ageing slowly and continuously over the last 100 years (Kinsella and Phillips 2005). This has provided the opportunity for anticipatory changes in policies and institutions – although even here, needed changes have not kept pace with the increases in longevity or our evolving understanding of institutions and approaches needed to create healthy ageing and optimise societal well-being in an ageing world. In the most developed countries, as defined by the UN, the proportion of the population aged 60 and over will grow by 7 per cent, from 21.8 per cent in 2010 to 28.8 per cent in 2030. However, in the less-developed countries, rates of ageing are much more rapid: overall, the proportion over age 60 will nearly double, from 8.6 per cent in 2010 to 14.2 per cent in 2030 (UN Population Division 2009). This is an average across regions. In Asia, Latin America, and the Caribbean, the percentages of people 60 and older will rise from 10 per cent in 2006 to 24 per cent in 2050. In contrast, in sub-Saharan Africa (SSA), the rise will be from 4.8 per cent to only 8.8 per cent. However, the absolute numbers of older persons in SSA will rise in the same period from 37 million to 155 million. The latter change will be the most rapid absolute increase of all regions of the world or for any other age group. As has been pointed out by Aboderin and Ferreira (2008), because of these very rapid changes, SSA will confront major challenges that differ from other regions, namely ensuring the security and well-being of this increasing number of older people. At the same time, there are opportunities from an ageing population that could be harnessed to enhance development and societal well-being in less developed countries. In Asian countries that are industrialised and/or rapidly maturing, the concerns are more focused on the implications of changing population age structures on workforce productivity, sustainability of social security systems, and economic growth, although there are issues in common with other regions of supporting the development of institutions that foster the benefits of population ageing.

Notably, as the population ages, the ratio of men to women in the population will likely decrease, since women have longer life expectancies than men (UN Population Division 2009). In 2007, there were already 70 million more women aged 60 or over than men worldwide, and twice as many women as men aged 80 or over (UNDESA 2007a). The aetiology of this gender differential in longevity needs to be understood so that men can benefit as much as women from increasing life expectancy. At the same time, the needs of older women, often differentially much poorer than men of the same age and more likely to have familial dependents, should be proactively focused on and supported in public policies.

All of these dramatic demographic shifts – in terms of increased life expectancy, higher ratios of old relative to young, and of women relative to men at older ages – have significant implications for future policies, institutions, systems, and for our preparing for the necessities as well as the opportunities of an ageing world. As discussed below, the public health success of increased longevity brings a need to add serious attention to health promotion and to the prevention and management of chronic diseases and conditions of ageing, superimposed on existing health concerns globally (Figures 21.2 and 21.3). If we do this, all ages will benefit.

Changing global health needs and patterns of illness associated with longevity and ageing

Global population ageing presents new challenges and necessities for public health, to ensure the health of populations as people live longer lives. First, there are new needs to prevent chronic diseases and conditions both across the life course and focused on age-specific

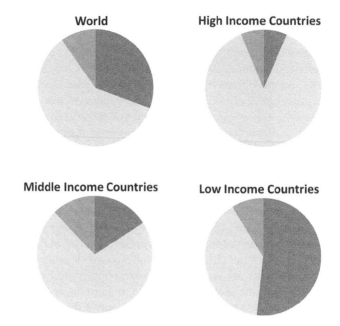

Figure 21.3 Proportion of deaths due to communicable and non-communicable causes, 2004. Dark grey – communicable diseases, including maternal and perinatal conditions and nutritional deficiencies; Pale grey – non-communicable conditions; Medium gray – injuries
Source: WHO Global Burden of Disease, Disease and Injury Regional Estimates for 2004; available at http://www.who.int/healthinfo/global_burden_disease/estimates_regional/en/ index.html.

vulnerabilities. Second, there is a need for recognition of new types of public health goals, including preserving active life expectancy during longer lives, and the addition of public health metrics appropriate to longer-lived populations. Third, there needs to be recognition of the environmental (physical and built) factors in health and independent living as people age and the particular needs to redesign environments, including cities, for ageing populations. Finally, there is a need for the redesign of social institutions to provide essential supports to those post-retirement, as well as to create new types of roles and opportunities for an ageing population to contribute to healthy ageing at the same time as contributing to the public good through remaining engaged. All of these factors are critical to health. The above-mentioned public health approaches that would support health and well-being in ageing would largely benefit all generations; recognition of this fact will permit the design of new kinds of win-wins for an ageing world, and strengthen our cross-generational social compact.

Developing countries have begun the epidemiological transition from predominance of infectious diseases to predominance of non-communicable diseases (Omran 1971), while developed countries have completed it (Figure 21.3). Already, in 2004, of the top ten causes of death in low-income countries, three were non-communicable chronic diseases: coronary heart disease (CHD), stroke and cerebrovascular disease, and chronic obstructive pulmonary disease (COPD); in middle-income countries, seven of the top ten were non-communicable (WHO 2008b); while in high-income countries, nine of the top ten were non-communicable.

Over the last century, non-communicable chronic diseases have become the major causes, worldwide, of mortality and, increasingly, of morbidity and disability. This has resulted from a confluence of factors: increasing life expectancy permitting the time for the progressive development of these diseases over the life course, and a dramatic increase in risk factors for chronic diseases – first in developed countries, and now globally. These risk factors are substantially those of shifting health behaviours: smoking, declining physical activity, and shifts in dietary intake, compounded by environmental risk factors such as air pollution. As these behavioural and environmental risks have been imported from developed to developing countries, and as we learn that community norms and social networks reinforce the uptake of adverse health behaviours, this puts into question whether, in fact, we should consider these risk factors and the resulting diseases 'non-communicable'; however, for the moment the terminology remains. Note in this regard that, in 1995, the global number of regular smokers among adults aged 15 and older had risen to 1.1 billion persons (Jha *et al.* 2002). In 1999–2004, 17.3 per cent of children aged 13–15, globally, regularly used a tobacco product, while 44.1 per cent were exposed to second-hand smoke in the home and 54.2 per cent in public places (Warren *et al.* 2006) (Figure 21.4). China itself now has one-third of all the smokers in the world, and 70 per cent of Chinese men smoke. Changes in diet in China exemplify changes worldwide, with the traditional Chinese diet, low in fat and vegetable-based, changing to one increasingly high in fat and meat-based. Declining physical activity in the face of industrialisation and urbanisation, and dietary patterns shifting to diets high in energy-dense foods, with high levels of saturated fats, added salt and refined sugars, and low in fruits and vegetables (WHO 2003a), are contributing to the increase globally in rates of overweight and obesity. Obesity itself increases risks of chronic diseases, particularly diabetes, hypertension, and cardiovascular diseases (CVD), independent of other effects of activity, diet, and smoking. Currently, at least 1 billion adults are overweight, including 300 million who are obese (WHO 2003b). Obesity prevalence ranges from less than 1 per cent in parts of Africa and Asia to approximately 80 per cent in

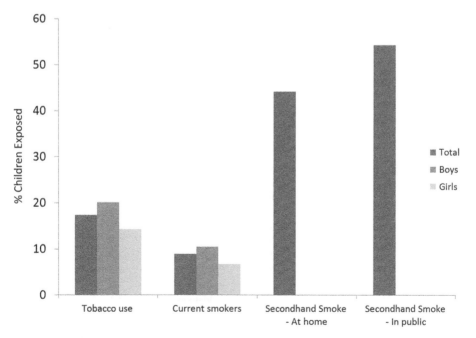

Figure 21.4 Smoking and tobacco use patterns among youth, aged 13–15, worldwide, 1999–2005.
Source: Warren et al. 2006.

Nauru (WHO 2008a) (Table 21.1). In many countries, undernutrition and obesity now co-exist. In Asia, for example, 22 per cent of children under age five are underweight (Black *et al.* 2008), 6 per cent of children aged 5–17 are overweight, and 1 per cent of children aged 5–17 are obese (WHO 2006). Smoking and high blood pressure have been shown to be responsible for the largest number of deaths in the US, followed by overweight/obesity, low physical activity, high dietary salt and trans-fats, and low dietary omega-3 fatty acids (Danaei *et al.* 2009). These modifiable risk factors, as noted below, are keys to prevention of non-communicable chronic diseases with ageing, and must be addressed in new and effective life-course approaches, at every age and stage of life, to promoting health during longer lives.

The behavioural risk factors – smoking, obesity, salt intake, and low physical activity – increase the risk of hypertension and diabetes. The latter two are increasing with advancing age in many populations and are growing health threats. In Tanzania, 25.4 per cent of men and 27.2 per cent of women had hypertension in 1987, but by 1998 this had increased to 41.1 per cent and 38.7 per cent, respectively (Addo *et al.* 2007). While hypertension was less common among rural residents, its prevalence has been increasing in all areas of Tanzania (Addo *et al.* 2007), with similar patterns observed worldwide (Cappuccio *et al.* 2004; Kearney *et al.* 2005). In parallel, and also directly tied to these risk factors, rates of diabetes are increasing worldwide. In

Table 21.1 Adult obesity prevalence. Top 10 countries with highest and lowest prevalence of obesity, by gender

	Women			*Men*	
Country	*% Overweight (BMI ≥25)*	*% Obese (BMI ≥30)*	*Country*	*% Overweight (BMI ≥25)*	*% Obese (BMI ≥30)*
Nauru	92.4	78.8	Nauru	96.6	83.2
Tonga	91.4	76.1	Cook Islands	92.6	69.5
Micronesia	90.1	72.9	Micronesia	92.1	66.2
Cook Islands	89.2	70.8	Tonga	90.3	60.7
Niue	85.0	61.0	Samoa	78.7	38.4
Samoa	82.1	57.3	Niue	78.5	36.8
Palau	82.4	55.0	United States	75.6	36.5
Kuwait	79.0	52.9	Argentina	73.1	31.4
Barbados	80.1	50.8	Palau	74.5	31.2
Trinidad & Tobago	77.0	46.1	Kiribati	73.2	29.8
CAR	18.5	1.3	Bangladesh	6.7	0.2
Burkina Faso	16.0	1.1	Zambia	7.5	0.1
DRC	13.3	0.8	Uganda	7.4	0.1
Vietnam	8.7	0.3	Rwanda	7.3	0.1
Nepal	8.0	0.2	Kenya	6.9	0.1
Bangladesh	5.4	0.2	DRC	4.8	0.1
Cambodia	9.3	0.1	CAR	7.2	0.1
Sri Lanka	6.0	0.1	Burundi	7.8	0.1
Eritrea	5.7	0.1	Vietnam	4.1	0.0
Ethiopia	3.3	0.0	Eritrea	3.1	0.0

Notes: DRC: Democratic Republic of Congo; CAR: Central African Republic. The WHO Global InfoBase compiles statistics from national and sub-national population surveys; BMI estimates are standardised by WHO to ensure comparability.
Source: Adapted from WHO Global InfoBase: overweight and obesity; available at https://apps.who.int/infobase/report.aspx.

2004, diabetes caused 1.14 million deaths, of which 20 per cent were in high-income countries, 34 per cent in low-income, and 46 per cent in middle-income countries (WHO 2008b). In Latin America, prevalence of diabetes among adults ranges from 1.2 per cent in parts of Chile, to 8.2 per cent in urban Argentina. The escalating impact can be seen by considering that, between 1980 and 1994, deaths from diabetes increased by 126 per cent in Andean Latin America. By 2025, the total number of people with diabetes in Latin America will exceed the number with diabetes in Canada and the US combined (Aschner 2002). In general, diabetes is more common in older adults, and in urban than rural areas (Bouguerra et al. 2007), although South Korea is a notable exception (Yoon et al. 2006). Chronic diseases including diabetes are equally and highly prevalent in rural and urban China. In South Africa, prevalence is low among the general population (5 per cent or less), but is up to 29–30 per cent among men and women aged 65 and older (Akinboboye et al. 2003). Throughout Africa, diabetes is more common among women than men, after adjusting for age (Akinboboye et al. 2003; Bouguerra et al. 2007); in Asia, diabetes is more common among men (Yoon et al. 2006). Diabetes and hypertension are strong, independent, and also interactive risk factors for heart disease and stroke. Smoking also predicts these diseases, as well as lung diseases (emphysema, lung cancer), peripheral vascular disease, and bladder cancer. In 1990, COPD was the sixth leading cause of death worldwide, responsible for 4.4 per cent of all deaths (WRI 1998); by 2004, COPD was the fourth leading cause of death worldwide, responsible for 5.1 per cent of all deaths (WHO 2008b).

Thus, all of these behavioural risk factors, along with obesity, hypertension, and diabetes, are risk factors for a host of non-communicable chronic diseases. As a result, the incidence and prevalence of a wide range of chronic conditions is increasing worldwide, including CVD, cancers, and COPD (Center et al. 2009; Emmanuel 1989; Gaziano 2008; Gupta et al. 2008; Kamangar et al. 2008; Okrainec et al. 2004). CVD has been increasing especially dramatically worldwide: between 1957 and 1987, mortality from coronary heart disease (CHD) increased from 1.98 per 1,000 to 5.01 per 1,000 among adults aged 60–64 in Singapore (Emmanuel 1989); and in India the proportion of deaths attributable to CVD increased from 21 per cent in 1984 to 25 per cent in 1998 (Gupta et al. 2008). The number of deaths due to coronary artery disease (CAD) is projected to increase by 46 per cent in established market economies, 108 per cent in China, 116 per cent in sub-Saharan Africa, 127 per cent in India, 141 per cent in Latin America, and 148 per cent in the Middle East between 1990 and 2020 (Okrainec et al. 2004). This increase in rates of CVD mortality has a global parallel with the rise in adverse risk factors. At the same time, where risk factors have been significantly decreased, such as in the US and Finland, analyses indicate that stroke and heart disease mortality rates have declined 30 to 60 per cent, with risk factor modification contributing to half of this decline and improved medical care contributing the other half (Hunnink et al. 1997; Goldman et al. 2001).

In addition, there are approximately 10 million new cases of cancer worldwide each year, excluding skin cancer (Center et al. 2009). Between 1983 and 2002, the incidence of colorectal cancer increased in Israel by 211 per cent among non-Jewish women, and 234 per cent among non-Jewish men; in Eastern Europe by 30 to 70 per cent among men and 23 to 40 per cent among women; in Shanghai by 50 per cent among adults; and in Hong Kong by 10 per cent among adults (Center et al. 2009). Between 1973 and 1997, incidence rates increased for prostate cancer worldwide and for esophageal and lung cancers in developing countries, while liver cancer incidence in developed countries has doubled over the past 30 years (Kamangar et al. 2008).

Consistently, the prevalence and mortality of so-called non-communicable chronic diseases and their risk factors increase with age – into the oldest ages. For instance, mortality due to CVD in Singapore in 1987 was 5.01 per 1,000 among adults aged 60–64 and 13.61 per 1,000 among adults aged 70 and over (Emmanuel 1989). The prevalence of hypertension in SSA is 20 per cent for adults aged 35 to 44, 50 per cent for age 45 to 54, and 80 per cent for women aged 65 and over (Addo *et al.* 2007). In the US, the age-standardised rate of hypertension among adults (aged 20 or older) is 30.4 per cent for women and 31.5 per cent for men , but among adults aged 65 and over, 75.3 per cent of women and 64.6 per cent of men have hypertension (CDC and NCHS 2009). That non-communicable diseases are ageing-associated is due to cumulative exposure to risk factors over the life course and the progressive increase in subclinical disease with increasing age, up to a threshold when this becomes clinically symptomatic as disease, often with disability, or death.

As a result of this chronic, progressive process of disease development, the highest prevalence of chronic, non-communicable diseases is in the older age groups. Notably, there has also been a rapid increase in non-communicable diseases in young and middle adulthood in developing countries, making it clear that the development of these major diseases is not limited to old age alone (Figure 21.5). The major shifts in lifestyle behaviours globally are probably part of the reason for the dramatic increase in chronic disease onset and death rates in young and middle-aged adults. The 2005 death rates for those 30 to 69 years, in a range of countries, are shown in Figure 21.5: these data make it clear that the development of major chronic diseases is having a substantial impact during working years, as well as in the oldest ages. These diseases, further, are not just affecting the rich. One example of this regards the implications of overweight and poor diets in China: they 'are becoming a greater burden for the poor than for the rich, with subsequent large increases in hypertension, stroke, and adult-onset diabetes. The related economic costs represent 4 to 8 per cent of the economy' (Popkin 2008: 1,064).

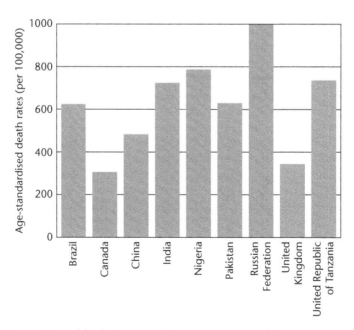

Figure 21.5 Non-communicable disease mortality among young adults
Source: WHO 2005.

Of course, non-communicable chronic diseases and geriatric conditions are not the only public health concern for an ageing world. Communicable diseases remain problematic in an ageing society. In many countries, chronic non-communicable diseases develop superimposed on already-existing communicable diseases, such as HIV, TB, and malaria, as well as conditions such as anaemia and/or undernutrition. With the successful treatment of communicable diseases such as HIV/AIDS, as well as population ageing, HIV is now becoming a chronic disease in many countries. As a result, our health systems need to address both prevention and care of HIV/AIDS as a chronic problem; design of health systems for prevention and care of non-communicable chronic diseases may increase the ability to care for communicable diseases as chronic problems, as well as be more effective, in a sustainable way, in their prevention. Further, health care providers and public health practitioners need to be attuned to recognise HIV/AIDS in the older age groups – because sexual activity of people living longer lives leads to greater risk of new HIV infection in older people. In the US in 2005, 29 per cent of all people living with HIV/AIDS were 50 or older (CDC 2008), and 19 per cent of all new AIDS diagnoses in the US were in adults aged 50 and older (CDC 2008). In Africa and Asia, approximately 5 per cent of people with AIDS were 50 and older, and in Australia and Germany, approximately 17 per cent were older adults (Knodel et al. 2003). HIV/AIDS in older adults may have less typical clinical presentations and require creative prevention strategies (Coon et al. 2003; Zingmond et al. 2003), as well as marking those potentially at greater risk of multi-morbid non-communicable diseases – in some cases as side effects of therapy. Further, prevention of HIV infection must include a focus on safe sex in the older age groups, as well as in younger persons. Prevention remains critical into the oldest ages, for HIV as well as other communicable diseases.

As chronic non-communicable diseases become more common, and are superimposed on prevalent, chronic communicable diseases, the likelihood of multi-morbidity increases overall, and is high in older adults. Multi-morbidity is the concurrent presence of more than one illness in an individual. Approximately 80 per cent of all older adults have at least one chronic condition, and older adults are often more likely to have two or more chronic conditions (Gijsen et al. 2001; Westaway 2010; Woo et al. 2007). For example, 73.7 per cent of men and 81.4 per cent of women aged 60 to 84 in South Korea have at least one chronic disease, and 37.6 per cent of men and 54 per cent of women have at least two chronic conditions (Woo et al. 2007). Multi-morbidity also increases with age: in Canada, 27.7 per cent of adults aged 25 to 44 have two or more conditions, compared with 63.4 per cent of those ages 65 and over (Fortin et al. 2005). Notably, the presence of non-communicable diseases can increase the risk of acquiring another non-communicable or a communicable disease, such as influenza or pneumonia, and of mortality from these. Further, where there is access to health care and medications, the challenges of treatment can add additional challenges to health, as well as benefits. The former results from polypharmacy, where older adults with multiple diseases are prescribed multiple medications. This can increase risk for adverse effects resulting from the medications themselves. Of concern, adherence to medication use declines when one is prescribed more than six medications.

Beyond chronic non-communicable and communicable diseases and their treatments, physiologic changes of ageing – sometimes independently and sometimes exacerbated by chronic diseases – can lead to geriatric conditions such as frailty, disability, and risk for other conditions such as falls. Furthermore, the likelihood of cognitive decline increases with age, primarily as a result of cerebrovascular diseases and/or Alzheimer's disease. All these health changes are risk factors, themselves, for loss of independence with ageing, with risk increasing in the presence of multiple health problems. Disability and dependency lead to requirements for supportive care, and environments to ameliorate or compensate for functional compromise.

The need for such approaches, both through community health promotion and community and institutional services, as well as through geriatrically informed health care and community-based health promotion, is compounded by social vulnerabilities that are associated with ageing such as widowhood and loss of income.

Despite stereotypes that envision older adults as dependent and frail, most older adults – at least in developed countries – describe themselves as being in good, very good, or excellent health: less them half have any disability, and generally less than a quarter describe themselves as dependent. In the US, less than 5 per cent of older adults reside in nursing homes. The educational level of the population predicts its active life expectancy, or the number of years lived without disability; thus, investing in childhood – and even life-long education – is a critical investment in healthy ageing. With ageing, health status becomes increasingly variable. Older adults are highly heterogeneous in terms of health and health needs, as are the types of prevention approaches that may be relevant. It is anticipated that the rise in obesity prevalence and other lifestyle changes may counteract some of the positive changes in health that have occurred with ageing. Overall, with increasing population longevity, the world's ageing population and the increase in chronic diseases must become additions to the public health pyramid and transform it into a rectangle (Figure 21.2b).

Public health must lead on prevention of chronic diseases in an ageing world

The major global public health goal for an ageing world is to prevent or delay the onset of disease and disability, or 'compress morbidity', into the latest points in the human lifespan, so as to increase the likelihood that longer lives include more years spent healthy. Despite expectations of prior generations that infirmity and incapacity were necessarily associated with ageing, it is now known that infirmity and incapacity are not inevitable in older ages. The new ability to differentiate ageing from disease is evidenced in the US by increasing rates of good-to-excellent health into oldest ages, and the significant declines in mortality in adults 65 and older from CVD and stroke since the 1950s. Broadly, there is convincing evidence that non-communicable diseases and geriatric conditions are preventable, to a significant degree, and that prevention works into the latest ages.

Adopting, globally, effective chronic disease prevention from birth and throughout the life course will be critical to laying the foundations for people living longer lives healthily. Further, as people age, the types of prevention needed expand and include primary, secondary, and tertiary prevention. Prevention into the oldest ages must include the maintenance of healthy behaviours, including adequate, healthful nutrition and physical activity, as well as protection from communicable diseases and prevention of smoking, hypertension, and diabetes. This will require multi-level approaches, from health literacy of individuals and changing societal norms regarding smoking and other health behaviours, to policies and global governance regarding contents of packaged foods and improved access to healthy foods. The worldwide rapid increase in non-communicable disease points to a need for new kinds of life-course approaches to their prevention. Prevention must start in earliest childhood and be applied throughout adulthood. It is clear that prevention – of smoking, hypertension, low physical activity, and poor diet – matters even into the oldest ages. Prevention, across the life course, must be developed at many levels. A basic one is ensuring individuals' knowledge and ability to maintain positive health behaviours. However, we recognise that environment matters at many levels, and must support and help create healthy behaviours through a variety of approaches. For example, new research indicates that thinking about chronic progressive diseases as 'non-communicable', while accurate in terms of the disease process, is not accurate in terms of risk factors. Although organ damage due to cardiovascular disease cannot be directly transmitted to another person, social norms are 'communicated' and lead to shared health practices among groups, including risk factors. Others not engaged in the practice can also be affected through social norms – such as by second-hand smoke. Thus, interventions need to be directed to social groups and communities, as well as individuals. Further, many of the causes of adverse health behaviours have to be resolved at structural, institutional, and even governance levels. One such approach involves designing our built environments, especially urban ones, to support physical activity and ensure availability of healthy foods; this has been formalised in the recommendations by the World Health Organization to create Global Age-Friendly Cities. Further, it is essential for the prevention of chronic diseases that we create global governance and corporate agreements, even legislation, to shift mass-produced food to healthier products which are significantly less energy dense and contain less carbohydrate, fat, and salt, and to decrease smoking and alcohol use.

Globally, improving and protecting our physical environment is also critical to health overall and to healthy ageing. Pollution and other environmental hazards can cause or worsen chronic diseases while environmental degradation, particularly in cities, contributes to increasing non-communicable disease rates and severity. Currently, up to 80 per cent of cities in Europe exceed WHO air quality standards, and in China, air pollution levels are up to six times higher than WHO standards (WRI 1998), with 90 per cent of cities having some serious degrees of air pollution. In total, 1.4 billion people live in urban areas with air pollution levels higher than WHO standards, which comprises just under half of the 3 billion urban residents worldwide (World Resources Institute 1988–99). Over the next 25 years, the urban population will increase to nearly 5 billion people, 90 per cent of whom will live in developing countries (UNFPA 2005). For every 10 mg/m^3 increase in airborne particulate matter, total mortality increases by 1 per cent, respiratory mortality increases by 3.4 per cent, and cardiovascular mortality increases by 1.4 per cent (Dockery and Pope III 1994). Worldwide, exposure to air pollution levels above the WHO standards may be responsible for up to 5 per cent of all urban deaths, and rising temperatures due to climate change are expected to make morbidity and mortality due to air pollution more severe (WRI 1998). Indoor air pollution, due to cooking fires and smoking, is also a major problem worldwide. In developed countries, air-tight houses can increase the concentration of indoor pollutants, making them more dangerous than outdoor air pollution, while in developing countries up to 80 per cent of energy needs are met by burning biological matter (WRI 1998). While adverse changes in the environment affect all ages, children and older adults, particularly those who are frail, are the age groups most immediately and adversely affected.

Further, with ageing, prevention of frailty and disability becomes critical, along with preventing falls, and reducing injuries and fractures. Such prevention will further minimise the risk of loss of independence or premature mortality, as well as preserve older peoples' ability to remain engaged and independent as long as possible. Remaining mentally and physically active and socially engaged are key approaches, at the population level, to preventing cognitive impairment, as well as disability, and supporting a positive quality of life. Social and environmental factors, the design of cities and access to transportation, and creation of social institutions that support engagement by older adults and offer income support will need to be created as part of an all-sector approach to support healthy and engaged ageing. It is essential that public health science be translated into clarity about prevention strategies and treatment approaches for every age group, by gender, and stratified by needs relevant to health status, so that a life-course approach to prevention spans and includes all age groups.

Overall, the public health approach to optimising health in ageing is built on a foundation of preventing both chronic non-communicable and communicable diseases. However, many other factors affect health in ageing, and need to be considered as additional, and important, components of a public health approach to supporting healthy ageing. These include access to health care and community services; prevention of geriatric conditions, including falls, frailty, and disability; and ensuring good housing and nutrition, adequate financial resources, social supports and networks, and meaningful engagement in community.

Social and economic factors modify health and well-being in ageing, and must be included in global health and prevention strategies. Increasing numbers of older adults live alone and in poverty, and at the same time are often responsible for support for other family members. In many rural areas, the major populations are older adults raising children, after those of working age migrate to cities. Older adults raising grandchildren require additional resources to support their well-being, as well as their ability to provide care. However, more than half of the world's population has no social security of any kind (ILO 2002). Worldwide, 30.2 per cent of men and 11.3 per cent of women aged 65 and older work for pay; the highest workforce participation for older men occurs in Africa, where 57.4 per cent still work, and for older women in Oceania, where 33.4 per cent still work (UNDESA 2007b). Overall, however, poverty among older adults is substantial. In Africa, up to 72 per cent of older adults living alone are poor and up to 90.2 per cent of older adults caring for children are poor (Kakwani and Subbarao 2005). Even in developed countries, elder poverty is high: nearly 30 per cent of urban older adults in the US live in poverty (Smeeding *et al.* 2008). The gender gap in survival – with greater numbers of women surviving into older age – exacerbates the challenges in old age for women. More than twice as many older women (19 per cent) as older men (8 per cent) live alone (UNDESA 2007a), and older women are significantly more likely to live in poverty than older men.

An ageing world: necessities and opportunities for global public health leadership

> The recommendations for action are organised according to three priority directions: older persons and development; advancing health and well-being into old age; and ensuring enabling and supportive environments. The extent to which the lives of older persons are secure is strongly influenced by progress in these three directions.
>
> (Madrid International Plan of Action on Ageing, 2002)

The ageing of the world is a success of medical care improvements, but even more so of public health activities. The challenge going forward is to develop the conditions in which people living longer lives spend that increased time healthy. The benefits to the world of being an ageing society can be substantial. This is discussed further, below. However, achieving these significant benefits will require investment in health and well-being with ageing, investing in education and health promotion of our children for their lifelong well-being, and in developing the health systems – both public health and medical care – that resolve threats to health by protecting the physical environment, ensuring healthy built environments and access to safe and healthy foods and water, and promoting activities which are essential to health promotion. It will also require the development of new kinds of roles and institutions for older adults to support their engagement in the community; roles that bring meaning and productivity in longer lives, and assurance of income support when people can no longer work. To do this will require creating new institutions, policies, and infrastructure for our changing demography. If this is achieved, then the benefits of ageing – for both developing and developed countries – can be realised.

There is concern that the financial needs of older adults will be harder to meet as the older population grows relative to the working population. There were nine working-age people for every adult aged over 65 in 2007, but by 2050 there will be only four working adults for each older adult (UN Population Division 2009). Similarly, the global ratio of parental support was four persons aged over 85 per 100 persons aged 50 to 64 in 2007, and by 2050 will be 12 per 100 (UN Population Division 2009). These ratios are expressed nationally as 'old-age dependency ratios'. These changing ratios are critical to address; however, it may be that how we frame the issue will determine which solution we can identify. It has been posited that the concept of old-age dependency ratios is anachronistic (Lutz et al. 2008), as in many countries only a minority of older adults have a disability, with 20 per cent or less dependent, and a significant proportion of older adults report being in good, very good, or excellent health. Further, the old-age dependency ratio, as constructed, does not take into account that there are significant benefits that older adults bring, or could bring, to society. These include traditional roles of responsibility for the well-being and continuity of the community and its traditions. In all societies, older adults serve as caregivers and financial providers. In 1995, older adults in Japan became net sources of financial transfers relative to other ages (Ogawa 2008); in Western countries, older adults transfer more resources to other generations than they receive. In South Africa, an experiment of providing old age pensions to selected groups of black women led to findings that the granddaughters of the women who received these income supplements gained more weight and were taller (Rowe et al. 2009), providing objective evidence of the intergenerational benefits of supporting the older generation.

Beyond financial support, older adults have historically had critical roles in society for transfer of many non-financial resources: as community glue and community watch, as carriers of history and values, and caregivers for their families. With the HIV/AIDS and drug epidemics, new roles and challenges have arisen. In many areas of the world, grandparents are raising grandchildren in ever greater numbers. In the US, 1.5 per cent of grandparents (30 per cent of whom are aged over 60) are primary caregivers for grandchildren and 6.1 per cent of grandchildren live with grandparent householders (US Census Bureau 2009), while in Africa, up to 61 per cent of orphans and 12 to 16 per cent of non-orphans live with grandparents (Bicego et al. 2003; UNICEF 2007). In Cambodia, 8.5 per cent of adults aged 50 or older had a son or daughter who died from AIDS in the previous five years; of these, 87.4 per cent were their primary caregivers and 78.8 per cent became caregivers of orphaned grandchildren (Knodel et al. 2006). These increasing roles for older adults raising grandchildren when parents are not present are a significant source of societal resilience in responding to the AIDS and other crises, but necessitate a variety of supports for these grandparents.

Society may need older adults to accept new roles and new kinds of responsibilities because they will be such a significant proportion of the population. To explore this, new roles are being developed for older adults, to harness the social capital of an ageing world in win-win ways. To date, these roles include both compensated and volunteer positions, designed ideally to help meet unmet societal needs and, simultaneously, promote the health and well-being of older adults themselves. Roles of particular interest are ones that meet the stage-relevant goals of older people to be generative (that is, to leave the world better for future generations) and ones that offer needed income support. One such approach, being developed in the US, is Experience Corps^{TM}, an evidence-based senior volunteer programme designed to bring a critical mass of older adults, after training, to improve the educational success of children in public schools, while being simultaneously a health promotion programme for the older adults, designed to effectively increase physical, cognitive, and social activity through social engagement and generativity (Freedman and Fried 1999; Fried *et al.* 2004a). Preliminary results of evaluations indicate that this evidence-based model, designed by gerontologists, early child educators, and public health professionals, improves the learning readiness and behaviour of children, reduces health risk factors, and improves intermediate measures of health, including cognitive function, of older volunteers (Carlson *et al.* 2009; Fried *et al.* 2004a; Rebok *et al.* 2004; Tan *et al.* 2006). This provides evidence both of the significant potential benefits of an ageing population, largely untapped at present, and of the value of investing in one generation in a way that will help all. These approaches, if designed effectively, should be able to contribute to a compression of morbidity and disability through social engagement, and redefine the now-anachronistic 'support-dependency ratio'. Many other types of roles for older adults in society can be developed, but should be designed to promote the health and well-being of the older adults, and to be generative through addressing important societal needs.

There are numerous additional ways in which longevity and the ageing of society has the potential to benefit all. Recent work indicates that increasing longevity is associated with increased wealth for countries. Although developing countries will be significantly challenged in adapting to population ageing due to the more rapid pace of ageing compared to developed countries, if appropriate policies and health promotion are advanced, they will likely benefit from increasing wealth as a result of this ageing. As stated by the Madrid Convention in 2002, this is critical to recognise, and should be a basis for population ageing being considered a key part of development agendas.

There are other ways in which investments in the needs of an ageing society are likely to benefit all. Certainly, this is the case for health systems, both public health and medical care, if designed to promote the health of older adults based on geriatric and public health principles. Such approaches have been developed to create age-appropriate and effective health promotion and prevention and chronic disease care that are cost-effective, and have improved outcomes, targeted to the health status and goals of the individual. However, geriatrically expert health systems are likely to provide excellent approaches for people of all ages. It is also the case for the recommendations of the World Health Organization's Global Age-Friendly Cities Project (WHO 2007). This work now involves more than 35 cities, addressing key areas so as to ensure that they 'support their residents as they age, [and] also tap the tremendous resources older people can offer' (Finkelstein *et al* 2008: 2). In the next 20 years, two-thirds of the world's population will be living in cities, and the populations of many cities will be ageing. Further, half of all cities will be rebuilt in this century. Doing such rebuilding with the needs of older adults in mind will be a cost-effective way to invest in the independence and well-being of older adults, and to create cities that have a higher quality of life for all. The key finding of the WHO Global Age-Friendly Cities project is that there are eight domains that must be addressed: housing, social participation, respect and social inclusion, civic participation and employment, transportation, outdoor spaces and buildings, community support and health services, and communication and information (WHO 2007). Additionally, minimising climate change and air pollution will also significantly benefit the health of older people and all people.

Finally, given older adults' vulnerabilities, they are also a group at high risk. This is true for risk associated with multi-morbidity, frailty, and disability, and risk from systems designed for care of relatively resilient individuals, such as many hospitals. This also applies to how we safeguard or sustain vulnerable older adults in the face of catastrophes and environmental extremes. Global public health approaches must be developed for an ageing world to protect this most vulnerable group from extremes of heat, likely to increase with climate change, and in the face of natural catastrophes, armed conflicts, and resulting forced migration. At present, those responding in humanitarian crises do not have mandates, expectations, or responsibilities to support and care for older adults. The rights of older adults globally must be affirmed, and social responsibility to bring public health to an ageing population must be addressed.

New metrics from an ageing world

As stated by Murray and Lopez, 'health trends in the next 25 years will be determined mainly by the ageing of the world's population …' (Murray and Lopez 1997a: 1,498). To understand these health trends, we will need metrics that help us better shape our ageing world to be an optimal one. For example, rather than just computing life expectancy, we also need to know estimates of morbidity-free and disability-free life expectancy (Katz *et al.* 1983; Murray and Lopez 1997b), or active life expectancy. We also need to change old age dependency ratios to measures that help us understand the benefits of an ageing population through the contributions that older adults make and through the health and independence associated with longevity in a country (Lutz *et al.* 2008), as well as those supports they receive. Such metrics will help us envision a positive future in an ageing world, as well as to plan more effectively to accomplish it and motivate necessary investment and policies.

In addition to new metrics, we will also need to tailor monitoring of health conditions, in order to understand how health status is evolving as the population ages, both in terms of the underlying causes of health status changes and in terms of the success of interventions. Such measures will need to include non-communicable chronic diseases and be flexible enough to permit understanding about how these conditions are superimposed on communicable (and often chronic) diseases, as well as on malnutrition or undernutrition; how they are compounded by conditions of ageing, including falls, frailty, disability, and dependency (Fried *et al.* 2004b); and the degree to which multiple health conditions are co-existing. Monitoring of key risk factors for health conditions will also be important. For the purposes of selecting targets for prevention, we must consider not just the population attributable risk of different risk factors, but the different cumulative impacts of these risk factors in causing multiple diseases. Finally, needs for primary, secondary, and tertiary prevention must be determined, and then met.

Beyond that, ultimately, as we increasingly have the opportunity to live longer lives, we must evolve our social compact to respect all age groups and how we each contribute to the positive definitions of being human, as well as realise the benefits of an ageing world.

As stated by the Madrid International Plan of Action on Ageing (2002):

> Population ageing is a universal force that has the power to shape the future as much as globalization. It is essential to recognize the ability of older persons to contribute to society by taking the lead not only in their own betterment but also in that of society as a whole. Forward thinking calls us to embrace the potential of the ageing population as a basis for future development.

References

Aboderin, I. and Ferreira, M. (2008) 'Linking ageing to development agendas in Sub-Saharan Africa: challenges and approaches', *Population Ageing*, 1(1): 51–73.

Addo, J., Smeeth, L., and Leon, D. A. (2007) 'Hypertension in Sub-Saharan Africa: a systematic review', *Hypertension*, 50: 1,012–18.

Akinboboye, O., Idris, O., Akinboboye, O., and Akinkugbe, O. (2003) 'Trends in coronary artery disease and associated risk factors in sub-Saharan Africans', *Journal of Human Hypertension*, 17: 381–7.

Aschner, P. (2002) 'Diabetes trends in Latin America', *Diabetes/Metabolism Research and Reviews*, 18: S27–31.

Bicego, G., Rutstein, S., and Johnson, K. (2003) 'Dimensions of the emerging orphan crisis in sub-Saharan Africa', *Social Science & Medicine*, 56(6): 1, 235–47

Black, R.E., Allen, L.H., Bhutta, Z.A., Caulfield, L.E., de Onis, M., Ezzati, M., Mathers, C., and Rivera, J. (2008) 'Maternal and child undernutrition 1', *The Lancet*, 371: 243–60.

Bouguerra, R., Alberti, H., Salem, L.B., Rayana, C.B., Atti, J.E., Gaigi, S., Slama, C.B., Zouari, B., and Alberti, K. (2007) 'The global diabetes pandemic: the Tunisian experience', *European Journal of Clinical Nutrition*, 61: 160–65.

Cappuccio, F.P., Micah, F.B., Emmett, L., Kerry, S.M., Antwi, S., Martin-Peprah, R., Phillips, R.O., Plange-Rhule, J., and Eastwood J.B. (2004) 'Prevalence, detection, management and control of hypertension in Ashanti, West Africa', *Hypertension*, 43: 1,017–22.

Carlson, M.C., Erickson, K.I., Kramer, A.F., Voss, M.W., Bolea, N., Mielke, M., McGill, S., Rebok, G.W., Seeman, T., and Fried, L.P. (2009) 'Evidence for neurocognitive plasticity in at-risk older adults: The Experience Corps Program', *Journal of Gerontology Series A: Biological Sciences and Medical Sciences*, 64A(12): 1, 275–82.

Castles, F.G. (2003) 'The world turned upside down: below replacement fertility, changing preferences and family-friendly public policy in 21 OECD countries', *Journal of European Social Policy*, 13(3): 209.

Center, M.M., Jemal, A., and Ward, E. (2009) 'International trends in colorectal cancer incidence rates', *Cancer Epidemiology, Biomarkers, and Prevention*, 18(6): 1,688–94.

Centers for Disease Control and Prevention (2008) *Persons Aged 50 and Older*, available at http://www.cdc.gov/hiv/topics/over50/index.htm (accessed 1 July 2009).

Centers for Disease Control and Prevention (CDC) and National Center for Health Statistics (NCHS) (2009) *CDC/NCHS Health Data Interactive: Hypertension, ages 20+: US, 1988–2006*, available at http://www.cdc.gov/nchs/hdi.htm (accessed 1 July 2009)

Central Intelligence Agency (CIA) (2009) *The World Factbook 2009*, available at http://www.cia.gov/library/publications/the-world-factbook/rankorder/2155rank.html (accessed 1 July 2009).

Coon, D.W., Lipman, P.D., and Ory, M.G. (2003) 'Designing HIV/AIDS social and behavioral interventions for the population of those 50 years and older', *Journal of Acquired Immune Deficiency Syndromes*, 33: S194–S205.

Danaei, G., Ding, E.L., Mozaffarian, D., Taylor, B., Rehm, J., Murray, C.J.L., and Ezzati, M. (2009) 'The preventable causes of death in the United States: Comparative risk assessment of dietary, lifestyle, and metabolic risk factors', *Public Library of Science Medicine*, 6(4): e10000058.

Dockery, D.W. and Pope III, C.A. (1994) 'Acute respiratory effects of particulate air pollution', *Annual Review of Public Health*, 15: 107–32.

Emmanuel, S.C. (1989) 'Trends in coronary heart disease mortality in Singapore', *Singapore Medical Journal*, 30: 17–23.

Finkelstein, R., Garcia, A., Netherland, J., and Walker, J. (2008) *Toward an age-friendly New York City: A findings report*, New York: The New York Academy of Medicine.

Fortin, M., Bravo, G., Hudon, C., Vanasse, A., and Lapointe, L. (2005) 'Prevalence of multimorbidity among adults seen in family practice', *Annals of Family Medicine*, 3: 223–8.

Freedman, M. and Fried, L.P. (1999) *Launching Experience Corps: Findings from a 2-year Pilot Project Mobilizing Older Americans to Help Inner-City Elementary Schools*, Oakland, CA: Civic Ventures.

Fried, L.P., Carlson, M.C., Freedman, M., Frick, K.D., Glass, T.A., Hill, J., McGill, S., Rebok, G.W., Seeman, T., Tielsch, J.M., Wasik, B., and Zeger, S. (2004a) 'A social model for health promotion for an ageing population: initial evidence on the Experience Corps® model', *Journal of Urban Health*, 81(1): 64–78.

Fried, L.P., Ferrucci, L., Darer, J., Williamson, J.D., and Anderson, G. (2004b) 'Untangling the concepts of disability, frailty, and comorbidity: implications for improved targeting and care', *Journal of Gerontology Series A: Biological Sciences and Medical Sciences*, 59: M255–M263.

Gaziano, T.A. (2008) 'Economic burden and the cost-effectiveness of treatment of cardiovascular diseases in Africa', *Heart*, 94: 140–44.

Gijsen, R., Hoeymans, N., Schellevis, F.G., Ruwaard, D., Satariano, W.A., and van den Bos, G.A.M. (2001) 'Causes and consequences of comorbidity: a review', *Journal of Clinical Epidemiology*, 54: 661–74.

Goldman, L., Phillips, K.A., Coxson, P., Goldman, P.A., Williams, L., Hunink, M.G., and Weinstein, M.C. (2001) 'The effect of risk factor reductions between 1981 and 1990 on coronary heart disease incidence, prevalence, mortality and cost', *Journal of the American College of Cardiology*, 38(4): 1,012–7.

Grant, J., Hoorens, S., Sivadasan, S., van het Loo, M., DaVanzo, J., Hale, L., Gibson, S., and Butz, W. (2004) *Low Fertility and Population Ageing: Causes, Consequences, and Policy Options*, Cambridge: Rand Europe.

Gupta, R., Joshi, P., Mohan, V., Reddy, K.S., and Yusuf, S. (2008) 'Epidemiology and causation of coronary heart disease and stroke in India', *Heart*, 94: 16–26.

Hunink, M.G., Goldman, L., Tosteson, A.N., Mittleman, M.A., Goldman, P.A., Williams, L.W., Tsevat, J., and Weinstein, M.C. (1997) 'The recent decline in mortality from coronary heart disease, 1980–1990: The effect of secular trends in risk factors and treatment', *JAMA*, 277(7): 535–42.

ILO (International Labour Organization) (2002) *Facts on Social Security*, Geneva: International Labour Office, available at http://www.ilo.org/public/english/protection/secsoc/downloads/events/factsheet.pdf (accessed 8 August 2009).

Jha, P., Ranson, M.K., Nguyen, S.N., and Yach, D. (2002) 'Estimates of global and regional smoking prevalence in 1995, by age and sex', *American Journal of Public Health*, 92: 1,002–06.

Kakwani, N. and Subbarao, K. (2005) *Ageing and Poverty in Africa and the Role of Social Pensions*, Brasilia: United Nations Development Programme and International Poverty Centre, available at http://www.undp-povertycentre.org/pub/IPCWorkingPaper8.pdf (accessed 1 July 2009).

Kamangar, F., Dores, G.M., and Anderson, W.F. (2008) 'Patterns of cancer incidence, mortality, and prevalence across five continents: defining priorities to reduce cancer disparities in different geographic regions of the world', *Journal of Clinical Oncology*, 24(140): 2,137–50.

Katz, S., Branch, L.G., et al. (1983) 'Active life expectancy', *New England Journal of Medicine*, 309(20): 1, 218–24.

Kearney, P.M., Whelton, M., Reynolds, K., Muntner, P., Whelton, P.K., and He, J. (2005) 'Global burden of hypertension: analysis of worldwide data', *The Lancet*, 365: 217–23.

Kinsella, K. and Phillips, D.R. (2005) 'Global ageing: the challenge of success', *Population Bulletin 60, No. 1*, Washington, DC: Population Reference Bureau.

Knodel, J., Watkins, S., and Van Landingham, M. (2003) 'AIDS and older persons: an international perspective', *Journal of Acquired Immune Deficiency Syndromes*, 33: S153–65.

Knodel, J., Zimmer, Z., Kim, K.S., and Puch, S. (2006) *The Impact of AIDS on Older-Age Parents in Cambodia*, Population Studies Center Research Report 06–594, Ann Arbor: University of Michigan, Institute for Social Research.

Lutz, W., Sanderson, W.C., and Scherbov, S. (2008) 'Global and regional population ageing: How certain are we of its dimensions?', *Journal of Population Ageing*, 1(1): 75–97.

Murray, C.J.L. and Lopez, A.D. (1997a) 'Alternative projections of mortality and disability by cause 1990–2020: Global Burden of Disease Study', *The Lancet*, 349: 1,498–504.

Murray, C.J. and Lopez, A.D. (1997b) 'Global mortality, disability, and the contribution of risk factors: Global Burden of Disease Study', *The Lancet*, 349: 1,436–42.

Ogawa, N. (2008) 'The Japanese elderly as a social safety net', *Asia-Pacific Population Journal*, 23(1): 105–13.

Okrainec, K., Banerjee, D.K., and Elsenberg, M.J. (2004) 'Coronary artery disease in the developing world', *American Heart Journal*, 148(1): 7–15.

Omran, A.R. (1971) 'The Epidemiologic Transition: A Theory of the Epidemiology of Population Change', *Milbank Memorial Fund Quarterly*, 29: 509–38.

Popkin, B.M. (2008) 'Will China's nutrition transition overwhelm its health care system and slow economic growth?' *Health Affairs*, 27(4): 1,064–76.

Rebok, G.W., Carlson, M.C., Glass, T.A., McGill, S., Hill, J., Wasik, B., Ialongo, N., Frick, K.D., Fried, L.P., and Rasmussen, M. (2004) 'Short-term impact of experience corps® participation on children and schools: results from a randomized pilot', *Journal of Urban Health*, 81(1): 79–93.

Rowe, J.W., Berkman, L.F., Binstock, R., Boersch-Supan, A., Cacioppo, J., Carstensen, L., Goldman, D., Fried, L., Jackson, J., Kohli, M., Olshansky, J., and Rother, J. (2009) 'Facts and fictions about an aging America', The Macarthur Foundation Research Network on an Ageing Society, *Contexts*, Fall, 8(4): 16–21.

Smeeding, T., Gao, Q., Saunders, P., and Wing, C. (2008) 'Elder poverty in an ageing world: conditions of social vulnerability and low income for women in rich and middle-income countries', Luxembourg Income Study Working Paper No. 497, available at http://www.lisproject.org/publications/liswps/497.pdf (accessed 1 July 2009).

Tan, E.J., Xue, Q.L., Li, T., Carlson, M.C., and Fried, L.P. (2006) 'Volunteering: a physical activity intervention for older adults – the experience corps ® program in Baltimore', *Journal of Urban Health*, 83(5): 954–69.

UNICEF (United Nations Children's Fund) (2007) *Young Lives: Statistical data on the status of children aged 0–4 in South Africa*, New York: UNICEF.

UNDESA (United Nations Department of Economic and Social Affairs) (2007a) *World Population Prospects: The 2008 Revision Population Database*, New York: UNDESA, available at http://esa.un.org/unpp/index.asp (accessed 1 July 2009).

UNDESA (United Nations Department of Economic and Social Affairs) (2007b) *World Economic and Social Survey 2007: Development in an Ageing World*, New York: UNDESA.

UNPD (United Nations Population Division) (accessed 2009) *World Population Prospects: 2006 Revision Population Database*, available at http://esa.un.org/unpp/ (1 July 2009).

UNFPA (United Nations Population Fund) (2005) *Population Issues: Meeting Development Goals*, available at http://149.120.32.2/pds/facts.htm (accessed 1 July 2009).

United States Census Bureau (2009) *American FactFinder*, available at http://factfinder.census.gov/ (accessed 24 June 2009).

Warren, C.W., Jones, N.R., Eriksen, M.P., and Asma, S. (2006) 'Patterns of global tobacco use in young people and implications for future chronic disease burden in adults', *The Lancet*, 367: 749–53.

Westaway, M.S. (2010) 'The impact of chronic diseases on the health and well-being of South Africans in early and later old age', *Archives of Gerontology and Geriatrics*, 50(2): 213–21.

Woo, E-K, Han, C., Jo, S.A., Park, M.K., Kim, S., Kim, E., Park, M.H., Lee, J., and Jo, I. (2007) 'Morbidity and related factors among elderly people in South Korea: results from the Ansan Geriatric (AGE) cohort study', *BMC Public Health*, 7: 10–19.

WHO (World Health Organization) (2003a) 'WHO/FAO release independent Expert Report on diet and chronic disease', *WHO News Releases*, 3 March, available at http://www.who.int/mediacentre/news/releases/2003/pr20/en/ (accessed 1 July 2009).

WHO (World Health Organization) (2003b) *Global Strategy on Diet, Physical Activity and Health: Obesity and Overweight*, Geneva: WHO, available at http://www.who.int/dietphysicalactivity/media/en/gsfs_obesity.pdf (accessed 1 July 2009).

WHO (World Health Organization) (2004) *Deaths and Injury Regional Estimates for 2004: World Bank Income Groups*, Global Burden of Disease (GBD), Geneva: WHO, available at http://www.who.int/healthinfo/global_burden_disease/estimates_regional/en/index.html (accessed 1 July 2009).

WHO (World Health Organization) (2006) *Fact Sheet: Obesity and Overweight*, Fact Sheet No. 311, Geneva: WHO, available at: http://www.who.int/mediacentre/factsheets/fs311/en/index.html (accessed 1 July 2009).

WHO (World Health Organization) (2007) *Global Age-friendly Cities: A Guide*, Geneva: WHO, available at http://www.who.int/ageing/publications/Global_age_friendly_cities_Guide_English.pdf (accessed 1 July 2009).

WHO (World Health Organization) (2008a) *The WHO Global InfoBase: Overweight and obesity (BMI)*, available at http://apps.who.int/infobase/report.aspx (accessed 1 July 2009).

WHO (World Health Organization) (2008b) *Fact Sheet: The Top Ten Causes of Death*, Fact Sheet No. 310, Geneva: WHO, available at http://www.who.int/mediacentre/factsheets/fs310/ (accessed 1 July 2009).

WRI (World Resources Institute) (1998) 'Linking environment and health: Introduction', in World Resources Institute, United Nations Environment Programme, United Nations Development Programme, and The World Bank, *World Resources 1998–99: Environmental Change and Human Health*, available at http://www.wri.org/publication/world-resources-1998–99-environmental-change-and-human-health (accessed 1 July 2009).

Yoon, K-H, Lee, J-H, Kim, J-W, Cho, J.H., Choi, Y.H., Ko, S-H, Zimmet, P., and Son, H-Y (2006) 'Epidemic obesity and type 2 diabetes in Asia', *The Lancet*, 368: 1,681–8.

Zingmond, D.S., Kilbourne, A.M., Justice, A.C., Wenger, N.S., Rodriguez-Barradas, M., Rabeneck, L., Taub, D., Weissman, S., Briggs, J., Wagner, J., Smola, S., and Bozzette, S.A. (2003) 'Differences in symptom expression in older HIV-positive patients: the veterans aging cohort 3 site study and HIV cost and service utilization study experience', *Journal of Acquired Immune Deficiency Syndrome*, 33: S84–S92.

Part V

Conflict, Violence, and Emergencies in Global Public Health

22

Conflict, Health, and Health Systems

A Global Perspective

Ronald J. Waldman and Margaret E. Kruk

The nature of armed conflict and, subsequently, its relation to health has changed a great deal during the past few decades. Whereas before the Second World War it was the norm for young men from different countries to dress in distinctive uniforms and to fight to the death to defend the honour of their respective countries, today it is quite rare. Today, most conflict is intra-statal and most of the 'dogs of war' (Shakespeare 1623) are unleashed not on rural battlefields, but in the very midst of cities, villages, and rural communities. While in the past armed combatants comprised the vast majority of casualties during periods of conflict, today as many as 90 per cent of deaths during times of conflict are incurred by the civilian population. While it remains important to tend to the needs of those fighters who are 'hors de combat' (the principal consideration that led to the formation of the International Committee of the Red Cross), it has become even more important, in terms of addressing the magnitude of human suffering, to address the humanitarian needs of civilian populations that may never have been explicitly involved in the conflict but have been caught up in it, quite unintentionally and through unfortunate circumstances. In this chapter, we will discuss the effects of conflict on health and on health systems, highlighting the evidence and debates in the field, as well as promising directions.

Conflict and public health

It may seem obvious, but it requires frequent restating: war and public health are incompatible pursuits (Toole, *et al.*, 1993). There are a number of reasons why societal violence may result in increased rates of mortality and/or morbidity in the general population and in specific high-risk subpopulations. These include, but are by no means limited to, increased injury and death from the direct results of the violence, such as physical trauma from bombs, land mines, and shootings. Yet, perhaps counter-intuitively, it is usually the 'indirect consequences' of conflict that are far more important contributors to the deterioration of the health status of the affected population. The strategic targeting of health facilities and hospitals by warring factions is a critical factor. The latter often leads to the absconment of professional health workers at all levels of the health system due to insecurity and perceived fear of, or actual, physical harm, which in turn serves as an important contributor to the absence of health services for the general population. This is compounded by looting, neglect of infrastructure, and the breakdown of the supply chain for drugs and vaccines, leaving clinics without essential medicines and supplies. Even when some essential health services remain, they are of substandard quality and unreliable. The result is increases in the incidence of and in deaths due to common illnesses such as pneumonia, diarrhoea, malaria, vaccine-preventable diseases, HIV/AIDS, tuberculosis, and other non-communicable chronic illnesses. For example, in the Democratic Republic of Congo, researchers found that most deaths were due not to violence but to preventable and treatable conditions, with more than 50 per cent of deaths attributable to fever and malaria, diarrhoea, respiratory infections, and malnutrition. Children under the age of five, who are especially vulnerable to these conditions, accounted for 45.4 per cent of all deaths even though they made up only 18.7 per cent of the survey sample (Coghlan *et al.* 2006).

Conflict also results in high rates of psychological trauma and associated depression, post-traumatic stress disorder, and anxiety. Despite their importance, mental health services have long been neglected in most conflict settings and the priority accorded to them by the international community has been woefully inadequate. Special mention should be made of the abhorrent practice of gender-based violence and its aftermath – sexual predation has been used as a weapon of war with impunity for centuries and its elimination should be a moral imperative for our time. Finally, the incompatibility of war and public health can extend well into the post-conflict period. Without a clear and coherent approach to the reconstruction of health systems and the provision of health services to a beleaguered population in an equitable, acceptable, and understandable manner, the damage caused by war can be prolonged until long after hostilities have ceased.

While various conflicts have led directly or indirectly to the formation of large international assistance organisations (e.g. the First World War – Save the Children Federation; the Second World War – International Rescue Committee; Biafra War of Secession – Médecins sans Frontières), relief efforts for beleaguered populations were for many years largely based on the good intentions of generous individuals and organisations rather than on a quantitative evaluation of needs. The study of public health in conflict and post-conflict settings can be said to have begun after the Cambodian genocide of 1975–9. Survivors fled to Thailand, where many were settled in the so-called 'death camps' of Sakeo and Khao-i-Dong. Epidemiological techniques were used to determine crude- and age-specific mortality rates (9.1/10,000 per day, highest in children aged four years and under) and the most frequent causes of death (febrile illnesses, presumed to be malaria) (Glass *et al.* 1980).

Further progress in developing a disciplined approach to public health during conflict was made in Somalia, from 1979–85. When armed conflict and inequitable land reform policies in the Ogaden region of Ethiopia, combined with the irredentist claims of the Somali government, led to the flight of hundreds of thousands of refugees into about 35 camps ranging from the north of Somalia to the south, a major, but largely unpublicised, international humanitarian relief effort was mounted. Under the leadership of the Ministry of Health of the Somali Democratic Republic, uniform guidelines for health and nutrition care were developed and, perhaps even more importantly, a centralised surveillance system for monitoring the health and nutrition status of the population was put into place. Regular reporting on conditions of major public health importance, including malnutrition, febrile illnesses, acute respiratory infections, acute watery diarrhoeal diseases and dysentery, and rash illnesses (a proxy for measles) was enforced, and allocations of pharmaceutical products were made from the Ministry of Health on the basis of the information provided. In this way, progress towards improving the health status of the population could be monitored, and untoward events, such as outbreaks of scurvy (Magan *et al.*

1983), hepatitis E, typhus, cholera, and other diseases could be quickly responded to and controlled.

The application of public health methods in conflict settings

Through these emergency events and others precipitated by conflict in Ethiopia, Mozambique, and Eastern Europe (especially in Bosnia) during the 1980s and the first part of the 1990s, an epidemiology of health in complex emergencies emerged (Toole and Waldman 1990,1993, 1997; Toole *et al.* 1988).

A number of key findings were found to characterise the public health needs of civilians affected by armed conflict. These included:

- Crude mortality rates of disastrous magnitude – as high as 10–15 times what became widely accepted as the 'emergency threshold' of one death per 10,000 population per day
- Mortality in the under-5 population consistently 2–3 times higher than that in the general population
- High suspected rates of maternal mortality, although levels of maternal morbidity and mortality were not clearly established, either due to inattention or to technical problems with their measurement
- High rates of preventable mortality and mortality due to common illnesses – measles was an especially lethal killer in emergency settings and required special attention, but diarrhoea, pneumonia, malaria (where endemic), and other vaccine-preventable diseases could also be important problems
- High prevalence of malnutrition: the quantity of relief rations was often inadequate, and their quality, especially in terms of micronutrients, could lead to major 'outbreaks' of micronutrient deficiencies (Magan *et al.* 1983; Malfait *et al.* 1993; Toole *et al.* 1988).

A turning point in the history of the practice of public health in conflict and post-conflict settings came in July 1994. Following the genocide in Rwanda and the ultimate ascendancy to power of the Rwandan Patriotic Front, a large number, perhaps a million, refugees, almost all of the Hutu ethnic group, fled to hastily assembled camps in Tanzania and Zaire (now the Democratic Republic of Congo). Traumatised by the events that had unfolded in their home country during the preceding months and terrorised to an extent by Hutu militia who urged continued resistance to the RPF, the refugees in the North Kivu province of Zaire were now subjected to an epidemic of cholera of unusual intensity. So bad were the conditions, and so insufficient the response, that epidemiologically derived estimates put crude mortality rates at appalling levels of 20–35 per 10,000 population per day. The situation was compounded by outbreaks of dysentery and meningitis, and by high rates of post-infectious malnutrition, ranging from 18–23 per cent, before it was brought under control during the second month. Out of a poorly estimated population of 500–800,000 nearly 50,000 individuals lost their lives during the relief effort, meaning that few, if any lives were saved (Goma Epidemiology Group 1995). Those who documented the events concluded that 'relief agencies must place increased emphasis on training personnel in relevant skills …' concluding that:

[M]ore attention to needs and capacities assessments, contingency planning, preparedness measures, and adoption of the most cost–effective interventions by UN agencies, NGOs and donor governments, including military contingents providing humanitarian assistance, would have resulted in better allocation of relief resources and, more importantly, could have saved even more human lives.

(Steering Committee of the Joint Evaluation of Emergency Assistance
to Rwanda 1996: 49)

Creating public health standards: the Sphere Project

The humanitarian relief community, especially the non-governmental organisations (NGOs), took the criticism to heart and responded aggressively to these recommendations. Training courses and degree programmes on public health in complex emergencies were developed and taught in a variety of settings. Perhaps most importantly, the Sphere Project, a set of basic principles of humanitarian assistance, standards of performance in health, nutrition, food and nutrition, water and sanitation, and shelter, as well as a training programme and a collaborative spirit, was developed. Together with alternative approaches to the improvement of the quality of care for those in need of humanitarian assistance in complex emergencies, the *Sphere Project Handbook* (currently being revised for the second time since its original publication in 2000) contributed to the transformation of the delivery of humanitarian assistance from a largely philanthropic, but relatively chaotic, set of activities to a more disciplined, methodical, systematic approach – one that recognised that civilian victims of war should not be passive recipients of charity but people with a right to relief interventions of acceptable quality. The 'science' of public health in conflict and post-conflict settings had not, and still has not, developed, and the evidence base for what works and what does not still needs substantial reinforcement, but the tragic outcomes documented in Goma are thought to have marked a turning point for the better.

The changing nature of conflict settings and implications for health

Still, in the past decade, as noted in the introductory remarks above, the nature of conflict and the conditions in which public health is practiced in its wake, have been drastically altered. Refugee camps, indeed refugees, are no longer the norm. Instead, prolonged low-intensity conflict has made the delivery of humanitarian assistance all the more difficult – large populations of people internally displaced (IDPs) by conflict receive no legal protection from the international community – unlike refugees, there are no conventions or treaties that govern their needs. In addition, many people caught up in today's conflicts are trapped 'in situ' – even though they are not displaced, their access to health, education, employment, and all other social services are severely limited.

From a technical standpoint, a number of significant changes have occurred, in an attempt to address the changing conditions and the recognition that a return to 'normal' life is likely to be an elusive goal for many combat-affected civilians, even after cessation of hostilities. New nutritional products, such as high-energy, low-protein milks and ready-to-use supplementary and therapeutic foods, have allowed feeding programmes and the treatment of severe malnutrition to be moved from clinical settings into the community. The magnitude of the HIV epidemic in some parts of the world, combined with the increased availability of antiretroviral drugs, have encouraged a greater focus on HIV/AIDS and on tuberculosis, two communicable diseases that had largely been ignored in humanitarian relief efforts only a few years ago. The control of these communicable diseases, and other priority health conditions, has been appropriately and progressively pushed down the medical system ladder, from hospital to clinic to health post, to within the community itself in order to enhance population access to these essential services. Importantly, two major health areas in great need of new technical interventions, reproductive health and mental health, have received significantly increased attention in recent years, although full agreement on what specific intervention packages should be implemented, and how they should be delivered, has eluded full consensus within the global relief community (Spiegel *et al.* 2010).

Technical considerations aside, perhaps the most important advance in current thinking about public health in conflict and post-conflict settings is that the health status of the population is not dependent on the actions of health practitioners alone, nor can the health sector aspire to achieve its objectives without the sincere and full adoption of a multisectoral approach. Security, for one thing, is paramount. A study conducted by the International Rescue Committee in the Democratic Republic of Congo in 2004 found both crude mortality rates and under-five mortality rates to be about twice as high in health zones that were experiencing violence as in those zones that were at relative peace. Although, of course, deaths attributable to violence were higher in the former, the majority of deaths in both groups were due to preventable and/or treatable diseases. The authors of the study concluded that 'improvements in security represent perhaps the most effective means to reduce excess mortality ...' (Coghlan *et al.* 2006: 50). How to achieve these improvements, whether through political pressure, diplomacy, or armed intervention, among other possibilities, is clearly beyond the usual scope of work of health professionals. However, advocacy for their achievement is critical and very much in line with the public health imperative of reducing morbidity and mortality by whatever means possible.

While public health and conflict may be for the most part incompatible, the practice of public health during the period of post-conflict societal rehabilitation is not. Just as non-health actors may be important in helping health practitioners expand coverage and access to health services during a conflict, fledgling governments in the post-conflict period must adopt new strategies that are intended not only to improve the health status of the population, but also to contribute to efforts to establish stable and legitimate political structures. The intended result of these efforts is to avoid a resumption of hostilities (the rate of conflict resumption following cease-fires is estimated to be greater than 50 per cent within five years) and, consequently, because of the adverse relationship between conflict and health, to save lives in the long term, as well as during the immediate post-conflict period (Collier *et al.* 2008).

A basic package of health services

The achievements of the Ministry of Public Health of Afghanistan (MoPH) over the past few years are a case in point. There, with the help of the international community, a Basic Package of Health Services (BPHS) was devised in 2005. The intent of the BPHS was to make a relatively small, manageable, affordable set of primary health care interventions available to as much of the population as possible at the earliest possible time following the establishment of a potentially legitimate government. The content of the BPHS was relatively non-controversial: its four principal components were maternal and newborn health care (including reproductive health services); child health and immunisation, including a focus on the content of the Integrated Management of Childhood Illnesses strategy and on a routine Expanded Programme on Immunization; the control of communicable diseases; and public nutrition. In addition, because of their importance in the setting of post-conflict Afghanistan, both mental health services and the management of disabilities received attention (Ministry of Public Health of Afghanistan 2005). Fundamentally, the BPHS established a 'social contract' between the government and the people, whereby the government promised to strive to make its content available at all public supported primary care health facilities throughout the country (a Basic Package of Hospital Services was adopted more recently). Importantly, the MoPH recognised that it did not have the human resources to effectuate the delivery of the promised services. Instead, it opted for a 'stewardship' role in health; that is, the Ministry took on the role of policy development and priority-setting, regulation, financing, administration, and, importantly, monitoring and evaluation. For the actual delivery of services, it chose, for the most part, to enter into contracts with NGOs. By providing the NGOs with financial incentives for reaching or surpassing pre-set targets, the MoPH has been able to make considerable progress toward the achievement of national objectives in the health sector and, by granting relative autonomy to the operational modalities of the NGOs, it has been able to bypass the administrative, logistical, and human resource problems that tend to place major burdens on public health systems in developing countries, whether conflict-affected or not (Ministry of Public Health of Afghanistan 2005).

Similar systems, all based on the Basic Package of Health Services, have been tried in post-conflict Cambodia (prior to Afghanistan) and in the Democratic Republic of Congo, south Sudan, and Liberia, subsequently. Although there is some healthy scepticism regarding the long-term viability of these systems, they seem to be potentially effective in the short term, at least. In Afghanistan, access to the BPHS has been extended to districts of the country in which more than 80 per cent of the population live. The number of functioning health facilities has grown from fewer than 500 in 2003 to more than 1,000, and the average number of visits to a health facility has increased from less than 0.3 to almost 1.0 per capita per year. Major gains have also been made in vaccination coverage, with major gains documented in infant mortality reduction (Loevinsohn and Sayed 2008). Of course, as has been said above, public health and conflict are closely related in an adverse sense, and in Afghanistan, as well as elsewhere, it can be shown that where insecurity is pervasive, access to health services, like population health status, suffers. As a result, progress in the eastern and southern provinces of Afghanistan, where civil strife continues and, in the past few years, has become more intense, has been slow (if present at all), and the ability of the MoPH to contract with NGOs to provide services in these areas is compromised.

Conclusion

To conclude, it should be asked, if relative peace is a pre-condition for a relatively well-functioning health system and, by extension, for improvement in the ability of a population to access health services, whether investments in the health sector are the most appropriate. Sadly, to this point, there is no clear evidence that supporting health personnel, clinical sites, prevention programmes such as vaccinations for children, the provision of pharmaceuticals, and so forth, makes a clear contribution to the ability of a country emerging from conflict to develop a stable and legitimate system of governance. There is no evidence to the contrary either – this is simply an issue that has not been measured. From a conceptual standpoint, given the valued role of health care in most societies and the public's expectation of government stewardship of health services, it is possible that provision of quality, reliable health services could signal a restoration of good governance to the population. This requires that governments be seen to take responsibility for the health sector. Instead, individual programme managers seem to remain mired within their own sectors: vaccination programmes measure the coverage they have achieved in getting BCG, DPT, and measles vaccines into the arms of children, not whether or not the services they are providing lowers levels of mistrust and suspicion of central authorities; the construction of clinics is frequently attributed to foreign donors or international organisations, not to the efforts of a young government to expand new and desperately needed services to a hurting population in an effort to build and to win over its confidence; the provision of clinical interventions is measured in terms of disease reduction, but not in terms of their contribution to political stabilisation and state-building. In short, the nature of conflict has changed, and recognition is growing that risk factors for poor health include the status of activities in the non-health sectors. However, the strategies utilised by health professionals, indeed the very objectives of health interventions, have not reflected that we live in a changed and ever-changing world. Until they do, not only will conflict and health continue to be incompatible, but the small gains that can be made in violent settings will continue to be short-lived and ephemeral. Public health action can make an important difference to the lives of many people around the world, and those unfortunate enough to have been caught up in violent settings through no fault of their own should be among them.

References

Coghlan, B., Brennan, R.J., Ngoy, P., Dofara, D., Otto, B., Clements, M., and Stewart, T. (2006) 'Mortality in the Democratic Republic of Congo: a nationwide survey', *The Lancet*, 367: 44–51.

Collier, P., Hoeffler, A., and Soderbom, M. (2008) 'Post-conflict risks', *Journal of Peace Research*, 45: 461–78.

Glass, R.I., Cates, W., Jr., Nieburg, P., Davis, C., Russbach, R., Nothdurft, H., Peel, S., and Turnbull, R. (1980) 'Rapid assessment of health status and preventive-medicine needs of newly arrived Kampuchean refugees, Sa Kaeo, Thailand', *The Lancet*, 1: 868–72.

Goma Epidemiology Group (1995) 'Public health impact of Rwandan refugee crisis: what happened in Goma, Zaire, in July, 1994?', *The Lancet*, 345: 339–44.

Loevinsohn, B. and Sayed, G.D. (2008) 'Lessons from the health sector in Afghanistan: how progress can be made in challenging circumstances', *JAMA*, 300: 724–6.

Magan, A.M., Warsame, M., Ali-Salad, A.K., and Toole, M.J. (1983) 'An outbreak of scurvy in Somali refugee camps', *Disasters*, 7: 94–6.

Malfait, P., Moren, A., Dillon, J.C., Brodel, A., Begkoyian, G., Etchegorry, M.G., Malenga, G., and Hakewill, P. (1993) 'An outbreak of pellagra related to changes in dietary niacin among Mozambican refugees in Malawi', *International Journal of Epidemiology*, 22: 504–11.

Ministry of Public Health in Afghanistan (2005) *A Basic Package of Health Services for Afghanistan*, Kabul: Ministry of Public Health in Afghanistan.

Shakespeare, W. (1623) Act 3, Scene 1, *Julius Caesar*, First Folio.

Spiegel, P., Checchi, F., Colombo, S., and Paik, E. (2010) 'Health-care needs of people affected by conflict: future trends and changing frameworks', *The Lancet*, 375: 341–5.

Steering Committee of the Joint Evaluation of Emergency Assistance to Rwanda (1996) *The International Response to Conflict and Genocide: Lessons From the Rwanda Experience*, London: Overseas Development Institute.

Toole, M.J. and Waldman, R.J. (1990) 'Prevention of excess mortality in refugee and displaced populations in developing countries', *JAMA*, 263: 3,296–302.

Toole, M.J. and Waldman, R.J. (1993) 'Refugees and displaced persons: War, hunger, and public health', *JAMA*, 270: 600–605.

Toole, M.J. and Waldman, R.J. (1997) 'The public health aspects of complex emergencies and refugee situations', *Annual Review of Public Health*, 18: 283–312.

Toole, M.J., Nieburg, P., and Waldman, R.J. (1988) 'The association between inadequate rations, undernutrition prevalence, and mortality in refugee camps: case studies of refugee populations in eastern Thailand, 1979–1980, and eastern Sudan, 1984–1985', *Journal of Tropical Pediatrics*, 34: 218–24.

Toole, M.J., Galson, S., and Brady, W. (1993) 'Are war and public health compatible?', *The Lancet*, 341: 1,193–6.

23

Ending Violence against Women
Essential to Global Health and Human Rights

Nancy Glass, Jacquelyn Campbell, Veronica Njie-Carr, and Terri-Ann Thompson

> Human rights are universal, violence against women has made human rights abuse universal.
>
> (Amnesty International, Women's Rights are Human Rights, 2004)

Introduction

This chapter provides a global picture of violence against women as a human rights violation that impacts the health, economics, and well-being of individuals, households, and society. It discusses the multiple, complex, and intersecting impact of violence on critical components of women's lives in the context of a human rights framework and examines the role of global leadership in ending violence against women.

Violence can occur against women or men, and be perpetrated by women or men. Globally, the vast majority of women experience violence at the hands of an intimate or ex-intimate partner or someone known to them; men most often experience violence from strangers. The level of violence differs between men and women. Tjaden and Thoennes (2000) found that in the US, women were 7–14 times more likely to be assaulted by male partners than males were by their women partners. Women are more likely to report ongoing fear and/or having changed their behaviours to accommodate a violent partner than men (Campbell 2002). Further, violence against women often takes place in a context of ongoing gender discrimination, as evidenced by higher rates of poverty and lower wages among women than their male counterparts, even for men and women with similar education and work experience (Riger *et al.* 2002). This economic discrimination significantly impacts women's ability to leave abusive relationships (Glass *et al.* 2008). This chapter's focus on violence against women within a human rights framework is critical because of the multiple and interrelated contextual factors involved in violence against women: higher levels of extreme violence and injury, fear, forced changes in victims' behaviours, and the poverty and discrimination that limits women's ability to live healthy, safe, and productive lives free of violence.

Global violence against women

Violence against women is a significant global issue. The *Multi-Country Study on Women's Health and Domestic Violence Against Women* (WHO 2005) used interviews from 24,000 women in 15 sites, both rural and urban, in ten countries representing diverse cultures (WHO 2005).[1] The WHO study highlighted the prevalence of physical and sexual violence, emotional abuse, and controlling behaviour by a current intimate partner or an ex-partner, as well as the lifetime prevalence of intimate partner violence (IPV). The study found that 15 to 71 per cent of ever-partnered women had experienced physical and/or sexual violence. Most settings reported 29 to 62 per cent, and significant variations between and within country (rural vs. urban) settings (WHO 2005). Reported lifetime prevalence of IPV was highest among women living in provincial (primarily rural) areas in the countries Bangladesh, Ethiopia, Peru, and Tanzania. The highest prevalence in the past year was reported in Tanzania at 54 per cent; Ethiopian women reported the highest prevalence (59 per cent) of ever experiencing sexual violence by an intimate or ex-intimate partner (WHO 2005). In most of the study settings, 30 to 56 per cent of women who reported experiencing violence by an intimate partner reported that the violence had been both physical and sexual.

A common misconception by policymakers and communities is that women are at greater risk of violence from a stranger rather than from an intimate partner, ex-intimate partner, or other men in their lives. The WHO study (2005) demonstrated that women in most of the ten participating countries reported that the greatest risk of violence came from a partner or ex-partner. For example, over 75 per cent of women aged 15 years or older who experienced violence reported that the violence was perpetrated by an intimate or ex-intimate partner. The only differences in this pattern were noted in urban Samoa and Brazil, where 40 per cent of violence was perpetrated by non-partners.

Impact of violence on women's health

Global studies have shown that, compared to women who have no history of violence, women who experience violence tend to report having impaired emotional, mental, general health, and social functioning, as well as increased suicidal behaviour (Ellsburg *et al.* 2008).

Reproductive health consequences of physical and sexual violence may include: infection with HIV (Dunkle *et al.* 2004) or other sexually transmitted infections (STIs) from infected perpetrators because of women's inability to negotiate condom use (Kalichman and Simbayi 2004), reduced access to/availability of resources such as post-exposure prophylaxis (PEP) or emergency contraceptive pills (ECP) following the sexual act (Heise and Elias 1995), and genital trauma from rape, which may contribute to increased risk of HIV transmission (Kim *et al.* 2003). Other potential physical effects include increased urinary tract infections, unwanted pregnancies (and subsequently unsafe abortions), and pregnancy complications or miscarriages (Gómez *et al.* 2009). A large percentage of rape and forced sex victims sustain fibroids and chronic pelvic pain (Letourneau *et al.* 1999), which require medical attention. The mental health consequences of both sexual assault and IPV often include depression, insomnia (and other symptoms consistent with post-traumatic stress disorder), and suicidal ideation (WHO 2005).

Globally, the economic imbalances between men and women and the high rates of IPV and sexual violence, with limited power to negotiate safe sex and condom use, have contributed to the disproportionate impact of HIV infection on women (Pronyk *et al.* 2006). As of 2007, over 15 million women were infected with HIV out of the 30.8 million adults living with the disease worldwide. The interrelationships between HIV infection and violence against women continue to be a growing concern for practitioners, researchers, and advocates working in the area of violence prevention. There is increasing evidence of direct and indirect pathways from violence against women to HIV, particularly in sub-Saharan Africa, where three persuasive, large studies show a direct relationship of IPV and HIV infection over and above other risk factors (Campbell *et al.* 2008). A recent study in the US showed a similar relationship, with 12 per cent of new HIV infections in women attributable to IPV (Sareen *et al.* 2009). In studies in which violence was not directly associated with HIV infection, violence was strongly associated with HIV risk factors such as multiple partners, transactional sex, early and coercive sexual debut, unprotected sex, and substance use (Karamagi *et al.* 2006; WHO 2005).

The interrelationships between HIV infection and violence against women can be clustered as follows:

(1) marital and non-marital rape or forced sex, particularly in countries with post-anarchy political instability such as Rwanda, the Democratic Republic of Congo, Sudan, and more recently, Zimbabwe (Human Rights Watch/Africa 1996; Kim *et al.* 2009);

(2) women and girls unable to negotiate protective measures such as the use of condoms because of socially constructed patriarchal systems (Greig *et al.* 2008) limiting women's power;

(3) children witnessing violence in the home or experiencing childhood violence, which may have long-term effects such as high-risk sexual behaviours during adolescent and young adult periods (Dunkle *et al.* 2004); and

(4) women who disclose their HIV status and experience violence from male partners because they are perceived to have been unfaithful or to have engaged in promiscuous behaviours.

Violence against women impacts households and society

Multiple interrelated and complex factors such as poverty and gender inequity constrain women's control over their lives (Odek *et al.* 2009). Gaining access to and control over income-generating activities would likely have positive benefits for women's health, link to social support, and improve well-being.

Studies conducted primarily in developing countries suggest that women who experience sexual violence tend to have poorer educational outcomes, limiting their future economic and decision-making opportunities. Non-consensual sex was significantly associated with lower chances of current school enrolment among males and females, lower educational attainment, and school progression delays (Hallman 2007). These results were more pronounced for females than for males. School-aged girls who were raped reported finding it more difficult to concentrate on studies after the assault, losing interest in school, and transferring or leaving school altogether (Human Rights Watch 2001).

Violent acts within an intimate relationship or perpetrated by a non-partner are propagated by social systems that allow men to control women in all aspects of their lives, stifling women's voices and limiting their choices to seek help within the family and larger community. Women bear the burden of the worst human rights violations, yet are limited in their agency to act. Particularly concerning is that within the context of such violence, some women believe and accept their husbands' right to punish them if they fail to perform their marital duties, and likewise accept forced sex (Lary *et al.* 2004). This social acceptance of gender power imbalances contributes to the impunity felt by perpetrators of violence against women.

Power imbalances are related to age differences, socio-cultural, and economic factors – particularly polygamous marriages and wife inheritance – which limit women's ability and control to negotiate preventive measures such as condom use (Greig *et al.* 2008). The tradition of wife inheritance among Luo women in western Kenya provides an example of power imbalance between women and men and socio-cultural factors that place women at risk for violence, stigma, and HIV/AIDS. Specifically, Luo widows must perform a cleansing ritual that includes sex with a cleanser prior to their integration into the community (Ambasa-Shisanya 2007). If the deceased spouse was HIV-infected, the professional cleanser is at risk for HIV; if the professional cleanser is HIV-positive, the widow is at risk as well. Limited research has addressed the role of cleansing rituals in the lives of widows, who/what influences the decision to participate and, most importantly, the role of these rituals in HIV transmission.

Understanding the relationship of violence against women to human rights

The concept of human rights asserts that every person has certain economic, social, and political rights by virtue of his or her humanity (International Council on Human Rights Policy 2005). The United Nations Universal Declaration of Human Rights (UDHR) goes well beyond these areas in defining human rights, and in its requirement of governments to take affirmative action to assure such rights, rather than simply refrain from infringing upon them (UN 1948).

The widely cited UDHR was influential in the development of international human rights laws. It declares that human rights apply to all human beings without distinction of gender, although it does not specifically address issues related to women or violence against women.

The first significant international recognition of women's rights as human rights was in 1979 – only 30 years ago – in the Convention on the Elimination of All Forms of Discrimination against Women (CEDAW). The CEDAW addresses the right of women to be free from trafficking and prostitution, but does not explicitly address IPV, sexual abuse, incest, or rape (UN 1979). It is important to note that the US is the sole industrialised nation in the world to have failed to ratify the CEDAW.

In the 1990s, there was further progress in the recognition of women's human rights with the adoption of a definition of gender-based violence (GBV) by the CEDAW Committee. The CEDAW was followed by the Declaration on the Elimination of Violence against Women (UN DEVAW 1993), the Vienna Declaration (UN World Conference on Human Rights 1993), and the Beijing Declaration and Platform for Action (UN Fourth World Conference on Women 1995). All three define violence against women, including violence within the family, as a human rights issue.

Violence against women is clearly a violation of the rights articulated in UDHR Article 3 (the right to personal security) and, in more severe cases, may also violate Articles 4 (slavery) and 5 (torture). In the more severe cases, in which there are ongoing patterns of physical and sexual violence, the perpetrator assumes rights and privileges that belong to the victim and thus lowers the status of the woman to less than that of a human being (Young and Maguire 2003). In the case of IPV, not only does the abusive partner or ex-partner inflict physical violence, sexual violence, and emotional abuse, but he also coercively controls the woman's environment, including income, housing, access to friends and families, work, food, children, culture, and sexuality. Insufficient governmental and institutional response from the criminal justice, health care, and social services systems are violations of women's rights and deny victims attempting to leave abusive situations of basic needs and living support.

The CEDAW, DEVAW, Beijing Platform, Vienna Declaration, and other documents represent tremendous accomplishments, and demonstrate that progress is being made in recognising violence against women as a component of human rights violations. While international human rights campaigns geared towards enhancing women's rights have gained momentum, application in the US of human rights concepts has evolved more slowly. The human rights framework has been regarded as irrelevant and inappropriate for 'advanced' democracies such as the US (DeFrancisco *et al.* 2003). Full application of the UDHR remains controversial in the US, as demonstrated by the failure of the US Congress to ratify the CEDAW, and the lack of a human rights court or forum. In addition, the US has focused its Bill of Rights and tradition on civil and political rights, such as the right to vote and to free speech, and has steadfastly opposed economic rights to housing, health care, and a living wage, seeing such rights as supportive of socialism or communism (DeFrancisco *et al.* 2003). The US views the rights of women to divorce and determine their reproductive capacity free from male involvement as 'anti-family' (Erwin 2006). In this context, US advocates for violence prevention, practitioners, and researchers have access to fewer resources than their global colleagues for developing, implementing, and evaluating violence prevention and intervention services and programmes within a human rights framework.

Implementing a human rights framework to address violence against women

The human rights framework (HRF) and its associated documents provide several important duties, principles, and standards that advocates for violence prevention, practitioners, and researchers could use for global changes in their response to violence against women. Programmes developed to respond to violence against women cannot be the only ones held accountable for designing and providing resources and programmes for women within the HRF. Other systems within communities, such as health care, criminal justice, and child welfare, must collaborate in applying a HRF.

The HRF goes beyond the passage of laws and policies. It also defines the *duties* of those responsible for development and implementation of laws and policies, the *principles* by which the framework will be implemented, and the *standards* to evaluate performance. The following sections are from an abridged version of the paradigm and analysis developed by the International Council on Human Rights Policy (2005) to describe the application of the HRF to governmental and non-governmental institutions.[2]

Many of the duties and principles of the HRF are already incorporated globally into governmental and non-governmental organisations' (NGOs') programmes. This provides an opportunity for programmes to build on their strengths and to more fully apply the duties, principles, and standards implicit in the HRF.

Duties

The HRF defines three duties for governments and NGOs (International Council on Human Rights Policy 2005), and is realistic, stressing that such duties are not without limits. Duties include respecting human rights, protecting human rights, and fulfilling human rights. Application of the framework is not a one-time event, but rather a complex, multi-level effort that evolves over several years, involving the coordination and integration of multiple systems within a community. Thus, communities and institutions are expected to plan and progressively implement advances, taking into account available resources and the understanding that human rights are interdependent and cannot be achieved all at once. Although many countries and communities have insufficient resources to implement all elements of the human rights framework, that is not an excuse to perform poorly in protecting women's rights. Instead, the maximum available resources need to be accessed and leveraged to fulfil these duties.

Principles

The HRF also has overarching principles that assist in the development and implementation of programmes and services. Within this framework, participation, non-discrimination (inclusion), accountability, and indivisibility of human rights are ingredients critical to the full realisation of principles. Individuals impacted by violence are entitled to participate in developing, implementing, and monitoring responses and services. They are entitled to engage critically with decisions that affect them and their families at individual, programmatic, and political levels. Programmes should be designed to include victims in their services, and to change policies and rules that limit the provision of services to certain victims. In low- and middle-income countries, where few resources exist for women, victims of violence need the opportunity to safely document the violence with local authorities without the risk of retaliation from the perpetrator(s) or authorities. Women are entitled to opportunities to 'speak truth to power' and to attain their own political power.

Standards

The four standards have been outlined within the framework to include: (1) availability, (2) accessibility, (3) acceptability, and (4) adaptability of services. Those responsible for implementing programmes can use these standards to evaluate their services for women and the larger community. Access must be provided to vital information about safety and resources linked to other services such as health care and criminal justice.

Incorporating the HRF outlined above is challenging and requires leadership and innovation in tandem with financial and workforce resources.

The way forward: global leadership on ending violence against women

President Obama highlighted the importance of global health in US diplomacy. The US remains both the largest funder of innovation in global health and the largest donor to care and support programmes – notably in the President's Emergency Plan for AIDS Relief (PEPFAR) and the Global Fund to Fight AIDS, Tuberculosis, and Malaria. However, these programmes have not been without problems. For example, the prevention efforts in PEPFAR were seen by many in the US and globally as ideologically hindered – forced to promote US agendas such as abstinence and the separation of HIV prevention from programmes for family planning and preventing violence against women. Nevertheless, there has been progress, and now all PEPFAR-funded programmes are required to include a gendered analysis of their programmes.

The International Violence against Women Act (I-VAWA) was reintroduced in the US Senate in February 2010. I-VAWA is a historic and unprecedented effort by the US to address violence against women globally. It directs the US government to create a comprehensive, five-year strategy to reduce violence in up to 20 diverse countries that have severe levels of violence against women. To achieve this goal, the I-VAWA[3] authorises more than $1 billion over five years in US government assistance to support international programmes that prevent and respond to violence against women.

I-VAWA acknowledges the intersection of health and human rights by funding health programmes and victim services, legal accountability, and a change of public attitudes towards perpetrators and victims. The I-VAWA is an opportunity to engage the global community and for the US to take leadership in protecting human rights by passing legislation and leading diplomatic, health, economic, and advocacy efforts to end the global plague of violence against women.

Notes

1 Participating countries were Bangladesh, Brazil, Ethiopia, Japan, Namibia, Peru, Samoa, Serbia and Montenegro, Thailand, and the United Republic of Tanzania (WHO 2005).
2 More in-depth information about the Human Rights Framework can be found in the International Council on Human Rights Policy, 2005.
3 Detailed information on the I-VAWA Act can be found at http://www.govtrack.us/congress/bill.xpd? bill=s110–2279.

References

Ambasa-Shisanya, C.R. (2007) 'Widowhood in the Era of HIV/AIDS: A Case Study of Slaya District, Kenya', *Journal of Social Aspects of HIV/AIDS*, 4(2): 606–15.

Campbell, J.C. (2002) 'Health Consequences of Intimate Partner Violence', *The Lancet*, 359: 1,331–6.

Campbell, J.C., Baty, M.L., Ghandour, R.M., Stockman, J.K., Francisco, L., and Wagman, J. (2008) 'The Intersection of Intimate Partner Violence Against Women and HIV/AIDS: A Review', *International Journal of Injury Control and Safety Promotion*, 15: 221–31.

DeFranciso, V.P., LaWare, M.R., Palczewski, C.H. (2003) 'The Home Side of Global Feminism: Why Hasn't the Global Found a Home in the U.S?', *Women and Language*, xxvi(1): 100–109.

Dunkle, K.L., Jewkes, R.K., Brown, H.C., Gray, G.E., McIntryre, J.A., and Harlow, S.D. (2004) 'Transactional Sex among Women in Soweto, South Africa: Prevalence, Risk Factors and Association with HIV Infection', *Social Science & Medicine*, 59: 1,581–92.

Ellsberg, M., Jansen, H.A., Heise, L., Watts, C.H., Garcia-Moreno, C., and WHO Multi-country Study on Women's Health and Domestic Violence against Women Study Team (2008) 'Intimate Partner Violence and Women's Physical and Mental Health in the WHO Multi-country Study on Women's Health and Domestic Violence: An Observational Study', *The Lancet*, 371(9,619): 1,165–72.

Erwin, P.E. (2006) 'Compelled to Safety: Victims of Domestic Violence at the Intersection of Criminal and Civil Courtroom Processes', *Dissertation Abstracts International, The Humanities and Social Sciences*, 67(4): 1,505.

Glass, N., Rollins, C., and Bloom, T. (2008) 'Expanding our Vision: Using the Human Rights Framework to Strengthen our Service Response to Female Victims of Male Intimate Partner Violence', in D. Whitaker and J.R. Lutzker (eds) *Preventing Intimate Partner Violence*, Washington, DC: American Psychological Association: 193–218.

Gómez, A.M., Spiezer, I.S., and Beauvais, H. (2009) 'Sexual Violence and Reproductive Health among Youth in Port-au-Prince, Haiti', *Journal of Adolescent Health*, 44(5): 508–10.

Greig, A., Peacock, D., Jewkes, R., and Msimang, S. (2008) 'Gender and AIDS: Time to Act', *AIDS*, 22 (Supplement 2): S35–S43.

Hallman, K. (2007) 'Sexuality, Reproductive Health and HIV/AIDS: Non-consensual Sex, School Enrolment and Educational Outcomes in South Africa', *Africa Insight*, 37(3): 454–72.

Heise, L.L. and Elias, C. (1995) 'Transforming AIDS Prevention to Meet Women's Needs: A Focus on Developing Countries', *Social Science & Medicine*, 40(7): 931–43.

Human Rights Watch (2001) *Scared at School: Sexual Violence in South African Schools*, New York: Human Rights Watch.

Human Rights Watch/Africa (1996) *Shattered Lives: Sexual Violence during the Rwandan Genocide and Its Aftermath*, Washington, DC: Human Rights Watch.

International Council on Human Rights Policy (2005) *Local Government and Human Rights: Doing Good Service*, Versoix: Switzerland.

Kalichman, S.C. and Simbayi, L. (2004) 'Sexual Assault History and Risks for Sexually Transmitted Infections among Women in an African Township in Cape Town, South Africa', *AIDS Care*, 16(6): 681–9.

Karamagi, C., Tumwine, J.K., Tylleskar, T., and Heggenhougen, K. (2006) 'Intimate Partner Violence against Women in Eastern Uganda: Implications for HIV Prevention', *BioMed Central Public Health*, 6: 284, available at http://biomedcentral.com/1471-2458-6-284 (accessed 20 January 2010).

Kim, A.A., Malele, F., Kaiser, R., Mama, N., Kinkela, T., Mantshumba, J.C., Hynes, M., De Jesus, S., Musema, G., Kayembe, P.K., Hawkins Reed, K., and Diaz, T. (2009) 'HIV Infection among Internally Displaced Women and Women Residing in River Populations along the Congo River, Democratic Republic of Congo', *AIDS Behaviour*, 13(5): 914–20.

Lary, H., Maman, S., Katebalila, M., McCauley, A., and Mbwambo, J. (2004) 'Exploring the Association between HIV and Violence: Young People's Experiences with Infidelity, Violence and Forced Sex in Dar es Salaam, Tanzania', *International Family Planning Perspectives*, 30: 200–206.

Letourneau, E.J., Holmes, M., and Chasendunn-Roarck, J. (1999) 'Gynecological Health Consequences to Victims of Interpersonal Violence', *Women's Health Issues*, 9: 115–20.

Odek, W.O., Busza, J., Morris, C.N., Cleland, J., Ngugi, E.N., and Ferguson, A.G. (2009) 'Effects of Micro-Enterprise Services on HIV Risk Behaviour among Female Sex Workers in Kenya's Urban Slums', *AIDS Behaviour*, 13: 449–61.

Pronyk, P.M., Hargreaves, J.R., Kim, J.C., Morison, L.A., Phetla, G., Watts, C., Busza, J., and Porter, J.D. (2006) 'Effect of a Structural Intervention for the Prevention of Intimate-partner Violence and HIV in Rural South Africa: A Cluster Randomised Trial', *The Lancet*, 368: 1,973–83.

Riger, S., Raja, S., and Camacho, J. (2002) 'The Radiating Impact of Intimate Partner Violence', *Journal of Interpersonal Violence*, 17(2): 184–205.

Sareen, J., Pagura, J., and Grant, B. (2009) 'Is Intimate Partner Violence Associated with HIV Infection among Women in the United States?' *General Hospital Psychiatry*, 31: 274–8.

Tjaden, P. and Thoennes, N. (2000) 'Prevalence and Consequences of Male-to-Female and Female-to-Male Intimate Partner Violence as Measured by the National Violence against Women Survey', *Violence Against Women*, 6(2): 142–61.

UN (United Nations) (1948) *Universal Declaration of Human Rights*, available at http://www.un.org/en/documents/udhr/ (accessed 20 January 2010).

UN (United Nations) (1979) *Convention on the Elimination of All Forms of Discrimination against Women* (CEDAW), available at http://www.un.org/womenwatch/daw/cedaw/text/econvention.htm (accessed 20 January 2010).

UN (United Nations) (1993) *Declaration on the Elimination of Violence against Women* (DEVAW), available at http://www.un.org/documents/ga/res/48/a48r104.htm (accessed 20 January 2010).

UN (United Nations) (1993) 'Vienna Declaration and Programme of Action', adopted by the World Conference on Human Rights, Vienna, 14–25 June.

UN (United Nations) (1995) *Fourth World Conference on Women*, available at http://www.un.org/womenwatch/daw/beijing/fwcwn.html (accessed 20 January 2010).

WHO (World Health Organization) (2005) *Multi-Country Study on Women's Health and Domestic Violence against Women: Summary Report of Initial Results on Prevalence, Health Outcomes and Women's Responses*, Geneva: WHO.

Young, S.L. and Maguire, K.C. (2003) 'Talking about Sexual Violence', *Women and Language*, 26(2): 40–52.

24

Protection of Children in Disaster and War

Neil Boothby and Alastair Ager

Introduction

In the field of global health, there is acute awareness of how context critically shapes what is feasible for practitioners to propose and communities to implement. This sensitivity to context has prompted some valuable learning across settings. Notably, the constraints created by a crisis, whether due to a natural disaster or a prolonged complex emergency, have inspired international actors who work on child protection to re-think the interventions that are used in stable, developed nations. These actors have identified the need for mechanisms that monitor and address threats to children in emergencies, as well as stage the construction of integrated systems of protection within the acute phase of the crisis. Recent work shows that it is possible to begin to build child protection systems that can withstand the pressures of conflict and displacement even during the initial phases of an emergency.

The 'Protective Environment Framework' was developed by the United Nations Children's Fund (UNICEF) as a basis to identify the key areas where actions can be taken to increase the protection available to children (Langren 2005).[1,2] The framework is broad enough to consider many potential influences on children's well-being, but has sufficient focus to frame clear actions that will promote protection in developing countries. The Protective Environment Framework, however, has seen limited application in situations of armed conflict, refugee migrations, and natural disasters. The lack of a systemic child protection framework has hampered efforts to plan and implement comprehensive protection responses for children in emergencies. It has resulted in ad hoc and (sometimes) anecdotal assessments that cannot be compared across communities, regions, or countries.

The Protective Environment Framework is presented here as a platform capable of bringing greater coherence to activities that strengthen child protection in wars, natural disasters, and refugee movements. Areas of the framework that need to be adapted – or, at least, flexibly applied – to systemically address child protection concerns in different types of emergencies are discussed. Key areas of focus for each of the eight framework elements are identified and key areas to be considered in emergency assessment and planning efforts are highlighted.

The protective environment and emergencies

The Protective Environment Framework specifies a range of factors that serve to protect children from risks and vulnerabilities in any given environment. These risks range from various types of exploitation to violence to family separation. It acknowledges the importance of actions that directly minimise these risks, such as peace dialogues aimed at ending conflict. However, while diplomacy and new policies are pursued, humanitarian agencies must seek to directly protect children in crisis settings through actions that 'shield' children from ongoing risks. Accordingly, it is on such actions that the framework focuses. Although the framework emphasises localised intervention, there is clearly a place for systemic change that in the long term fosters a protective culture. There are eight key elements identified in the framework of the 'protective environment for children' (UNICEF 2006):

Elements of the Protective Environment for Children

Monitoring and reporting

Governmental commitment to fulfilling protection rights

Protective legislation and enforcement

Attitudes, traditions, customs, behaviour, and practices

Open discussion and engagement with child protection issues

Children's life skills, knowledge, and participation

The capacity to protect among those around children

Services for recovery and reintegration

Application of the 'protective environment' elements in settings of humanitarian response will require generic adaptations. First, humanitarian actors must overcome the tendency to limit their assessment of the impact of a given crisis on children to their immediate environment, rather than looking at the whole scope of potential vulnerabilities and community dynamics. Assessment should always take into account wider concerns that interact with crisis-related risks. Primary among these are social and economic conditions that:

- Risk the commoditisation of children as economic units at a young age
- Lead to extreme gender division and inequity
- Shape childhood and adolescence in other harsh and exploitative ways.

Second, a humanitarian crisis may provide unique opportunities to introduce significant positive change within one or more of the framework's components. Recent examples of how crises created an occasion to improve protective environments include the Asian tsunami and end of political conflict in Aceh (reflecting action particularly around 'Governmental commitment to fulfilling protection rights' and 'The capacity to protect among those around children'), as well as 'Form 8' reform on rape and gender-based violence in Darfur (reflecting changes in 'Protective legislation and enforcement'). These examples demonstrate how a crisis can allow communities and governments to prioritise protection, given what has happened.

Third, the *intent* of the government and other parties in responding to a conflict will be a key consideration in developing protection responses for refugee and internally displaced populations (Inter-agency Standing Committee 2002; Slim and Eguren 2004). If authorities are committed to protecting the rights of refugees or displaced persons (including children), collaboration and capacity-building to create protective mechanisms in a society are realistic options, even if official systems are weak and technical competence low. In contrast, if one or both parties are resistant, abusive, or directly involved in human rights violations, coercive denunciation of behaviour that harms children may serve as a core advocacy strategy, and substitution of assistance and services will be required.

Fourth, it is important to consider personal and political intent at multiple levels: community, district, provincial, and national. Even in Darfur – where the national government promotes widescale violence and human rights abuses – opportunities to promote a protective environment for children were identified at the state level (Bremen *et al.* 2007).

And fifth, it is important to focus on how a range of groups may be benefiting from a conflict. These may include:

- Governments
- Militia fighters
- Economic elites
- Members of the diaspora outside conflict zones.

Attention to hard-to-reach – and sometimes forgotten groups – may be a key to securing protective responses for children, as it forces consideration of structural and other factors at the root of all major protection risks.

Areas of emergency focus

This section outlines key considerations and areas of focus for each of the framework's eight elements. It also highlights some key planning concerns for implementing the framework in conflict settings.

Monitoring and reporting

Monitoring and reporting are key to the development of critical areas of humanitarian action, including effective targeting of humanitarian resources, keeping abreast of child rights' trends, promoting informed advocacy regarding key risks and vulnerabilities, and establishing evidence regarding successful interventions. Minimally, governments, United Nations (UN) bodies, or participating non-governmental organisations (NGOs) should establish a child protection monitoring and reporting system capable of capturing short-term changes and long-term trends. Assessment and programme planning need to address key operational challenges to developing such a system, which may include:

- How to capture the breadth of information required
- How to ensure proper trend analyses
- How to feed back effectively the information that has been captured to policymakers and those who implement programmes
- How to ensure coverage within and beyond established displaced persons camps

- How to appropriately train personnel for data collection and collation, deploy them, and cope with security issues
- How to address problems of retribution to reporting agencies
- How to ensure confidentiality and cope with possible risks to victims
- How to define the role of government or other duty barriers in data collection.

There is a current 'divide' between protection and human rights information collection in UN field operations that reflects the global debate regarding the definition of these two interconnected fields as separate entities. This divide appears to have brought few benefits to the reporting and monitoring of child protection issues which so clearly straddle the two (OIOS 2006). The former, protection, focuses on the documentation of individual cases for legal follow-up and redress, and requires a monitoring and reporting system based on narrative reporting of individual incidents. It is staff- and time-intensive – and not designed to achieve comprehensive coverage or to yield aggregate data on child rights violations. The latter, human rights, seeks information for strategic planning, protection programming, and political advocacy; these needs are better met through surveys designed to establish incidence (number of child rights violations taking place at a given time) or prevalence (percentage of child population whose rights are violated) rates. To date, child protection surveys of these kinds are not standard practice.

Commitment of authorities to fulfilling protection rights

Government commitment to respecting, protecting, and fulfilling child protection is an essential element of a protective environment. In emergency situations, efforts to obtain commitments from authorities to fulfil child protection rights must often be extended to the government and other duty barriers. In situations of armed conflict, these will include other parties to the conflict and armed groups that influence or control populations in remote areas of the country or in internally displaced persons (IDP)/refugee camps. Even if acknowledgment of and negotiations with other political–military actors is difficult or forbidden, obtaining the commitment of all 'duty barriers' to adhering to child rights standards is an important objective.

Mandated and non-mandated international agencies often assume roles in emergencies that place them in positions of serving as 'de facto' or 'on-the-ground' authorities. This takes place, for example, when peacekeeping missions are undertaken, and when the UN or NGOs assume lead management roles or engage in direct service delivery in refugee or displaced persons camps. Their commitment and capacity to child protection must be assessed and developed as well.

There are enormous protection challenges when government authorities or another party to a conflict is wilfully instigating or refusing to prevent human rights violations. Intentional human rights abuse requires protective activities that are aimed at authorities and/or other duty barriers. Key modes of protection action may include denunciation (pressing authorities through public discourse into meeting their obligations) to accomplish policy change objectives, for example, and substitution (directly providing services to victims of violations) to accomplish assistance and support needs. In contrast, if authorities are not directly engaged in rights violations, protection actions may include persuasion (convincing authorities through private dialogue) or mobilisation (engaging leaders, political bodies, or states that have the capacity to influence authorities to satisfy their obligations), and empowering national/local structures to carry out their functions to protect and assist affected populations (Slim and Eguren 2004).

Harsh economic conditions and longstanding social and cultural factors play significant roles in promoting – or undermining – protective environments for children. The commitment of governments and other duty barriers to actively address the economic and social dimensions of a crisis is essential. Within governments, ministries of labour and social (and cultural) welfare may be well positioned to address social and economic phenomena and practices related to child protection, including street children, abandoned babies, female circumcision, domestic violence, and sexual exploitation, among other issues. Often these ministries will be among the most marginalised within a government, and will lack financing, infrastructure, and training. They often are not operational, and their presence will be limited to national and state capitals. If the goal is development of institutions to establish mechanisms for the long term, clearly these and other key ministries will need to play significant roles.

Protective legislation and enforcement

An adequate legislative framework designed to protect children from abuse, and its implementation and enforcement, are essential elements of a protective environment. The absence of these safeguards in emergencies may be symptomatic of a general lack of procedural protections, absence of multisectoral support services, and laws that already negatively impact women and vulnerable children. They may be highlighted even more during an emergency, along with other protection concerns, such as a lack of redress for human rights crimes.

Many countries and communities around the globe have formal and informal systems of justice, and the adequacy of protective legislation and enforcement needs to be examined across these interrelated systems. Traditional justice systems, for example, may operate at the community level, and deal with civil disputes and personal affairs, including domestic violence. Judgments are often decided by a council of elders or other local leaders, and cases are sometimes brought to them without contact with the police or any formal justice structures. Many crimes committed by children or against them may be handled by such a system. Community courts often focus on restorative justice, compensation to victims, and community service, rather than imprisonment or other formal punishments. Conflict and forced migration may disrupt these informal justice systems; however, the individuals that served on them remain important potential resources for protection within IDP and refugee camps.

Other types of informal courts include those sanctioned by government authorities. They, too, may operate at town, district, or regional levels, and deal directly with minor criminal, civil, and personal cases through the application of both customary law and general principles of formal justice. Sanctioned informal courts are used to ease the caseload of the formal justice system, and are thus often the first step in judicial action. Many offenses involving children will fall under the jurisdiction of these types of informal courts. It is important to assess whether or not such courts are readily trusted by the community. In politically or ethnically divided settings, they may be perceived to be highly biased because individuals serving on them are often appointed by or affiliated with government or enemy authorities.

Attitudes, traditions, customs, behaviour, and practices

Family, kinship, tribal, and, at times, feudal relationships are part of complex socio-economic systems that maintain order and assign roles and responsibilities to all members of society. Of particular interest to a protective environment perspective are the expectations made of children, and the features of community life that may be considered protective (or harmful) to them.

A strong commitment to family is an important feature of potential security and stability for children, for instance. The widespread practice of informal 'adoption' of orphaned or separated children is usually a key indication of the strength of kinship obligation to protect and care for children, and should be part of an early situational assessment. Family stability is also linked with a strong sense of the need for moral education, and a clear concern for children to be provided with clear moral precepts and example. There is also a range of social and religious customs – from alms giving, to youth groups, to traditional conflict resolution procedures – that are potentially protective, as well. Expectations and obligations of protecting one's kin – widely cited as a frequent occurrence in the context of emergencies – also point to social bonds that serve protective functions.

Protection assessments need to ascertain the extent to which a given emergency has disrupted the capacity of communities to fully utilise a wide range of intricate social mechanisms that have previously been used to maintain social cohesion within and between villages. Accordingly, it usually makes sense to consider means of supporting or, where they have completely failed, re-establishing traditional mechanisms that have a protective value.

There are likely to be other features of community life which – shaped by harsh physical and economic conditions and deeply engrained cultural attitudes and practices – appear profoundly hostile to the welfare of children. Two major concerns that require careful assessment and response in emergencies are the commoditisation of children as a source of labour, and the control of girls (and their sexuality) through marked gender disparity.

The commoditisation of children as economic units may be exacerbated by war, famine, and confinement in displaced and refugee camps. Children – especially girls – may be required to remain home for longer periods of time to care for younger siblings. Females may also be expected to assume dangerous roles, such as firewood collection in hostile environments outside of subsidised camps, because such duties would be even more threatening to males. Although emergencies may severely challenge household livelihoods, longstanding cultural norms and values regarding childhood – and especially children's roles in the household economy and gender expectations – will need to be strategically addressed in emergency settings.

A similar analysis is required on gender disparity and the subjugation of women. The role of girls in the household economy is a special concern, as is their engagement in the broader labour market. Access to education, informal education opportunities, and other potentially protective activities should be routinely assessed. Female circumcision, early marriage, toleration of domestic abuse, and marginalisation of women from decision-making all point to the engrained nature of attitudes maintaining the vulnerability of women and girls. When these and other harmful practices are widespread, strategies more sophisticated than 'awareness raising' are necessary to address such longstanding, socially sanctioned patterns.

Open discussion and engagement with protection issues

Community dialogue is an essential component of humanitarian response assessments, and is especially important in situations of armed conflict when responding to the needs of children. There are many aspects of a crisis that members of the affected population are likely to know more about than outside agencies, including, for instance:

- Nature and timing of the threats they confront
- Mindset and habits of those who threaten them
- Resources within the community
- History of previous threats and coping mechanisms
- Practical possibilities for resisting threats
- Optimal linkage between the community and agency responses.

Assessments need to take into account that some protection issues will be more openly discussed by community members than others, and not assume the problem does not exist because people say it does not. Communities may show a willingness to discuss conflict-related rape or child soldiers, for instance, while domestic violence and child labour remain taboo. At the same time, a natural disaster or armed conflict often prompts people to look critically at their previous attitudes and practices. In Pakistan, for example, open dialogue with traditional Afghan leaders about their desire to continue to have women and girls treated by female doctors led to the establishment of home-based schools for refugee girls – institutions which were subsequently evaluated to be superior learning environments compared to 'formal' schools established in camps (Rugh 2000). Participatory assessment methods in northern Uganda enabled displaced women to discuss domestic violence and rape in a manner that resulted in the establishment of prevalence rates and women's ranking of these concerns as their top protection–assistance priorities (Boothby *et al.* 2007B). Good practice is also emerging on how to engage children in analyses of their own protection and well-being concerns (Boothby *et al.* 2007a).

Authorities' willingness to engage in earnest dialogue on key child protection should be taken into account when determining what routes will be pursued to secure commitments to child protection. Some milestones to consider include:

- Have authorities begun to discuss and analyse social phenomenon, such as street children, from a protection perspective? Or do they limit discussion to economics and security?
- Are they open to the issue of rape and children associated with fighting groups? Or are they silent because of the implications of acknowledging such concerns?
- Have authorities signalled a willingness to hold their own police or soldiers accountable for child rights violations? Or do they deny their involvement in such incidents?

Children's life skills, knowledge and participation

Children are less vulnerable to abuse when they are aware of their right not to be exploited, or of services available to protect them. With the right information, children can draw upon their knowledge, skills, and resilience to reduce their risk of exploitation.

Access to education provides protection. Or does it? This advocacy refrain is only true when schools are physically safe and emotionally healing environments. During emergencies, adverse teacher–student ratios often soar to even higher levels, already harsh disciplinary practices deteriorate into public humiliation and corporal punishment, peer teasing may worsen into overt bullying, and boys and girls may be at greater risk for sexual exploitation than ever before. How to ensure these core protective ingredients are in place is a key assessment concern.

Core protective factors in schools include:

- Adequate teacher–student ratios
- Elimination of humiliation, bullying, and corporal punishment
- Safeguards against sexual abuse and exploitation.

A review of education in emergencies suggests that school enrolment rates do not always drop in an emergency; sometimes they actually increase (Bremer *et al.* 2007; IRC 2006). Key factors influencing enrolment include:

- History of enrolment previous to emergency
- Short-term economic survival needs
- Safety and distance to schools
- Presence or absence of funding for emergency education
- Fees levied by teachers and/or school committees.

Finally, youth often actively engage in the political discourse regarding the current crisis, and have strong feelings about what has happened to their communities and what lies ahead. While such participation may be valuable and broadly welcomed, particular attention during an emergency needs to be paid to the political manipulation of children in schools, religious institutions, youth groups, and other social networks.

The capacity to protect among those around children

Parental capacity to protect their children may be seriously compromised by conflicts, famines, and natural disasters. Crisis-affected families are often in a weaker position to provide material support for their children, and may be too overburdened with survival concerns to provide adequate emotional support as well. Forced migration and economic pressures often require women to assume work roles that involve longer separations from their children than is normal. The stress on families is exacerbated by the disruption or collapse of traditional livelihood strategies, which can include food collection, seasonal migration, and raising livestock. The protective capacities of other important people within the community are also likely to have been undermined by shifts in power and fragmentation of structures. Traditional leaders may no longer be able or willing to negotiate cessations of military action; religious leaders may encourage violence rather than tolerance; health care facilities may not consistently represent a protective space for children; and schools may become indoctrination vehicles for political factions, or even recruitment grounds.

An assessment of the protective capacities within a given community needs to focus on how the emergency has affected:

- Family livelihoods
- Gender, labour, and child care roles
- Teachers' roles, corporal punishment, indoctrination, and recruitment in schools
- Roles of traditional and religious leaders and their commitments to child protection.

Services for recovery and reintegration

The eighth – and final – element of the 'protective environment' involves direct services for children who have experienced protection violations. While other elements of the protective environment are focused on prevention, this element considers what resources are available to support children when prevention activities have failed. Government services are key in this area; however, the often limited capacity and reach of governments – coupled with the comparatively ample financial resources afforded to international actors – usually results in NGO delivery of the majority of recovery and reintegration services.

While there are occasions when the development of recovery and reintegration services without government involvement is warranted, support to authorities who are willing to fulfil child protection commitments, but lack the capacity to do so, is essential. Some NGOs view humanitarian assistance as non-political and refrain from supporting duty barriers. Yet research in emergency settings has consistently found that services and projects that never link to broader government systems (when such systems exist) have little to no impact on long-term protective environments (Chae *et al.* 2007; Paul 1999; UNICEF/ADAP 2006).

Resolving the good practice paradox

There is an old Scottish farmers' adage: if you try to catch two rabbits at the same time you are likely to lose both. Applied to an emergency response scenario – if one agency tries to provide urgent services to vulnerable groups, and at the same time tries to promote systemic solutions to child protection needs, the agency is likely to fail at both, and children are likely to suffer as a result.

A better way to resolve the good practice paradox is to promote a protection strategy that supports multiple actors' engagement in different and complementary actions within the eight elements of the protective environment framework. Simply put, the good practice paradox may be resolved through:

- Understanding the mandates, programming capacities, priorities, and expertise of the agencies and organisations on the ground
- Determining how agencies can best combine actions to meet critical needs rapidly and promote long-term solutions
- Actively coordinating these varied and complementary actions.

Mandated organisations, such as UNICEF and UNHCR, will most likely be required to both play leadership roles in planning and promoting systemic responses to child protection concerns, and also take on supportive roles for NGO engagement in recovery and reintegration services. Taking the lead strategic role will require UN emergency protection staff capable of undertaking situational analyses, making links with authorities, ensuring monitoring and reporting systems evolve, and using child protection data to influence policies and programmes. Expertise on vulnerable groups of children will be required, as well; however, this technical expertise should be used to inform (and coordinate) NGO actions, rather than to engage in direct service delivery.

Notes

1 Here we will use the UNICEF definition of children as anyone 18 years or younger.
2 For the purpose of this chapter, we examine child protection from an abuse, exploitation, and exposure to violence perspective, but do not include important work done in the areas of child health and nutrition. Our examination also looks at measures that promote children's physical and emotional well-being, provide them with equal access to basic services and safeguard their legal and human rights.

References

Boothby, N., Ager, A., and Ager, W. (2007) *A Guide to the Evaluation of Psychosocial Programming in Emergencies*, New York: UNICEF.
Boothby, N., Ager, A., Wessells, M., and Stark, L. (2007) 'How Do We Know What Works in Protection? Building the Evidence Base', presentation to the Washington Network on Children and Armed Conflict, Washington, DC, 1 May.
Bremer, M., Ager, A. and Boothby, N. (2006) *Situation Analysis of Child Protection in Darfur, Report Submitted to UNICEF*, New York: UNICEF.

Chae, S., Taylor, R. and Douglas, A. (2007) 'Youth Engaged in Service: A Visionary Strategy for Post-Conflict Recovery', working draft, *Innovations in Civic Partnership*.

Inter-Agency Standing Committee (IASC) (2002) *Growing the Sheltering Tree: Protecting Rights Through Humanitarian Action, Programmes and Practices Gathered From the Field*, Geneva: Inter-Agency Standing Committee.

Landgren, K. (2005) 'The Protective Environment: Development Support for Child Protection', *Human Rights Quarterly*, 27: 214–48.

Office of Internal Oversight Services (OIOS) (2006) *Independent Review of Monitoring and Reporting (MRM) for Children and Armed Conflict (CAAC): Executive Summary*, New York: United Nations.

Rugh, A. (2000) *Home-Based Girls' Schools in Balochistan Refugee Villages: A Strategy Study*, Islamabad: Save the Children.

Slim, H. and Eguren, L.E. (2004) *Humanitarian Protection: A Guidance Booklet*' (pilot version), London: Active Learning Network for Accountability and Performance in Humanitarian Action (ALNAP).

UNICEF (United Nations Children's Fund) (2007) *Children in Conflict and Emergencies*, available at http://www.unicef.org/protection/index_armedconflict.html (accessed 23 September 2007).

UNICEF and ADAP (United Nations Children's Fund and Adolescent Development and Participation Programme) (2005) 'Global Strategic Planning Consultation on Adolescent Programming in Emergency and Transition', report on meeting in Geneva, Switzerland, 28–30 November.

25

Nutrition in Emergencies

Indicators and Reference Levels

Helen Young

Introduction

> There is no best indicator, best measure of an indicator, or best analysis of an indicator in a generic sense. The definition of 'best' depends ultimately on what is most appropriate for the decision that must be made.
>
> (Habicht and Pelletier, 1990: 1519)

There is a long history of using nutritional or anthropometric indicators to gauge the severity of food insecurity, famine, and nutritional emergencies dating back to the 1960s in Biafra and India. A decade later, in the 1970s, nutrition surveys in emergencies had become increasingly common and guidelines on nutritional surveys and nutrition programmes in emergencies were subsequently published (de Ville de Goyet *et al.* 1978; Peel, 1977). In acute emergency contexts, high prevalences of acute malnutrition have been and continue to be associated with high death rates, and are understood to reflect the severity of the crises. However, in the past decade it appears that prevalence levels of acute malnutrition in emergencies have fallen compared to earlier decades. For example, a review of 298 surveys submitted to the Refugee Network Information System (RNIS) between 1992 and 1994 found that prevalence levels of acute malnutrition ranging from 20 per cent up to 50 per cent were common in emergencies in Angola, Liberia, Rwanda/Burundi, and Somalia, with the number of reports of acute malnutrition even higher in southern Sudan (up to 80 per cent) (Borrel and Salama 1999).

In contrast, in more recent crises it has been unusual for prevalence rates to exceed 30 per cent, and in many regions including southern Africa, Asia and Latin America it is rare for the prevalence of acute malnutrition to exceed even 10 per cent. The highest prevalence rates tend to be found in East Africa, particularly among pastoralist populations living in the more remote arid lands of northern Uganda, Kenya, Somalia, and Ethiopia, who also tend to suffer higher mortality rates.[1]

To determine the severity of malnutrition in a community, the prevalence of low weight-for-height or anthropometric wasting may be compared with predefined reference levels (prevalence ranges). For example, Table 25.1 shows the classification system published in the World Health Organization (WHO) guidelines. This shows that a prevalence of between 10 per cent and 15

Table 25.1 Nutritional indicators

Indicators	Abbreviation	Definition
Prevalence of wasting	Low WH	Per cent below minus 2 Z score weight-for-height (% < −2 WHZ)
	Low MUAC[1]	Per cent below MUAC cut-offs
Global Acute Malnutrition	GAM	Per cent below minus 2 Z score weight-for-height *AND* oedema (% < −2 WHZ)
Severe Acute Malnutrition	SAM	Per cent below minus 3 Z score weight-for-height *AND* oedema (% < −3 WHZ)
Prevalence of stunting	Low HA	Per cent below minus 2 Z score height-for-age (% < −2 HAZ)
Prevalence of underweight	Low WA	Per cent below minus 2 Z score weight-for-age (% < −2 WAZ)
Prevalence of chronic undernutrition in non-pregnant and non-lactating women of reproductive age (15–49 years)	Low BMI	Per cent below cut-offs for Body Mass Index (weight/height^2).

1 The unadjusted measurement of mid-upper arm circumference (MUAC) is an indicator of lean body mass and wasting.
Source: Young, H. and S. Jaspars 2009.

per cent acute malnutrition is classified as a serious situation, and above 15 per cent is considered critical (WHO 2000). Anthropometric reference levels provide a basis for establishing goals for management and policymaking, for example, as a guide to interpret prevalence of malnutrition. The levels also help to inform and improve accountability in decision-making, particularly in emergency or famine situations, and increasingly are being used in more developmental contexts. Reference levels are also known as thresholds, trigger thresholds, benchmarks, or norms, and all refer to a comparison against which an indicator can be examined or gauged (Mathys 2007; Van der Heide *et al.* 2007).

The aim of this chapter is to review the use of anthropometric indicators, their cut-off points, and the reference levels used in emergencies. It is largely based on a more in-depth review by Young and Jaspars (2009). The next section broadly considers the use of anthropometry and anthropometric indicators, differentiating between the use of anthropometry as applied to individuals, or to communities. The chapter then reviews the main anthropometric indicators, their reference levels, and their application in emergency assessments and programme management, including their strengths and limitations.

Use of anthropometry

The use of anthropometry varies depending on whether it applies to individuals (e.g. for identifying malnourished children), or whether it applies to communities and wider populations (as an indicator to gauge the severity of a nutritional emergency).

The type and severity of anthropometric deficit in an individual is classified using nutritional indices and their cut-off points (Table 25.1). Indices are constructs from measurements which relate an observed measurement to its counterpart in a reference population. For example, an individual child's weight is compared with the median weight of healthy children of the same height, known as the reference population.

Among children, the three most commonly used anthropometric indices relating to body size and composition are Weight-for Height (WH), Height-for-Age (HA), and Weight-for-Age (WA).

Box 25.1 Aetiology of wasting and stunting

Wasting occurs as a result of recent rapid weight loss, or a failure to gain weight within a relatively short period of time. In addition, disease (especially diarrhoea and measles) also leads to weight loss and wasting. Wasting is more common in infants and younger children, often during the stage when complementary foods are being introduced and children are more susceptible to infectious diseases. Wasting is reversible in the short term as children may gain weight, and often occurs on a seasonal basis as a result of a seasonal hunger gap or higher disease incidence.

Stunting, indicating short stature or failure to achieve full growth potential, implies long-term and cumulative influences of inadequate nutrition and/or repeated infections such as diarrhoea. Deficiencies of micronutrients (particularly vitamin A, iron, and zinc), as well as macronutrients, play a significant role in stunting.

Stunting prevalence increases progressively from immediately after birth until reaching a plateau at around 24 months, a result of which is that stunting prevalence is lower among younger children as compared with older children. A high prevalence of stunting among older children is reflective of their past nutrition, but may also indicate conditions currently experienced by younger children in that same community. Similar stunting prevalence can have a several-fold difference in the prevalence of severe wasting (Black *et al.* 2008).

An index has biological meaning; an indicator represents the application or use of an index, usually in conjunction with a cut-off point, for making an assessment (in this case, of malnutrition). Indicator cut-off points focus on the lower end of the frequency distribution, and at the extremes, which in turn provide case-definitions for the nutritional deficits such as wasting (low WH) and stunting (low HA) (see Box 25.1). For example, WH Z scores below −2 distinguish children who are anthropometrically wasted. WH is the nutritional index, and −2 Z scores is the cut-off point. Nutritional indices are used to construct nutritional indicators: the per cent of individuals in the population below the cut-off point.

Technically, cut-off points can be defined on the basis of either statistical criteria, risk of physiological dysfunction, and/or prescriptive criteria (Pelletier 2006). For example, the new WHO Multi-Reference Growth Standards (MRGS) are based on prescriptive criteria, which seek to define how children should grow rather than simply describe how they do grow (UN IASC and SCN 2009). The use of a growth standard (in contrast to simply reference data or a reference population) involves value or normative judgments. Although the MRGS are prescriptive, the cut-off of < −2 SD is based on statistical probability, for instance, 2.5 per cent of children in the reference population fall below this cut-off.

Selecting the appropriate anthropometric indicator

The choice of a particular nutritional indicator depends on what type of decision-making is being informed through its analysis. This means that the selection of a particular indicator – the nutritional index and cut-off point – should reflect the objectives of their use in a particular situation and context, such as:

- Identifying past and current risk, and/or predicting future risk (an increase in wasting in a population may identify present and future risk, whereas an increase in stunting in the population identifies past risk). The use of prevalence of wasting as an indicator of mortality risk has been recommended for emergency-affected populations where it is not practical to estimate mortality rates directly (Mason 2002; Nieburg *et al.* 1992).

- Targeting – selecting individuals or populations for nutritional intervention, including both curative (treatment of malnutrition) and preventative interventions (delivery of food assistance).
- Response decisions – predicting benefit from an intervention, or measuring impact.

The decisions to be made in emergency contexts are likely to be very different from the decisions to be made in non-emergency and more developmental contexts. National emergencies are usually declared by sovereign states, who request help from the international community. The causes vary from natural disasters including earthquakes (Haiti and Chile, 2010), floods and tsunamis, to complex emergencies involving civil conflict, famine, drought, and food insecurity (which are often linked with governance failures and may be protracted in nature). In the non-emergency contexts, issues of chronic malnutrition and underlying causes will feature more prominently, whereas in the emergency phases the emphasis from public health and food security responders will be on determining the severity of acute food insecurity. The technically best indicators are likely to vary markedly according to these different uses.

Nutritional indicators and their reference levels

Nutritional indices measure different things and they produce different and conflicting proportions of the population categorised as underweight, stunted, or wasted. Table 25.1 shows examples of the nutritional indices and nutritional indicators reviewed in this chapter.

Weight-for-height

WH reflects body weight in relation to height. Acute malnutrition includes both wasting, or low WH, and nutritional oedema.[2] Any child with bilateral oedema has severe acute malnutrition (SAM), even if the WH is above −2 SD. If they are less than <−2 SD WH, they have moderate acute wasting or moderate acute malnutrition (MAM). The term Global Acute Malnutrition (GAM) includes all children with moderate wasting, severe wasting, or oedema, or any combination of these conditions.

WH is the preferred nutritional indicator for emergencies because it is indicative of severe recent or current events; for example, acute food insecurity or famine, and outbreaks of disease, such as diarrhoea or measles. WH, as well as Mid-Upper Arm Circumference (MUAC) and weight change, are good indicators for reflecting seasonal, for example, short-term changes, in food intake and disease.

For these reasons, WH is the index of choice for all situations which involve short-term nutritional-response actions, such as screening for emergency interventions, while also being important as a warning of impending food insecurity. An additional reason why WH is the preferred index in emergencies is because it does not need an estimation of the child's age, which may be difficult to verify in emergency settings where mothers or other carers may not know precisely or have a record of their child's date of birth on a health card, birth certificate, or similar document.

In more stable (non-emergency or post-emergency) settings, wasting prevalence is often higher for young children (< 24 months) as compared with older children because it is this younger age group who tend to be affected by the natural cessation of breastfeeding and introduction of complementary foods, the latter of which may increase risk of disease through increased exposure to pathogens and loss of immunity previously imparted by breast-milk.

If the prevalence of low WH increases in a given population, and there is a greater relative increase in wasting among older children than younger children, this may suggest a different causality. It is possible that the increasing prevalence among older children is a result of wider population food insecurity which would affect older as well as younger children. For this reason, it is crucially important that prevalence of WH is reported separately for older (85 cm and above) and younger (< 85 cm) children.

Body shape also influences prevalence estimates of low WH; children with long limbs (lower Sitting Height to Standing Height Ratio or SSR) tend to be taller and have a lower WH than children with higher SSR values. Studies in Somalia and Ethiopia found that older pastoralist children (85 to 110 cm) tended to have longer limbs (lower SSRs) as compared with agrarian children, which generated higher prevalence estimates of low WH among pastoralists as compared with agrarian children. These differences were less apparent among younger children (< 85 cm). Low WH and low MUAC produced similar estimates among agrarian groups but among pastoralists the WH estimate was significantly higher than the MUAC (Myatt *et al.* 2009). However, there have been no studies indicating the functional outcomes associated with low WH among older 'pastoralist children', such as risk of dying or disease, and therefore it would be wrong to conclude that they were less at risk simply as a result of their body shape.

Studies of the relationship between malnutrition and mortality found that WH is the least effective predictor of mortality (Pelletier 1991). This can be explained in part by the fact that most studies examining the relationship between malnutrition and mortality found a low prevalence of GAM, although they were not conducted in emergency contexts and, furthermore, only looked at long-term mortality risk (up to 24 month follow-up periods), while WH is likely to be a better predictor of short-term risk. In addition, several studies compared moderate GAM (< 80 per cent WH) with severe stunting (low WA < 60 per cent), which are different categories of malnutrition, and hence not always comparable.

There are three different accepted sources of WH reference levels. These include first, *selective feeding decision-making frameworks*; second, *classification of situations according to nutritional risk*; and third, *food security and famine classification systems*. The origins of these reference levels are a mix of recommendations from expert meetings and research-based papers focused on improving accountability in decision-making (Young and Jaspars 2009).

Selective feeding decision-making frameworks

The earliest classification systems were developed by Oxfam GB as a tool to determine the need for selective feeding programmes in emergency settings, and similar reference levels were later adopted by Médecins Sans Frontières (MSF), the office of the United Nations High Commissioner for Refugees (UNHCR), and the WHO (Lusty and Diskett 1984; MSF 1995; WHO 2000). These reference levels were based on the prevalence levels and other conditions found in refugee camps in Cambodia, Uganda, Sudan, Somalia, and Ethiopia from the 1970s onwards. They combined prevalence levels of acute malnutrition with the presence or absence of a number of 'aggravating factors' (including crude mortality above 1/10,000/day, an epidemic of measles and a high prevalence of respiratory or diarrhoeal disease, poor sanitation environment, unreliable food distribution system), so that the reference level for taking specific actions is adjusted for the presence of certain factors which can quickly make malnutrition worse.

Table 25.2 Reference levels for classification of severity of acute malnutrition in a community (< -2 Z scores, or oedema)

	Usual/Acceptable	Worrying/Poor	Serious	Critical
WHO 1992	<5%*	5–9%	10–14%	>15%
SCN/RNIS 2004		5–8%	>10%	

Source: WHO Report on the Consultation on Rapid Nutrition Assessment in Emergencies 1992 and WHO The Management of Nutrition in Major Emergencies 2000.

Classification of situations according to nutritional risk

The two main nutritional risk classification systems currently utilised are the Refugee and Nutrition Information System/Nutrition Information in Crisis Situations (RNIS/NICS) and the WHO classification (Table 25.2). The RNIS/NICS pioneered a system designed to report and track the nutritional situation of refugees and displaced populations around the world. Emergencies are classified into five categories of nutritional risk, reflecting a deteriorating nutritional situation based on GAM prevalence and an analysis of underlying causes (food, health, and care) and adequacy of response. The RNIS/NICS reference levels have been altered since they were first proposed, with a decline in the most severe nutritional risk category (from > 40 per cent to > 10 per cent).

The WHO classification system is currently the most widely accepted classification for determining whether a population is experiencing an 'emergency'.

Food security and famine classification systems

Several concurrent attempts to develop food security classification systems were developed to make decision-making more accountable, and to agree upon a definition of famine to cut short the continual politicised debates as to whether a famine was occurring, such as occurred in Sudan (1998), Malawi (2002), and Ethiopia (2000) (Darcy and Hoffman 2003; Howe and Devereux 2004). A declaration of famine is an acknowledgement of humanitarian crises which generally requires an international humanitarian response. Until such a crisis is declared, governments may be unwilling to seek or accept aid from donors and aid agencies, which can seriously impede and delay any response. These classification systems are therefore intended to improve the objectivity of the analysis, and timeliness of the response.

While there is broad consensus that WH is a good indicator of recent and current nutrition, the debate over the use of WH reference levels continues. The use of fixed reference levels was rejected by the Sphere Minimum Standards of Disaster Response (2003) guidelines in favour of a more contextual analysis of trends in nutritional status, underlying causes, and seasonal influences (The Sphere Project 2003). This is in part because the significance of a given level of wasting is a function of the prevalence of stunting, disease incidence, and background mortality rates.

There has also been considerable debate over whether to use fixed or relative reference levels in populations who regularly suffer 'emergency' levels of acute malnutrition, such as the pastoralist populations described earlier. However, these higher levels of acute malnutrition are also associated with higher mortality rates, and there is a danger of 'normalising' these higher rates just because they are seen more frequently.

Methodologically, there is also a problem in that there are no standard indicators or agreed-upon methods with which to measure or assess underlying causes of malnutrition, or the aggravating factors described above. There is, in addition, the challenge of taking account of seasonal trends in all three groups of underlying causes of malnutrition, which influence seasonal patterns of malnutrition, morbidity, and mortality. Unless these are recognised and understood it will be difficult to assess the impact of a given emergency.

Mid-upper arm circumference (MUAC)

MUAC is the preferred indicator for case definitions of wasting based on a cut-off of 115 mm (as recommended by WHO/UNICEF in 2009). Prior to this, agencies have used a cut-off of below 11 cm for admission to therapeutic feeding programmes[3] (Prudhon 2002; MSF 1995).

A meta-analysis of previous studies indicates that MUAC is the best predictor of short-term mortality (Pelletier 1991). Because MUAC is not adjusted for the height or weight of a child, it increases with age (and height and weight) by about 2 cm between one and five years of age. For this reason, a given MUAC cut-off is biased towards younger children. This age effect partly accounts for its superior mortality-predicting power.

The prevalence of low MUAC (< 115 mm) is similar (based on the new WHO child growth standards) to the prevalence of SAM (< -3 WHZ). At this extreme cut-off point, numbers are small and confidence intervals wide. For this reason, it is difficult to develop reference levels. However, it has been recommended in the past that a prevalence of 1 per cent SAM is indicative of excess mortality and should be used to guide appropriate programmatic responses (Mason 2002).

Height-for-age

An elevated prevalence of low height-for-age (HA) – or stunting – is indicative of specific risks, including mortality, morbidity, poorer school performance, decreased work capacity, and increased risk of adult morbidity and early death. The term 'chronic malnutrition' is often used to describe low HA, in part because height deficits occur as a result of a long-term process.

WHO has proposed reference levels for low HA and also low WA for the purposes of classifying ranges of worldwide prevalences. These simply reflect a convenient statistical grouping of prevalence levels from different countries (WHO Expert Committee 1995: 209).

Low HA has been closely associated with socio-economic status and poverty in the longer term, and a more recent study has shown a graded response of HA to different categories of food security among children aged one to 24 months (Saha et al. 2009). Similar stunting prevalence can have a several-fold difference in the prevalence of severe wasting.

Interpretation of low HA of an individual child depends crucially on the age range of the children; for younger children, low HA reflects a continuing process of failing to grow, while for older children it reflects past nutrition and a state of 'having failed to grow'.

Weight-for-age

Underweight is the term used to describe low WA, with cut-offs of minus 3 Z scores for severe underweight, and minus 2 Z scores for moderate and severe underweight status. Low WA can indicate either wasting (low WH), or more commonly, stunting (low HA). For this reason, WA is known as a composite index and its interpretation at both the individual and population level is not as clear-cut as wasting and stunting, given it reflects both long-term changes in the nutrition of the individual or population, and short-term recent changes captured by WH.

For the purposes of interpretation, it is more useful to consider wasting and stunting separately rather than in this combined index because they each reflect a different physiological

Table 25.3 Classification of worldwide prevalence ranges of low height-for-age and low weight-for-age among children under five years

Prevalence group	Prevalence ranges (% of children < −2 Z Scores)	
	Low height-for-age (stunting)	Low weight-for-age (underweight)
Low	< 20	< 10
Medium	20–29	10–19
High	30–39	20–29
Very high	>= 40	>= 30

Source: WHO Expert Committee 1995.

condition which is not distinguished by the underweight indicator (Black *et al.* 2008). WA is widely used by WHO and UNICEF in monitoring trends in the global prevalence of underweight, and is also one of the Millennium Development Goal (MDG) indicators. Reference levels for the classification of WA prevalence have been proposed by WHO (Table 25.3), although they are in less frequent use than the HA reference levels.

A deterioration in HA and WA can be used as confirmation of worsening food security, and can also be used for monitoring long-term trends, measuring impact over time, and for advocacy purposes to raise awareness about the nutritional situation and appropriate policy responses.

Body mass index

Cases of frank starvation among adults are one of the most visible characteristics of acute famine, observations of which have been widely recorded. Degrees of underweight among adults (chronic energy deficiency or chronic undernutrition) are categorised on the basis of Body Mass Index (BMI) measured on non-pregnant and non-lactating women of reproductive age (15–49 years).

The advantages of BMI as a nutritional indicator for adults are that it reflects fat and protein stores, and is correlated with increased risk of low birth-weight babies and mortality. However, it is difficult to measure, particularly among the stooping elderly who cannot stand up straight, thereby influencing measurements; is prone to age-related changes; and is modified by body shape (ratio of sitting height to standing height). Nevertheless, evidence strongly suggests that a serious decline in the mean and prevalence of low BMI is almost certainly associated with serious declines in food insecurity.

In nutritional emergencies, low BMI has been used in the screening and selection of admissions of adults into therapeutic feeding centres (Collins *et al.* 2000). In general, nutrition

Table 25.4 WHO BMI classification

Type and level of nutritional problem	BMI range (kg/m^2)
Obese	> 30.0
Overweight	25.0–29.9
Normal	18.5–24.9
Mild thinness	17.0–18.49
Moderate thinness	16.0–16.99
Severe thinness	< 16.0

Source: WHO Expert Committee 1995.

Table 25.5 BMI reference levels recommended by WHO

Low prevalence (warning sign, monitoring required):	5–9% of population with BMI < 18.5 (kg/m^2)
Medium prevalence (poor situation):	10–19% < 18.5 (kg/m^2)
High prevalence (serious situation):	20–39% < 18.5 (kg/m^2)
Very high prevalence (critical situation)	>=40% with BMI < 18.5 (kg/m^2)

Source: WHO Expert Committee 1995.

surveys of adults in emergencies are less common than surveys among infants and young children because infants and young children suffer higher mortality than adults (apart from older children), and are more vulnerable to all types of malnutrition. Surveys of adults have been used in helping to determine the degree to which a whole population has been affected by undernutrition.

Several factors other than nutritional status influence BMI, including body shape, height decline with age, and seasonal fluctuations in weight. The RNIS/NICS recommend adjusting for body shape differences as indicated by the SSR by applying the Cormic Index when comparing the BMI of different populations to account for body shape differences (Collins *et al.* 2000).

Reference levels for the interpretation of low BMI (< 18.5) (Table 25.5) are somewhat arbitrary and reflect the distribution of BMI in developing countries in the mid-1990s. More recent analysis has shown prevalence levels to be higher with ranges from 10 per cent to 19 per cent in most countries (Black *et al.* 2008).

Conclusions

Use of anthropometry for largely curative interventions (which take place after the malnutrition has occurred) is very different from a population-based approach – aimed at improving the nutritional situation of affected populations rather than individuals. The former requires a good case-definition with high sensitivity and low specificity for identifying children most likely to die, while the latter requires a broader population-based statistic that reflects the entire population distribution.

In conclusion, to be useful, an anthropometric classification system needs to be simple and take account of the type of growth failure, its severity, duration, and magnitude, and needs to be agreed upon and endorsed by key stakeholders. This review has shown that this is not always possible and each indicator has particular drawbacks or limitations, which need to be understood in the interpretation of reference levels.

While reference levels help decision-makers to qualify the severity of a nutritional situation, the challenge remains to correctly identify the underlying causes – are they food-, health-, or care-related? It is crucial that public health factors and seasonal patterns of disease, care, and food insecurity are also taken into account. The scale of the analysis is also a crucial factor; often, extremely high rates are confined to a specific localised area or population, and significant geographic variations occur which necessitates careful targeting of interventions. On the other hand, not all emergencies are characterised by increases in acute malnutrition. For example, among refugees and returnees in Kosovo and neighbouring countries, the level of acute malnutrition remained well below 5 per cent throughout the crisis in 1999. In some situations, micronutrient deficiency diseases may be a greater public health priority than acute malnutrition. For example, in Afghanistan between 2000 and 2003, outbreaks of scurvy were reported while levels of acute malnutrition remained relatively low. However, in almost all emergency situations, there will be an increase in nutritional risk as a result of either a deterioration in general public health, food insecurity, and/or a disturbance in social or care-giving behaviours.

Notes

1 Mason *et al.* reviewed data on acute malnutrition and mortality in the Greater Horn region (Eritrea, Ethiopia, Kenya, Somalia, southern Sudan, and Uganda) for the period 2000–06, drawn from 900 nutrition surveys of children. On average, the wasting prevalence for pastoral children was 17 per cent compared to 10 per cent for agriculturalists or mixed livelihoods. In bad years, the prevalence of acute malnutrition among pastoralists often rose to 25 per cent or higher, but for agriculturalists rarely rose above 15 per cent (Mason *et al.* 2008).

2 Nutritional or bilateral pitting oedema is the retention of intracellular fluid, particularly in the feet, ankles, and lower limbs and is an indicator of kwashiorkor. All children with bilateral pitting oedema are regarded as being severely acutely malnourished irrespective of their WH.

3 Therapeutic Feeding Programmes treat infants and children who are severely malnourished.

References

Black, R.E., Allen, L.H., Bhutta, Z.A., Caulfield, L.E., de Onis, M., Ezzati, M., Mathers, C., and Rivera, J. (2008) 'Maternal and Child Undernutrition: Global and Regional Exposures and Health Consequences', *The Lancet*, 371(9,608): 243–60.

Borrel, A. and Salama, P. (1999) 'Public Nutrition from an Approach to a Discipline: Conern's Nutrition Case-studies in Complex Emergencies', *Disasters*, 24(4): 326–42.

Collins, S., Duffield, A., and Myatt, M. (2000) *Adults: Assessment of Nutritional Status in Emergency-Affected Populations*, Administrative Committee on Coordination/Sub-Committee on Nutrition, New York: United Nations.

Darcy, J. and Hoffman, C.-A. (2003) *According to Need? Needs Assessment and Decision Making in the Humanitarian Sector*, Humanitarian Policy Group Report 15, London: Overseas Development Institute.

Howe, P. and Devereux, S. (2004) 'Famine Intensity and Magnitude Scales: A Proposal for an Instrumental Definition of Famine', *Disasters*, 28(4): 353–72.

Lusty, T. and Diskett, P. (1984) *Oxfam's Practical Guide to Selective Feeding Programmes: Oxfam Practical Guide No 1*, Oxford: Oxfam.

Mason, J. (2002) 'Lessons on Nutrition of Displaced People', *Journal of Nutrition*, 132(7): 2096S–2103S.

Mason, J.B., Chotard, S., Dietrich, M., Oliphant, N., Smith, E., Rivers, J., Hailey, P., and Mebrahtu, S. (2008) 'Fluctuations in Wasting in Vulnerable Child Populations in the Greater Horn of Africa', in *Working Papers in International Health and Development, No. 08–02*, New Orleans: Department of International Health and Development, Tulane University.

Mathys, E. (2007) *Trigger Indicators and Early Warning and Response Systems in Multi-Year Title II Assistance Programs*, Washington, DC: Food and Nutrition Technical Assistance Project.

MSF (Médecins Sans Frontières) (1995) *Nutrition Guidelines*, Paris: Médecins Sans Frontières.

Myatt, M., Duffield, A., Seal, A., and Pasteur, F. (2009) 'The Effect of Body Shape on Weight-for-Height and Mid-upper Arm Circumference Based Case Definitions of Acute Malnutrition in Ethiopian Children', *Annals of Human Biology*, 36(1): 5–20.

Nieburg, P., Person-Karell, B., and Toole, M.J. (1992) 'Malnutrition-mortality Relationships among Refugees', *Journal of Refugee Studies*, 5(3/4): 247–56.

Peel, S. (1977) *Selective Feeding Procedures: Oxfam Practical Guide No 1*, Oxford: Oxfam.

Pelletier, D.L. (1991) *Relationships between Child Anthropometry and Mortality in Developing Countries: Implications for Policy, Programs, and Future Research*, Monograph 12: Cornell Food and Nutrition Policy Programme.

Pelletier, D. (2006) 'Theoretical Considerations Related to Cutoff Points', *Food and Nutrition Bulletin*, 27(4 Supplement Growth Standard): S224–36.

Prudhon, C. (2002) *Assessment and Treatment of Malnutrition in Emergency Situations*, Paris: Action Contre la Faim.

Saha, K.K, Frongillo, E.A., Alam, D.S., Arifeen, S., Persson, L.A., and Rasmussen, K.M. (2009) 'Household Food Security is associated with Growth of Infants and Young Children in Rural Bangladesh', *Public Health Nutrition*, 138(7): 1,383–90.

Sphere Project (2003) *Humanitarian Charter and Minimum Standards of Disaster Response: 2004 revised edition*, Oxford: Oxfam.

UN IASC (United Nations Inter-Agency Standing Committee) and Standing Committee on Nutrition (SCN) (2009) *Fact Sheet on the Implementation of 2006 WHO Child Growth Standards for Emergency*

Nutrition Programmes for Children aged 6–59 Months, available at http://oneresponse.info/Global Clusters/Nutrition/Pages/default.aspx (accessed 18 May 2010).

Van der Heide, C.M., Brouwer, F., Bellon, S., Bockstaller, C., and Garrod, G. (2007) *Review of Approaches to Establish Reference Levels to Interpret Indicators*, Wageningen: Wageningen University.

de Ville de Goyet, C., Seaman, J., and Geijer, U. (1978) *The Management of Nutritional Emergencies in Large Populations*, Geneva: World Health Organization.

WHO (World Health Organization) (2000) *The Management of Nutrition in Major Emergencies*, Geneva: WHO, United Nations High Commissioner for Refugees, International Federation of Red Cross and Red Crescent Societies, World Food Programme.

WHO (World Health Organization) Expert Committee (1995) *Physical Status: The Use and Interpretation of Anthropometry. WHO Technical Report Series 854*, Geneva: WHO.

Young, H. and Jaspars, S. (2009) *Review of Nutrition and Mortality Indicators for the Integrated Food Security Phase Classification (IPC) Reference Levels and Decision-making*, Geneva and Rome: United Nations Standing Committee on Nutrition and The Integrated Food Security Phase Classification (IPC) Global Partners.

26

Water and Conflict

Moving from the Global to the Local

Erika Weinthal and Avner Vengosh

> The challenge of securing safe and plentiful water for all is one of the most daunting
> challenges faced by the world today ... Our experiences tell us that environmental stress
> due to lack of water may lead to conflict and would be greater in poor nations.
> (UN Secretary General Ban Ki-moon speaking at the World Economic Forum,
> Davos, Switzerland, 24 January 2008)

Water and conflict

Water is vital for human existence, but unlike other natural resources such as energy, there
are no substitutes. For large segments of the world's population, the procurement of clean,
plentiful water is a daily struggle. The United Nations (UN) estimates that by 2025, more
than 2.8 billion people worldwide will be living in countries that are water-stressed – that is,
when available freshwater resources per capita falls below 1,700 cubic meters per year (FAO
2007). Freshwater resources are, moreover, unevenly distributed both geographically and
temporally (see Figure 26.1); the Middle East and North Africa (MENA) region, in particular, is one of the most water-scarce areas in the world (World Bank 2007). With 5 per cent
of the world's population, it contains less than 1 per cent of the world's available fresh water
(Al-Jayyousi 2004). Expected population growth for 2025, according to Sowers *et al.*
(2010), will further increase the level of water stress in the MENA, as water availability
per capita is likely to decrease in the range of 30 to 70 per cent. Most MENA countries will
then be under the definition of 'absolute water scarcity' (i.e. less than 500 m^3/year/capita)
(Sowers *et al.* 2010). With the world's largest population, China also faces comparable levels
of water scarcity (757 m^3/year/capita) in its northern region, where 42 per cent of the
population lives, but which only has access to 14 per cent of the country's water (UNDP
2006: 136–7).

By the end of the twentieth century, it was thus widely assumed that water scarcity would be
a driver of conflict between nation states, especially in the arid regions of MENA. World leaders
such as former UN secretary-general, Boutros Boutros-Ghali, famously warned, 'the next war in
the Middle East will be fought over water, not politics' (Vesilind 1993: 53). The *Economist*,
furthermore, predicted in 1999 that '[w]ith 3.5 billion people affected by water shortages by

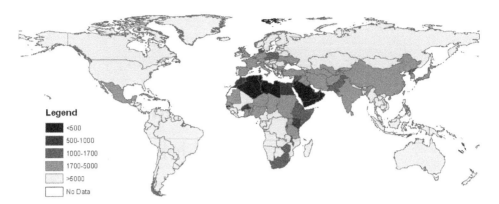

Figure 26.1 Global total actual renewable water resources per capita (m³/year) in 2005
Source: Adapted from AQUASTAT database, available at http://www.fao.org/nr/water/aquastat/dbase/index.stm; figure © Brittany R. Merola.

2050, conditions are ripe for a century of water conflicts'. The empirical evidence, however, has yet to support such prophecies. Rather, when it comes to water resources at the interstate level, cooperation is much more ubiquitous. The historical record shows that states rarely if ever go to war over water; in parsing more than 1,800 state-to-state water interactions in trans-boundary basins between 1946 and 1999, Wolf *et al.* (2003) demonstrated that none have led to formal war. Yet such encouraging findings should not obscure the fact that the '[MENA] region has a striking absence of inclusive and comprehensive international water agreements on its most significant trans-boundary water courses' (World Bank 2007: 80). The Nile River Basin, which is shared by ten countries and inhabited by approximately 150 million people, for example, has a long history of tension (e.g. Egypt-Sudan conflicts in the 1950s). In spite of current progress with the Nile Basin Initiative (World Bank 2007: 83), Egypt – the dominant downstream riparian (i.e. water user along the river) – continues to appropriate more than 90 per cent of the Nile River.

With the maturation of the field of water conflict and cooperation, the notion of impending water wars has come to be better understood as a 'myth' rather than a 'reality' (Bencala and Dabelko 2008). This is not to say that tensions do not exist among states regarding their shared and limited water resources, but rather there is a growing realisation that the source of conflict is emanating from disagreements within a country due to a lethal combination of population growth, unsustainable water withdrawals, lack of adequate water management, weak institutions, and pressure for economic development (e.g. see Wolf 2007). The Pacific Institute's Water Conflict Chronology indicates that between 2000 and 2009, most occurrences of water conflict were at the sub-national level, of which nearly half were development disputes. Examples in 2009 include hundreds of Mumbai residents in India protesting water cuts that resulted in one person being killed and dozens injured, and violent clashes in Ethiopia over access to water in the Somali border region.

The purpose of this chapter is twofold. First, we seek to delineate some of the major challenges states face concerning the provision of water at the sub-national level that include, for example, urbanisation, deteriorating water quality, climatic change, and food security. Second, in response to these challenges, we survey some of the prevailing solutions proposed for addressing water scarcity and improving water quality – for example, privatisation, dam construction, water transfer schemes, desalination, and land purchases. In doing so, we describe how policy solutions that ostensibly aim to augment water supplies and expand delivery can have unintended negative effects that alter the terms of access to water resources, negatively affect human livelihoods, and pit certain segments of the population against their own governments and/or transnational actors. As such, these conflicts at the sub-national level differ from those between states. Most notably, a broader constellation of actors, including communities, environmental activists, non-governmental organisations (NGOs), multinational corporations, and international lending organisations, are involved in the battle to determine appropriate technological and policy solutions for the provision of water. Furthermore, while issues of scarcity and questions of access continue to underlie tensions at the sub-national level, increasingly these battles have also raised issues pertaining to water quality, equity, and public participation (Conca 2005, 2006).

Urbanisation and water privatisation

Approximately 1 billion people do not have access to safe water and 2.5 billion people lack access to proper sanitation (UNDP 2006). Five to 10 million people, moreover, die each year from water-related diseases and/or inadequate sanitation (Wolf 2007). Many low- and middle- income countries (LMIC) experience a vicious cycle in which high rates of population growth and accelerated urban expansion place additional pressure on both surface and groundwater resources, causing their depletion and contamination. This in turn reduces the capacities of communities to provide safe water and sustain economic development. Surface water is typically affected by biological contamination, particularly in areas with poor sanitation and lack of sewage treatment. Groundwater can be contaminated by man-made sources associated with sewage leakage and agriculture, but can also be affected by naturally occurring contaminants such as arsenic (e.g. Bangladesh, Hossain, 2006), fluoride (e.g. East Africa, Meenakshi and Maheshwari, 2006), and radionuclides (e.g. Jordan, Vengosh et al., 2009).

One of the primary challenges governments and their populations face when it comes to urban expansion is how to best augment water supplies and address poor water quality. This problem of lack of access to safe water and sanitation is especially acute with the rise of mega-cities in the developing world – for instance, Mexico City, Dhaka, São Paulo, Bangkok – that are inhabited by more than 10 million people. As of 2005, there were 18 mega-cities worldwide, but as rural populations continue to relocate to urban areas, by 2025 this number is predicted to reach 27 (Tortajada 2008). Most of these mega-cities are in LMIC and entail a patchy conglomeration of illegal and legal settlements sprouting up on the outskirts of large cities. On the one hand, in the absence of direct access to tap water in their homes, the poor are often forced to pay more for water (which often does not meet government standards), through purchases from private vendors. On the other, urban growth not only places new pressure on dilapidated infrastructure and weak institutional capacity, but has also led to the over-exploitation and degradation of surrounding water resources, such as in Pakistan and Bangladesh (Richards 2002; Tortajada 2008).

In short, these mega-cities, as well as other major urban centres around the world, will require huge investments to extend water supply and sanitation to meet the needs of expanding populations. For instance, in 2002 it was estimated that Mexico would require $1.7 billion per year for water supply and sanitation investments (Tortajada 2008: 152). One such option for improving water supply and services is privatisation in which water is treated like any other commodity and sold according to its market value. Simply put, the architects of water privatisation argue that foreign capital is vital for upgrading systems and refurbishing infrastructure. Already a large number of countries have experimented with turning over control of their urban water resources to private companies, including Argentina, Bolivia, Brazil, Chile, India, Indonesia, Jordan, Kenya, Mexico, Morocco, Nigeria, the Philippines, Poland, South Africa, Turkey, and Zambia (Richards 2002: 12). Yet, for multinational corporations to agree to make such large capital investments upfront, they often raise the price of services to recoup these initial costs.

The critics of privatisation, in response, claim that that the global movement to privatise public utilities disenfranchises local populations and harms the environment; rather, they see access to clean water as a basic human right and belonging to the people (Shiva 2002). For the poor then, a jump in the price of water pushes it further out of their reach. This right to water, they note, has been recognised in a number of non-binding UN resolutions and declarations, including the 2002 General Comment 15 by the UN Committee on Economic, Social and Cultural Rights, which states '[t]he human right to water entitles everyone to sufficient, safe, acceptable, physically accessible and affordable water for personal and domestic uses' (United Nations 2002). Moreover, some countries such as South Africa have enshrined this right in their constitutions to guarantee the entire population 'access' to sufficient water with the goal of a minimum allowance of 50 L per person per day (Greeff 2003).

Because water privatisation fundamentally changes communities' access to water and/or makes water services prohibitively expensive, its commodification has increasingly been linked to conflict at the sub-national level (Bencala and Dabelko 2008). This is particularly the case when privatisation is carried out in a non-transparent manner with little or no public participation (Conca 2005). The most well-known case in which violence has erupted in response to the privatisation of the supply and distribution of drinking water was in Cochabamba, Bolivia. In 1999, the Bolivian government negotiated a contract for the sale of its entire water system, including all industrial, agricultural, and residential systems, to a foreign-led consortium – Aguas del Tunari – a joint venture owned by Bechtel (US) and Edison SPA (Italy). Facing a sharp price hike in the water bill, in April 2000, an unlikely alliance of farmers, environmentalists, neighbourhood associations, labour unions, and middle-class professionals swarmed onto the streets to protest the sale of the city's water system. Massive protests left one person dead and dozens injured. Soon afterwards the government was forced to cancel the contract with Aguas del Tunari (for details, see Baer 2008).

Alternative water resources and their limitations

Urbanisation, moreover, has shifted demands for water use away from the agricultural sector, which in many LMIC, as in the MENA, commands on average 70 to 90 per cent of available water, towards the domestic sector (Sowers et al. 2010). The shift in water supply from the agricultural to the domestic sector not only forces the urban population to vie for water with the rural sector, but is problematic given the stricter standards for water quality.

Owing to the depletion and contamination of existing water resources, many countries are thus exploring alternative water resources to meet the growing demands of their urban populations, and to mollify their agricultural sectors. These include 'new water' generated by desalination (for drinking water) and treated wastewater (for the agriculture sector). In arid and semi-arid areas of MENA and south-west USA, 'fossil' groundwater is becoming an important resource that offers a substitute for traditional replenished water resources. The generation of new water, however, requires huge capital investments and high technical capacity that are typically not available in many resource-poor countries. Currently, desalination occurs mainly in countries like the USA, Spain, and Israel, as well as oil-rich countries such as Saudi Arabia and the other Gulf states in the Middle East. The ability of low-income countries to adopt these technologies is largely dependent on external investments and the active involvement of multinational consortiums. Future development of desalination is likely to encourage privatisation of the water sector that has in most cases been controlled by the state. Given that the cost of tap water generated from desalination is expected to be significantly higher (i.e. the cost for one cubic metre in a large reverse osmosis desalination plant varies from $0.60 to $1.00), the introduction of desalination in poor, water-scarce countries is likely to increase the gap between the rich and poor, and could spark similar conflicts between communities, governments, and multinational corporations over who controls access to and the delivery of limited water resources.

A second alternative water resource is the recycling of wastewater for the agricultural sector through adequate treatment to remove all contaminants from sewage effluents. This again requires large capital investments and advanced technologies. Inadequate treatment of sewage could become a large health issue, particularly if such wastewater is used to irrigate for crops like lettuces and other greens. It could also cause major contamination of underlying aquifers (e.g. the Gaza Strip, Weinthal *et al.* 2005). Consequently, sustainable utilisation of treated wastewater requires a high performance of treatment systems coupled with adequate water quality monitoring, which are not always available in low-income countries.

The third option is mining fossil groundwater from aquifers that were replenished during previous wet climate conditions. Fossil groundwaters in the MENA region, for example, are derived from the Nubian Sandstone Basins in Libya, Egypt, Saudi Arabia, and Israel. In response to a deepening water crisis, the Jordanian government, for instance, contracted a French company to pump fossil groundwater from the Disi aquifer in southern Jordan to Amman, to meet demand from the growing urban population for drinking water in conjunction with the diminishment and salinisation of replenished aquifers in Jordan. Mining fossil groundwater is, however, possible only for the short term. At the same time, the use of fossil groundwater presents a whole new array of problems related to water quality. For example, one study has highlighted the problem of the quality of fossil groundwater from the Disi aquifer in Jordan, having found high levels of naturally occurring radium in the water that exceed international drinking water standards by many-hundred percent. High levels of radium in drinking water have severe health implications; the presence of this carcinogenic element in groundwater has potential health risks for millions that consume similar groundwater in the MENA countries (Vengosh *et al.* 2009).

Virtual water and conflict

One of the main achievements of nation states over the course of the twentieth century has been to harness the world's rivers to support economic development and broaden agriculture. Yet, in many countries, the current water supply is no longer sufficient to expand crop cultivation and simultaneously preserve a sufficient level of water for domestic consumption and industrial growth. Mounting water scarcity has caused many countries to import food to supply their rapidly growing populations. For example, all countries in the MENA region except Syria are net importers of food (World Bank 2007: 10). At the same time, many of the MENA countries export food, particularly to Europe, during the winter. This import and export of food, Tony Allan (2001) has argued, is a form of virtual water in which water is essentially embedded in food such as water-intensive commodities like wheat.

The import of 'virtual water' has allowed countries to indirectly address water scarcity and alleviate political tension around diminishing water resources (Sowers *et al.* in press). Yet rich countries, such as the water-scarce countries in the Gulf region, along with other countries in Asia with large populations that are also poor in water resources (e.g. China, South Korea, and India), have nonetheless begun to produce food overseas in countries where production costs are much lower and land and water are plentiful (Von Braun and Meinzen-Dick 2009). Since the mid-2000s, such countries have been buying up farmland throughout Africa and Asia to produce food directly or to lease land for crop cultivation.

These land deals provide a further glimpse into the changing nature of water conflicts – whereby conflicts over water scarcity are transferred away from the countries that are water-stressed to those that are bounteous in land and water. In particular, these acquisitions of land by outsiders underscores the fragility of property rights in many low-income countries, where top-down policies that change access to land and water resources may foster political instability, as poor people are pushed off their farmland that has provided the basis for their subsistence. Specifically, conflicts may arise when local communities perceive that they are not reaping any of the benefits of these land deals and instead have lost land without adequate compensation. In Madagascar, political protest that led to the overthrow of the government in 2009 was precipitated by the leasing of arable land to the South Korean conglomerate, Daewoo, for food production (*The Economist* 2009). Further conflict may ensue over access to land, as many of the deals have taken place in countries already riven by conflict such as Pakistan and Sudan (Martin 2008). For instance, Egypt, Jordan, Kuwait, Qatar, Saudi Arabia, South Korea, and the United Arab Emirates (UAE) have all signed agricultural deals with Sudan between 2008 and 2009.

Dams and development

Over the course of the twentieth century, countries have also relied upon dam construction for storage purposes to augment their water supplies and for hydroelectricity production. Yet dams, like other policy decisions that alter rules of access, hold the potential to stir conflict when they restrict prior water allocations of both communities and states. Dams already have a long history of eliciting social protest because their construction not only involves the inundation of large patches of pristine natural environment, but also the resettlement of populations and the loss of cultural heritage sites.

Whereas large dam construction has slowed and come to a halt in many high-income countries, it remains a poignant source of contention elsewhere, as governments struggle to provide both adequate water and electricity to their populations (Conca 2005; Khagram 2004). The government of Turkey, for example, has undertaken its Southeastern Anatolia Project, which is one of the largest dam projects in the world. While this project has brought greater prosperity and massive agricultural development to eastern Turkey, it has halved the water flow in the other parts of the Euphrates River, severely affecting the quantity and quality of the river in the downstream counties of Syria and Iraq (Beaumont 1996).

Populations that have experienced the direct brunt of dam construction are those that live in the path of flooding caused by dam projects. The World Commission on Dams reports that dam projects have displaced between 40–80 million people. The Three Gorges Dam Project on the Yangtze River in China has resulted in the forced relocation of over a million people. Paradoxically then, the state in its role as an agent of development, ends up becoming the foe of those very segments of the population that it has set out to assist through harnessing the variable flows of large rivers for hydroelectricity production. This is especially the case when projects are introduced in a non-transparent manner in which the human and environmental impacts are overlooked. Thus, the threat of displacement in India from the Narmada Dam

Project has led to mass demonstrations at the local level against both the Indian government and international lending agencies (Khagram 2004).

Climate change, population growth, and conflict

Lastly, many of the climate models predict that global warming will increase the recurrence of droughts and exacerbate water scarcity in arid and semi-arid regions and, at the same time, that water-rich regions will experience an intensification of precipitation and higher frequencies of floods (Christensen *et al.* 2007). For low-lying coastal regions, sea-level rise induced from global warming will contribute to the inundation of these coastal regions. Other models also suggest that population growth will contribute to an increase in global water scarcity (Vörösmaty *et al.* 2007). Under both scenarios, global water scarcity is likely to intensify, and the unequal distribution of water resources among and within states is likely to deepen (Figure 26.1).

Climate change, as a result, has been linked to conflict over water through several pathways. In particular, major flooding and/or worsening water scarcity might foster large-scale population migrations that could induce changes in demographic balances internally. More so, populations that originally inhabited coastal zones are likely to migrate inland (e.g. low-lying areas of Bangladesh). Others may migrate from rural communities into urban environments due to inadequate agriculture infrastructure and lack of water or from arid to temperate zones. In eastern Syria, for example, prolonged drought (2006–09) without effective interventions has affected 1.3 million people, and the loss of the 2008 harvest has accelerated migration to urban areas ('water refugees') in which 40–60,000 families have migrated in response to the drought and increased levels of extreme poverty (United Nations 2009).

Conclusion

To recap, many conflicts surrounding water resources at the onset of the twenty-first century are taking place at the sub-national level rather than between nation states and concern the question of what is the appropriate path of development for states and their societies. The issue of whether water is an economic commodity versus a human right, in particular, is likely to continue to exacerbate the split between pro-development interests and human rights and anti-poverty activists. Managing climate change impacts will also force states to reconsider what is the best path for ensuring access to safe and sufficient water resources. In water-scarce areas then, the absence of appropriate adaptive measures to address the combination of high population growth, increasing water demands, diminishing water resources, and their contamination will continue to negatively affect global human health.

References

Al-Jayyousi, O. (2004) 'Water Scarcity in the WESCANA Region: Threat to or Prospect for Peace?', in *The Conservation and Sustainable Use of Freshwater Resources in West Asia, Central Asia and North Africa*, Third IUCN World Conservation Congress, Bangkok, Kingdom of Thailand, 17–25 November.

Allan, J.A. (2001) *The Middle East Water Question: Hydropolitics and the Global Economy*, London: I. B. Tauris.

Baer, M. (2008) 'The global water crisis, privatisation, and the Bolivian water war', in J.M. Whiteley, H. Ingram, and R. Perry (eds) *Water, Place, and Equity*, Cambridge, MA: MIT Press.

Beaumont, P. (1996) 'Agricultural and environmental changes in the upper Euphrates catchment of Turkey and Syria and their political and economic implications', *Applied Geography*, 16(2): 137–57.

Bencala, K.R. and Dabelko, G.D. (2008) 'Water wars: Obscuring opportunities', *Journal of International Affairs*, 61(2): 21–33.

Christensen, J.H., Hewitson, B., Busuioc, A., Chen, A., Gao, X., Held, I., Jones, R., Kolli, R.K., Kwon, W.-T., Laprise, R., Magaña Rueda, V., Mearns, L., Menéndez, C.G., Räisänen, J., Rinke, A., Sarr. A., and Whetton, P. (2007) 'Regional Climate Projections', in S. Solomon, D. Qin, M. Manning, Z. Chen, M. Marquis, K.B. Averyt, M. Tignor, and H.L. Miller (eds) *Climate Change 2007: The Physical Science Basis. Contribution of Working Group I to the Fourth Assessment Report of the Intergovernmental Panel on Climate*, Cambridge and New York: Cambridge University Press.

Conca, K. (2005) *Governing Water: Contentious Transnational Politics and Global Institution Building*, Cambridge, MA: MIT Press.

Conca, K. (2006) 'The new face of water conflict', *Navigating Peace*, Washington, DC: Woodrow Wilson International Center for Scholars.

Economist (2009) 'Sin aqu a non', *The Economist*, 11 April, 59.

FAO (Food and Agriculture Organization) (2007) *Coping with Water Scarcity: Challenge of the Twenty First Century*, available at http://www.fao.org/nr/water/docs/escarcity.pdf (accessed 23 March 2010).

Greeff, L. (2003) 'Towards free basic water', in *Grab for Water? Different Strategies to Solve the Global Water Crisis*, Berlin: Heinrich Böll Stiftung.

Hossain, M.F. (2006) 'Arsenic contamination in Bangladesh: an overview', *Agriculture, Ecosystems & Environment*, 113: 1–16.

Khagram, S. (2004) *Dams and Development: Transnational Struggles for Water and Power*, Ithaca, NY: Cornell University Press.

Martin, A. (2008) 'The food chain: Mideast facing choice between crops and water', *New York Times*, 21 July, p. A1.

Meenakshi and Maheshwari, R.C. (2006) 'Fluoride in drinking water and its removal', *Journal of Hazardous Materials*, 137(1), 456–63.

Pacific Institute, 'Water Conflict Chronology', available at http://www.worldwater.org/conflict.html (accessed 22 March 2010).

Richards, A. (2002) 'Coping with water scarcity: the governance challenge', Institute on Global Conflict and Cooperation, Policy Paper No. 54, available at http://www.repositories.cdlib.org/igcc/PP/PP54 (accessed 23 March 2010).

Shiva, V. (2002) *Water Wars: Privatisation, Pollution, and Profit*, Cambridge, MA: South End Press.

Sowers, J., Vengosh, A., and Weinthal, E. (2010) 'Climate change, water resources, and the politics of adaptation in the Middle East and North Africa', *Climatic Change*, DOI: 10.1007/s10584-010-9835-4.

Tortajada, C. (2008) 'Challenges and realities of water management of megacities: The case of Mexico City metropolitan area', *Journal of International Affairs*, 61(2): 147–66.

UN (United Nations) (2002) 'Substantive issues arising in the implementation of the international covenant on economic, social, and cultural rights: General comment no. 15', Committee on Economic, Social and Cultural Rights, Twenty-ninth session, Geneva, 11–29 November.

UN (United Nations) (2009) *Syria Drought Response Plan*, available at http://ochaonline.un.org/humanitarianappeal/webpage.asp?Page=1810 (accessed 23 March 2010).

UNDP (United Nations Development Programme) (2006) *Human Development Report 2006, Beyond Scarcity: Power, Poverty and the Global Water Crisis*, New York: United Nations Development Programme.

Vengosh, A., Hirschfeld, D., Vinson, D.S., Dwyer, G.S. Raanan, H., Rimawi, O., Al-Zoubi, A., Akkawi, E., Marie, A., Haquin, G., Zaarur, S., and Ganor, J. (2009) 'High naturally occurring radioactivity in fossil groundwater in the Middle East', *Environmental Science and Technology*, 43(6): 1,769–75.

Vesilind, P.J. (1993) 'Water: The Middle East's critical resource', *National Geographic*, 183(5): 38–70.

Von Braun, J. and Meinzen-Dick, R. (2009) 'Land grabbing by foreign investors in developing countries: Risks and opportunities', International Food Policy Research Institute, Policy Brief No. 13, Washington DC: International Food Policy Research Institute.

Vörösmaty, C.J. Green, P., Salisbury J., and Lammers R.B. (2007) 'Global water resources: Vulnerability from climate change and population growth', *Science*, 289: 284–8.

Weinthal, E., Vengosh, A., Marie, A., Gutierrez, A., and Kloppmann, W. (2005) 'The water crisis in the Gaza Strip: Prospects for remediation', *Ground Water*, 43: 653–60.

Wolf, A.T. (2007) 'Shared waters: Conflict and cooperation', *Annual Review of Environmental Resources*, 32: 241–69.

Wolf, A.T., Yoffe, S.B., and Giordano, M. (2003) 'International waters: Identifying basins at risk', *Water Policy*, 5: 29–60.

World Bank (2007) *Making the Most of Water Scarcity: Accountability for Better Water Management Results in the Middle East and North Africa*, Washington, DC: World Bank.

Part VI

Global Public Health Policy and Practice

27

Global Health Diplomacy

Ilona Kickbusch and Chantal Berger

Introduction

This chapter will be concerned mainly with the new field of global health diplomacy, and focuses on health diplomacy as it relates to health issues that transcend national boundaries and are global in nature. It also discusses the challenges at hand and how they are being addressed by different actors at different levels of governance.

Global health is one of the areas in which a new approach to diplomacy in the twenty-first century is most manifest. The term refers to 'those health issues which transcend national boundaries and governments and call for actions on the global forces and global flows that determine the health of people. It requires new forms of governance at national and international levels which seek to include a wide range of actors' (Kickbusch and Lister 2006: 7). It differentiates itself from other commonly used terms such as international health and public health in that 'global health, adopted broadly over the past decade, is meant to transcend past ideological uses of international health to imply a shared global susceptibility to, experience of, and responsibility for health' (Birn 2009: 63).

As new trans-border health challenges need to be resolved jointly by countries working together, health is moving further beyond the purely technical realm and is becoming a critical element in foreign policy, security policy, and trade agreements. This represents a shift from an approach in which international health is mainly considered in the context of development policy, and measures its results in the resource flow from North to South, to one where global health transcends borders and is marked by a sense of collective responsibility for health. As a consequence of this globalisation of health, national health problems can no longer be dealt with in isolation, but rather call for coordinated and cooperative global health efforts. Today, multilateral health negotiations matter, as they touch upon national and economic interests and reflect the tension between national sovereignty and global collective action, as well as those between expansive business interests and the protection of the health of vulnerable groups. Simple classifications of policy and politics – domestic and foreign, hard and soft, or high and low – no longer apply.

With a rapidly changing global context, a shift in patterns of disease, an improved understanding of the social and economic determinants of health, and a diversity of institutional actors, the global health landscape has changed considerably over recent years. There is a need to manage health risks that spill into and out of every country, to address the broader determinants of health from a whole of government perspective, and to involve, both formally and informally, a broader range of actors and interests, bringing together state and non-state actors.

The changing nature of global health diplomacy

Diplomacy is frequently referred to as the art and practice of conducting negotiations (Berridge 2005), and is generally still understood to mean the conduct of international relations through the intervention of professional diplomats from ministries of foreign affairs on issues of 'hard power', initially war and peace, and later economics and trade. In recent years, however, there has been an increase in the number of international agreements on 'soft issues', such as the environment and health. It is now increasingly recognised that even some of these softer issues can have significant 'hard' ramifications on national economies (Kickbusch *et al.* 2007).

Diplomacy today acknowledges the importance assigned to 'soft power' and 'smart power' strategies. There is an increasing recognition that certain 'global public goods' need to be negotiated and ensured, and that international regimes formed to coordinate behaviour among countries as in the area of trade and economic development need to be complemented by others in areas such as environment and health.

As a part of this diplomatic trend, international negotiation has experienced a new pattern of political behaviour, moving from bilateral to multilateral diplomacy. With the former referring to the more classical type of bilateral diplomacy directed primarily towards the conduct of relations on a state-to-state basis, multilateral diplomacy exhibits a change in these traditional relationships. As of 1919, a completely novel form was added to the institutional repertoire of states, namely the multipurpose, universal membership organisations, firstly the League of Nations, then, after World War II, the United Nations. Multilateral international diplomacy involves the art of building and managing coalitions before, during, and after negotiations on a particular issue across national boundaries – frequently within the context of international organisations. In particular, the twenty-first century diplomacy structure is highly complex, with a multitude of actors, issues, roles, and values. In the past, it was enough for a nation to look after itself – today that is no longer sufficient. As Heine (2006) states: 'the model of an international system based purely on independent states has been replaced by one in which the nation-state is still a key component, but by no means the only one' (Heine 2006: 4).

The term 'global health diplomacy' aims to capture these multi-level and multi-actor negotiation processes that shape and manage the global policy environment for health. Ideally, global health diplomacy results in three key outcomes:

(1) it helps to ensure better health security and population health outcomes for each of the countries involved (thus serving the national and the global interest),
(2) it helps to improve the relations between states and strengthens the commitment of a wide range of actors to work to improve health, and
(3) it provides an understanding of health as a common endeavour to ensure health as a human right and a global public good with the goals to deliver results that are deemed fair 'for all' (i.e. reducing poverty, increasing equity).

Global health diplomacy brings together the disciplines of pubic health, international affairs, management, law, and economics, and focuses on negotiations that shape and manage the global policy environment for health. Its content areas include: (1) negotiating for public health across boundaries in health and non-health fora, (2) global health governance, (3) foreign policy and health, and (4) developing national global health strategies.

Global health governance

The global health landscape has changed considerably in recent years, and the number of organisations dealing with health issues has increased exponentially. The rise in public–private partnerships, donors, funds, and other actors have all contributed to the diversification of actors in the global health arena.

A major part of global health diplomacy takes place within the United Nations specialised agency for health – the World Health Organization (WHO) – but the range of actors and settings has expanded rapidly. This includes venues such as the World Trade Organization (WTO), the World Bank, regional organisations, and new organisations such as global alliances, global funds, and global forums.

Classical international health governance is structured on the understanding that governments have primary responsibility for the health of their people and are able, in cooperation with other states, to protect their populations from health risks. Today, there are not only an increasing number of trans-border risks, but there is also a growth in the number and degree of influence of non-state actors in health governance. As such, health governance in an era of globalisation is marked by an ever-changing landscape of actors that enter into changing alliances, partnerships, and agreements. Additional or new forms of health governance are needed in order to effectively respond to new global health challenges (Dodgson *et al.* 2002). Global health governance is thus the conscious creation, shaping, steering, strengthening, and use of international and transnational institutions and regimes of principles, norms, rules, and decision-making procedures (Krasner 1983) to organise the promotion and protection of health on a global scale.

Increasingly, negotiations on global health matters are not only conducted between public health experts representing health ministries of nation states, but also include a growing array of other national actors and major players in the global arena such as NGOs, the private sector, academia, and foundations. At the beginning of the twenty-first century, health concerns demonstrate most of the governance challenges in a globalised world. These modern negotiations have become characterised by unstructured pluralism and an imbalance of power among a variety of actors. International organisations such as the WHO are no longer the extension of national policies – they change them, bundle them, and sometimes provide the groundwork for national legislation. The Framework Convention on Tobacco Control (FCTC) and the International Health Regulations (IHR) are classic examples.

Health and foreign policy

We are witnessing an increased role of health in global and foreign affairs, including, in particular, trade and security, as exemplified in the SARS epidemic and fears of biological terrorism. Health is now part of the G8 summits, the UN General Assembly, and poverty reduction strategies. In what he calls the 'Copernican shift in global health', Alcazar (2008: 11) illustrates that 'globalization takes the issue of health from the relative obscurity in which it found itself, especially in developing countries, and brings it to the front page where it is featured not as health as we know it, but as global health in combination with foreign policy, which we are still struggling to define'. Furthermore, Fidler (2007: 53) remarks that 'historically, public health has predominantly been a domestic policy concern but developments over the last decade have forced public health experts and diplomats to think of health *as* foreign policy, namely public health as important to states' pursuit of their interests and values in international relations'.

Foreign policy has been defined as 'the strategy or approach chosen by the national government to achieve its goals in relation with external entities. This includes decisions to do nothing' (Hudson 2008: 12). Traditional functions of foreign policy are increasingly becoming challenged with new realities. Fidler identifies four functions of foreign policy in order of high politics (security concerns) to low politics (economic well-being and development): (1) ensuring national security, (2) protecting national economic power and well-being, (3) fostering development of strategically important regions and countries, and (4) supporting human dignity (Fidler 2006: 54). Cooper (2003: 85) observes that nowadays, 'the objective of foreign policy is taken to be peace and prosperity rather than power and prestige'. Priorities have shifted where health is now the focus of diplomacy.

Throughout the twentieth century, public health was generally categorised as a development or human dignity issue with low-politics implications. But the post-Cold War period has demonstrated that public health today features more frequently and intensively in all of foreign policy's basic functions. Foreign policymakers are increasingly confronted in their traditional areas of operation with health-related issues, problems, and crises. For example, on the national security function, health has manifested itself in the form of threats from biological weapons, proliferation, and bioterrorism. Furthermore, debates concerning the impact of international trade and investment on public health demonstrate public health's importance to the state's pursuit of its economic interests. The traditional 'wealth leads to health' notion has been challenged by the 'health leads to wealth' argument.

Health policy can no longer remain purely national. Interdependence in a globalised world has created its own dynamic, and health is a key element. Foreign policy and diplomacy offer important tools to deal with the increasing interdependence and thus serve as extensions to national policy efforts. Making use of these tools to reorient health and foreign policies in ways that align national interest with the diplomatic, epidemiological, and ethical realities of a globalised world could thus substantially contribute to the protection and promotion of global health. The problem is that, so far, health 'has not been at the heart of foreign policy theory or practice and perhaps not even at the margins' (Fidler 2007: 243) – although today the degree of foreign policy attention devoted to health is historically unprecedented. What is thus needed is what has come to be termed as 'health foreign policy' and 'health diplomacy', that is, new developments bringing together diplomatic negotiating skills with public health expertise. Such alignment also requires governments to overcome 'fragmented policy competencies in national governance systems' (Drager and Fidler 2007: 162) and to widen the content and concept of diplomacy to include issues such as health, but also environment and trade.

The commitment of global health as a foreign policy issue manifested itself in the Oslo Declaration – *Global Health: A Pressing Foreign Policy Issue of our Time*, launched in 2007 by the ministers of foreign affairs of Brazil, France, Indonesia, Norway, Senegal, South Africa, and Thailand.

> In today's era of globalization and interdependence there is an urgent need to broaden the scope of foreign policy. We believe that health is one of the most important, yet still broadly neglected, long-term foreign policy issues of our time [...] We have therefore agreed to make impact on health a point of departure and a defining lens that each of our countries will use to examine key elements of foreign policy and development strategies, and to engage in a dialogue on how to deal with policy options from this perspective.
>
> (Amorim *et al.* 2007: 1,373)

Foreign policy and diplomacy no longer reside solely with the traditional diplomats, but also include a wide range of other state and non-state actors (Barston 2006). Today's minister of health has a dual responsibility: to promote his or her country's health and to advance the health interests of the global community. In addition, diplomats no longer just have to talk to other diplomats. Rather, they need to interact with NGOs, the private sector, scientists, advocates, and the media, since all these actors are now heavily involved and implicated in the negotiating process (Kickbusch *et al.* 2007).

Developing national global health strategies

A few countries are beginning to address global health more consistently at the national level by mapping activities in global health across all government sectors, establishing new mechanisms of coordination within government, and developing a 'national global health strategy', frequently at the initiative of the international department in the ministries of health. Health diplomacy initiatives in Switzerland and the UK prove to be good examples of the recognition and application of these changing realities.

The first such policy document comes from Switzerland, where a joint strategic approach to global health was developed by the Departments of the Interior (represented by the Swiss Federal Office of Public Health) and the Department of Foreign Affairs. This document, *Agreement on Foreign Health Policy Objectives*, was presented to the Swiss Federal Council (the government cabinet) in October 2006. It brings together three major strands of global health action that generally run in parallel with little coordination or are even in competition with one another. This includes the activities within the health sector that address normative health issues, international agreements and cooperation, global outbreaks of disease and pandemics; the commitment to health in the context of assistance towards development; and the policy initiatives in other sectors – such as foreign policy and trade. It emphasises the commitment of Switzerland to human rights and defines five priorities in foreign health policy: the health of the Swiss population, the coherence between national and international health policy, the strengthening of international health cooperation, the improvement of the global health situation, and the strengthening of the Swiss commitment as host country to WHO and to major health industries.

The United Kingdom established a national global health strategy which offers the second example of a government-based strategy. Adopted in 2008, the strategy is based on the premise that health is a human right and global public good. It aims to bring together the UK's foreign relations, international development, trade, and investment policies, all of which have an effect on global health. Five areas of action are identified: (1) better global health security, (2) stronger, fairer, and safer systems to deliver health, (3) more effective international organisations, (4) stronger, freer, and fairer trade for better health, and (5) strengthening the way we develop and use evidence to improve policy and practice. The strategy also abides by several principles such as equity within and between countries, health as an agent for good in foreign policy, learning from other countries' policies and experience, tackling health challenges that begin outside the UK border, and working in partnership with other governments, multilateral agencies, civil society, and businesses.

These strategies have come in response to the increasing need to address the crossroads between national and global health policy. Many other countries are now working on similar strategies to advance global health by establishing links between various sectors.

Conclusion

We are at a turning point in health policy: the nature of twenty-first century health – the global health society – calls for a radical change of mindset and a reorganisation of how we govern health in the twenty-first century. There has been a significant change in the health debate, where health is seen as an investment, a collective global challenge, and a human right in need of ethics and values. Health is now becoming a driving force.

Global health diplomacy is a constantly developing field, with a need for conceptual development, capacity building, and practical training programmes. Training[1] aims to bring together diplomatic and health professionals to understand their common interests in health as foreign policy. It is clear that the growing concern for multilateral cooperation on critical global health problems requires purposeful engagement in learning across these two sectors. There is a need to include non-governmental actors, philanthropy, and the private sector in this exciting new field of study. The aim is to bring these actors together in one venue and develop some of the negotiation skills necessary to effectively function in today's complex health landscape.

Globalisation demands more effective collective action by governments, civil society, and business. This in turn leads to new organisations, networks, processes, agreements, and norms. What is critical is managing the interfaces between these new actors, and the dynamics between overlapping fields.

Note

1 The Global Health Programme at the Graduate Institute of International and Development Studies, Geneva, has over the last three years successfully run a series of Executive Courses on Global Health Diplomacy: three courses in Geneva in June 2007, 2008, and 2009, a course in Beijing in August 2009 with a pre-course in cooperation with the World Health Organization (WHO) in Geneva in 2008, a course in Nairobi in September 2009, and two courses in partnership in the US in Washington DC, USA (CDC, UCSF) in 2008, and in Ottawa, Canada in 2009 (CSIH). Each of these experiences has brought new ideas, perspectives, and lessons learned to the process of developing the field. For more information see www.graduateinstitute.ch/globalhealth.

References

Alcazar, S. (2008) 'The Copernican Shift in Global Health', *Global Health Programme, Graduate Institute of International and Development Studies*, Working Paper no. 3.

Amorim, C., Douste-Blazy, P., Wirayuda, H., Store, J., Gadio, C., Dlamini-Zuma, N., and Pibulsonggram, N. (2007) 'Oslo Ministerial Declaration–global health: a pressing foreign policy issue of our time', *The Lancet*, 369(9,570): 1373–8.

Barston, R. P. (2006) *Modern Diplomacy*, New York: Pearson Longman.

Berridge G. R. (2005) *Diplomacy: Theory and Practice*, London and New York: Palgrave, Macmillan.

Birn, A. E. (2009) 'The stages of international (global) health: Histories of success or successes of history?' *Global Public Health*, 4(1): 50–68.

Cooper, R. (2003) *The breaking of nations: Order and chaos in the 21st century*, New York: Atlantic Monthly Press.

Dodgson, R., Lee, K., Drager, N. (2002) 'Global Health Governance: A conceptual review', *World Health Organisation, Department of Health and Development*, Discussion Paper no. 1.

Drager, N. and Fidler, D. (2007) 'Foreign Policy, trade and health: At the cutting edge of global health diplomacy', *Bulletin of the World Health Organization*, 85(3): 162.

Fidler, D. (2006) 'Health as foreign policy: Harnessing globalization for health', *Health Promotion International*, 21(Supplement 1): 51–8.

Fidler, D. (2007) 'Reflections on the revolution in health and foreign policy', *Bulletin of the World Health Organization*, 85(3): 243–4.

Heine, J. (2006) 'On the Manner of Practising the New Diplomacy', Canada: The Centre for International Governance Innovation, Working Paper no. 11.

Hudson, V. (2008) 'The history and evolution of foreign policy analysis', in S. Smith, A. Hadfield, and T. Dunne, *Foreign Policy: Theories, Actors, Cases*, New York: Oxford University Press.

Kickbusch, I. and Lister, G. (2006) *European Perspective on Global Health: A Policy Glossary*, Brussels: European Foundation Centre.

Kickbusch, I., Silberschmidt, G., and Buss, P. (2007) 'Global health diplomacy: the need for new perspectives, strategic approaches and skills in global health', *Bulletin of the World Health Organization*, 85(3): 230–32.

Krasner, S. (ed.) (1983) *International Regimes*, New York: Cornell University Press.

Switzerland Department of Foreign Affairs (2006) *Agreement on foreign health policy objectives*, 9 October 2006, available at http://www.bag.admin.ch/themen/internationales (accessed 27 September 2009).

United Kingdom (2008) *Health is Global: A UK Government Strategy 2008–13*, available at www.dh.gov.uk/publications (accessed 27 September 2009).

28

The Politics of Global Aid

Peter Muennig and Celina Su

International aid refers to the transfer of funds from one entity or government to another across borders. In global public health, even aid is contentious. Tensions surround how much aid is necessary, how it should be used, and even whether it should be given at all. These tensions arise not only because aid to poor countries is often poorly used, but also because it may, sometimes, do more harm than good. For instance, the Democratic Republic of the Congo has been a major recipient of aid for many decades and has deteriorated in most measures of development over that time. In other cases, though, aid seems to have played a major role in developing nations' literacy, health, and economic well-being. South Korea, one of the world's richer economies, was largely built on aid. In this chapter, we will take a critical look at the key arguments and bodies of evidence of each of these schools of thought.[1]

Different types of aid

International aid may take the form of an American citizen or foundation writing a cheque to Doctors Without Borders or the Red Cross. This is sometimes called *humanitarian aid* because such funding often supports programmes to alleviate immediate human suffering. Aid may also take the form of a government transferring cash aid or goods, like helicopters to another government. This is often called *bilateral aid* because it goes from one governmental party to another. An intergovernmental organisation like the World Bank can also provide funding for a project in Rwanda. This form is often called *multilateral aid* because organisations such as the World Bank are funded by many different nations. Finally, many scholars consider remittances – aid sent from expatriate workers back to their families at home – as a form of large-scale, 'informal', international aid (Maimbo and Ratha 2005). This chapter will only discuss formal aid.

Both bilateral aid and multilateral aid are often called 'official direct assistance' (ODA). Usually, aid takes the form of a grant, but it can also take the form of a loan or smaller shipments of in-kind goods, for example, tents and non-perishable foods in post-earthquake Pakistan. Humanitarian aid is usually delivered through non-governmental organisations (NGOs), or small, typically non-profit, organisations that deliver services directly to communities.

The objective of international aid

The most commonly stated objective of international aid is not explicitly geared for public health interventions, but *economic development*. This economic development is usually phrased in terms of gross domestic product (GDP) growth, financial stability, and poverty reduction (Easterlin 1974). According to one logic, once financial health is established, the government can then afford public health and education services. However, others have questioned whether it is reasonable to expect that 6.5 billion people driving cars, using air conditioning, and generating large amounts of consumer waste is a viable vision for a healthy future.

Amartya Sen and Martha Nussbaum have proposed that *human development* be emphasised instead. They argue that economic development is valuable, but that people also cherish the right to education, a long and healthy life, political participation, and other 'capabilities' (Sen 1999). Sen, in particular, points to many examples in which economic development has little relation to health and longevity. For instance, many countries have achieved comparable or superior life expectancy and literacy rates to the United States while still ranking among the poorer nations on earth. On the other hand, China's rapid rise as an economic superpower has unleashed public health disasters like cancer clusters due to unregulated pollution and mass poisonings due to unsafe baby food products, alongside relatively less growth of educational institutions for its rural poor (Wu *et al.* 1999). As a result, China has experienced a slower rate of gain in life expectancy during its meteoric rise in economic development than it did during its years of brutal communist suppression (WHO 2000).

Such critiques led the United Nations to develop the Human Development Index (HDI) in 1990, a measure of growth on three scales: the economy, literacy, and life expectancy. Human development scholars argue that well-rounded development will best occur via investments in education and health. The aid required for economic growth might take the form of infrastructure projects (e.g. dams and roads) coupled with mandates for market reforms, such as privatisation of public utilities. The aid required for human development might take the form of investments in schools and public health, leaving the economic development up to the host country.

A very brief history of US aid

The massive destruction seen in Europe, Asia, and North Africa during the Second World War created strong incentives for new intergovernmental institutions aimed at peacekeeping and financial cooperation. The leading economic powers formed the United Nations, which was primarily charged with creating dialogue between nations in order to stem wars. They also formed the International Bank for Reconstruction and Development, commonly known as the World Bank, which was charged primarily with rebuilding Europe. Finally, the International Monetary Fund (IMF) was formed to reduce the chance of another global recession, one of the many major factors thought to precipitate the war.

Following the Second World War, colonial powers began a slow process of decolonisation in countries such as Senegal and India. Poor nations were given autonomy and aid, but were left with little by way of institutions, such as banks or ministries. Without adequate economic, social, or political structures in place to absorb and distribute the aid, development was slow-moving.

Further, the effectiveness of aid programmes themselves was compromised by political concerns: US policymakers framed Cold War era aid in terms of American security as well as economic largesse. By the 1950s, the United States and the Union of Soviet Socialist

Republics (USSR) began to see governments run by dictatorship as preferable to those adopting the other side's political economy,[2] whether in the form of reigning ethos or allegiance. For instance, in 1954, the United States overthrew a Jeffersonian-based democratic government in Guatemala in part because the government was left-leaning (Schlesinger and Kinzer 1982).

Though this situation continued through the 1960s, the Kennedy administration in the United States did set out to win the hearts and minds of people in poor nations (democratic or otherwise) with a good deal of development aid. Citizens of wealthy nations contributed to this agenda as well, leading to a decade of unprecedented giving. However, by the end of the decade, only modest economic or human development had actually taken place.

The 1970s saw the formation of the Organization of the Petroleum Exporting Countries (OPEC) (Barsky and Kilian 2002). These were generally poor Middle Eastern countries with poorly formed institutions themselves. However, they were able to coordinate spikes in oil prices worldwide (primarily with the intent of punishing the United States for assisting Israel). The plan worked, but it mostly hurt developing nations that could not afford the high oil prices. Moreover, the OPEC countries did not have mature banks, and had to deposit their newfound riches in the banks of the Western countries they meant to punish. These banks, overflowing with petrodollars, then lent the money back to poor nations with interest so that they could buy more fuel. The end result of this vicious cycle was skyrocketing debt in poor nations.

In the 1980s, Ronald Reagan and Margaret Thatcher were respectively elected to power in the United States and the United Kingdom. Their administrations enacted what is now known as the 'Washington Consensus', or a set of economic mandates attached to aid dollars by multinational organisations (such as the World Bank/IMF), including reducing expenditures on government services (e.g. education, health, and transportation), privatising government agencies, and removing trade barriers (Williamson 1993). These 'structural adjustment programmes' led to currency devaluation, recessions, and social changes from which many countries have not yet recovered. Structural adjustment did help to reduce the debt burden, which by the 1980s led to a net flow of money from poor nations to rich nations in the form of interest payments. However, it also caused the virtual disappearance of the middle class, most of whom were government employees, in poor nations (Gaidzanwa 1999; Moghadam 1999).

The 1990s brought the end of the Cold War, and there was thus less incentive for the United States and its allies to provide ODA. This, coupled with the burgeoning HIV/AIDS epidemic (worsened by the impact of structural adjustment on public health infrastructure), resulted in declines in life expectancy in many sub-Saharan African nations. Still, the decade also saw the stellar rise of formerly impoverished nations in Asia, a rise mostly attributed to investments in agriculture and education.

The 2000s saw the rise of humanitarian aid, with the world's two richest men – Bill Gates and Warren Buffet – pooling resources to form the largest charitable organisation yet. Other forms of private giving increased, as did ODA. China's powerful manufacturing engine, coupled with unparalleled consumer spending in the United States, led to an enormous rise in commodity prices. China, eager to fuel its manufacturing engine, turned to poor nations that were rich in mineral resources (such as Sudan and Zambia), often exchanging ODA for access to these resources (Michel *et al.* 2009). Moreover, China has been willing to go where few aid agencies dare, tapping into war-torn areas and highly corrupt governments alike.

While this chapter focuses on non-military aid, it should be noted that since 2000, the US has once again significantly increased aid in the name of national security, especially in the Middle East (Root 2008). Such military aid has primarily consisted of cash transfers and large credits for the purchase of US-made weapons and equipment.

Current international giving

The United States is the largest donor overall, but this is because it is the world's largest economy. As a percentage of its gross national product (GNP), the US ranks towards the bottom of the industrialised nations, providing about 0.2 per cent (UN 2006). This is well below the official target set by the United Nations of 0.7 per cent of GNP. The only nations that actually meet this goal are Sweden, Luxembourg, Norway, and the Netherlands, which tend to donate between 0.8 and 1 per cent of their GNP. However, if aid provided directly by US citizens is added to the overall figure, the US rises to the top of the list.

Models of global aid for public health

Development and public health experts have forwarded several dominant models of thinking on how global aid should *ideally* improve global health.

One model assumes no specific prescriptions for public health, rather, it dictates a model *methodology* for decision-making. The model argues that policy decisions (to allocate global aid in ways that will maximise public health) are best made via the *ex ante* approach (Harsanyi 1953). In this approach, one is asked to imagine that he or she is making decisions prior to being born into the world, for example, without knowing whether you will become a hungry villager in rural Malawi or a well-fed head-of-state.

Now, imagine further that you are asked to allocate $30 billion in aid on Earth. While $30 billion is not enough to solve the world's problems, it could make a dent in suffering if used properly. One way of using it is via *cost-effectiveness analysis*. Imagine we had the following list:

1. Sanitation projects $0.50 per life saved.
2. School projects $0.75 per life saved.
3. Vaccination projects $1 per life saved.
4. Bed nets $3 per life saved.
5. Primary medical care $15 per life saved.
6. HIV/AIDS testing and treatment $300 per life saved.

We could invest our $30 billion in the poorest areas without clean water, schooling, or vaccination and save well over 30 billion lives. Alternatively, we could focus the same funding on primary medical care and save 2 billion lives. If we invested in HIV/AIDS treatment, we might save 100 million lives. Finally, we could ignore the list altogether and invest in dams in Africa, nuclear power plant construction in South Africa, or a transnational super-highway through Southeast Asia. The latter projects could save or could take lives over the long run, but it is safe to assume that they would not be ideal investments if our objective is to maximise health.

The reality is that aid money is more likely to be spent on the above priorities in reverse, with significantly more money going to dams than to sanitation projects. Some of these 'sub-optimal' investments may actually be ideal for certain countries or localities. For instance, a country that has achieved reasonable vaccination rates and has invested in schools may need roads and power plants. Likewise, a locality with very high rates of tuberculosis and HIV/AIDS will perhaps benefit more from medical clinics than an area that is afflicted with diseases that can be prevented with public health measures, such as diarrhoea and malaria. Context is the most important factor in international aid.

Other reasons for ignoring the above list of priorities include: overriding political priorities, ethical concerns, or lack of clear information (on the part of the donor, the recipient requesting the funding, or both).

Political concerns often top the list. The World Bank was once the world's largest funder of dams internationally. Now it is China. In both cases, the money was, and still is, often donated or lent for political reasons. The Chinese government has become one of the major sources of aid in Southeast Asia and Africa alike, in the hopes of acquiring rights to timber, oil, or minerals. The World Bank continues to fund large infrastructure projects despite also funding studies showing that dollars invested in schools would be a preferred investment.

Ethical concerns also play a large role. For instance, the anthropologist Paul Farmer argues that the 'reigning ideologies' of public health favour 'efficiency over equity' (Farmer 2004: 18). While not denying that cost-effectiveness is an important life-saving tool, Farmer argues that it is wrong for a treatment to be seen as 'cost-effective in New York, but not in Siberia' (Farmer 2004: 131). Applying this to the above *ex ante* perspective, Farmer essentially argues that we should refuse the $30 billion and instead demand that all resources be distributed with preferential treatment for the poor who need it most.

Finally, a lack of information often plays a role in funding decisions, as well. Small NGOs too often invest in tertiary care hospitals to treat diseases like cholera when latrines are needed instead (Dichter 2003). Few NGOs and donors prioritise appropriate technology utilisation.

Some development experts argue that aid agencies have conducted enough *ex ante* exercises and analyses, and that human development is best achieved via heavy investments in schooling and agriculture (Strauss and Thomas 1998). The idea is that education and nutrition build human capital, the platform needed for economic development. Schooling also confers important survival skills – humans adapt to a harsh ecological niche via cognition. Investments in schools and agriculture may be one important reason why so many Asian nations have undergone rapid human development. It is difficult, however, to parse out the relative contributions of investments in schools and the agricultural reforms (or 'green revolutions') that occurred at the same time.

A second model, forwarded by the economist Jeffrey Sachs, proposes that aid projects be pooled in such a way that they synergise (Sachs 2006). For instance, in addition to a full stomach, learning is best achieved if students have a safe home environment, are healthy, have employment, and have a means of transport to school. It differs from the model described above in that it does not isolate or prioritise specific programmes and projects. This approach is typified by the Bolivar Health Center in the 1960s or the recent Millennium Villages Project (Geiger 2002).

This model has been derided by William Easterly as 'Utopian Social Engineering'. He argues that outsider meddling in others' practices are doomed to failure, equating it with 'IMF/World Bank-sponsored comprehensive reforms called "structural adjustment"' (Easterly 2006: 14). He points out that Professor Sachs has forwarded 449 interventions, but in trying to get any one accomplished, '[p]lanners are distracted by doing the other 448 interventions' (Easterly 2006: 6).

A final dominant model utilises an institutional approach to policymaking, to emphasise not the specific public health programmes to be implemented, but the ways in which local knowledge, incentives, and reform can be brought together for effective service delivery. For instance, one project in a poor county in Brazil managed to break through entrenched bureaucracy and cronyism to dramatically increase vaccination rates and public health service provision. It did so by creating competition between local governments on measures of efficacy and paying workers high wages for what was seen as important work, among other reforms. The downside of this approach is that it is difficult to bring to different cultural and development contexts.

Aid is harmful

A number of researchers and aid officials have come to believe that aid is harmful. This line of reasoning gained prominence in the 1960s with Milton Friedman and Peter Bauer. For instance, Friedman has argued that foreign aid 'strengthened governments that were already too powerful' (1991: 3). By this, he meant that aid was encouraging public investment rather than private, thereby limiting 'free trade' and economic growth. While ODA is the primary target of most critics, humanitarian aid provided by NGOs has also come into question (Carapico 2000; Gugerty *et al.* 2000).

Humanitarian assistance

One common argument regarding humanitarian assistance is that aid abdicates governments from their rightful responsibilities (Rahman 2006). If enough organisations are providing vaccinations, schooling, and primary health care, then the recipient government comes to believe that it no longer needs to provide these services. If true, this is problematic for a number of reasons. First, NGOs, which tend to be smaller in size and capacity, do not have the reach of governments. Therefore, a lot of poor areas will be left without service or serviced by a now neglected Ministry of Health. Second, NGOs tend not to coordinate with one another. Thus, when many NGOs provide schooling or health services, there is no way of ensuring that staff are trained in a consistent manner. Local curricula are replicated from scratch for each NGO, resulting in highly variable quality of service delivery and wasted resources. Third, different NGOs have very different missions, with many having religious backing. This can turn parents away when, for instance, a Christian organisation sets up a school in a predominantly Muslim area. Finally, humanitarian aid is highly dependent upon charitable trends in developed nations and foreign economic fluctuations. Given that the donors do not have their own children in these schools, there is little incentive to make sure that they remain viable.

Responding to such concerns, some NGOs have moved to work more closely with recipient governments. For instance, a health NGO might work through the Ministry of Health to improve coordination and service delivery. However, when delivered this way, such aid essentially becomes ODA, which has also been judged as harmful by some, especially in contexts with little governmental democratic accountability.

Official direct assistance

As with funding from smaller organisations, ODA can foster dependency, corruption, and poor governance. Dambisa Moyo argues that the responsibility for development be handed back to governments so that they can take charge of their own destiny (2009). Moyo's objective is to restate and update the ideas of Bauer and Easterly. For instance, she details hypothetical links between ODA and corruption. She argues that with market reform and autonomy, poor countries can naturally undergo economic development. Moyo sees debt forgiveness as a major source of this harm (because it provides the temptation to apply for loans and steal the proceeds) and sees stipulations attached to loans as problematic because 'conditionalities carry little punch' (Moyo 2009: 52).

The idea that ODA is harmful has also been forwarded by activists, who argue that financial interventions from the International Monetary Fund and the World Bank have done more harm than good (Klein 2001). They point out that during the 1997 Asian financial crisis, China, the one country that ignored the advice of the World Bank and the IMF, emerged from the crisis unscathed; the rest languished in recession for many years. Likewise, they place the blame for the Argentinean financial crisis of 1999 on the IMF. However, unlike Moyo, activists generally see the imposition of free market reforms (e.g. via the Washington Consensus) as the fundamental problem rather than the solution. For instance, they argue that free market reforms are only facially neutral, if at all. Moreover, they argue that reforms are often structured in ways that protect subsidies in the US and Europe, even as they require that poor nations rid themselves of similar subsidies. In contrast to Moyo, many activists argue that the solution is to forgive debt, terminate the use of donor-oriented and time-limited projects, allow for flexible budgets, and invite participatory decision-making.

Aside from this anecdotal evidence that aid produces harm, there is a body of research to support the claims of naysayers. For example, Hadjimichael (1995) and Reichel (1995) find a negative relationship between savings and aid, and Boone (1996) claims that aid has largely financed consumption rather than investment.

Generally, such researchers argue that free market and trade-oriented reforms will foster economic development, in contrast to human development-oriented approaches that empha-sise schools and public health projects (such as latrines and water purification projects). These studies, however, are largely based on weak ecological data. While the biggest aid recipients in sub-Saharan Africa have a dismal record of economic growth and human development, it is difficult to know whether aid recipients do poorly because they were weakly governed to begin with (and thus in the need for aid), or whether they experienced continued decline precisely because they received aid. Some organisations, such as Oxfam, have argued that 'trade not aid' approa-ches will fail until wealthy countries open their markets to poor ones, and so long as poor countries lack the infrastructure or markets needed to take advantage of trade opportunities (Watkins 2002).

Aid is poorly managed

Other development and health experts argue that global aid is not inherently harmful, rather, the key challenge lies in allocating aid in helpful, context-appropriate ways. While there are few comprehensive studies, development projects are often criticised both for mismanagement and for introducing disruptions and wage disparities to the local economy (Gasper 2000). Here, we provide one anecdote of the challenges faced in the field. One mid-sized aid project in the Sudan sought to hire a new Kenyan worker to conduct fieldwork and to help with adminis-trative tasks. The organisation, funded by the United States Agency for International Development (USAID), sought to hire a local person. Since there were no skilled locals available, the NGO settled for an African national, a Kenyan.

The organisation pays Western wages, a king's fortune to a Kenyan. This worker already owned a large business bought with past aid jobs, and was busy with the task of running it. Therefore, despite the fact that the foreign workers were putting in 80-hour weeks, the new hire demanded a 9-to-5 job and a light workload and got it. Of course, the ideal situation for many NGOs would be to have a highly trained and motivated local workforce who knew the landscape and culture and worked for local wages. That way, more aid can be delivered more effectively. The reality is too often the exact opposite of this ideal.

Management at all levels is a major challenge. The world's most highly trained managers tend not to want to work in poor nations for low wages. It is therefore difficult to recruit or even train good managers for aid work. This does not stop many aid agencies from hiring expensive consultants who are often unfamiliar with the local context, and who dole out advice that the aid agency has little capacity to incorporate.

Aid is misused

Too often, one-size-fits-all policies are applied with disastrous results both by ODA and humanitarian organisations. On the ODA side, critics point to how IMF officials imposed structural adjustment programmes, originally developed with rich nations in mind, onto poor nations that the decision-makers had, in many cases, never even visited. Such trends have led some practitioners to argue for sets of 'good' practices rather than donor-dictated 'best' ones (Feek 2007).

A persistent problem is the use of inappropriate technology. In 2009, the World Health Organization, among others, initiated a drive for universal primary health care in poor nations. While it is true that many nations can and should invest in primary health care, the poorest nations do not yet have the public health infrastructure in place. As a result, funding for primary health care systems will largely be spent treating illnesses that would have never happened if clean water, sanitation, vector control, and vaccination programmes were in place.

There is little question that aid can be better used, but the solutions are not easy to come by. There is not yet a clear cure for corruption, even in democratic nations. Moreover, ODA is still largely driven by political agendas, and humanitarian aid is driven by donor priorities, rather than the priorities of the governments receiving the aid.

All is well, just send more

In the three decades following the Korean War, South Korea received more aid from the US than any other country in the history of international aid. South Korea is now one of the most powerful nations on earth, both economically and in terms of its human capital. So too, some argue, could be nations in sub-Saharan Africa if only the aid package were large enough. Such critics assert that donor governments have consistently failed to meet the 0.7 per cent of GDP giving targets established at the United Nations General Assembly in 1970 (Hirvonen 2005).

While there are staunch camps, each with their strong beliefs about aid, the reality is that they are probably all partially correct. There are likely some countries that cannot absorb aid, there are leaders who would steal it, and others who would put it to good use. This highlights one of the most enduring problems associated with aid: the human tendency to overgeneralise a valuable hypothesis.

Notes

1 For more in-depth reading, see Amartya Sen's *Development as Freedom*, Paul Collier's *The Bottom Billion*, and 'Development in Dangerous Places' at the *Boston Review* http://bostonreview.net/BR34.4/ndf_development.php.
2 Here, we define 'political economy' simply, as the system of relationships between the state and political institutions, the market and other economic structures, laws, and civil society.

References

Barsky, R.B. and Kilian, L. (2002) 'Oil and the macroeconomy since the 1970s', *Journal of Economic Perspectives*, 18: 115–34.

Boone, P. (1996) 'Politics and the effectiveness of foreign aid', *European Economic Review*, 19 (3): 279–329.

Carapico, S. (2000) 'NGOs, INGOs, GO-NGOs and DO-NGOs: Making Sense of Non-Governmental Organizations', *Middle East Report*, 214: 12–15.

Dichter, T. (2003) *Despite Good Intentions: Why Development Assistance to the Third World Has Failed*, Amherst, MA: University of Massachusetts Press.

Easterlin, R. (1974) 'Does economic growth improve the human lot? Some empirical evidence', in P.A. David and M.W. Reder (eds), *Nations and Households in Economic Growth*, New York: Academic Press.

Easterly, W.R. (2006) *The White Man's Burden: Why the West's Efforts to Aid the Rest Have Done So Much Ill and So Little Good*, New York: Penguin Press.

Farmer, P. (2004) *Pathologies of Power: Health, Human Rights, and the New War on the Poor*, Berkeley, CA: University of California Press.

Feek, W. (2007) 'Best of practices?', *Development in Practice*, 17: 653–5.

Friedman, M. (1991) *Economic Freedom, Human Freedom, Political Freedom*, available at http://www.cbe.csueastbay.edu/~sbesc/frlect.html (accessed 29 July 2009).

Gaidzanwa, R. (1999) *Voting With Their Feet: Migrant Zimbabwean Nurses and Doctors in the Era of Structural Adjustment*, Uppsala: Nordic Africa Institute.

Gasper, D. (2000) 'Anecdotes, Situations, Histories-Varieties and Uses of Cases in Thinking about Ethics and Development Practice', *Development and Change*, 31: 1,055–83.

Geiger, H.J. (2002) 'Community-oriented primary care: A path to community development', *American Journal of Public Health*, 92: 1,713–6.

Gugerty, M., Kremer, M., Center, L., and Floor, T. (2000) *Outside Funding of Community Organizations: Benefiting or Displacing the Poor?*, National Bureau for Economic Research (NBER), Working Paper No. W7896, Cambridge, MA: NBER.

Hadjimichael, M.T.D, Ghura, D., Mulheisen, M., Nord, R., and Ucer, E.M. (1995) *Sub-Saharan Africa: Growth, Savings, and Investment 1986–93*, Occasional Paper 118, Washington, DC: International Monetary Fund.

Harsanyi, J.C. (1953) 'Cardinal utility in welfare economics and in the theory of risk-taking', *The Journal of Political Economy*, 61: 434.

Hirvonen, P. (2005) *Stingy Samaritans: Why Recent Increases in Development Aid fail to Help the Poor*, New York: Global Policy Forum, available at http://www.globalpolicy.org/home/240/45056.html (accessed 1 March 2010).

Klein, N. (2001) 'Reclaiming the commons', *New Left Review*, 9: 81–9.

Maimbo, S. and Ratha, D. (2005) *Remittances: Development Impact and Future Prospects*, Washington, DC: World Bank Publications.

Michel, S., Beuret, M., and Woods, P. (2009) *China Safari: On the Trail of Beijing's Expansion in Africa*, New York: Nation Books.

Moghadam, V. (1999) 'Gender and globalization: Female labor and womens mobilization', *Journal of World Systems Research*, 5: 367–88.

Moyo, D. (2009) *Dead Aid*, New York: Farrar, Straus and Giroux.

Rahman, S. (2006) 'Development, democracy and the NGO sector: Theory and evidence from Bangladesh', *Journal of Developing Societies*, 22: 451.

Reichel, R. (1995) 'Development aid, savings and growth in the 1980s: A cross-sectional analysis', *Savings and Development*, 19: 279–96.

Root, H. (2008) *Alliance Curse: How America Lost the Third World*, Washington, DC: Brookings Institution Press.

Sachs, J.D. (2006) *The End of Poverty: Economic Possibilities for Our Time*, New York: Penguin.

Schlesinger, S. and Kinzer, S. (1982) *Bitter Fruit: The Story of the American Coup in Guatemala*, New York: Doubleday and Company.

Sen, A. (1999) *Development as Freedom*, New York: Knopf.

Strauss, J. and Thomas, D. (1998) 'Health, nutrition, and economic development', *Journal of Economic Literature*, 36: 766–817.

UN (United Nations) (2006) *United Nations Millennium Project: Offical Development Assistance in 2005*, available at http://www.unmillenniumproject.org/press/07.htm (accessed 21 December 2009).

Watkins, K. (2002) 'Last chance in Monterrey: Meeting the challenge of poverty reduction', Oxfam Briefing Paper No. 17, Oxford: Oxfam International.

Williamson, J. (1993) 'Democracy and the "Washington Consensus"', *World Development*, 21: 1,329–36.

WHO (World Health Organization) (2000) *World Health Report 2000—Health Systems: Improving Performance*, Geneva: WHO, available at http://www.who.int/whr/2000/en/index.html (accessed 24 July 2008).

Wu, C., Maurer, C., Wang, Y., Xue, S., and Davis, D.L. (1999) 'Water pollution and human health in China', *Environmental Health Perspectives*, 107: 251–6.

29

Global Tobacco Control Policy

Heather Wipfli and Jonathan M. Samet

While the health risks of tobacco smoking have been known for decades, the pandemic of tobacco use continues. There are now an estimated 1.3 billion smokers worldwide, along with hundreds of millions more who use oral tobacco products (WHO 2008). The attributable disease burden is enormous – about 6 million premature deaths worldwide each year – and is projected to grow substantially across the twenty-first century (WHO 2002). While the global tobacco epidemic continues to grow, great progress has been made in tobacco control in some countries, primarily in North America and Western Europe, where smoking rates have dropped by about 50 per cent over the last four decades; mortality rates from several smoking-caused diseases, including lung cancer and coronary heart disease (CHD), are declining; and smoke-free initiatives are protecting non-smokers from inhaling second-hand smoke (SHS). The World Health Organization's (WHO) Framework Convention on Tobacco Control (FCTC), a global public health treaty incorporating best practices in tobacco control, now provides a foundation for other regions to follow.

This chapter provides an overview of global tobacco control policy. After reviewing the global burden of disease caused by smoking, the chapter focuses on evidence-based approaches to controlling tobacco use and describes the process through which the FCTC was developed. The chapter ends with a consideration of the policy challenges that remain. The chapter can only briefly consider the many elements of this broad topic; for greater depth, we recommend the historical perspectives on the epidemic and the tobacco industry provided by Kluger and Brandt in their books (Brandt 2007; Kluger 1996), the comprehensive reviews of health effects provided in the US surgeon-general's reports (US DHHS 2004, 2006), the monograph series published by the US National Cancer Institute, and publications of the WHO Tobacco Free Initiative (TFI), including the recent MPOWER reports (WHO 2008, 2009). The journal *Tobacco Control* provides up-to-date coverage of research and news.

Background: the global burden of tobacco use and disease

Patterns and practices of tobacco use vary around the globe. Cigarette use began to rise in high-income countries in the early 1900s after the newly industrialised and centralised tobacco industry instituted its effective marketing methods. Fortunately, the peak of tobacco consumption has passed in most high-income countries, where male and female prevalence rates have been declining for decades. In 2008, the percentage of Americans who smoke cigarettes dropped below 20 per cent, while teen smoking fell to the lowest levels in over 15 years (CDC 2008b). Similarly, prevalence rates in the United Kingdom reached 22 per cent in 2008 (ASH 2008). In many Northern, Southern, and Western European countries, the prevalence of smoking in men has also fallen over the past 25 years (Peto and Lopez 2004). As a consequence, lung cancer deaths in men decreased in many European countries between 1985 and 2000 (Boyle *et al.* 2003).

Around the world, tobacco use patterns vary by income level and location. Many low- and middle-income countries have lagged approximately 40 years behind high-income countries. The rise in tobacco prevalence in low- and middle-income countries was largely due to the complete transformation, centralisation, and further globalisation of the tobacco industry between 1970 and 1998, and the active search for new markets as a result of declining tobacco use in high-income countries. Because of industry penetration and aggressive marketing, smoking prevalence rates among men in many middle-income countries approached and exceeded 50 per cent by 2000.

Men in Asia have had particularly high cigarette smoking rates. In some Asian countries (China, South Korea, and Japan, for example), a majority of men have long been cigarette smokers, reflecting the widespread acceptability of smoking and its ingrained social roles. A majority of all young men in China still become persistent smokers in a country with an estimated 350 million smokers (Liu *et al.* 1998; Niu *et al.* 1998; Peto *et al.* 1999). In India,

Table 29.1 Adverse effects from exposure to tobacco smoke

Health effect	SGR 1984	SGR 1986	EPA 1992	Cal/EPA 1997	UK 1998	WHO 1999	IARC 2004	Cal/EPA* 2005	SGR 2006
Increased prevalence of chronic respiratory symptoms	Yes/a	Yes/a	Yes/c	Yes/c	Yes/c	Yes/c		Yes/c	Yes/c
Decrement in pulmonary function	Yes/a	Yes/a	Yes/a	Yes/a		Yes/c		Yes/a	Yes/c
Increased occurrence of acute respiratory illnesses	Yes/a	Yes/a	Yes/a	Yes/c		Yes/c		Yes/c	Yes/c
Increased occurrence of middle ear disease		Yes/a	Yes/c	Yes/c	Yes/c	Yes/c		Yes/c	Yes/c
Increased severity of asthma episodes and symptoms			Yes/c	Yes/c		Yes/c		Yes/c	Yes/c
Risk factor for new asthma			Yes/a	Yes/c				Yes/c	Yes/c
Risk factor for SIDS				Yes/c	Yes/a	Yes/c		Yes/c	Yes/c
Risk factor for lung cancer in adults		Yes/c	Yes/c	Yes/c	Yes/c		Yes/c	Yes/c	Yes/c
Risk factor for breast cancer for younger, primarily postmenopausal women								Yes/c	
Risk factor for nasal sinus cancer								Yes/c	
Risk factor for heart disease in adults				Yes/c	Yes/c			Yes/c	Yes/c

Yes/a = association; Yes/c = cause.
SGR 1984: US Department of Health and Human Services (1984); SGR 1986: US Department of Health and Human Services (1986); EPA 1992: US Environmental Protection Agency (1992); Cal/EPA 1997: California Environmental Protection Agency and Office of Environmental Health Hazard Assessment (1997); UK 1998: Scientific Committee on Tobacco and Health and HSMO (1998); WHO 1999: World Health Organization (1999); IARC 2004: International Agency for Research on Cancer (2004); Cal/EPA 2005: California Environmental Protection Agency and Air Resources Board (2005); SGR 2006: US Department of Health and Human Services (2006).
*Only effects causally associated with SHS exposure are included.
Source: Adapted from Samet *et al.* 2009.

approximately 51 per cent of men and 10 per cent of women use some form of tobacco, totalling an estimated 250 million tobacco users (Reddy and Gupta 2004).

Globally, 40 per cent of smokers live in just four countries; China, India, Indonesia, and Russia. China, with 20 per cent of the world's population, produces and consumes about 30 per cent of the world's cigarettes. However, even the small countries are targets for the tobacco industry.

Efforts to reduce tobacco use are based on irrefutable evidence that it causes death and disease in humans. The diseases caused by smoking include those sites directly reached by inhaled smoke and sites affected by circulating or excreted tobacco smoke components or metabolites. The list of diseases caused by smoking is extensive. It includes specific diseases of most organ systems: major categories include cancer, cardiovascular disease, and chronic obstructive pulmonary disease, as well as adverse reproductive outcomes (Hecht and Samet 2007). A now-substantial body of evidence has also identified diseases and other adverse effects caused by passive smoking (Table 29.1).

Global estimates from 2002 placed the mortality burden from smoking at over 6 million deaths annually. Lung cancer deaths exceeded 1 million, but the largest contributors were deaths from cardiovascular and respiratory diseases (Table 29.2). The main diseases by which smoking prematurely kills people differ across the world because of varying background rates of disease (e.g. tuberculosis). However, regardless of geography, approximately 50 per cent of persistent tobacco smokers will die prematurely from their addiction (Peto and Lopez 2004).

Fundamental tobacco control approaches

Modern tobacco control efforts largely date back to the 1962 Royal College Report in the UK and first US surgeon-general's report in 1964, both entitled 'Smoking and Health' (Royal College of Physicians of London 1962; US Department of Health Education and Welfare

Table 29.2 Projected global tobacco-caused deaths, by cause, 2015 baseline scenario

Cause	Tobacco-caused deaths	
	Number (millions)	*Per cent of total*
All causes	6.43	100
Tuberculosis	0.09	1
Lower respiratory infections	0.15	2
Malignant neoplasms	2.12	33
Trachea, bronchus, lung cancers	1.18	18
Mouth and oropharynx cancers	0.18	3
Esophagus cancer	0.17	3
Stomach cancer	0.12	2
Liver cancer	0.10	2
Other malignant neoplasms	0.34	5
Diabetes mellitus	0.13	2
Cardiovascular diseases	1.86	29
Ischemic heart disease	0.93	14
Cerebrovascular disease	0.52	8
Other cardiovascular diseases	0.24	4
Respiratory diseases	1.87	29
COPD	1.76	27
Digestive diseases	0.20	3

Source: Adapted from Mathers and Loncar 2006.

1964). These reports concluded that cigarette smoking is causally related to lung cancer, and recommended action to control its use. National experiences have since generated an extensive evidence base that documents the most effective policy approaches.

Taxation

Increasing the price of tobacco through higher taxes has been found to be the single most cost-effective way to decrease consumption and encourage users to quit (WHO 2008). Increasing tobacco taxes by 10 per cent generally decreases consumption by 4 per cent in high-income countries and by about 8 per cent in low- and middle-income countries (WHO 2008). Higher taxes are most effective for reducing smoking by the young and the poor. It has been estimated that a 70 per cent increase in the price of tobacco could prevent up to a quarter of all smoking-related deaths worldwide (WHO 2008).

Tobacco taxes are generally accepted by the public and policymakers. However, the tobacco industry fights against tax increases with economic arguments, including the proposal that higher taxes decrease government revenues and hurt the poor, who are more likely to smoke. Although the impact of taxes is slightly higher in low- and middle-income countries, experience has shown that government revenues still do not decrease for the short term after a tax increase. In South Africa, for example, every 10 per cent increase in excise tax on cigarettes has been associated with an approximate 6 per cent increase in cigarette excise revenues (WHO 2008). Tax increases can also benefit the poor if they are used to help smokers quit and allow them to reallocate money to essential goods, increase their productivity, and decrease their medical costs. More recently, the revenues raised by tobacco taxes have been used to fund tobacco control and other health and social programmes. In Thailand, for example, an earmarked tax on tobacco and alcohol is used to fund the Thai Health Foundation, which carries out health promotion activities throughout the country.

The industry often argues that higher taxes will lead to greater smuggling. In 2002, it was estimated that around one quarter of internationally traded cigarettes entered the black market, making cigarettes the world's most widely smuggled legal consumer product (WHO 2002). However, tax differentials between countries are a relatively small part of the smuggling problem and the costs of improved law enforcement and border security to control the problem only add up to a fraction of the additional revenue that could be earned from taxes. In 2000, for example, governments around the world were estimated to lose out on collecting US $25–30 billion annually in tax revenue due to cigarette smuggling (Jha and Chaloupka 2000).

Indoor smoking bans

The widespread movement to restrict indoor smoking began in the 1980s with credible scientific evidence on passive smoking and disease risk and powerful conclusions on the causation of disease by the US surgeon-general and various organisations (US DHHS 1986). This movement gained momentum throughout the 1990s. In 1999, California became the first state in the US to become completely smoke-free in all public places; now, ten years later, over 70 per cent of the US population is covered by comprehensive smoke-free legislation (American Nonsmokers' Rights Foundation 2006). In 2005, Ireland became the first country to ban smoking in all public places, and a growing number of countries have followed.

The speed at which new comprehensive smoke-free policies have been passed is due in large part to the popularity of complete bans among the public, and the evidence base showing that smoke-free legislation is effective in reducing exposure and improving the health of non-smokers, as well as reducing consumption levels and encouraging cessation among smokers (US DHHS 2006). Moreover, evidence from experience with the growing number of public smoking bans indicates that smoke-free legislation does not negatively affect revenues of the hospitality industry (Scollo et al. 2003).

As early as the 1970s, the industry was aware that policies restricting or ending smoking in public places would severely undermine the social acceptability of smoking and create an environment that would foster cessation and discourage young people from starting (Drope and Chapman 2001). The industry has criticised the scientific evidence and attempted to retain controversy regarding the health effects of second-hand smoke (SHS), the extent of exposures, and the effectiveness and costs of controlling it (Drope et al. 2004). Recently, the tobacco industry has resisted complete bans by promoting a strategy of 'accommodation' built on the idea that extensive ventilation and air cleaning can allow both smokers to smoke and non-smokers to have clean air. Scientific evidence, however, indicates that such ventilation strategies are unable to remove the toxic components of SHS from the air (Samet et al. 2005).

Health warnings and mass media campaigns

Fifty years after the US surgeon-general concluded that smoking causes lung cancer, relatively few tobacco users worldwide fully understand the health risks associated with their addiction. The extreme addictiveness and the range of health dangers have not been effectively communicated to the public (WHO 2008). Strong health warnings on tobacco packaging and counter-advertising campaigns have been found to be effective in educating the public and convincing users to quit (National Cancer Institute 2008).

Health warnings on cigarette packages were among the very first governmental strategies employed to inform the public about the dangers of tobacco use. In the 1960 and 1970s, a number of countries required health warnings reading 'Caution: Cigarette smoking may be hazardous to your health' to be placed on all cigarette packages. In the mid-1980s, health warnings were revised in a number of countries to include disease specific warnings such as 'Smoking causes lung cancer, heart disease, emphysema, and may complicate pregnancy'. In 2000, Canada became the first country to require that graphic images be included on all warning labels.

By 2005, cigarette packages in virtually every country carried health warnings, yet the size, number, and manner of presentation differed notably between countries (Hammond et al. 2006). The WHO recommends that to be effective, warnings should be large, clear and legible, include both pictures and words in the principal languages of the country, cover at least half of the pack's main display areas, and describe specific illnesses caused by tobacco use (WHO 2008). Evidence indicates that health warnings on tobacco packages increase awareness of the risks of smoking; in addition, the use of pictures of disease have a greater impact than words alone, and are critical in reaching the large number of illiterate people in the world. Pictures have been found to be especially effective in conveying messages to the children of tobacco users, who are the most likely to start using tobacco (WHO 2008).

The tobacco industry has tried to avoid and weaken health warning proposals for decades. Initially, the industry focused on keeping warnings as general and inconspicuous as possible. More recently, the industry's opposition to health warning legislation has had less to do with the content of the message than the required size and placement of the warnings and the impact that they may have on the overall look of cigarette packs. An infamous industry quote by Ludo Cremers, divisional vice president of marketing for Brown and Williamson Tobacco Corp. reads, 'If they reject your pack, they reject your brand' (Adams 2002). The industry has argued that by disrupting the image of their packaging, the warnings violate trademark provisions. In Europe, the industry sued the European Commission (EC) in the European Court of Justice (ECJ), claiming that by allowing EU countries to adopt graphic health warnings the EC had violated their trademark rights. The ECJ ruling upheld the right of states to adopt graphic health warnings (European Court of Justice 2002).

Counter-advertising campaigns, although expensive, are another way to inform the public about the harms of tobacco use. The US Centers for Disease Control and Prevention (CDC) recommends that governments generally spend US $2–4 per person annually on anti-tobacco health communication (WHO 2008). In some low-income countries, this investment will likely have to be shared with non-governmental partners.

Advertising bans

Throughout the first half of the twentieth century, tobacco was heavily advertised in high-income countries. The advertising was intended to associate cigarettes with youth, freedom, glamour, and sex appeal. Restrictions on tobacco product advertising first began in the 1960s, when a number of countries banned advertisements on television. A few countries, such as Sweden, Norway, Finland, and Singapore, have had comprehensive bans in place since the 1970s, while most high-income countries have increasingly restricted tobacco advertising across more and more media (Saffer 2000). Most recently, efforts to denormalise tobacco use have focused on removing tobacco use and product placement from films. Until the late 1990s, most low- and middle-income countries had not followed with similar, broad bans on advertising.

Banning advertising is an effective policy to reduce tobacco use, but evidence suggests that the bans must be comprehensive. Most econometric studies have found that increased expenditure on advertising increases demand for cigarettes, while banning advertising leads to a reduction in consumption (Andrews and Franke 1991; Lynch and Bonnie 1994; National Cancer Institute 2008; Roemer 2003). The World Bank reviewed the international evidence regarding the effects of cigarette advertising and concluded that advertising increases cigarette consumption, and that legislation ending advertising would reduce consumption provided that it is comprehensive, covering all media and uses of brand names and logos (Jha and Chaloupka 1999). Partial advertising bans allow the tobacco industry to focus on other unbanned mediums, such as newspapers and the internet, or to convert advertising expenditures to sponsorship of events such as races, sports, and music festivals.

The tobacco industry uses a number of arguments against advertising bans. One frequent argument is that advertising is targeted at current smokers to switch brands, it does not affect overall consumption, and it does not entice youngsters to start smoking. However, industry documents from the early 1970s confirm that advertising has 'a statistically significant effect on the expansion of sales' (McGuiness and Cowling 1975: 327), and youth are crucial to replace ageing and dying smokers. The US industry also defended the argument that it has the right to market a legal product all the way to the US Supreme Court, which in 2000 ruled in favour of the industry (US Supreme Court 2001). The industry also argues that tobacco advertising makes a significant contribution to the economies in which it operates. In 2003, cigarette companies spent $15.2 billion on advertising and promotional expenses in the US (CDC 2009). The money spent on advertising not only encourages tobacco use but also creates a more favourable media environment for the industry and prevents hostile editorial comment. A

1978 industry survey in the US concluded that: 'advertising revenue can indeed silence the editors of American magazines' (Smith 1978: 31).

Cessation services

To have an immediate impact on the smoking-attributable disease burden, tobacco control strategies need to include effective cessation modalities. One consistent finding among tobacco users in high-income countries is their desire to quit. The majority (67 per cent) of cigarette smokers in Britain say they want to stop smoking (Office for National Statistics 2009). In the US, the proportion of current everyday smokers who tried to quit in 2007 was 53.1 per cent among persons aged 18–24 years, 39.9 per cent among those aged 25–44 years, 38.1 per cent among those aged 45–64 years, and 25.3 per cent among those aged over 65 years (CDC 2008a). In 2007, the success rate of smoking cessation among young American adults was 8.5 per cent compared to 5.0 per cent in older adults (Messer et al. 2008). Since 2002, former smokers have outnumbered current smokers in the US (CDC 2008b).

However, cessation rates in low- and middle-income countries remain very low. In China, for example, less than 11 per cent of smokers have ever tried to stop smoking, and only 2 per cent have succeeded (Yang et al. 2001). However, data indicate that a majority of current youth smokers in low- and middle-income countries want to stop smoking and have already tried to quit, although very few youth who currently smoke have ever attended a cessation programme (Global Youth Tobacco Survey Collaborating Group 2002).

Current treatment options include various methods, from simple medical advice to pharmacotherapy, along with telephone help lines and counselling. However, the options available to smokers vary greatly depending on their country. The WHO recommends that three treatment types be included in national tobacco control efforts: (1) tobacco cessation advice incorporated into primary health care services; (2) easily accessible and free quit lines; and (3) access to low-cost pharmacological therapy (WHO 2008).

A global approach: the framework convention on tobacco control and MPOWER

By the mid-1990s, social, economic, and political globalisation began to have an ever-greater impact on national tobacco control efforts. In Singapore, for example, the effectiveness of the advertising ban in place since 1970 began to weaken as advertising from neighbouring Malaysia increasingly crossed the border via electronic media. There was also a growing awareness about the growing public health tragedy on the rise as a result of the global assault by transnational tobacco companies. It became increasingly clear to tobacco control advocates that exporting national experiences from high-income countries to low- and middle-income countries was not enough to counter an unregulated global tobacco industry.

In 1994, at the 9th World Conference on Tobacco or Health, a resolution was passed calling on the WHO to initiate negotiations on an international tobacco treaty. Only two years later, the WHO member states answered this call and adopted, by consensus, a resolution leading towards accelerated multilateral negotiations on a framework convention on tobacco control and possible relating protocols (WHO 1999). The FCTC process marked the first time that the member states of the WHO enacted the organisation's power to negotiate and sign a binding treaty aimed at protecting and promoting public health. It also represented the first time that states cooperated worldwide to respond to the causation of avoidable chronic disease.

The FCTC was developed as a scientific, evidence-based approach to tobacco control. The World Bank's 1999 publication *Curbing the Epidemic*, which identified the cost-effective interventions that enhance revenues and promote health, provided perhaps the single most important tool in preparing for the negotiations (Jha and Chaloupka 1999). The FCTC working group, created to consolidate the scientific evidence for the convention, cited the World Bank report as the empirical evidence supporting the demand-reduction strategies proposed (WHO 2006).

The FCTC negotiations took place between 2000 and 2003. Six formal negotiating sessions were held during the period, in addition to regional negotiating sessions and technical conferences. Over 170 states participated in at least one of the negotiating sessions. Throughout the negotiations, WHO, NGOs, and individual states held seminars on technical aspects of the convention and distributed information to delegates. The technical seminars and the distribution of information over the years evolved into what Dr Derek Yach, former WHO executive director for Non-Communicable Disease and Mental Health, has called 'the best university of global tobacco control' (Simpson 2003).

In May, 2003, the WHO member states unanimously adopted the FCTC final text. Many universal elements of national tobacco control policy became core provisions of the FCTC final text, including a comprehensive ban on tobacco advertising, promotion, and sponsorship; a ban on misleading descriptors that convince smokers that certain products are safer than standard cigarettes ('lights'); and a mandate to place rotating warnings that cover at least 30 per cent of tobacco packaging, with encouragement for even larger, graphic warnings.

The FCTC entered into force in February 2005 after 40 countries had ratified the treaty. By mid-2009, over 160 nations had ratified the treaty, making it one of the most widely accepted UN treaties. Governments around the world have adopted new tobacco control measures to better align themselves with the treaty's goals. New Zealand, for example, increased its health warning to come into compliance with the FCTC, and the Indian parliament responded to the FCTC by passing the Cigarettes and Other Tobacco Products Act of 2003. Many countries, however, still lack the political will and domestic capacity to effectively implement the treaty.

Building on the FCTC process, WHO released its first 'Report on Control of the Tobacco Epidemic', entitled 'MPOWER', in 2008 (WHO 2008). MPOWER stands for a set of six key tobacco control measures that reflect and build on the policy approaches embedded within the WHO FCTC and that were outlined above. The initial report, which surveyed tobacco control policies worldwide, concluded that no country has carried out all of the tobacco control measures necessary to forestall illness and that only 5 per cent of the world's population resides in countries fully protecting residents with any one of the crucial measures to reduce smoking rates. The second MPOWER report released in 2009 found only slight progress over the first year that MPOWER was implemented (WHO 2009).

Future challenges

Despite progress within many countries and at the international level, there is still much work to be done in addressing the global tobacco epidemic. Having made national commitments to tobacco control, as evidenced by ratification of the FCTC, most low- and middle-income countries still do not have the national infrastructure and resources in place to effectively implement the called-upon measures. Even in some countries where the necessary infrastructure does exist, the needed resources have not been obligated to prevent further tobacco-related death and disease among their own populations.

Experiences in several countries show that a few trained and committed tobacco control professionals can have substantial impact. However, within many low- and middle-income countries there is not even one individual working full-time on tobacco control, and public health capacity in general is too often weak (Samet *et al*. 1998). All countries must build a core of tobacco control professionals and institutions that will sustain tobacco control initiatives for decades to come. A number of capacity-building programmes have been carried out throughout the world, but the development of technological infrastructure to sustain in-country programmes is needed.

Further research is needed in a number of countries on the applicability and effectiveness of a range of internationally promoted policies. For example, in India, a tax increase may simply prompt smokers to switch from higher cost cigarettes to far cheaper bidis. Longer-term research initiatives need to focus on the cessation and harm reduction issues. In regards to cessation, traditional approaches to the packaging and marketing of pharmacological products for smoking cessation will not be viable for the majority of smokers who are poor, live in low- and middle-income countries, and cannot afford the treatments that have been developed. Even if they could afford the products, they lack awareness and understanding of how they could help with cessation. Different cultural norms and economic realities will necessitate altered delivery mechanisms that are appropriate locally, as has been the case in high-income countries.

Many tobacco control advocates remain highly sceptical of the potential benefits and pitfalls of harm reduction, including global regulation and product testing. Product testing strategies might be feasible in countries like the US, where tobacco is largely used in the form of manufactured cigarettes and only a few companies sell cigarettes. By contrast, there are numerous products in India for which testing methods have not yet been developed and for which the test compounds and biomarkers have not been established. Replacing cigarette smoking with oral tobacco products has been proposed as a method of reducing health risks among cigarette smokers. Swedish snus, a moist snuff low in tobacco-specific nitrosamines, has received particular attention because it has been widely used in Sweden, apparently with little increase in population risks for cancer and cardiovascular disease (Roosaar *et al*. 2008). However, there is concern that strategies to introduce lower-risk products will diminish efforts to promote prevention and cessation. Despite these challenges, science-based guidance will be needed in the regulation and communication about the diverse tobacco market in the future, and the unfolding US regulatory experience through the Food and Drug Administration (FDA) will undoubtedly inform any future global regulatory system.

Towards a tobacco-free world

Effective tobacco control policy approaches have resulted in declining smoking rates in many countries, smoke-free cities, states, and countries, and an international treaty, ratified by most nations, that obligates tobacco control. These remarkable outcomes were driven by credible scientific evidence, a global industry in need of regulation, strong champions, and information-sharing between countries at multiple levels.

Fundamental questions related to the impact of globalisation on health and to the responsibility for governance are perhaps no better illustrated than in the case of tobacco. Lessons learned from the tobacco control story can, and should, be used to inform control strategies for other emerging chronic disease epidemics, including obesity. At the same time, much hard work lies ahead to continue to change behaviour and social norms around tobacco. The health and economic benefits of tobacco control will depend on the effective implementation of comprehensive policy approaches in all countries, including higher taxes, indoor smoking bans, effective warning labels, large mass media, and comprehensive bans on tobacco advertising, including smoking on television and in films. Such policies and programmes will prevent youth from starting to smoke, drive the demand for effective cessation products, and lead us to achieve the full health and economic gains of tobacco control. With its nations working together, the world can end the tobacco problem.

References

ASH (Action on Smoking and Health) (2008) *Essential Information 01: Smoking Statistics: Who Smokes and How Much*, London: ASH.

Adams, B. (2002) 'B&W CEO Reveals Plans for Company', *Business First of Louisville*, 6 May 2002, available at http://louisville.bizjournals.com/louisville/stories/2002/05/06/daily9.html (accessed 26 March 2010).

American Nonsmokers' Rights Foundation (2006) *Summary of 100% Smokefree State Laws and Population Protected by 100% U.S. Smokefree Laws*, available at http://www.no-smoke.org/pdf/SummaryUS PopList.pdf (accesed 18 February 2009).

Andrews, R.L. and Franke, G.R. (1991) 'The determinants of cigarette consumption: a meta-analysis', *Journal of Public Policy and Marketing*, 10(1): 81–100.

Boyle, P., d'Onofrio, A., Maisonneuve, P., Severi, G., Robertson, C., Tubiana, M., and Veronesi, U. (2003) 'Measuring progress against cancer in Europe: has the 15% decline targeted for 2000 come about?' *Annals of Oncology*, 14(8): 1,312–25.

Brandt, A.M. (2007) *The Cigarette Century: The Rise, Fall, and Deadly Persistence of the Product That Defined America*, New York, Basic Books.

CDC (Centers for Disease Control and Prevention) (2008a) 'Cigarette smoking among adults: United States, 2007', *MMWR Morbidity and Mortality Weekly Report*, 57(45): 1,221–6

CDC (Centers for Disease Control and Prevention) (2008b) 'Smoking-attributable mortality, years of potential life lost, and productivity losses: United States, 2000–2004', *MMWR Morbidity and Mortality Weekly Report*, 57(45): 1,226–8.

CDC (Centers for Disease Control and Prevention) (2009) *Fact Sheet: Tobacco Industry Marketing*, available at http://www.cdc.gov/tobacco/data_statistics/fact_sheets/tobaccoindustry/marketing/index.htm (accessed 25 March 2010).

Drope, J. and Chapman, S. (2001) 'Tobacco industry efforts at discrediting scientific knowledge of environmental tobacco smoke: a review of internal industry documents', *Journal of Epidemiology and Community Health*, 55(8): 588–94.

Drope, J., Bialous, S.A., and Glantz, S.A. (2004) 'Tobacco industry efforts to present ventilation as an alternative to smoke-free environments in North America', *Tobacco Control*, 13(Supplement 1): i41–i47.

European Court of Justice (2002) *Judgment of the Court on the Validity and Interpretation of Directive 2001/37/EC – Manufacture, Presentation and Sale of Tobacco Products*, available at http://curia.europa.eu/jurisp/cgi-bin/gettext.pl?lang=en&num=79978789C19010491&doc=T&ouvert=T&seance=ARRET (accessed 25 March 2010).

Global Youth Tobacco Survey Collaborating Group (2002) 'Tobacco use among youth: a cross country comparison', *Tobacco Control*, 11(3): 252–70.

Hammond, D., Collishaw, N.E., and Callard, C. (2006) 'Secret science: tobacco industry research on smoking behaviour and cigarette toxicity', *The Lancet*, 367(9,512): 781–7.

Hecht, S.S. and Samet, J.M. (2007) 'Cigarette smoking', in W.M. Rom, *Environmental and Occupational Medicine*, 4th edn, Philadelphia, PA: Wolters Kluwer/Lippincott Williams & Wilkins.

Jha, P. and Chaloupka, F.J. (1999) *Curbing the Epidemic: Governments and the Economics of Tobacco Control*, Washington, DC: World Bank.

Jha, P. and Chaloupka, F. (eds) (2000) *Tobacco Control in Developing Countries*, Washington, DC and New York: World Bank and World Health Organization.

Kluger, R. (1996) *Ashes to Ashes: America's Hundred-Year Cigarette War, the Public Health, and the Unabashed Triumph of Philip Morris*, New York, Alfred A. Knopf.

Liu, B.Q., Peto, R., Chen, Z.M., Boreham, J., Wu, Y.P., Li, J.Y., Campbell, T.C., and Chen, J.S. (1998) 'Emerging tobacco hazards in China: 1. Retrospective proportional mortality study of one million deaths', *British Medical Journal*, 317(7,170): 1,411–22

Lynch, B.S. and Bonnie, R.J. (1994) *Growing Up Tobacco Free: Preventing Nicotine Addiction in Children and Youths*, Washington, DC: Institute of Medicine, National Academy Press.

McGuiness, T. and Cowling, K. (1975) 'Advertising and the aggregate demand for cigarettes', *European Economic* Review, 6 (3): 311–28.

Mathers, C.D. and Loncar, D. (2006) 'Projections of global mortality and burden of disease from 2002 to 2030', *PLoS Medicine*, 3(11): e442.

Messer, K., Trinidad, D.R., Al-Delaimy, W.K., and Pierce, J.P. (2008) 'Smoking cessation rates in the United States: a comparison of young adult and older smokers', *American Journal of Public Health*, 98(2): 317–22.

National Cancer Institute (2008) 'The role of the media in promoting and reducing tobacco use', *Tobacco Control Monograph No. 19., Bethesda, MD: U.S. Department of Health and Human Services, National Institutes of Health, National Cancer Institute*.

National Cancer Institute (2009) *Tobacco Control Monograph Series: Public Health Issues in Smoking and Tobacco Use Control*, available at http://cancercontrol.cancer.gov/tcrb/monographs/index.html (accessed 9 February 2009).

Niu, S.R., Yang, G.H., Chen, Z.M., Wang, J.L., Wang, G.H., He, X.Z., Schoepff, H., Boreham, J., Pan, H.C., and Peto, R. (1998) 'Emerging tobacco hazards in China: 2. Early mortality results from a prospective study', *British Medical Journal*, 317: 1423–4.

Office for National Statistics (2009) *Opinions Survey Report No.40: Smoking-Related Behaviour and Attitudes*, 2008/09, Newport, South Wales: Office for National Statistics.

Peto, R., Chen, Z.M., and Boreham, J. (1999) 'Tobacco: the growing epidemic', *Nature Medicine*, 5(1): 15–7.

Peto, R. and Lopez, A.D. (2004) 'The future worldwide health effects of current smoking patterns', in P. Boyle, N. Gray, J. Henningfield, J. Seffrin and W. Zatonski, *Tobacco: Science, Policy and Public Health*, Oxford: Oxford University Press.

Reddy, K.S. and Gupta, P.C. (eds) (2004) *Report on Tobacco Control in India*, Mumbai: Ministry of Health & Family Welfare.

Roemer, R. (2003) *Legislative Action to Combat the World Tobacco Epidemic*, Geneva: World Health Organization.

Roosaar, A., Johansson, A.L., Sandborgh-Englund, G., Axell, T., and Nyren, O. (2008) 'Cancer and mortality among users and nonusers of snus', *International Journal of Cancer*, 123(1): 168–73.

Royal College of Physicians of London (1962) *Smoking and Health: Summary of a Report of the Royal College of Physicians of London on Smoking in Relation to Cancer of the Lung and Other Diseases*, London: Pitman Medical Publishing Co.

Saffer, H. (2000) 'Tobacco advertising and promotion', in P. Jha and F. Chaloupka, *Tobacco Control in Developing Countries*, New York: Oxford University Press.

Samet, J.M., Yach, D., Taylor, C., and Becker, K. (1998) 'Research for effective global tobacco control in the 21st century: report of a working group convened during the 10th World Conference on Tobacco or Health', *Tobacco Control*, 7(1): 72–7.

Samet, J.M., Bohanon, H.R. Jr., Coultas, D.B., Houston, T.P., Persily, A.K., Schoen, L.J., Spengler, J., Callaway, C.A., and ASHRAE's Environmental Tobacco Smoke Position Document Committee (2005) *ASHRAE Position Document on Environmental Tobacco Smoke*, Atlanta, GA: American Society of Heating Refrigeration and Air Conditioning.

Samet, J.M., Neta, G.I., and Wang, S.S. (2009) 'Secondhand smoke', in M. Lippmann, *Environmental Toxicants: Human Exposures and Their Health Effects*, 3rd edn, Hoboken, NJ: John Wiley.

Scollo, M., Lal, A., Hyland, A., and Glantz, S. (2003) 'Review of the quality of studies on the economic effects of smoke-free policies on the hospitality industry', *Tobacco Control*, 12(1): 13–20.

Simpson, B.W. (2003) 'Smoke Out!', *The Magazine of the Johns Hopkins Bloomberg School of Public Health*, 26–35.

Smith R.C. (1978) 'The magazines' smoking habit', *Columbia Journalism Review*, 16: 29–31.

US DHHS (US Department of Health and Human Services) (1986) *The Health Consequences of Involuntary Smoking: A Report of the Surgeon General*, Washington, DC: US Department of Health and Human Services, Public Health Service, Office on Smoking and Health.

US DHHS (US Department of Health and Human Services) (2004) *The Health Consequences of Smoking: A Report of the Surgeon General*, Atlanta, GA: US Department of Health and Human Services, Centers for Disease Control and Prevention, National Center for Chronic Disease Prevention and Health Promotion, Office on Smoking and Health.

US DHHS (US Department of Health and Human Services) (2006) *The Health Consequences of Involuntary Exposure to Tobacco Smoke: A Report of the Surgeon General*, Atlanta, GA: US Department of Health and Human Services, Centers for Disease Control and Prevention, Coordinating Center for Health Promotion, National Center for Chronic Disease Prevention, and Health Promotion, Office on Smoking and Health.

US Department of Health Education and Welfare (1964) *Smoking and Health: Report of the Advisory Committee to the Surgeon General*, Washington, DC: US Government Printing Office.

US Supreme Court (2001) *Lorrillard Tobacco Company v. Reilly*, 533 U.S. 525, 121 S.Ct. 2404. 150 L.Ed.2d 532.

WHO (World Health Organization) (1999) *Towards a WHO Framework Convention on Tobacco Control*, WHA52.18, Geneva: WHO.

WHO (World Health Organization) (2002) *World Health Report: Reducing Risks, Promoting Healthy Life*, Geneva: WHO.

WHO (World Health Organization) (2006) *Report of the Open-Ended Intergovernmental Working Group on the WHO Framework Convention on Tobacco Control*, A/FCTC/COP/1/2, Geneva: WHO.

WHO (World Health Organization) (2008) *WHO Report on the Global Tobacco Epidemic, 2008: The MPOWER Package*, Geneva: WHO.

WHO (World Health Organization) (2009) *WHO Report on the Global Tobacco Epidemic, 2009: Implementing Smoke-Free Environments*, Geneva: WHO.

WHO (World Health Organization) and Tobacco Free Initiative (n.d.) *Tobacco Free Initiative (TFI) Publications*, available at http://www.who.int/tobacco/resources/publications/en/ (accessed 9 February 2009).

Yang, G., Ma, J., Chen, A., Zhang, Y., Samet, J.M., Taylor, C.E., and Becker, K. (2001) 'Smoking cessation in China: findings from the 1996 national prevalence survey', *Tobacco Control*, 10(2): 170–74.

30

Global Nutrition

Complex Aetiology Demands Social as well as Nutrient-Based Solutions

Joanne Csete and Marion Nestle

Introduction

Nutrition is crucial to the course of chronic and infectious illness and other aspects of human health and well-being. In resource-constrained and wealthy countries alike, poor nutritional status contributes to the leading causes of morbidity and mortality. Nutrition should be an important element of health policy-making, programmes, and education in all countries, but often is not. This chapter reviews, briefly and selectively, global data on the nutritional status of populations, consequences of malnutrition, results of programmes designed to address malnutrition, and the challenges that remain.

Here, *malnutrition* refers to conditions that typically result from excessive, deficient, or unbalanced intake of essential nutrients, often complicated by illness. Malnutrition includes *overnutrition*, usually due to overconsumption of *macronutrient* (protein, fat, carbohydrate) calories and manifested as obesity. *Undernutrition* (protein-energy) is manifested as stunting (low height for age), wasting (low weight for height), and underweight (low weight for age). Undernutrition is often accompanied by deficiencies of essential vitamins and minerals (*micronutrients*). *Food insecurity*, which is closely related to malnutrition, means lack of access to sufficient food for an active and healthy life, whether at the level of individuals, households, or communities (FAO 2006).

Prevalence and consequences of malnutrition

Protein-energy undernutrition

The conditions of stunting, wasting, and being underweight are highly prevalent in the world, especially among young children. Sub-Saharan Africa has the highest regional prevalence of childhood stunting and wasting (Table 30.1). South Asia is the most nutritionally deficient Asian sub-region, with an estimated 40 per cent prevalence of stunting and 5.7 per cent severe wasting (Black *et al.* 2008: 245). India alone has an estimated 61 million young children who are stunted (Black *et al.* 2008: 246). Globally, over 177 million young children are stunted, and over 19 million are severely wasted. The proportion of young children who were underweight

Table 30.1 Prevalence of childhood undernutrition, 2005

Region	<5 children (millions)	% stunted (95% confidence interval)	% severely wasted (95% CI)	% underweight (95% CI)	Low birthwt (% <2500 g)
Africa	141,914	40.1 (36.8–43.4)	3.9 (2.2–5.7)	21.9 (19.8–24.0)	14.3
Asia	356,879	31.3 (27.5–35.1)	3.7 (1.2–6.2)	22.0 (18.5–25.6)	18.3
Latin America	56,936	16.1 (9.4–22.8)	0.6 (0.2–1.0)	4.8 (3.1–6.4)	10.0
All 'developing countries'	555,729	32.0 (29.3–34.6)	3.5 (1.8–5.1)	20.2 (17.9–22.6)	16.0

Stunting = height/age < 2 SD; severe wasting = weight/height; underweight = wt/age < 2 SD; standard deviations based on WHO child growth standards http://www.who.int/childgrowth/standards/en/.
Source: Black *et al.* 2008.

declined from 32 to 27 per cent from 1990 to 2006 in 71 low-income countries, but the smallest decline was in sub-Saharan Africa (UNICEF 2007).

A low body-mass index (BMI), defined as the weight of an individual (in kg) divided by the square of height (in m^2), indicates undernutrition in adults. Women are considered undernourished with a BMI below 18.5 kg/m^2. Over 20 per cent of women of child-bearing age in sub-Saharan Africa, South Asia, and Southeast Asia have BMIs below this threshold (Black *et al.* 2008: 244), and 40 percent of women aged 15–49 in India and Bangladesh.

The consequences of protein-energy undernutrition are dire; it underlies some 3.5 million deaths per year and 35 per cent of morbidity among young children (Black *et al.* 2008: 243), and is the single most important determinant of the global burden of disease (Caulfield *et al.* 2004). Among young children, the risk of death increases significantly with the degree of undernutrition; severe wasting has an overall mortality odds ratio of about 9.4 and severe stunting about 4.1 (Black *et al.* 2008: 247). Evidence from several countries suggests a direct relationship between undernutrition in early childhood and poor performance in school or cognitive function later in childhood (Victora *et al.* 2008).

Undernutrition has intergenerational causes and consequences. Young children who are stunted tend to have short stature as adults. Pregnant women of short stature face elevated risk of requiring caesarean sections (Black *et al.* 2008: 244), a risk factor for maternal and neonatal death where health services are inadequate. Low BMI among pregnant women is associated with intrauterine growth restriction (Black *et al.* 2008: 244), which is strongly linked to low birth-weight. Low birth-weight, in turn, is associated with neonatal morbidity and mortality, impaired growth and poor cognitive development (UNICEF/WHO 2004). In short, undernutrition puts millions of children at risk of death in young childhood, makes them more susceptible to serious illness, and impairs their capacity for educational attainment.

Micronutrient undernutrition

Vitamin and mineral (micronutrient) deficiencies are widespread in adults and children in many countries. Among the most important of these are the following.

Vitamin A: An estimated 190 million children under the age of five (about one-third of all under-five children) and 19 million pregnant women, or about 15 per cent, are vitamin A-deficient, the vast majority in sub-Saharan Africa and South Asia (WHO 2009a).

This deficiency impairs the immune response to many infectious diseases, contributing to the premature death of an estimated 1 million young children annually (UNICEF and Micronutrient Initiative 2004). Severe vitamin A deficiency causes xerophthalmia and blindness.

Iron-deficiency anaemia: About 1.62 billion people in the world suffer from anaemia (based on haemoglobin levels); the prevalence is highest among pre-school children (47.4 per cent) and pregnant women (41.8 per cent) (de Benoist *et al.* 2008). Anaemia in pregnant women contributes to risk of maternal death, and anaemia in children to impaired cognitive development (Black *et al.* 2008: 249).

Iodine: Iodine deficiency is the most prevalent cause of brain damage in the world (WHO 2009b). Children born to women with severe iodine deficiency are at high risk of mental retardation. Even mild iodine deficiency among pregnant women can cause intrauterine growth restriction and impaired foetal brain and motor development. Some 38 million newborns per year are at risk of mental impairment because of iodine deficiency (Micronutrient Initiative 2009).

Overnutrition

The World Health Organization (WHO) defines obesity and overweight as 'abnormal or excessive fat accumulation that may impair health', as measured by BMI: overweight is a BMI of 25 or above and obesity is a BMI of 30 or above (WHO 2009c: 1). By these definitions, an estimated 1.6 billion adults were overweight in 2005, and some 400 million were obese. By 2015, about 2.3 billion adults are projected to be overweight and over 700 million obese (WHO 2009c: 1). An estimated 20 million children under the age of five were overweight in 2005. Obesity is increasing rapidly in the global South, particularly in urban areas. From the mid-1980s to about 2005, obesity prevalence increased threefold in low- and middle-income countries exposed to 'Western' diets (Hossain *et al.* 2007). Obesity and undernutrition co-exist within single communities and even within families in many countries, constituting a 'dual burden' (Caballero 2005: 1514).

Overweight and obesity in adults are associated with a high risk of cardiovascular disease, the world's most frequent cause of death; diabetes, which WHO projects to double as a cause of mortality by 2016; musculoskeletal disorders; and some cancers (WHO 2009c). Based on disability-adjusted life years (DALYs), obesity accounts directly for about 16 per cent of the global burden of disease (Hossain *et al.* 2007: 213). Obesity in children is ushering in a previously unimaginable global epidemic of type 2 diabetes in adolescents, and is associated with cardiovascular disease risk factors as well as psychosocial problems (Ebbeling *et al.* 2002).

Causes of malnutrition

Undernutrition

It is tautological that nutritional outcomes are related to diet on an immediate level, but the aetiology of undernutrition is complex. Figure 30.1, an adaptation of the widely used United Nations Children's Fund (UNICEF) framework on causes of child malnutrition, suggests several levels of causation. Diet as an immediate cause of undernutrition is mediated by infectious illnesses such as diarrhoea and the high energy demands of fever. One intermediate factor is the lack of access to adequate water and sanitation and to affordable, good-quality health care that characterises many communities at risk of undernutrition.

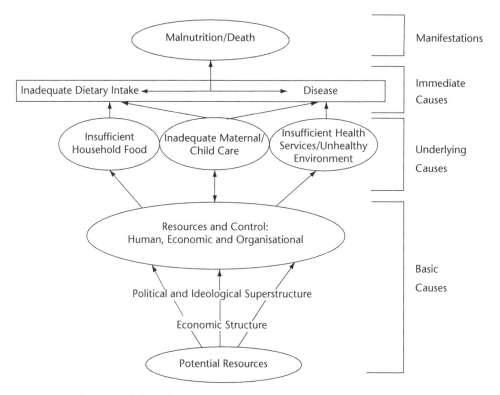

Figure 30.1 Causes of child malnutrition: UNICEF framework
Source: UNICEF 1990.

Food insecurity

Food insecurity is a function of poverty. The Food and Agricultural Organization's (FAO) count of 'hunger' or individual food insecurity topped 1 billion for the first time in 2009 (FAO 2009). The increase to 1.02 billion from the 2008 estimate of 915 million (up from 873 million in 2004–06) was explained by lower household income due to the global recession, as well as historically high staple food prices (FAO 2009). Sub-Saharan Africa and South Asia have the highest proportions of food-insecure people. Until 2007, most food-insecure persons were rural dwellers of countries of the global South, including landless farm families (Pinstrup-Andersen and Cheng 2007). With the recession of 2008–09, the majority of food-insecure people may still be rural, but millions of the newly food-insecure were poor urban-dwellers who lost low-paying jobs in recession-affected sectors (FAO 2009; Natsios and Doley 2009). Food riots occurred in more than 50 countries by mid-2008 (von Braun 2008), mostly in urban areas.

Although world food production has outpaced population growth since the 1980s (Holt-Giménez 2008), food prices have risen. Among the factors behind the price rise are increasing global demands for grain-intensive meat and dairy products (Natsios and Doley 2009), as well as diversion of grain crops to the production of biofuels (von Braun 2008). Many small farmers in food-insecure countries are not linked to global markets and do not easily benefit from higher food prices (von Braun 2008).

Child care and infant feeding

Breastfeeding is well-known to convey immunological benefits to young children, protect against pathogens, and sustain good growth and cognitive development. Exclusive breastfeeding for the first six months of life is recommended by the WHO, but only about half of children under the age of two months in the global South are exclusively breastfed, and under 30 per cent from age two to five months (Black *et al.* 2008). Complementary foods added to breast-milk after six months must contain sufficient protein, energy, and micronutrients to meet a rapidly growing child's needs. Much stunting and wasting occurs in children from age six to twelve months and is linked to suboptimal complementary feeding (Black *et al.* 2008).

Breastfeeding and complementary feeding are undermined by poverty, women's lack of decision-making autonomy, unsupportive workplace conditions (Pelto *et al.* 2003), and aggressive marketing of manufactured infant foods. The International Code of Marketing of Breastmilk Substitutes, a voluntary code of conduct approved by nearly all United Nations (UN) member states, forbids marketing practices such as making unjustified health claims about infant formula, providing free samples to new mothers, and making donations to health professionals (WHO 1981). While 71 countries have incorporated some elements of the Code in national law (UNICEF 2009), it is still widely violated (Aguayo *et al.* 2003; IBFAN 2007). Breastfeeding promotion efforts were somewhat stymied by the recognition that HIV can be transmitted through breastfeeding (Labbok *et al.* 2004). Research has since shown that exclusive breastfeeding can minimise HIV transmission and may be the best option for many women with HIV (WHO 2006).

Overnutrition

The global obesity epidemic is linked to the 'nutrition transition' – a shift from undernutrition to overnutrition usually associated with economic development (Popkin 2007). Nutrition transitions most likely to result in obesity include a combination of dietary change – increased consumption of foods high in saturated fat and sugar (the 'Western diet') – and decreased physical activity (Popkin 2003). An enormous increase in the consumption of sweetened beverages since the mid-1970s has contributed significantly to rapid global weight gain (Popkin 2007). The lowest-income people in the lowest-income countries are unlikely to be overweight, but in middle-income countries, lower-income people are at high risk of obesity since nutrient-rich, low-fat diets are usually more expensive in middle-income countries than cheap, energy-dense fast foods (Caballero 2005).

The marketing clout of large multinational food producers and retailers has successfully promoted the consumption of high-fat and sweetened foods and drinks (Popkin 2007). Food marketing expenditures in Southeast Asia, for example, tripled to US $6 billion from 1984 to 1990 (Chopra *et al.* 2002: 954). Since eating habits and tastes are formed in childhood, marketing processed and sweetened foods to children can be an effective sales strategy. Fast food chains locate their outlets near schools and link marketing to movies and toys for children (Ebbeling *et al.* 2002; Nestle 2007). Marketing of sweetened drinks and junk food in schools is a pervasive practice in the US and parts of Europe (Ebbeling *et al.* 2002; Nestle 2007), and there is every reason to suppose it will continue to be replicated elsewhere.

Addressing malnutrition

Undernutrition

UN member states committed to pursuing the goal of reducing 'hunger' by half from 1990 to 2015 as part of the Millennium Development Goals (MDG). Progress will be measured by estimating the proportion of under-five children who are underweight for age and the percentage of people consuming a minimum level of calories (MDG Monitor 2009). The goal does not mention micronutrient undernutrition or obesity.

In 2008, the Child Undernutrition Study Group, an eminent expert body, conducted a comprehensive review of interventions for which there was some evidence of effectiveness. The Group concluded that evidence justified implementation of several interventions in all countries where child undernutrition is a significant problem: for children – breastfeeding and complementary feeding promotion, vitamin A supplementation and salt iodisation, treatment of severe wasting, and zinc in management of diarrhoea; and for women of child-bearing age – iron, folate, and calcium supplementation, smoking cessation, and reduction of exposure to indoor air pollution (Bhutta *et al.* 2008). By a different criterion – the reduction of child mortality – optimal breastfeeding is judged to be the most effective investment that countries can make, and improved complementary feeding the third most effective (insecticide-treated bed nets for malaria prevention is second) (Labbok *et al.* 2004).

Although not mentioned in the MDG, micronutrient deficiencies have become a priority for major donors. They are the low-hanging fruit of nutritional challenges, lending themselves to technical solutions that do not necessarily involve improving access to food, reducing poverty, or addressing social determinants of malnutrition. As of 2005, 34 countries had iodised virtually all table salt, which effectively protects against iodine deficiency, and 60 countries had significantly increased availability of iodised salt since 1995 (UNICEF 2007). Trends in vitamin A deficiency are more difficult to discern, but there is some indication that serum retinol levels improved among pre-school children from 1995 to 2009 (WHO 2009a), probably linked to large-scale supplement distribution. From 1999 to 2005, the number of children receiving supplements rose fourfold (UNICEF 2007). Iron deficiency anaemia, however, has been less amenable to such rapid improvement. Available data do not reveal consistent trends, but all surveys reviewed by WHO indicate very widespread anaemia in all regions (de Benoist *et al.* 2008: 12) despite efforts at iron fortification of staple foods.

The Global Alliance for Improved Nutrition (GAIN), a 'public–private partnership' focused on creating markets for micronutrient-fortified foods, may be the world's largest single programme targeting undernutrition, as it is supported by the Gates Foundation, many food companies, bilateral donors, WHO and UNICEF (GAIN 2009a). As of 2008, GAIN estimated that 99 million women and children were consuming fortified staples as a result of its work (GAIN 2009b). A promising initiative in some settings has been 'home fortification', using low-cost sachets of micronutrient-rich powders or 'sprinkles' containing iron that can be added to meals (Micronutrient Initiative 2009). Sustainability of supply and affordability of these products present challenges.

With regard to childhood protein-energy undernutrition, prevention is of course desirable, but immediate treatment of severe undernutrition, especially childhood wasting, is urgent to avert death. The treatment of severe wasting has been transformed since 2000 by use of energy-rich, micronutrient-dense, ready-to-use therapeutic foods (RUTF) (WHO *et al.* 2007). WHO lauds RUTF as a means of enabling severely wasted children to be treated effectively without expensive hospitalisation (WHO *et al.* 2007). The most widely used RUTF, a micronutrient-fortified groundnut and milk paste (WHO *et al.* 2007), is so calorie-dense that it is not surprising that adding it to a child's diet quickly reverses wasting, but sustaining the cost-effective provision of RUTF and preventing relapse of children when they have finished RUTF regimens are ongoing problems.

As noted above, enabling women to breastfeed optimally would avert childhood mortality and undernutrition better than any other single measure. The momentum behind global programmes in this area has declined recently, perhaps in response to the combined effects of confusion about HIV and breastfeeding, unrelenting marketing of infant formula by manufacturers, and 'message burnout' after decades of promotion (Labbok *et al.* 2004). Several studies have demonstrated the effectiveness of providing individual or group-based support to encourage exclusive breastfeeding of young children and optimal complementary feeding (Bhutta *et al.* 2008), but only rarely can these programmes be sustained at a level that can counter the marketing might of formula companies (IBFAN 2007).

Ultimately, in addition to access to affordable, good-quality health services, combating undernutrition depends on access to a nutritious and varied diet, something that, as the MDG concludes, is closely linked to reducing poverty. Although a complete discussion of approaches to reducing food insecurity is beyond the scope of this overview, it is worth noting a renewed debate about supporting agricultural production in food-insecure areas, an important element of food security. Green Revolution approaches for Africa have been boosted by a major investment in this area by the Gates Foundation (2009). Critics argue that while yields of wheat and rice increased markedly in response to Green Revolution breakthroughs in the 1960s and 1970s, they came at the price of environmental devastation, as they require high levels of pesticides and petroleum-based fertilisers, and encourage export agriculture and industrial-scale monoculture (Holt-Giménez *et al.* 2006). Such approaches also undermine traditional eco-systems based on varied crops and animal husbandry (Oxfam International 2009; Shiva 2000).

Overnutrition

Efforts to prevent obesity must address both diet and physical activity – the two parts of the obesity equation – and must reach people as early in life as possible (Nestle and Jacobson 2000). Ebbeling and colleagues (2002: 478) concluded that in the US and UK behavioural and educational interventions were overwhelmed by 'adverse environmental factors', of which the most adverse was extravagantly funded marketing of fast food and soft drinks, especially in schools. This conclusion echoes Nestle's (2007) analysis of aggressive marketing in the US of high-energy, nutrient-poor foods passed off as 'healthful' while powerful food industry lobbyists in Washington work to weaken government dietary guidelines and marketing regulations. Food company sponsorship of children's television programmes is largely forbidden in Norway, Sweden, and Finland (Kaiser Family Foundation 2004). Such a measure seems unlikely in the US and other countries in which state interference with private commerce is politically unpalatable.

WHO's Global Strategy on Diet, Physical Activity and Health was designed to address the growing disease burden associated with overnutrition (WHO 2004). The Strategy cites the food industry as a 'partner' with governments in fighting obesity and suggests that it 'consider introducing new products with better nutritional value' and 'practice responsible marketing ... especially to children' (WHO 2004, para 61). A 2003 WHO background report meant to contribute to the Global Strategy recommended that added sugars comprise less than 10 per cent of daily calorie intake. Following pressure from the Bush Administration, with its close ties to the sugar industry, that recommendation did not appear in the Global Strategy (Nestle 2007: 379). Some experts have criticised the Global Strategy for depicting the food industry as an ally (Chopra *et al.* 2002) and recommend binding regulations on food marketing along the lines of the Framework Convention on Tobacco Control (Chopra and Darnton-Hill 2004).

Conclusion

Both undernutrition and overnutrition are closely linked to poverty. Even in wealthier communities, the poorest people are most constrained in acquiring nutritious food. Malnutrition is an intransigent problem with no simple solution. Most nutrition interventions are not linked coherently to anti-poverty programmes or well-integrated into health programmes (Morris *et al.* 2008). On the global health agenda, most aim only to improve diet; they intervene at the level of immediate causes and are not linked to basic or even intermediate determinants of nutrition outcomes.

As globalisation opens doors for new solutions to worldwide health problems, it also increases the reach and power of multinational corporations. Every element of the complex causation of malnutrition cannot be addressed in all programmes, even by large multilateral bodies, but it should not be too much to expect that national and multilateral authorities pay attention to the actions and motives of for-profit food companies. More assistance is needed to translate the voluntary Breastmilk Code into national law and to support countries in prosecuting offenders. More countries should follow the lead of Sweden, Norway, and Finland in establishing legally binding restrictions on unethical advertising of unhealthy foods to children.

Improving food security will always be challenging, particularly since it affects both rural people who depend on marginal land and fragile soils and the growing millions of urban poor (Oxfam 2009). The kind of food production compatible with good nutritional and environmental outcomes is the subject of vigourous debate. Proponents of small-scale, low-input agriculture argue that it can feed the world by sustainably feeding each corner of it (Chappell 2007); agribusiness has a different view. The debate may be tipped when important donors such as the Gates Foundation – with over US $60 billion in assets and a hands-on approach to giving (Black *et al.* 2009) – enter the scene. The world may never know the full potential of eco-friendly low-input agriculture if assistance to food-insecure countries is dominated by a vision of narrow and corporatised technical solutions to address complex social, economic, and environmental challenges.

Successful approaches to reducing malnutrition require leadership that is independent, evidence-based, and multidisciplinary. The independence of nutrition research and policy has been too often compromised by ties to the food industry or agribusiness (Lesser *et al.* 2007; Nestle 2007:116–20). The vision of nutrition science for reducing malnutrition has not often enough taken into account the full range of constraints faced by the poor, leading some nutritionists to call for approaches to malnutrition that take better account of social, environmental, cultural, and political determinants of nutrition outcomes (Cannon and Leitzmann 2005). Finally, effective solutions are unlikely to suggest themselves without meaningful participation in nutrition decision-making by those who live every day with nutritional deprivation.

References

Aguayo, V.M., Ross, J.S., Kanon, S. and Ouedraogo, A.N. (2003) 'Monitoring compliance with the International Code of Marketing of breastmilk substitutes in West Africa: Multisite cross sectional survey in Togo and Burkina Faso', *British Medical Journal*, 326: 127–30.

Bhutta, Z.A., Ahmed, T., Black, R.E., Cousens, S., Dewey, K., Guigliani, E., Haider, B.A., Kirkwood, B., Morris, S.S., Sachdev, H.P.S. and Shekar, M. (2008) 'What works? Interventions for maternal and child undernutrition and survival', *The Lancet*, 371: 417–40.

Bill & Melinda Gates Foundation (2009) *Agricultural development strategy overview*, available at http:// www.gatesfoundation.org/agriculturaldevelopment/Documents/agricultural-development-strategy-overview.pdf (accessed 15 August 2009).

Black, R.E., Allen, L.H., Bhutta, Z.A., Caulfield, L.E., de Onis, M., Essati, M., Mathers, C., and Rivera, J. (2008) 'Maternal and child undernutrition: Global and regional exposures and health consequences', *The Lancet*, 371: 243–60.

Black, R.E., Bhan, M.K., Chopra, M., Rudande, I., and Victora, C.G. (2009) 'Accelerating the health impact of the Gates Foundation', *The Lancet*, 373: 1584–5.

Caballero, B. (2005) 'A nutrition paradox – underweight and obesity in developing countries', *New England Journal of Medicine*, 352: 1,514–16.

Cannon, G. and Leitzmann, C. (2005) 'The new nutrition science project', *Public Health Nutrition*, 8: 673–94.

Caulfield, L.E., de Onis, M., Blössner, M., and Black, R.E. (2004) 'Undernutrition as an underlying cause of child deaths associated with diarrhea, pneumonia, malaria and measles', *American Journal of Clinical Nutrition*, 80: 193–8.

Chappell, M.J. (2007) 'Shattering myths: Can sustainable agriculture feed the world?', *Food First Backgrounder*, 13(3), available at http://www.foodfirst.org/files/pdf/backgrounders/bgr.100107final.pdf (accessed 12 August 2009).

Chopra, M. and Darnton-Hill, I. (2004) 'Tobacco and obesity epidemics: Not so different after all?', *British Medical Journal*, 238: 1,558–60.

Chopra, M., Galbraith, S. and Darnton-Hill, I. (2002) 'A global response to a global problem: The epidemic of overnutrition', *Bulletin of the World Health Organization*, 80: 952–8.

de Benoist, B., McLean, E., Egli, I., and Cogswell, M. (eds) (2008) *Worldwide Prevalence of Anaemia: 1993–2005*, Geneva: World Health Organization.

Ebbeling, C.B., Pawlak, D.B. and Ludwig, D.S. (2002) 'Childhood obesity: Public-health crisis, common sense cure', *The Lancet*, 360: 473–82.

Food and Agricultural Organisation of the United Nations (FAO) (2006) *Food Security (Policy Brief Issue No. 2)*, Rome: FAO, available at ftp://ftp.fao.org/es/ESA/policybriefs/pb_02.pdf (accessed 5 August 2009).

FAO (Food and Agricultural Organization of the United Nations) (2009) *More people than ever are victims of hunger*, press release, available at http://www.fao.org/fileadmin/user_upload/newsroom/docs/Press%20release%20june-en.pdf (accessed 12 August 2009).

GAIN (Global Alliance for Improved Nutrition) (2009a) *GAIN partnerships*, available at http://www.gainhealth.org/partnerships (accessed 13 August 2009).

GAIN (Global Alliance for Improved Nutrition) (2009b) *GAIN project results*, available at http://www.gainhealth.org/performance/project-results (accessed 13 August 2009).

Holt-Giménez, E. (2008) *The world food crisis: What's behind it and what we can do about it*, Oakland, CA: Institute for Food and Development Policy, available at http://www.foodfirst.org/files/pdf/PB%2016%20World%20Food%20Crisis.pdf (accessed 12 August 2009).

Holt-Giménez, E., Altieri, M.A. and Rosset, P. (2006) *Ten reasons why the Rockefeller and the Bill and Melinda Gates Foundations' Alliance for another green revolution will not solve the problems of poverty and hunger in sub-Saharan Africa*, Oakland, CA: Institute for Food and Development Policy, available at http://www.foodfirst.org/files/pdf/policybriefs/pb12.pdf (accessed 13 August 2009).

Hossain, P., Kawar, B. and El Nahas, M. (2007) 'Obesity and diabetes in the developing world: A growing challenge', *New England Journal of Medicine*, 356: 213–15.

IBFAN (International Baby Food Action Network) (2007) *Breaking the Rules, Stretching the Rules*, Kuala Lumpur: IBFAN-ICDC.

Kaiser Family Foundation (2004) *The role of media in childhood obesity* (issue brief), Washington, DC: Kaiser Family Foundation, available at http://www.kff.org/entmedia/upload/The-Role-Of-Media-in-Childhood-Obesity.pdf (accessed 11 August 2009).

Labbok, M.H., Clark, D. and Goldman, A.S. (2004) 'Breastfeeding: Maintaining an irreplaceable immunological resource', *Nature Reviews Immunology*, 4: 565–72.

Lesser, L.L., Ebbeling, C.B., Goozner, M., Wypij, D. and Ludwig, D.S. (2007) 'Relationship between funding source and conclusion among nutrition-related scientific articles', *PLoS Medicine*, 4(1): e5, 0041–8.

Micronutrient Initiative (2009) *Together we can end hidden hunger: Annual report 2007–2008*, Ottawa: Micronutrient Initiative, available at http://www.micronutrient.org/CMFiles/MI-AnnualReport07-EN.pdf (accessed 12 August 2009).

Millennium Development Goal (MDG) Monitor (2009) *Eradicate extreme hunger and poverty (MDG Goal Monitor)*, available at http://www.mdgmonitor.org/goal1.cfm (accessed 11 August 2009).

Morris, S.S., Cogill, B. and Uauy, R. (2008) 'Effective international action against undernutrition: Why has it proven so difficult and what can be done to accelerate progress?', *The Lancet*, 371: 608–21.

Natsios, A.S. and Doley, K.W. (2009) 'The coming food coups', *Washington Quarterly*, 32: 7–25.

Nestle, M. (2007) *Food politics: How the Food Industry Influences Nutrition and Health*, rev. edn, Berkeley, CA: University of California Press.

Nestle, M. and Jacobson, M.F. (2000) 'Halting the obesity epidemic: A public health policy approach', *Public Health Reports*, 115: 12–24.

Oxfam International (2009) *Investing in poor farmers pays: Rethinking how to invest in agriculture* (briefing paper), London: Oxfam, available at http://www.oxfam.org.uk/resources/policy/trade/downloads/bp_129_investing_in_poor_farmers.pdf (accessed 13 August 2009).

Pelto, G.H., Levitt, E. and Thairu, L. (2003) 'Improving feeding practices: Current patterns, common constraints and the design of interventions', *Food and Nutrition Bulletin*, 24: 45–82.

Pinstrup-Andersen, P. and Cheng, F. (2007) 'Still hungry: One eighth of the world's people do not have enough to eat', *Scientific American*, 297: 96–103.

Popkin, B.M. (2003) 'The nutrition transition in the developing world', *Development Policy Review*, 21: 581–97.

Popkin, B.M. (2007) 'The world is fat', *Scientific American*, 297: 60–7.

Shiva, V. (2000) *Stolen Harvest: The Hijacking of the Global Food Supply*, Cambridge, MA: South End Press.

UNICEF (United Nations Children's Fund) (1990) *Strategy for Improved Nutrition of Children and Women in Developing Countries*, New York: UNICEF.

UNICEF (United Nations Children's Fund) (2007) *Progress for children: a world fit for children*, New York: UNICEF, available at http://www.unicef.org/publications/files/Progress_for_Children_No_6_ revised. pdf (accessed 13 August 2009).

UNICEF (United Nations Children's Fund) (2009) *Annual report of the executive director: Progress and achievements against the medium-term strategic plan*, available at http://www.unicef.org/about/ execboard/files/09-9-Annual_Report_2009_-_13_April_-JI-final.pdf (accessed 14 August 2009).

UNICEF (United Nations Children's Fund) and the Micronutrient Initiative (2004) *Vitamin and mineral deficiency: A global damage assessment report*, available at http://www.micronutrient.org/CMFiles/PubLib/Report-67-VMD-A-Global-Damage-Assessment-Report1KSB-32420080-9634.pdf (accessed 12 August 2009).

UNICEF (United Nations Children's Fund) and WHO (World Health Organization) (2004) *Low birthweight: Country, regional and global estimates*, New York: UNICEF, available at http://www.unicef.org/publications/files/low_birthweight_from_EY.pdf (accessed 14 August 2009).

Victora, C.G., Adair, L., Fall, C., Hallal, P.C., Martorell, R., Richter, L. and Sachdev, H.S. (2008) 'Maternal and child undernutrition: Consequences for adult health and human capital', *The Lancet*, 371: 340–57.

von Braun, J. (2008) *Responding to the world food crisis: Getting on the right track*, Washington, DC: International Food Policy Research Institute, available at http://www.ifpri.org/publication/responding-world-food-crisis-getting-right-track (accessed 11 August 2009).

WHO (World Health Organization) (1981) *International Code of Marketing of breastmilk substitutes*, Geneva: WHO, available at http://whqlibdoc.who.int/publications/9241541601.pdf (accessed 4 August 2009).

WHO (World Health Organization) (2004) *Fifty-Seventh World Health Assembly: Global strategy on diet, physical activity and health, Resolution 57.17*, Geneva: World Health Organization, available at http://apps.who.int/gb/ebwha/pdf_files/WHA57/A57_R17-en.pdf (accessed 11 August, 2009).

WHO (World Health Organization) (2006) *Consensus statement from the WHO HIV and infant feeding technical consultation*, Geneva: WHO, available at http://www.who.int/child_adolescent_health/documents/if_consensus/en/index.html (accessed 14 August 2009).

WHO (World Health Organization) (2009a) *Global prevalence of vitamin A deficiency in populations at risk, 1995–2005*, Geneva: WHO, available at http://whqlibdoc.who.int/publications/2009/9789241598019_eng.pdf (accessed 13 August 2009).

WHO (World Health Organization) (2009b) *Micronutrient deficiencies: Iodine deficiency disorders*, available at www.who.int/nutrition/ (accessed 11 August 2009).

WHO (World Health Organization) *Obesity and overweight*, available at http://www.who.int/mediacentre/factsheets/fs311/en/print.html (accessed 15 August 2009).

WHO (World Health Organization), World Food Programme, United Nations System Standing Committee on Nutrition, and United Nations Children's Fund (2007) *Community-based management of severe acute malnutrition: A joint statement*, Geneva: WHO, available at http://www.who.int/nutrition/topics/Statement_community_based_man_sev_acute_mal_eng.pdf (accessed 14 August 2009).

31

Health Communication

A Catalyst to Behaviour Change

Jane T. Bertrand, Alice Payne Merritt, and Gary Saffitz

Health communication is a vehicle to improve health, save lives, and change social norms. It has become so much a part of the cultural landscape globally that those exposed and influenced may not even realise they are being targeted for a public health intervention.

For example, for five seasons, viewers in South Africa were riveted by *Tsha Tsha*, an award-winning TV serial drama that featured (among other characters and topics) the joys and sorrows of a beautiful and talented young woman as she learns that a former boyfriend is HIV positive, confronts her own HIV status, and valiantly fights the stigma of the disease within her own family and community. Children in this same country tune into *Takalani Sesame* (the localised version of *Sesame Street*), where Kami, the sero-positive Muppet, increases awareness of HIV, helps children cope with the loss of a parent, and models acceptance of persons living with HIV. For more than four decades, communication has been central to the international family planning movement, serving as a catalyst to improve social norms around family size, educate populations to the range of methods, and create demand for local services via almost every known channel of communication. Shy adolescents in Peru wanting to learn about sexuality, contraception, and male/female relationships can go online to get the basics from Isabela, *la Consejera Virtual* (the virtual counsellor). Radio and TV spots broadcast throughout rural Indonesia alert farmers to the dangers of avian influenza and instruct them in 'report, burn, and bury' procedures. Community-based interventions help communities to deal with a host of health challenges with collective action; in Malawi, a non-governmental organisation (NGO) programme mobilised grandmothers in relation to HIV to take advantage of their status as 'wise women' in the community. The list of such interventions is nearly endless.

Health communication is also part of the landscape in resource-rich countries, although it is less ubiquitous, in part because of the prohibitive cost of television and billboard advertising and the absence of international donor funding that supports much of the health communication in poorer countries. In the United States, topics frequently in the media include cancer, diabetes, obesity, and heart disease (Kaiser Family Foundation 2008). Much of this health communication is driven by the commercial sector capitalising on direct-to-consumer promotion of pharmaceuticals and building demand for healthy lifestyle products including diets, fitness, beauty, and health foods. During the 2009 outbreak of swine flu (H1N1 virus), the 'health

---

Box 31.1 Channels used in health communication programming (adapted from Salem *et al.* 2008)

Mass media:

- Broadcast (TV, radio at national or regional level: public service announcements, talk shows, call-in shows, serial dramas, diaries, magazine or variety formats, animated cartoons, music videos, songs and jingles, celebrity endorsements)
- Print material (newspaper/magazine advertising, news coverage, direct mail, decision-making aides for clients and providers, comic books, photonovelas, pamphlets, flyers, posters, transit signs, billboards)

Electronic communication:

- Internet web sites
- Social media (e-forums, blogs, chat rooms, Facebook, Twitter)
- Distance learning
- CD-ROMs
- Mobile phone programmes

Community-based channels:

- Community mobilisation, group interaction (meetings, rallies)
- Outreach activities by programme staff and community members
- Live performances (street theatre, puppet shows, talent shows, contests)
- Community media (newspapers, local radio)

Interpersonal communication/counselling:

- Between provider/client, teacher/student, parent/child, or among peers
- Client counselling, telephone hotlines, instruction, informal discussion groups

---

communication team' included the anchors of the major news channels and the president of the United States.

Health communication falls into four main categories (see Box 31.1): (1) mass media, (2) community-based interventions, (3) interpersonal communication/counselling (IPC), and (4) electronic media. This chapter outlines what lies behind the health communication programming that is now ubiquitous worldwide. For additional reading, see Shiavo (2007) and Parker and Thorson (2009).

The evolution of health communication programmes over time

The approach to health education that emerged in the mid-twentieth century emphasised relatively dry information, presented in posters and pamphlets that 'preached' good behaviour: what to eat, how often to brush one's teeth, how much sleep to get, and related topics that had students watching the clock for the next class. In these early days, most mass media campaigns consisted of late night public service announcements (PSAs) covering a range of topics, which aired on the few network affiliates when most people were sleeping.

By contrast, today's health communication is very dynamic. In countries worldwide, today's youth with internet access can find programming that uses Web 2.0 technology to create fun, interactive experiences designed to make them a part of the subject matter. Sources such as YouTube provide information delivered in an entertaining format – though with no controls on the factual accuracy of the information.

Over the last half century, health communication has evolved through at least four periods.

(1) The clinic era, based on a medical care model and the notion that if people knew where services were located, they would find their way to the clinics. Health communication consisted largely of a more traditional patient education approach accompanied by the use of instructional materials.
(2) The field era, a more visible and participatory approach with emphasis on outreach workers, community-based distribution, and a variety of information, education, and communication (IEC) materials distributed in conjunction with programmes.
(3) The social marketing era, developed from the commercial concept that consumers will buy the products they want (often at subsidised prices). Promoting brands stimulated the demand side while convenient access expanded the supply side.
(4) The strategic behaviour change communication era, founded on behavioural science models focused on individuals, communities, and organisations, and emphasising the need to influence social norms and policy environments to facilitate individual and social change (Piotrow et al. 2003).

Designing effective programmes

What makes communication strategic? Box 31.2 outlines the characteristics of strategic communication that allow programmes to achieve their objectives.

Although different organisations may use a slightly different framework, the process for designing a programme is very similar, whatever the subject matter, country, or audience. In the Center for Communication Programs (CCP) at the Johns Hopkins Bloomberg School of Public Health (JHBSPH), we have identified five key steps necessary to design an effective programme, which we designate as the 'P Process':

(1) Analysis: determine severity and causes of problems; identify factors inhibiting or facilitating desired changes; develop a problem statement; carry out formative research; conduct a participation analysis; carry out a social and behavioural analysis; assess communication and training needs;
(2) Strategic Design: establish communication objectives; develop programme approaches and positioning; determine channels; prepare an implementation plan; develop a monitoring and evaluation plan;
(3) Development and Testing: develop concepts, materials, messages, stories, and prototypes; test with stakeholders and audience representatives, conduct in-depth pre-testing; revise concepts, messages, materials based on findings; retest (if needed) and make final adjustments before replication, printing, and final production;
(4) Implementation and Monitoring: produce and disseminate campaign; train trainers, key providers, and field workers; mobilise key participants; manage and monitor the programme; adjust the programme based on monitoring findings; and

(5) Evaluation and Re-planning: measure outcomes and assess impact; disseminate results; determine future needs; revise/redesign the programme. These 'P Process' steps are depicted in Figure 31.1.

Planners find it useful to articulate the 'pathways' by which a health communication programme will achieve its objectives in the form of a conceptual framework. The pathways diagram allows different stakeholders to understand from the start what the programme is trying to achieve and what intermediate steps will be necessary to reach specific outcomes. It identifies three distinct and interrelated domains of communication that work in concert to create a more comprehensive approach to creating and sustaining change. These include: Communication within the Social/Political Environment to impact on policies and structures that create more supportive environments; Communication within the Service Delivery System to improve the quality, access, and effectiveness of interactive communication/counselling between the health care system and users; and Communication to Individuals and Communities to positively impact on social norms, community involvement, and health behaviours.

The conceptual framework also provides an invaluable point of reference in defining the indicators to be used to evaluate its effectiveness. Figure 31.2, for example, illustrates a pathways framework relevant to a health communication programme for HIV prevention.

Box 31.2 Elements of strategic communication

1. Results-oriented: designed to achieve specific behavioural objectives
2. Science-based (research and theory): uses data from multiple sources and communication theory to guide design
3. Client-centered: starts with the client's interests and works backwards to design programmes that address them
4. Participatory: has stakeholders participate in the design and engages the audience in an interactive manner
5. Benefit-oriented: emphasises the advantages of adopting a particular behaviour or product
6. Service-linked: directs the audience to the relevant services (e.g. clinic, testing site, distribution post)
7. Advocacy-related: encourages acceptance of the behaviour or product among peers and creates a positive attitude among decision-makers, policymakers, and leaders
8. Expanding to scale: goes beyond pilot programmes or boutique projects to reach major segments of the intended audience
9. Multiple reinforcing channels: replicates consistent messages, often under a unifying theme/umbrella, across the different channels outlined in Box 31.1.
10. Quality programming: utilises well-qualified professionals to produce/design and disseminate the communication, as well talented actors, where applicable, which can compete with commercially produced materials
11. Programmatically sustainable: fully involves local health and communication professionals/organisations that are able to replicate the process in future rounds of programming
12. Cost-effective: reaches large numbers of the intended audience at an acceptable cost; results in acceptable cost per unit of change.

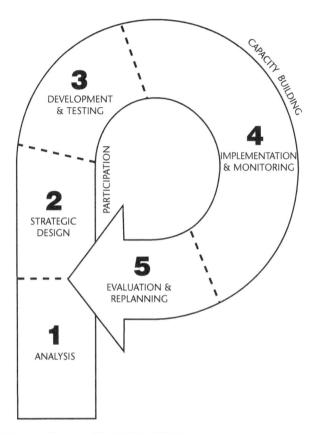

Figure 31.1 The P Process (designed by CCP/JHBSPH)
Source: HEALTH COMMUNICATION PARTNERSHIP (HCP) 2003.

Using research to guide health communication programming

Those unfamiliar with health communication may fail to appreciate the extent to which research guides the design and implementation of health programming. What looks like an entertaining spot on TV or attractive message in print is often the result of significant investments of time and resources in research.

Three types of research/evaluation guide this process.

(1) Formative research establishes the epidemiology of the health issue, including the socio-demographic characteristics of those most affected. This type of information is invaluable in segmenting the population, so that the programming can focus on those most at risk or best placed to enact change (for example, in many countries, women are the ones that use contraceptives, but husbands may be the key decision-makers). Formative research can measure current levels of knowledge, attitudes, self-efficacy, and behaviour with regard to a given health issue, which guides planners in deciding the key intervention strategies and messages for the programme. It also identifies the channels through which the target group receives its information and persons that are credible on a

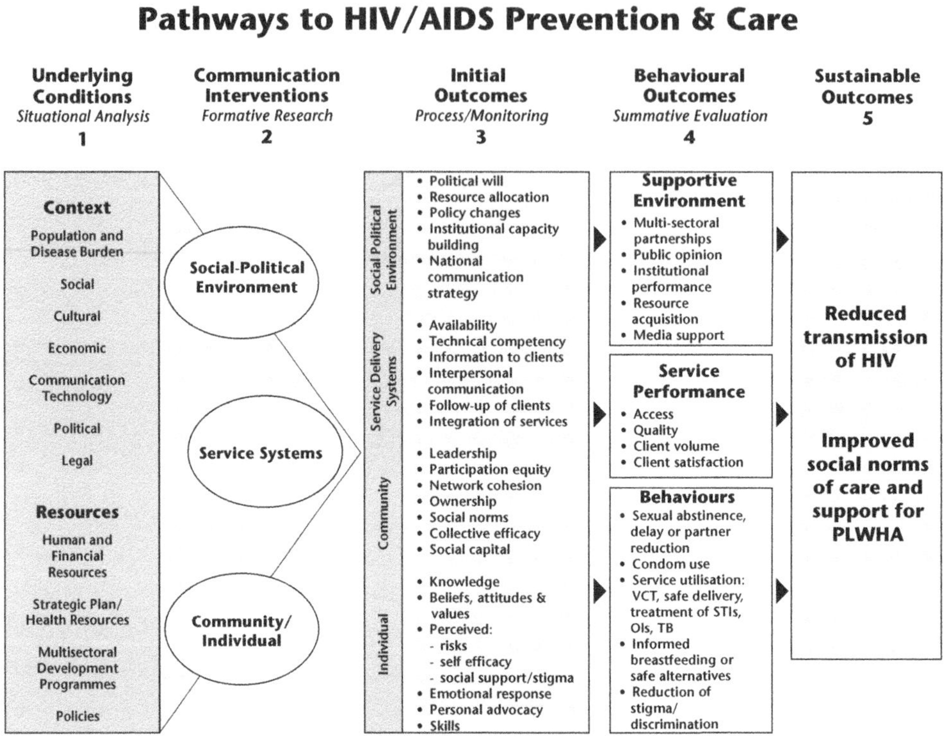

Pathways to HIV/AIDS Prevention & Care

Figure 31.2 Illustrative 'pathways' framework that shows how an HIV communication programme is expected to achieve its objectives

particular topic. Of particular importance, formative research identifies the barriers to behaviour change. For example, why is it that a given population has very high levels of knowledge of a given problem (e.g. HIV), but does not change behaviours accordingly?

(2) Process evaluation serves to determine whether the programme – once launched – is proceeding according to plan. The results are important in making mid-course corrections. For a particular programme or intervention, the evaluator measures one or more of the following components (adapted from Saunders *et al.* 2005):

- Fidelity to the plan of action
- Dose delivered by programme implementers (e.g. quantity of messages seen or heard, number of channels through which messages were seen/heard)
- Reach/participation rate among intended audience
- Dose received via different channels (or extent of exposure through a single channel); assessment of the quality of the interaction
- Satisfaction among intended audiences to different programme components
- Recruitment and maintenance of participants in the programme
- Context, including environmental influences and spill-over from other programmes.

(3) Summative evaluation measures results: Did change occur consistently with the objectives of the programme? To what extent is this change attributable to the health communication intervention? Did more change occur among some subgroups than

others (e.g. by gender, education, place of residence)? And what was the cost per unit of change (cost-effectiveness)? Summative evaluation can range from the very simple (e.g. tracking service statistics in the wake of a campaign to see if service utilisation or sales increased) to the very complex. Evaluators wishing to demonstrate cause-and-effect relationships employ experimental and quasi-experimental designs to test their hypotheses, although the use of observational studies with strong analytic techniques (e.g. propensity scoring, structural equations) is on the rise.

The investment in research is often related to available resources. Multi-million dollar programmes devote a significant portion of their budget (often 10–15 per cent) to research and evaluation, to ensure that they 'get it right' and to document the change they are able to achieve. It is now standard practice to use both qualitative and quantitative methods in designing and evaluating health communication programmes. Even small-scale, low-budget programmes find some means of conducting research that will help to improve programme effectiveness.

The role of entertainment education (E-E)

Everybody loves a good story. The laughter and tears, joy, and misery of drama captivate and entertain. When entertainment is combined with education, it can have a powerful role in influencing peoples' attitudes and perceptions. Entertainment formats portray people in different situations, faced with different choices, struggling with family and community pressures, weighing their options and making decisions – sometimes with good outcomes but sometimes not.

Entertainment-education tends not to be prescriptive (i.e. it does not tell the audience what to do). Rather, it portrays characters in real-life situations, interacting with friends, wives, husbands, lovers, bosses, parents, and others. E-E is based on Albert Bandura's social learning theory, which postulates that people can change their own attitudes and behaviours by being exposed to role models acting out different behaviours and consequences (Singhal et al. 2006). Audiences identify with different characters and follow their plights. In doing so, they are able to observe them react to situations, process decisions, grapple with conflictive feelings, and take action – for better or worse. Through these stories, viewers or listeners are able to appreciate first-hand the consequences of risk taking. The problems related to public health lend themselves well to this format: alcoholism, unprotected sex, stigma from HIV, domestic violence, death from childbirth, to name a few. The audience internalises these situations and comes to understand the implications of risky actions. These characters can become such 'personalities' that their very names conjure up health promotion themes. Thanks to a highly popular radio programme in Tanzania about a lecherous old man named Fataki who seeks the sexual favours of young girls, 'Fataki' is a commonly used term on the streets of Dar Es Salam to refer disparagingly to the sugar-daddy syndrome.

E-E can take many different formats: TV and radio dramas, music videos, folk songs, street theatre, puppetry, variety shows, and contests, among others. It has increasingly become a major part of contemporary health communication programming. One of the first efforts was the Archers' radio drama in England, focused on agricultural practices and communities. Simplemente Maria in Peru was a classic that aired in 1969; thousands of illiterate domestic servants were so inspired by Maria's climb to fame that they enrolled in classes to learn to read and to sew. Many consider Miguel Sabido of Mexico to be the father of modern-day soap operas for health and social causes; his telenovelas drew unprecedented numbers of Mexicans to view emotionally compelling drama, laced with social messages (e.g. on family planning). In the late 1980s, the runaway Mexican hit song, *Détente*, by teen stars Tatiana and Johnny met with astounding success, topping the charts in multiple Latin America countries – all for a song that encouraged teens to delay sexual debut. Two decades later, *Scrutinize* is alerting youth in South Africa to the risks of HIV, using an edgy animated character and a hip hop beat.

E-E can also strike a more serious note. Reality radio has become popular in a number of sub-Saharan African countries. The producers of 'Radio Diaries' work with people living with HIV and AIDS to help them recount their real-life stories of their struggle to cope with their disease and the stigma it brings. Such programmes give voice to those affected by HIV, and also humanise the disease ('giving AIDS a face'), thus creating a more sympathetic climate for people living with HIV and AIDS.

Evidence of the effectiveness of health communication programmes

Several researchers have addressed the question of health communication campaigns and their impact on behaviour across multiple health topics (Hornik 2002). As Snyder (2007) reports, the level of effectiveness of health campaigns that include use of the mass media and avoid coercion have an average effect size of five percentage points ($r = 0.05$). That is, if 60 per cent of the target population performed the desired behaviour before the campaign, the percentage post-campaign would be 65. The level of effect size depends in part on the specific behaviour that is promoted. Based on the available literature, seatbelt campaigns ($r = 0.15$), dental care ($r = 0.13$), and adult alcohol reduction ($r = 0.11$) have had the greatest success rates, whereas youth drug and marijuana campaigns have had the least success ($r = 0.01$–0.02). Topics that fall in between include family planning ($r = 0.06$), youth smoking prevention ($r = 0.06$), mammography screening ($r = 0.04$), adult smoking prevention ($r = 0.04$), and tobacco prevention campaigns ($r = 0.04$).

For new topics, it is possible to anticipate relative success rates by examining characteristics of the behaviour (Snyder 2007). Across health issues, campaigns promoting the adoption of a behaviour that is new to the individual, or the replacement of an old behaviour with a new one (e.g. switching from whole milk to 1–2 per cent milk), have a greater success rate than campaigns aiming to cease an unhealthy behaviour people are already doing or preventing commencement of a risky behaviour (such as unsafe sex in relation to HIV prevention).

One innovative approach to evaluating the effectiveness of a communication programme is to look simultaneously at the multiple programmes operating in a given population, rather than to tease out the effects of a single programme as if it operated in a vacuum. In South Africa, researchers evaluating the effects of HIV communication measured exposure to the 19 most important HIV communication programmes and 17 different HIV behavioural outcome variables. They were able to determine the percentage of the population exposed to each of the different programmes ('reach' of the programmes), as well as to link exposure to a given programme to specific behavioural outcomes. For example, condom use was 7 percentage points higher among viewers of a TV serial drama *Tsha Tsha*, controlling for a large number of socio-demographic variables and exposure to the other HIV-related programmes with propensity score analysis (Kincaid *et al.* 2008).

Although one hears the claim that it is difficult to capture the effects of communication programmes, in fact the methodology for doing so is quite advanced (Babalola and Kincaid 2009). However, the cost of conducting such evaluation is substantial (some would say prohibitive).

Example of an effective health communication programme: pandemic flu preparedness in Egypt

The recent programme on pandemic flu preparedness in Egypt illustrates how the different concepts above come together into an intervention that can reach millions of people with life-saving information. This example related to avian influenza (AI) is particularly relevant, in that this condition was virtually unknown to the majority of the population in Egypt before the campaign.

Box 31.3 Changing lives through health communication – pandemic flu preparedness in Egypt

While the emergence of avian influenza (H5N1) has had a significant impact on many countries, three countries – Indonesia, Vietnam, and Egypt – account for 76 per cent of all human cases worldwide. To date, Egypt has recorded 50 cases of human infection with 22 deaths. These statistics underscore the reality in Egypt, where raising poultry is a backyard business and almost 30 per cent of all families raise their own chickens, contributing to 13–14 per cent of their household's total monthly income.

The strategic health communication response to the early outbreaks among poultry and then humans was led by the Ministry of Health, with technical support from the Communication for Healthy Living Project and donor support from the United States Agency for International Development (USAID).

It began with the development of a National AI Communication Strategy, which established an orchestrated campaign designed to offer credible, timely, and clear information to both avoid panic and enhance community understanding of actions that can be taken to protect birds and humans from further spread. Message themes during these initial campaigns focused on the modes of infection transmission, hygiene and safe preparation of poultry for consumption, keeping children safe through distancing from birds, and proper handling and caging of poultry. Interventions included television ads and a wide range of printed materials targeted to households (with and without live poultry), school children, and to and through a network of 16,000 independent pharmacists under the Ask Consult brand, who are often the front line information providers for community health issues. Consumer fliers, Q&A booklets, fact sheets, and posters were distributed through the Ministry of Health's 5,000 community clinics, community outreach programmes, community NGOs, and the Ask Consult pharmacies. In addition, an AI hotline was established for reporting human and bird infections.

The reach of these first campaigns was strong, reaching 85 per cent of Egyptian households after the first two days of the launch, and indicating a tremendous need for reliable information on the flu outbreak (Figure 31.3A). Further analysis identified that, while the awareness of AI was relatively high and the perception of risk was relatively high, the perception of susceptibility of this risk was relatively lower. While the public acknowledged the very real threat, they believed 'it won't happen in my backyard', or 'it won't affect me or my family' (Figure 31.3B). In addition, bio-security measures were relatively weak and inconsistent.

Jane T. Bertrand, Alice Payne Merritt, and Gary Saffitz

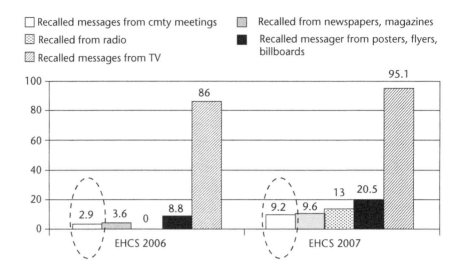

☐ Recalled messages from cmty meetings   ▨ Recalled from newspapers, magazines

▦ Recalled from radio   ■ Recalled messager from posters, flyers, billboards

▨ Recalled messages from TV

Figure 31.3A   Trend in reach of campaign
Sources: Egyptian Health Communication Survey, June (n = 4052, 15–49 adults in 21 governorates) Egyptian Health Communication Survey, Dec 2007 (n = 3770, 15–49 adults in 21 governorates).

	Perceived threat	**Individual efficacy**	
		Low	High
	Low	Not concerned Not confident **38%**	Not concerned but confident **50%**
	High	Concerned Not confident **53%**	Concerned & Confident **65%**

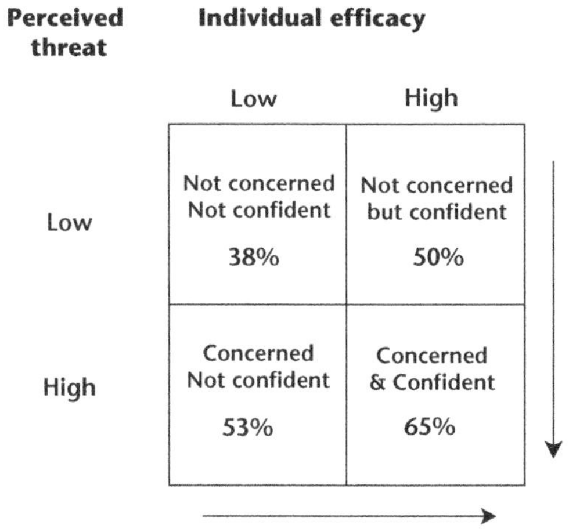

Figure 31.3B   Percent who reported 2+ protective actions in past 3 months by audience segment

A new community-based approach was needed to create more realistic risk perceptions, and improve knowledge and motivation to address the threat. Based on lessons learned from the initial campaigns, an AI Free Village Programme was created, which mobilised communities to do voluntary mapping (surveys and assessments), door-to-door messaging, peer-to-peer role modelling, and government and NGO outreach programmes. This combination of mass media and more immediate and targeted community mobilisation helped to create greater change in caging practices and protective behaviours (Figures 31.3C and 31.3D).

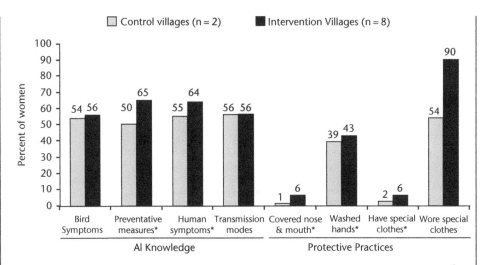

Figure 31.3C All knowledge and protective practices in intervention vs. control villages[1], 2008

Notes: [1] All villages recive media-based national communication exposure. Intervention villages also receive support for local CDA/NGO and outreach activity.

Sources: MVHS III 2008, n = 3171 married women, aged 15–49 in Fayoum & Minya governorates, *p<.0001.

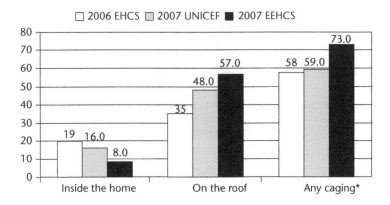

Figure 31.3D Trends in caging practices

Note: * Consistent (all the time) plus intermittent (caging at certain times).
Sources: Egyptian Health Communication Survey, June 2006 (n = 4052, 15–49 adults in 21 governorates).
UNICEF Avian Flu Survey, Feb 2007 (n = 4009, 15+women in 12 governorates).
Egyptian Health Communication Survey, Dec 2007 (n = 3770, 15–49 adults in 21 governorates).

Further study of the results suggested that the intervention villages had a greater rate of change than those that did not participate in the AI Free Villages programme (Figure 31.3E). In addition, there was a measurable dose effect, where the greater the number of messages recalled was correlated with a greater amount of change (Figure 31.3F).

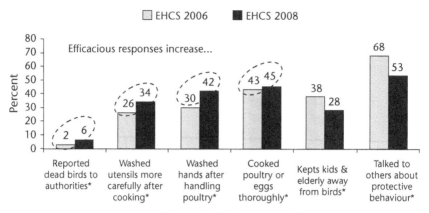

Figure 31.3E   Trends in protective behaviours 2006–2008
Sources: Egyptian Health Communication Survey, June 2006 (n = 4052, 15–49 adults in 21 governorates); Egyptian Health Communication Survey, Jan 2008 (n = 3770, 15–49 adults in 21 governorates); Chi-square, *p<.001.

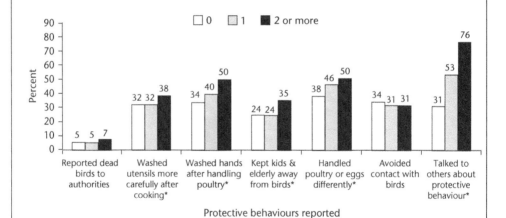

Figure 31.3F   Protective behaviours reported since campaign began, by number of campaign messages recalled
Sources: Egyptian Health Communication Survey, June 2008 (n = 3770, 15–49 adults in 21 governorates).

The Egypt programme identified several key success factors behind the AI communication interventions, including: multi-sectoral action involving diverse and complementary partners; multi-level implementation operating at the national, community, and household/individual levels; a tangential benefit that builds on other practices that define health competency (such as hand-washing at appropriate times); and a dynamic approach that allows for innovation and change as the disease mutates and changes.

Health communication programmes have evolved markedly in recent decades, reaching audiences with programmes that captivate attention, change social norms, and save lives through improved health behaviours. Health communication can have the greatest effect when multiple communication channels are used to promote change that enables communities, health services, and other environments. Developing a strategic approach to guide programmes, utilising effective communication design steps, and integrating research into key stages of programme development maximises social and behaviour change. The ubiquity of health communication programmes in countries worldwide attests to the power of this intervention.

References

Babalola, S. and Kincaid, D.L. (2009) 'New Methods for Estimating the Impact of Health Communication Programs', *Communication Methods and Measures*, 3(1): 61–83.

Hornik, R.C. (ed.) (2002) *Public Health Communication: Evidence of Behavior Change*, Mahwah, NJ: Lawrence Earlbaum Associates.

Kaiser Family Foundation and Project for Excellence in Journalism (2008) *Health News Coverage in the US Media, January 2007–June 2008*, Washington, DC: Kaiser Family Foundation and Project for Excellence in Journalism.

Kincaid, D.L., Parker, W., Johnson, S., Schierhout, G., Connolly, C., and Pham, V.T.H. (2008) *AIDS Communication Programs, HIV Prevention, and Living with HIV/AIDS in South Africa, 2006*, Pretoria: John Hopkins Health and Education South Africa.

Parker, J.C. and Thorson, E. (eds) (2009) *Health Communication in the New Media Landscape*, New York: Springer.

Piotrow, P.T., Rimon, J.G.II, Payne Merritt, A., and Saffitz, G. (2003) *Advancing Health Communication: The PCS Experience in the Field*, Baltimore, MD: Johns Hopkins Bloomberg School of Public Health Center for Communication Programs.

Salem, R.M., Bernstein, J., Sullivan, T.M., and Lande, R. (2008) 'Communication for Better Health', *Population Reports*, Series J, No. 56, Baltimore: INFO Project, Johns Hopkins Bloomberg School of Public Health.

Saunders, R.P., Evans, M.H., and Praphul, J. (2005) 'Developing a Process-Evaluation Plan for Assessing Health Promotion Program Implementation: A How-To Guide', *Health Promotion Practice*, 6(2): 134–47.

Schiavo, R. (2007) *Health Communication: From Theory to Practice*, San Francisco, CA: Jossey-Bass.

Singhal, A., Papa, M.J., Sharma, D., Pant, S., Worrell, T., Muthuswamy, N., and Witte, K. (2006) 'Entertainment Education and Social Change: The Communicative Dynamics of Social Capital', *Journal of Creative Communications*, 1: 1–18.

Snyder, L. (2007) 'Health Communication Campaigns and their Impact on Behavior', *Journal of Nutrition Education and Behavior*, 39: S32–S40.

Part VII

Global Public Health
and Development

32

Tracking Development Assistance for Health, 1990 to 2007[*]

Nirmala Ravishankar, Katherine Leach-Kemon, and Christopher J.L. Murray

Introduction

The past decade witnessed a rapid rise in development assistance for improving health in low- and middle-income countries. The emergence of several new global health players from outside the traditional nexus of bilateral agencies, multilateral organisations, and development banks that dominated the international aid scene in previous decades has accompanied this growth in resources. The dramatic increase in global health financing and the recipients of these dollars have garnered much attention from global health experts and have resulted in great speculation about the effectiveness of aid (Farmer and Garrett 2007; Farrar 2007; Garrett 2007; Moyo 2009; Scheiber *et al.* 2007) and the impact of new global health initiatives (Brugha *et al.* 2002; Lim *et al.* 2008). Currently, many anticipate a decline in funding levels as a result of the global recession (Kaiser Family Foundation 2008; Marmot and Bell 2009; McNeil 2009; UN News Service 2008).

Prior to this study, existing research revealed little about the exact magnitude of development assistance for health (DAH), who was financing it, how much it had grown over time, and where it was going. Most studies have only examined aid from donor governments and multilateral organisations (Ethelson *et al.* 2004; Narasimhan and Attaran 2003; OECD 2008; OECD, 200-; Powell-Jackson *et al.* 2006; Waddington *et al.* 2005) and have failed to capture important private sources of funding. A few attempts have been made to measure the size of DAH, but these typically offer single-year snapshots (Kates *et al.* 2006; Sridhar and Batniji 2008), or cover a relatively small number of years and have not been updated (Michaud 2003; Michaud and Murray 1994).

Timely and reliable information on DAH is a global public good. Government officials in developing countries and donor nations alike can use these data for evidence-based policymaking and planning. The data also are needed by policymakers in recipient countries, taxpayers in donor countries, and activists worldwide to monitor whether donors are honouring their financial commitments and stated priorities. Understanding how financial aid flows into the health system is also an essential part of evaluating the impact and cost-effectiveness of DAH.

---

[*] This chapter is adapted from Ravishankar *et al.* 2009.

Tracking development assistance of health

The Institute for Health Metrics and Evaluation (IHME) has launched a multiyear effort to track DAH, developing a comprehensive system to examine global health resources. In our inaugural 2009 study, we sought to monitor the volume of health aid to low- and middle-income countries, and to understand its nature and composition by generating valid, reliable, and comparable estimates of DAH. IHME will update these estimates annually. Our approach to tracking DAH is built around measuring flows from major global health actors, which we refer to as global health channels of assistance (see Box 32.1). These channels are institutions and agencies whose main purpose is providing development assistance.

We defined DAH as all financial and in-kind contributions from global health channels that aim to improve health in developing countries. Financial contributions include all payments on health grants and loans. In-kind contributions refer to the cost of delivering health services, supplying drugs and medical supplies, providing technical assistance, generating global public goods such as disease surveillance, and administering grants and loans.

Because our goal was to measure development assistance for the health sector and not for all sectors that influence health, we excluded aid to sectors such as water and sanitation as well as humanitarian aid. We counted disbursements rather than commitments because the former represent the actual funds that flowed from donors to recipient countries, while the latter represent funds that are likely to flow over multiple years in the future. We included all concessionary loans, which charge either no interest or a rate lower than the current market rate. Our estimates do not take loan repayments into account.

We used numerous data sources to estimate DAH. To measure DAH flowing through bilateral agencies, global health initiatives, the European Commission, development banks, and the United Nations agencies, we relied on sources such as the Organisation for Economic Co-operation and Development (OECD), annual reports, audited financial statements, and databases obtained via organisations' web sites and personal correspondence. For private sources, we used data from the United States Agency for International Development (USAID), the Bill & Melinda Gates Foundation (BMGF), the Foundation Center, annual reports, audited financial statements, web sites, personal communications, and tax returns.

Box 32.1 Global health channels of assistance tracked

- Bilateral aid agencies in 22 member countries of the Development Assistance Committee of the Organisation for Economic Co-operation and Development (OECD-DAC)
- European Commission (EC)
- The World Health Organization (WHO)
- The United Nations Children's Fund (UNICEF)
- The United Nations Population Fund (UNFPA)
- The Joint United Nations Programme for HIV/AIDS (UNAIDS)
- The World Bank, including the International Development Association (IDA) and the International Bank for Reconstruction and Development (IBRD)
- The Asian Development Bank (ADB)
- The Inter-American Development Bank (IDB)
- The African Development Bank (AfDB)
- US-based private foundations, including the Bill & Melinda Gates Foundation (BMGF)
- US-based non-governmental organisations (NGOs)

Tracking DAH from 1990 to 2007 proved to be a formidable task for many reasons. First, there are no integrated databases containing high-quality data on health disbursements from private foundations worldwide or the health activities of non-governmental organisations (NGOs). Second, before reaching its final destination, whether it is a health centre or an NGO in a developing country or a research laboratory in a US university, DAH often flows through multiple intermediaries, increasing the risk that the same dollar could be counted multiple times. Third, lack of transparency in aid reporting was one obstacle to measuring DAH. Many bilateral donors failed to fully report disbursements, aid recipients, and project descriptions. Lack of transparency was more severe in earlier years of the study period, which makes it difficult to understand how the volume, recipients, and objectives of DAH changed over time. The methods we devised to address these challenges have been published in the *Lancet* (Ravishankar *et al.* 2009).

Trends in development assistance for health, 1990 to 2007

By channel of assistance

Figure 32.1 presents the total envelope of DAH by year, disaggregated by channels of assistance. It is hard to miss the dramatic rise in total health assistance from 1990 to 2007 in the graph. Between 1990 and 2007, DAH quadrupled in volume from $5.6 billion to $21.8 billion. The figure also shows that the rate of growth was not constant over those years. Health assistance grew gradually in the 11 years from 1990 to 2001, roughly doubling from $5.6 billion to $10.9 billion. It took only six years for it to double again, from $10.9 billion in 2001 to $21.8 billion in 2007.

A multitude of actors have managed these global health dollars during the past 18 years: bilateral agencies, regional development banks, the two arms of the World Bank – the International Development Association (IDA) and the International Bank for Reconstruction

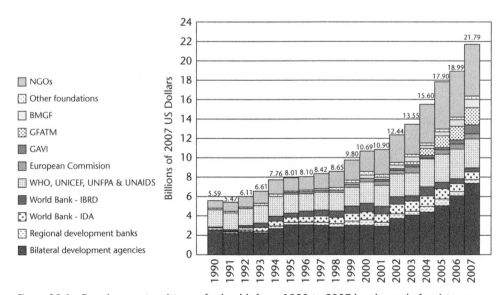

Figure 32.1 Development assistance for health from 1990 to 2007 by channel of assistance
Source: IHME DAH Database

and Development (IBRD) – the United Nations (UN) agencies, the European Commission (EC), the Global Alliance for Vaccines and Immunisation (GAVI), the Global Fund to Fight Aids, Tuberculosis and Malaria (GFATM), the Bill & Melinda Gates Foundation (BMGF), and other US-based foundations.

Tracking the flow of DAH by channel of assistance reveals dramatic changes in the institutional architecture of global health over the years. The share of health aid from bilateral agencies decreased from 46.8 per cent in 1990 to 27.1 per cent in 2001, and then increased in subsequent years to 34 per cent in 2007. The percentage of total health assistance flowing from UN agencies decreased from 32.3 per cent in 1990 to 14 per cent in 2007. The World Bank and regional banks accounted for 21.7 per cent of total health assistance at their relative peak in 2000. That percentage dropped to 7.2 per cent by 2007. GFATM and GAVI scaled up rapidly from less than 1 per cent of health assistance each in 2002 to 8.3 per cent and 4.2 per cent, respectively, in 2007. BMGF as a channel peaked in 2007 at 3.9 per cent of health assistance. The share of resources flowing through NGOs increased from 13.1 per cent of health assistance in 1990 to 24.9 per cent in 2006, the last year for which we have reported data for the NGOs (NGOs' contribution to DAH in 2007 was projected). For each channel of assistance, the graph shows the total financial and in-kind health-related contributions, net of any transfers to other channels also tracked by IHME. For example, bilateral agencies' grants to GAVI were subtracted from bilateral agencies' disbursements to avoid double-counting.

Each channel of assistance has markedly different priorities and approaches. As the distribution of DAH changes and shifts in favour of different actors, the manner in which DAH is delivered also changes. As one of the increasingly prominent global health initiatives, GAVI's goal is to increase vaccination coverage and reduce child mortality in developing countries by mobilising long-lasting funding, purchasing and distributing vaccines, providing technical assistance, and strengthening health systems. GFATM was founded in 2002 as a fund for increasing developing countries' access to new life-saving treatments for HIV/AIDS, tuberculosis, and malaria. In addition, the activities of US NGOs, which contribute a major share of DAH, run the gamut. The activities of the top 20 US NGOs ranked by overseas health expenditures (see Table 32.1) provide a window into the diverse activities of the nearly 1,000 US NGOs in our study. Their programmes include supplying donated drugs and medical equipment, implementing prevention programmes, sending medical volunteers to developing countries, training health workers, and working in the area of research and development for new health technologies.

By source of funding

Figure 32.2 presents the data shown in Figure 32.1 from a different perspective, revealing the funding sources that have fuelled the growth in DAH from 1990 to 2007. Contributions from donor governments accounted for nearly two-thirds of total DAH flowing to developing countries. As a per cent of total, their contributions ranged from 60 per cent to 76 per cent in the years covered by the study. The US government was the single largest donor of public DAH during this entire time period. Other big donors included the governments of the UK, Japan, Germany, France, the Netherlands, Canada, Sweden, Norway, and Italy.

Figure 32.2 also shows that private sources of funding were responsible for a growing share of total health assistance, from 19 per cent in 1998 to 26.7 per cent in 2007. BMGF as a source includes both BMGF's contributions as a channel of assistance and the expenditures

Table 32.1 NGOs registered in the US with highest cumulative overseas health expenditures from 2002 to 2006

Rank	NGO	Overseas health expenditure	Total overseas expenditure	Per cent of revenue from private sources	Per cent of revenue from in-kind contributions
1	Food For The Poor	1492.3	3137.0	91.0	80.4
2	Population Services International	1250.3	1275.6	10.7	0.1
3	MAP International	1196.8	1210.2	99.8	96.4
4	World Vision	826.1	3150.4	73.5	28.6
5	Brother's Brother Foundation	785.8	1158.6	99.9	99.0
6	Feed The Children	706.9	2044.5	96.9	82.6
7	Catholic Medical Mission Board	699.0	746.6	99.6	93.0
8	Project HOPE	583.6	635.6	89.6	69.2
9	Medical Teams International	568.8	698.8	98.5	89.0
10	Management Sciences for Health	515.5	617.6	11.1	0.0
11	United Nations Foundation	505.9	726.9	86.1	9.6
12	Catholic Relief Services	498.1	2547.9	37.3	2.0
13	Interchurch Medical Assistance	462.6	466.6	89.6	85.6
14	Direct Relief International	431.8	507.1	99.9	91.7
15	PATH	389.5	444.1	92.2	0.0
16	The Carter Center	378.2	472.3	94.1	45.4
17	International Medical Corps	338.7	354.1	52.1	42.8
18	Pathfinder International	269.6	301.0	20.9	0.9
19	Save the Children	229.1	1229.1	48.4	1.9
20	National Cancer Coalition	226.6	242.4	100.0	93.1

Data for 2007 have not been released yet. Expenditure is expressed in millions of real 2007 US$.

from other channels financed by BMGF. Counted this way, BMGF is one of the largest sources of privately financed health assistance. All private charitable donations as well as private giving from US-based foundations besides BMGF are included in the 'other' category.

Contributions from private corporations to US-based NGOs constitute another large component of privately financed health assistance. In-kind donations of drugs and medical equipment from pharmaceutical companies are included in this category. The value of these donations may be inflated due to accounting methods used by US NGOs discussed later in this chapter.

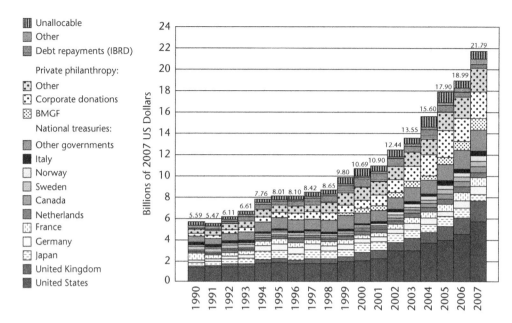

Figure 32.2 Development assistance for health from 1990 to 2007 by source of funding

Note: Funds from channels for which we were unable to find disaggregated revenue information and inter-agency transfers from non-DAH institutions are included in 'unallocable'. 'Other' refers to interest income, currency exchange adjustments, and other miscellaneous income.

Source: IHME DAH Database.

In addition to contributing to the expansion of global health financing, donors have influenced the arena through their funding preferences. Figure 32.3 shows how the governments of the US and the UK channelled a large fraction of DAH through NGOs and recipient governments in 2007. Countries such as Italy and France preferred to channel much of their funding through GFATM and GAVI in 2007. This graph also illustrates how lack of transparency – epitomised by some governments' failure to fully report the recipients of their aid – prevents us from fully understanding where these donors invested their dollars. In terms of reporting on aid recipients, the US government ranked the worst in 2007, failing to specify a recipient for more than 30 per cent ($1.79 billion) of its aid.

Figure 32.4 illuminates BMGF's funding priorities. BMGF's investments reflect its prioritisation of global health research through its funding of universities and research institutions. BMGF also has helped shape the global health agenda through its financing of public–private initiatives for global health, including GFATM, GAVI, and various product-development partnerships.

By type of assistance

Our estimates of DAH not only include financial assistance but also in-kind flows. Figure 32.5 reveals that in-kind donations accounted for nearly 40 per cent of DAH in 2007. In-kind donations are grouped into two categories. The first – programme management, research, and technical assistance – includes all expenditures by UN agencies on health programmes, the costs

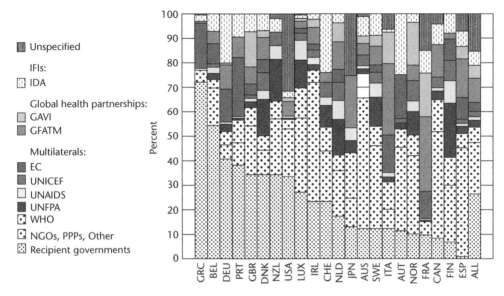

Figure 32.3 Channel-wise composition of publicly financed DAH by donor in 2007

Note: The composition of DAH from the 22 member countries of the OECD-DAC is shown. AUS = Australia, AUT = Austria, BEL = Belgium, CAN = Canada, CHE = Switzerland, DEU = Germany, DNK = Denmark, ESP = Spain, FIN = Finland, FRA = France, GBR = United Kingdom, GRC = Greece, IRL = Ireland, ITA = Italy, JPN = Japan, LUX = Luxembourg, NLD = the Netherlands, NOR = Norway, NZL = New Zealand, PRT = Portugal, SWE =Sweden, USA = United States.

Source: IHME DAH Database.

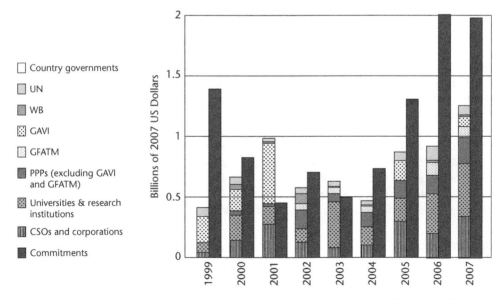

Figure 32.4 BMGF's global health commitments and disbursements from 2000 to 2007

Note: The multishaded bars represent disbursements and the gray shaded bars show commitments. 'Universities and research institutions' includes universities, NGOs, foundations, and government institutions in low-, middle-, and high-income countries with a research focus. 'Country governments' include all non-research oriented government agencies.

Source: IHME DAH Database of BMGF global health grants.

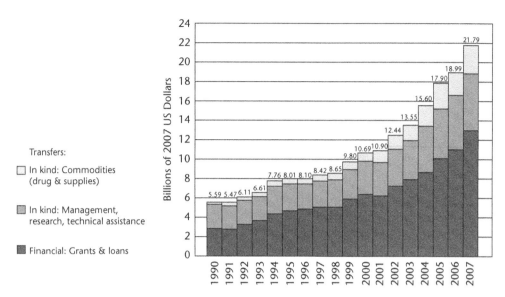

Figure 32.5 Development assistance for health from 1990 to 2007 by type of assistance
Source: IHME DAH Database.

incurred by loan- and grant-making institutions for providing technical assistance and pro-gramme management, and expenditures by NGOs net of any commodities delivered. Donated drugs and other commodities comprise the second component of in-kind transfers and are shown separately.

The surprisingly large volume of in-kind health aid raises several questions both about how in-kind transfers are valued and what their opportunity costs are. First, the true value of drug donations to recipients in developing countries may be less than the book value that US-based NGOs recorded in the US tax returns and USAID data used in this analysis. The value of donations to recipient communities also may be less due to the mismatch between the drugs and supplies and local health needs, and the fact that some of these products may have a short shelf life (Reich *et al*. 1999).

Second, the hiring of international experts from donor countries to administer health programmes and provide technical assistance has often been decried as 'phantom aid' by many aid advocacy groups. Whether dollars spent paying staff at global health institutions constitutes a waste of global health resources or is the necessary cost for generating much-needed knowledge, policy guidance, and training is a research question in its own right regarding the cost-effectiveness of this mode of development assistance.

By health focus

Given current debates about disease-specific vertical programme support and general health system support, we analysed the volume of development assistance earmarked for three priority diseases among donors – HIV/AIDS, tuberculosis, and malaria – as well as support for sector-wide approaches and health-systems strengthening. We were unable to identify the health focus of all DAH, however, as some donors and channels of assistance failed to provide project descriptions. In 2007, for example, we were able to obtain project-level information for $13.8 billion out of $21.8 billion of total DAH.

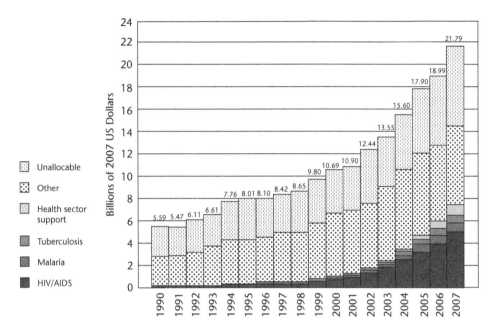

Figure 32.6 Development assistance for health from 1990 to 2007 for HIV/AIDS, tuberculosis, malaria, and health sector support

Note: 'Unallocable' corresponds to DAH for which we did not have project-level information on disease focus.

Source: IHME DAH and project databases.

The trends in Figure 32.6 show that disbursements for HIV/AIDS grew, first gradually from $0.2 billion in 1990 to $0.7 billion in 2000, and then more rapidly to $4.9 billion in 2007. Development assistance for tuberculosis and malaria remained small in comparison: $0.6 billion and $0.7 billion, respectively, in 2007. However, resources for malaria showed substantial increases, beginning in 2005.

Promoting the use of new and cost-effective health technologies to prevent and treat HIV/ AIDS, tuberculosis, and malaria has emerged as a leading global health priority in recent years. In 1999, WHO warned that six diseases, including HIV/AIDS, tuberculosis, and malaria, were the primary causes of death worldwide and disproportionately affected developing countries (WHO 1999). Prioritisation of these diseases can be traced to the 2000 G8 Summit in Okinawa (Ministry of Foreign Affairs of Japan 2000a) and the Abuja Declaration on HIV/AIDS, Tuberculosis, and Other Related Infectious Diseases in 2001 (Organization of African Unity 2001). The creation of GFATM, with the express mandate to use innovative mechanisms to mobilise public and private funds and ensure that they are used effectively, was another manifestation of this commitment.

Given the extensive amount of attention given to HIV/AIDS by donors, recipient country governments, public–private partnerships, and multilateral institutions, it is surprising that DAH for HIV/AIDS only represented about one-third of disease-allocable DAH and one-quarter of total DAH in 2007 (CNN 2003; GFATM 2009; Ministry of Foreign Affairs of Japan 2000b; Organization of African Unity 2001; UK Prime Minister's Office 2005; UN 2001).

Development assistance for tuberculosis and malaria is small in comparison to flows for HIV/ AIDS. Given the differential allocation of resources among these three diseases, one might expect these funding patterns to reflect the relative health impact attributable to these three diseases. Disease burden, or the impact of ill health in terms of premature death, is measured here in terms of total disability-adjusted life years (DALYs). This measurement takes into account both years of life lost due to death and years lived with disability (Murray and Lopez 1996). While current burden estimates show that malaria and tuberculosis account for 4.9 per cent of total burden of disease in low- and middle-income countries, compared to 4.1 per cent for HIV/AIDS, funding for malaria and tuberculosis was only 6.3 per cent of total DAH compared to 22.7 per cent for HIV/AIDS in 2007 (WHO 2008).

Figure 32.6 also shows health sector support funds mobilised through partner coordination mechanisms, which amounted to $0.9 billion in 2007. In 2005, many bilateral donors signed the Paris Declaration on Aid Effectiveness, which, among other policy recommendations, called for increased use of recipient countries' financial systems and sector-wide approaches to development assistance (OECD 2005). Despite the large number of donor government signatories and bilateral agencies' targeted programmes for health sector support (UK DFID 2007), the volume of these flows remained low. Measuring aid for health sector support is one way to monitor donors' implementation of the Paris Declaration principles. Future updates of DAH will provide a means to assess the impact of newer, related initiatives, such as the International Health Partnership, on funding levels for health sector support (International Health Partnership 2009).

By geographic focus

The volume of aid received by low- and middle-income countries varies considerably, both in the aggregate and in ratio to the country's population. Figures 32.7 and 32.8 show the top ten recipient countries in terms of total global health dollars and per capita global health dollars received between 2002 and 2007. The first list of top health aid recipients consists of the most populous developing countries (India, China, Indonesia, and Pakistan); African countries that have attracted large amounts of health assistance through the US President's Emergency Plan for AIDS Relief (PEPFAR) and GFATM (Uganda, Ethiopia, Tanzania, Zambia, and Kenya); and one that fits both descriptions (Nigeria). The second list of countries receiving the highest amount of health dollars per person is comprised of small island nations (Micronesia, Tonga, Sao Tome and Principe, the Solomon Islands, Samoa, and Cape Verde) and countries with small populations (Zambia, Namibia, Suriname, and Guyana).

The two figures also show the channels through which these countries received external aid for health. The World Bank, GFATM, and the US government are the primary channels of health aid in the first list. The composition is more varied in the second list and reflects the continuing strength of ties between donor countries and their ex-colonies and protectorates as well as modern geopolitical and economic considerations. For example, Australia and the Netherlands are the biggest donors of health aid to their erstwhile colonies, Solomon Islands and Suriname, respectively. Micronesia, which entered a compact of free association with the US in 1986, receives almost all its health aid from the US, and, as a result, ranks higher than all other countries in per capita DAH funding. Japan, Tonga's largest donor, is the primary consumer of Tongan exports (Ministry of Foreign Affairs of Japan 2008).

Notwithstanding historical, economic, and political links, it is worth asking if the current distribution of health dollars reflects health needs across countries. While the detailed analysis required to answer this question is beyond the scope of this chapter, we examine the correlation between DAH and the burden of disease as a first approximation.

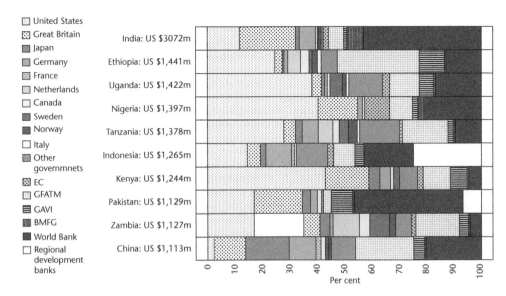

Figure 32.7 Top ten recipients of development assistance for health from 2002 to 2007, disaggregated by channel of assistance

Note: The amount of DAH received by each country in real 2007 US$ is shown alongside the name of the country. Only DAH allocable by country is reflected in the figure.

Source: IHME DAH Project Database.

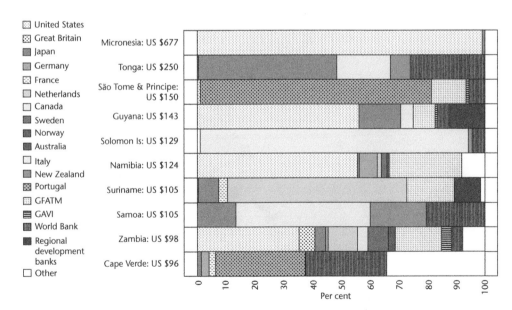

Figure 32.8 Top ten countries in terms of per capita development assistance for health received from 2002 to 2007, disaggregated by channel of assistance

Note: The amount of DAH received by each country in real 2007 US$ is shown alongside the name of the country. Only DAH allocable by country is reflected in the figure.

Source: IHME Project Database and UN World Population Database.

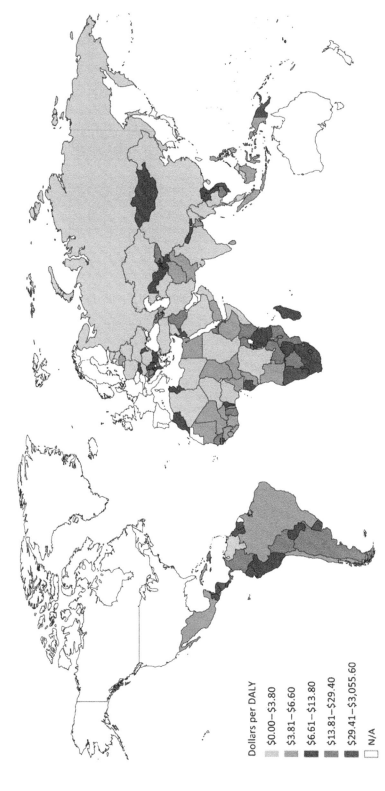

Figure 32.9 World map of development assistance for health

Dollars per DALY
$0.00–$3.80
$3.81–$6.60
$6.61–$13.80
$13.81–$29.40
$29.41–$3,055.60
N/A

Computation of the correlation coefficient between health assistance and disease burden by year showed that the correlation had risen from 0.6 to 0.8 between 1997 and 2007. The drive to fund HIV/AIDS, tuberculosis, and malaria programmes appears to be channelling global health dollars to areas of higher burden than ever before. Figure 32.9 shows a map of health aid per unit of disease burden for total health assistance. The map gives a more nuanced picture of the relationship between DALYs and DAH, however, showing tremendous variation in health aid per DALY across regions and within regions. We also calculated the correlation between per capita health aid and per capita GDP; it was near zero until the mid-1990s, but it has

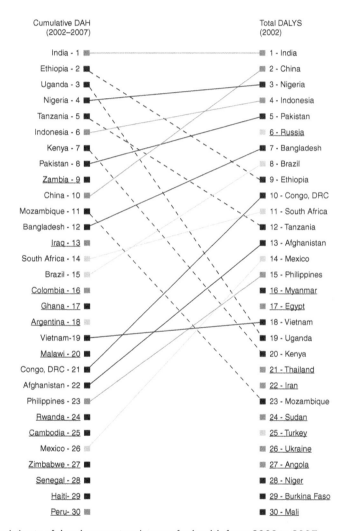

Figure 32.10   Top 30 country recipients of development assistance for health from 2002 to 2007, compared with top 30 countries in terms of all-cause burden of disease in 2002

Note: Low-, lower-middle-, and upper-middle-income countries are shown with black, grey, and light grey markers and arrows, respectively. Countries in either column that received a rank lower than 30 in the other column and are, therefore, unmatched in the figure, are underlined. Only DAH allocable by country is reflected in the figure.

Source: IHME Project Database and WHO Burden of Disease Database.

decreased steadily from –0.1 in 1999 to –0.3 in 2007. This suggests that poorer countries are receiving increasing amounts of health aid.

Figure 32.10 presents another perspective on the same question of how DAH compares with burden of disease. The top 30 recipients of health aid are ordered by rank in the left column, while countries are ranked in decreasing order of burden on the right. India topped both lists. Some high-burden countries, such as China, Brazil, and Bangladesh, had a much higher rank on the burden list than on the health aid list. In other words, they received much less assistance than would be expected given their disease burden. The situation was the reverse in Ethiopia, Uganda, Tanzania, Kenya, and Mozambique, all of which received more funds than would be expected given their disease burden. All five countries received health aid from PEPFAR from 2004 to 2007.

Countries that appeared in one list and not the other are underlined. On the left are countries that are in the top 30 in terms of aid received but are not among the top 30 in terms of disease burden. Zambia, Iraq, Colombia, Ghana, Argentina, Malawi, Rwanda, Cambodia, Zimbabwe, Senegal, Haiti, and Peru fall in that category. All of them, with the exception of Argentina, are either low- or lower-middle-income countries. On the right side are countries that have high burdens by global standards but are not the top recipients of aid. This describes the situation in Russia, Myanmar, Egypt, Thailand, Iran, Sudan, Turkey, Ukraine, Angola, Niger, Burkina Faso, and Mali, all of which, with the exception of Russia and Turkey, are either low- or lower-middle-income countries. Colombia is an important ally of the US in the war against drugs, while the US military's efforts in Iraq may contribute to its high ranking on the DAH list.

In sum, these results indicate that country allocation of DAH appears to be driven by many considerations beyond the burden of disease, including historical, political, and economic relationships between certain donors and recipient countries.

The map reflects international boundaries in 2006. Since DALY data were only available for 2002, we used this as a proxy for burden in all subsequent years. Countries that received zero DAH over the study period and countries with zero or missing burden data are not shown. DAH received is shown in millions of real 2007 US$.

Conclusion

This study carefully documents a trend widely recognised in the field of global health, namely that development assistance for improving health in developing countries has expanded significantly in the last 18 years. The study provides the first systematic and comprehensive estimates of the total envelope of health aid from both public and private sources from 1990 to 2007.

Global health resources have more than quadrupled from 1990 to 2007, with the rate of growth accelerating beginning in 2002. The increase in aid for health has been fuelled by a huge expansion of dollars for HIV/AIDS, but other areas of global health also have grown dramatically. The influx of resources has come not only from public sources but also from private philanthropy. Our findings reveal that DAH is composed not only of financial flows, but also of sizeable shares of in-kind resources.

The expansion of resources for global health, especially in the past ten years, has been accompanied by a major change in the institutional landscape, with channels such as GFATM, GAVI, and US NGOs commanding a steadily larger share of DAH. The share of DAH routed through organisations such as the UN system and the World Bank have shrunk over time. The growing influence of GFATM, GAVI, and US NGOs – each of which possesses unique approaches to development work – has changed the way the bulk of DAH is delivered. Furthermore, these trends in aid flows have created a competitive model of funding, which runs the risk of undermining the critical role of the UN agencies as trusted neutral brokers between the scientific and technical communities on the one hand and developing country governments on the other.

While aid for HIV/AIDS, tuberculosis, and malaria accounts for a significant part of the expansion in resources, there have been large increases in other areas of health as well. While there is much rhetoric about increasing funds transferred to developing countries through general health sector support, the data suggest that it remains a very small part of health aid – less than 5 per cent in 2007. The disconnect between the rhetoric about the importance of shifting to sector support and the reality, as captured in these results, highlights the importance of data on the actual flows.

Examining the distribution of health assistance across countries reveals a complex picture. It appears that countries with a higher disease burden, and poorer countries, are on the whole receiving more health assistance than their healthier and wealthier counterparts. However, this relationship is far from being completely predictable. At the same level of disease burden, countries received remarkably different amounts of health aid. Historical, economic, and political factors that are unrelated to health also determine which developing countries donor governments favour.

Timely and reliable information on global health resource flows is crucial for policymaking and planning at the national level. The need for timelier reporting of commitments and disbursements by institutions is only reinforced in this time of global recession and financial turmoil. It is also needed for monitoring whether donors are honouring their commitments, for fostering greater transparency in aid reporting, and for accurately evaluating the impact of global health interventions. As the debate on aid effectiveness intensifies, careful documentation of the magnitude of global health resources can serve as a foundation for an evidence-based debate. For example, the data are currently being used to investigate what developing country governments do with their own resources when they receive increased health aid. IHME is committed to providing an annual assessment of DAH as a resource for an enhanced debate on the role of development aid in improving global health.

References

Brugha, R., Starling, M. and Walt, G. (2002) 'GAVI, The First Steps: Lessons for the Global Fund', *The Lancet*, 359(9,304): 435–8.

CNN (Cable News Network) (2003) *Bush's State of the Union Speech* (29 January), available at http://www.cnn.com/2003/ALLPOLITICS/01/28/sotu.transcript/ (accessed 3 June 2009).

Ethelston, S., Bechtel, A., Chaya, N., Kantner, A. and Vogel C.G. (2004) *Progress and Promises: Trends in International Assistance for Reproductive Health and Population, 2004*, Washington, DC: Population Action International.

Farmer, P. and Garrett, L. (2007) 'From "Marvelous Momentum" to Health Care for All: Success is Possible with the Right Programs', *Foreign Affairs*, 86: 155–61, available at http://www.foreignaffairs.org/20070301faresponse86213/paul-farmer-laurie-garrett/from-marvelous-momentum-to-health-care-for-all-success-is-possible-with-the-right-programs.html (accessed 11 March 2009).

Farrar, J. (2007) 'Global Health Science: A Threat and an Opportunity for Collaborative Clinical Science', *Nature Immunology*, 8(12): 1,277–9.

Garrett, L. (2007) 'The Challenge of Global Health', *Foreign Affairs*, 86: 14, available at http://www.foreignaffairs.org/20070101faessay86103/laurie-garrett/the-challenge-of-global-health.html (accessed 11 March 2009).

GFATM (Global Fund to Fight AIDS, Tuberculosis, and Malaria) (2009) *History of the Global Fund*, available at http://www.theglobalfund.org/en/history/?lang=en (accessed 3 June 2009).

International Health Partnership (2009) *Welcome to IHP+*, available at www.internationalhealthpartnership. net (accessed 1 September 2009).

Kaiser Family Foundation (2008) 'HIV/AIDS /Global Financial Crisis could Harm HIV/AIDS Funding, Piot Says', *Kaiser Daily HIV/AIDS Report*, 29 October, available at http://www.globalhealthreporting. org/article.asp?DR_ID=55258 (accessed 11 March 2009).

Kates, J., Morrison, J.S. and Lief, E. (2006) 'Global Health Funding: A Glass Half Full?' *The Lancet*, 368(9,531): 187–8.

Lim, S.S., Stein, D.B., Charrow, A. and Murray, C.J. (2008) 'Tracking Progress Towards Universal Childhood Immunisation and the Impact of Global Initiatives: A Systematic Analysis of Three-dose Diphtheria, Tetanus, and Pertussis Immunisation Coverage', *The Lancet*, 372(9,655): 2,031–46.

McNeil, D.G. Jr. (2009) 'Global Fund is Billions Short', *The New York Times*, 2 February, available at http://www.nytimes.com/2009/02/03/health/research/03glob.html?_r=2 (accessed 11 March 2009).

Marmot, M.G. and Bell, R. (2009) 'How Will the Financial Crisis Affect Health?', *British Medical Journal*, 338: b1314.

Michaud, C. (2003) *Development Assistance for Health: Recent Trends and Resource Allocation*, Boston, MA: Harvard Center for Population Development.

Michaud, C. and Murray, C.J. (1994) 'External Assistance to the Health Sector in Developing Countries: A Detailed Analysis, 1972–90', *Bulletin World Health Organization*, 72(4): 639–51.

Ministry of Foreign Affairs of Japan (2000a) *Okinawa international conference on infectious diseases*, Tokyo: Ministry of Foreign Affairs of Japan, available at http://www.mofa.go.jp/policy/economy/summit/2000/ infection.html (accessed 3 June 2009).

Ministry of Foreign Affairs of Japan (2000b) *The Okinawa International Conference on Infectious Diseases Chair's Summary*, available at http://www.mofa.go.jp/policy/economy/summit/2000/genoa/infection1. html (accessed 3 June 2009).

Ministry of Foreign Affairs of Japan (2008) *Japan-Tonga Relations*, available at http://www.mofa.go.jp/ region/asia-paci/tonga/ (accessed 3 June 2009).

Moyo, D. (2009) *Dead Aid: Why Aid is Not Working and How There is a Better Way for Africa*, New York: Farrar, Straus and Giroux.

Murray, C.J.L. and Lopez, A.D. (eds) (1996) *The Global Burden of Disease: A Comprehensive Assessment of Mortality and Disability from Diseases, Injuries, and Risk Factors in 1990 and Projected to 2020*, Cambridge, MA: Harvard University Press on behalf of the World Health Organization and the World Bank.

Narasimhan, V. and Attaran, A. (2003) 'Roll Back Malaria? The Scarcity of International Aid for Malaria Control', *Malaria Journal*, 2: 8.

Organization of African Unity (2001) *Abuja Declaration on HIV/AIDS, Tuberculosis and Other Related Infectious Diseases*, available at http://www.un.org/ga/aids/pdf/abuja_declaration.pdf (accessed 3 June 2009).

OECD (Organisation for Economic Co-operation and Development) (2005) *Paris Declaration on Aid Effectiveness*, available at http://www.oecd.org/dataoecd/11/41/34428351.pdf (accessed 1 September 2009).

OECD (Organisation for Economic Co-operation and Development) (2008) *Focus on Aid to Health*, available at http://www.oecd.org/document/44/0,3343, en_2649_34469_24670956_1_1_1_1,00.html (accessed 11 March 2009).

OECD (Organisation for Economic Co-operation and Development) (200-) *International Development Statistics (IDS): Online Databases on Aid and Other Resource Flows*, available at www.oecd.org/dac/stats/ idsonline (accessed 2 December 2008).

Powell-Jackson, T., Borghi, J., Mueller, D.H., Patouillard, E. and Mills, A. (2006) 'Countdown to 2015: Tracking Donor Assistance to Maternal, Newborn, and Child Health', *The Lancet*, 368(9,541): 1,077–87.

Ravishankar, N., Gubbins, P., Cooley, R.J., Leach-Kemon, K., Michaud, C.M., Jamison, D.T., and Murray, C.J.L. (2009) 'Financing Global Health: Tracking Development Assistance for Health from 1990 to 2007', *The Lancet*, 373: 2,113–24.

Ravishankar, N., Gubbins, P., Cooley, R.J., Leach-Kemon, K., Michaud, C.M., Jamison, D.T., and Murray, C.J.L. (2009) *'Financing Global Health 2009: Tracking Development Assistance for Health*. Seattle: Institute for Health Metrics and Evaluation, available at http://www.healthmetricsandevaluation.org/resources/policyreports/2009/financing_global_health_0709.html (accessed 28 September 2010) .

Reich, M.R., Wagner, A.K., McLaughlin, T.J., Dumbaugh, K.A. and Derai-Cochin, M. (1999) 'Pharmaceutical Donations by the USA: An Assessment of Relevance and Time-to-Expiry', *Bulletin of the World Health Organization*, 77(8): 675–80.

Schieber, G.J., Gottret, P., Fleisher, L. K. and Leive, A.A. (2007) 'Financing Global Health: Mission Unaccomplished', *Health Affairs*, 26(4): 921–34.

Sridhar, D. and Batniji, R. (2008) 'Misfinancing Global Health: A Case for Transparency in Disbursements and Decision Making', *The Lancet*, 372(9,644): 1,185–91.

UK DFID (UK Department for International Development) (2007) *Working Together for Better Health*, London: Department for International Development, available at http://www.dfid.gov.uk/Documents/publications/health-strategy07-evidence.pdf (accessed 1 September 2009).

UK Prime Minister's Office (8 July 2005) *Africa: An Historic Opportunity*, available at http://www.number10.gov.uk/Page7880 (accessed 3 June 2009).

UN (United Nations) (2001) *Secretary General Proposes Global Fund for Fight against HIV/AIDS and Other Infectious Diseases at African Leaders Summit*, press release, issued 26 April, available at http://www.un.org/News/Press/docs/2001/SGSM7779R1.doc.htm (accessed 3 June 2009).

UN (United Nations) News Service (2008) 'Financial Crisis Threatens Push to Boost Global Health, Says Top UN Official', *United Nations News Centre*, 12 November, available at http://www.un.org/apps/news/story.asp?NewsID=28911&Cr=financial&Cr1=crisis (accessed 11 March 2009).

Waddington, C., Martin, J. and Walford, V. (2005) *Trends in International Funding for Malaria Control*, prepared for the Roll Back Malaria Partnership, London: HLSP Institute.

WHO (World Health Organization) (1999) *Leading Infectious Killers*, available at http://www.who.int/infectious-disease-report/pages/graph5.html (accessed 3 June 2009).

WHO (World Health Organization) *GBD 2004 Summary Tables*, available at http://www.who.int/entity/healthinfo/global_burden_disease/DALY7%202004.xls (accessed 3 June 2009).

33

Global Blindness and Visual Impairment

Alfred Sommer

Definition and magnitude of the problem

An estimated 38 million people are blind by the World Health Organization (WHO) definition of central acuity of less than 20/400 (Resnikoff *et al.* 2004). But this severely underestimates the impact of ocular disease on societal productivity. Many important tasks, from reading to driving, to mending fish nets, require vision of 20/60 or better. The global estimate of those who are visually impaired or blind exceeds 135 million, most of whom are incapacitated by their disability and unable to fully participate in economic and development activities to the degree they otherwise might (Resnikoff *et al.* 2004). This impact is magnified by the need, by many of those who are visually impaired, for the assistance of sighted caregivers, which further deprives the economy of individuals who might otherwise contribute more effectively to development. More than half of all blindness is avoidable, and most avoidable blindness occurs among poor people in the least developed regions of the world. Not surprisingly, there is a direct correlation between per capita GDP and the prevalence of blindness (Figure 33.1) (Ho and Schwab 2001).

Cataract

The single greatest cause of avoidable blindness is unoperated cataract. In most underdeveloped regions (and poor populations of wealthy countries), unoperated cataract accounts for roughly half of all blindness. A cataract is simply an opacification of the lens of the eye, which commonly increases with aging. In some populations, as in many areas of India, cataracts develop a decade or so earlier than they do in other countries. Exposure to ultra-violet light, tobacco use, frequent diarrhoea, and poor nutrition may play a role. As a result, visual impairment often forces otherwise vigorous individuals to lose their jobs. Many also suffer a loss of social standing (Frick and Foster 2003; Javitt *et al.* 1983).

The crux of the problem is not so much the formation of cataracts, but the fact that ophthalmic surgeons are performing too few cataract operations to meet the population's needs. In recent years a new metric has been devised to capture the potential magnitude of this imbalance: the Cataract Surgical Rate (CSR), expressed as the number of cataract operations performed each year per million people in the population. While one might expect modest variation in the CSR appropriate for different populations (depending, in part, on the age at

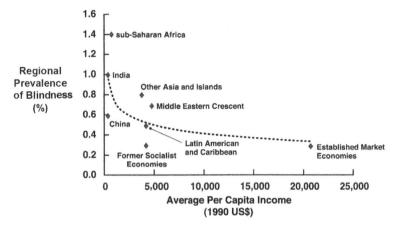

Figure 33.1   Prevalence of blindness in relation to per capita income
Source: Adapted from Ho and Schwab 2001.

which visually disabling cataract first occurs), CSR rates appear to be roughly similar across most populations in which adequate surgical services exist to meet demand. The CSR of high-income countries (the US, Europe, Japan) hovers around 4,000 to 5,000. In contrast, the CSR in much of sub-Saharan Africa and East Asia is only a tenth as great, dooming 90 per cent of those in need of cataract surgery from ever receiving it (Table 33.1) (Foster 2001).

People lack access to cataract surgeons because there are too few surgeons in their country; existing surgeons live and work in desirable urban centres far removed from the rural country-side; surgeons charge more than poor patients can afford; or the surgeons are inefficient, having not yet adopted techniques that would permit them to do far more procedures in the same amount of time. Each of these constraints is critical; some are even solvable.

India is a marvellous example of the strides that can be made with government commitment and inspired ophthalmic leadership. In the 1980s, India had a huge backlog of unoperated cataract blindness. As can be seen from Table 33.2, the CSR was estimated at 500. But in the late 1970s and early 1980s, remarkable insights and initiatives radically changed the situation. First, systems were developed for streamlining surgery, by assigning lower-skilled (and lower-paid) staff to carry out much of the activities previously performed by an ophthalmologist or nurse. By employing two or more operating tables in each operating room, support staff could

Table 33.1 Cataract surgical rates (CSR)

	Population (millions)	Cataract Operations (millions)	CSR (per million population per year)
N. America	300	1.65	5,500
N. Europe	400	1.60	4,000
Australia/ Japan	150	0.08	5,300
India	1,000	3.1	3,100
China	1,250	0.6	500
Africa	650	0.2	300

Table 33.2 Change in CSR: India (cataract operations per million population per year)

1980	500
1990	1,000
2000	3,000
2005	4,500

prepare patients for surgery and help them off the table after the surgery was completed. The surgeon moves from table to table doing only what the skilled surgeon is uniquely skilled to do. A second transforming event was the widespread introduction of intraocular lenses (IOLs) at the time of surgery. Previously, patients around the globe depended upon unsightly, distortion-inducing 'post-cataract' spectacles to correct the optical error induced by the removal of their lens. Once IOLs became standard in wealthier countries, the number of cataract operations rose dramatically, as patients sought intervention earlier in the course of their disease. But those early IOLs were (and in the West, remain) extremely expensive, costing on average well over US$300. Formative research in India revealed that patients were far more motivated to seek cataract surgery if they met a 'satisfied customer' (a fellow villager who was satisfied with their cataract surgical outcome). It was clear that patient satisfaction was vastly increased when the cataract was replaced with an intraocular lens, but the costs of such lenses were many times the total cost of affordable surgery for most Indians. In response, special manufacturing facilities were built to produce intraocular lenses locally, in India, which were sold for only US$5 a piece. This dramatically increased both patient satisfaction and their ability to afford modern cataract surgery.

Researchers also discovered that patients were generally willing to contribute roughly two months' wages towards the cost of cataract surgery – something they could not afford if they waited until they were blind and unemployed. Earlier surgery became the norm. A number of hospitals established schemes by which some of the payment of wealthier patients helped subsidise the costs of caring for poorer patients. Finally, with the help of a large loan from the World Bank, and support from the International Lions Club's 'SightFirst' programme, the Indian government helped to underwrite part of the costs of cataract surgery for the poor. The result has been a dramatic, eightfold increase in the number of cataract operations performed in India each year, raising the CSR to nearly 4,000 – the same as in wealthier market economies.

China is a distressing contrast to India's experience. Over the past 25 years, the quality of cataract surgery in China has increased dramatically, but not nearly as much as its cost, which has risen nearly a hundredfold. As a result, the number of cataract operations in China has barely increased at all, the CSR remains very low, and the prevalence of blindness has gone up an estimated 3 per cent (in contrast, the prevalence of blindness in India is estimated to have fallen by 25 per cent) (Resnikoff *et al.* 2004). India and China are both capable of training adequate numbers of high-quality cataract surgeons, though only in India has the population truly benefited.

Africa (and the rural and poor populations of many developing countries) suffers from a different problem entirely: a dramatic paucity of trained ophthalmologists. Most of the wealthy world has roughly one ophthalmologist per 20,000 population; India has one per 100,000. However, the ratio in sub-Saharan Africa is even worse, at an estimated one per million. To make matters worse, those few ophthalmologists predominantly live and work in the major cities, and unlike the subcontinent, the rural population of Africa is more dispersed, and the transportation infrastructure less developed. It is therefore more difficult for Africans to reach ophthalmic surgeons, even if they wished to. One could say that the real ratio of ophthalmol-ogists for rural Africa is more like one ophthalmologist per 10 million people (in reality no ratio can meaningfully capture the paucity of resources in countries where there are literally no ophthalmologists working in rural areas). A variety of individuals and organisations in the 'West' regularly organise 'ophthalmic missions' of highly trained ophthalmologists to work for weeks, or occasionally months, in underserved rural areas. While these clearly benefit the few patients with whom they come in contact, their impact on blindness rates is negligible.

Some better-off developing countries like Indonesia, with its 1,000 trained ophthalmolo-gists, suffer a CSR barely higher than that of Africa, because nearly all the ophthalmologists live and work in the country's five major cities (author's personal observation, January 2009).

Exactly how the cataract blindness problem in Africa (and other underserved areas of the globe) will be solved in one, or even two generations, remains a mystery, unless a radically different paradigm is applied: training and supervising large numbers of cataract 'technicians' to perform the surgery needed in the rural countryside. These would be mature health workers who have been taught and are capable of performing high-quality surgery (largely a technical skill) without having to first spend eight to ten years in formal university education and medical and surgical training (which, perversely, would also qualify them to migrate to urban areas of wealthier African nations or to higher-paying jobs in high-income countries).

Solving the problem of unoperated cataract is not beyond the scope of existing science – it is purely an issue of political will, leadership, and adoption of the appropriate technology, training, and management.

Trachoma

Trachoma is the leading infectious cause of blindness and is primarily present in poor, unhygienic environments. It is caused by repeated re-infection, usually between young children and between children and their mothers, with *Chlamydia trachomatis*. A single or a few such infections are generally innocuous. But repeated re-infection, which elicits repeated inflamma-tion and eventually scarring of the inner aspects of the upper lids, causes the upper eyelids and lashes to rub against the cornea. Resulting trauma and exposure of the cornea leads to corneal ulceration, scarring, and blindness.

One of the most fascinating factors about trachoma is just how closely it is related to development. Trachoma, and resultant blindness, was once common throughout the (now) developed world; indeed, some of the earliest, most famous eye hospitals (Moorfields Eye Hospital in London, the Massachusetts Eye and Ear Infirmary in Boston) were established to care for trachoma patients (Taylor 2008). One of the most dreaded examinations undergone by would-be immigrants to the US at Ellis Island was the search for active trachoma; if present, the individual was barred from entry. Almost magically, trachoma disappeared 'spontaneously' from the Western world as hygiene standards improved in tandem with (sometimes very modest) increases in development and rising socio-economic status.

Indonesia offers a modern, 'Eastern' example of this same phenomenon. During the 1950s the Indonesian government trained over 200 'eye nurses' to do nothing but trichiasis surgery (meant to prevent the scarred trachomatous lids from turning inward and rubbing against the cornea). By 1976, 20 years later, these specially trained eye nurses had all been reassigned to general duties in rural health clinics, because active, inflammatory trachoma had disappeared spontaneously. The same occurred in Saudi Arabia and Thailand, as roads reached once impoverished, rural areas, not only stimulating modest development but also presumably raising local levels of hygiene.

Today, we know that washing a child's face with water, once or twice a day, dramatically reduces their risk of infection and active, inflammatory trachoma. We also know that a clean environment reduces the population of eye-seeking flies, which in some environments are an important mode of transmission of infection. Even more recently, Pfizer developed a near-wonder drug, Zithromax (azithromycin), which, when given to an entire community once or twice a year, dramatically reduces the rates of infection and disease (Schachter *et al.* 1999; Taylor *et al.* 1985; West *et al.* 1995, 1996). While azithromycin was originally quite expensive, Pfizer pledged to make the drug freely available to those countries that could effectively use it through the International Trachoma Initiative (ITI). The drug is now off-patent and available at lower cost.

These new insights and tools have spurred a common global goal for achieving the eradication of blinding trachoma as a major public health problem by the year 2020 (GET 20/20). The common template employs a coordinated, comprehensive strategy of Sanitation/Antibiotics/Face washing/and Environmental cleanliness (SAFE). Pfizer donates the drug to countries that need it through a programme funded in collaboration with the Edna McConnell Clark Foundation (the ITI – which is now housed at the Task Force for Child Survival and Development in Atlanta). Many philanthropic organisations are contributing to the costs of the SAFE programme, while local and international NGOs provide technical assistance. Success depends largely, however, on local, national 'ownership' to ensure coordinated approaches and facilitation of needed services.

A number of fascinating and critical questions remain. First, will this global programme, that must be owned and directed by local governments, receive sufficient support and attention to achieve the GET 20/20 goal? If economic development occurs, will this be sufficient to achieve the goal on its own, or, conversely, can the goal of elimination be achieved in the absence of at least some degree of development? Only time – and concerted attention – will tell.

Vitamin A deficiency (xerophthalmia)

Vitamin A deficiency is a major cause of childhood blindness in poor populations throughout the developing world, precisely because poor populations can not afford diets adequate in vitamin A (meat, eggs, and dairy products). Instead, poor children rely for their vitamin A on inadequate amounts of coloured vegetables and fruits (spinach, papaya, carrots), which contain beta-carotene, a molecule that can be converted, in the gut, to vitamin A. Unfortunately, the conversion of beta-carotene in the diet to vitamin A is extremely inefficient; much less efficient than had previously been thought. It turns out that there is simply not enough vitamin A and beta-carotene in the food supplies of Africa, Asia, and Latin America to meet their populations' needs (West *et al.* 2002).

An estimated 6 million individuals develop night blindness, and half a million become permanently blind every year (primarily young children) (West 2002). Despite this tragedy, ministers of health were initially reluctant to deploy the modest resources needed to counter the problem, because they felt compelled to concentrate what limited resources they had on programmes that saved children's lives. With the discovery that improving vitamin A status dramatically reduced child mortality, the global health community embraced improvement in vitamin A status, as this single intervention could simultaneously prevent half a million cases of blindness and as many as a million deaths each year (Sommer and West 1996). The primary approach to improving vitamin A status in most developing countries is the periodic administration of two cents' worth of vitamin A to every child twice or three times a year, an intervention judged by the World Bank and the Copenhagen Consensus to be among the most cost-effective of all health interventions. Other means of improving vitamin A status are under development; these include fortifying processed foods with vitamin A, getting mothers to add vitamin A (and other micronutrients) to the food they feed their children ('point of use fortification'), and increasing the concentration and bio-availability of beta-carotene in dietary staples through traditional horticultural techniques (corn, sweet potato), and bioengineering ('golden rice').

Once countries become wealthier, the amount of vitamin A (and other micronutrients) in the average diet improves, though some estimates suggest that even wealthy, Western nations require ongoing fortification of common dietary staples to achieve required levels of intake and status.

Onchocerciasis

The other significantly blinding disease of the tropics is onchocerciasis (river blindness), which is largely limited to sub-Saharan Africa and parts of Latin America. It is caused by a worm, *Onchocerca volvulus*, which is transmitted through the bite of black flies that breed along the banks of fast-moving streams. Because these breeding sites are often situated in agriculturally productive valleys, their abandonment, as being 'valleys of the blind', became an enormous impediment to development. Because of the economic impact of river blindness, its control became the first major health programme to be supported by the World Bank.

One of the hardest hit areas, a multi-country zone initially around the Upper Volta region, became the site of the highly successful Onchocerciasis Control Programme (OCP), where transmission was all but eliminated through the sophisticated use of biodegradable larvicides that dramatically reduced the concentration of black flies. This remains a continuing success.

Unfortunately, in other affected areas of Africa, the streams are smaller and often covered by foliage, precluding efficient spraying with insecticides. Instead, a remarkable drug, Mectizan (ivermectin), is used to treat the disease in whole communities, which reduces the burden in each person who receives the drug and reduces the transmission between individuals (the black fly is less likely to become infected by biting an individual less capable of infecting it). Mectizan had originally been developed and produced by Merck for the agricultural market (it kills heart worm in dogs, among other uses). It was subsequently shown to be safe in humans and highly effective in reducing the concentration of microfilaria in infected patients. The microfilaria – the tiny offspring of the adult macrofilaria that exist in nodules throughout the body – are what reach the eye and cause blindness. Further, the drug only needs to be taken once a year. Unfortunately, it needs to be taken for many years, because Mectizan does not kill the adult worms (there is no safe and effective macrofilaricide), and each adult female produces over a million microfilaria every year. Recognising that those who needed the medication could never afford to purchase it, Merck dramatically agreed to donate 'all the drug that's needed for as long as it's needed'. National programmes have come together to organise 'community-directed distribution programmes'. With continuing World Bank support and community 'ownership', annual Mectizan distribution has dramatically suppressed infection and the risk of blinding sequelae, but these will need to be continued for many years to come, or until such time as a safe and effective macrofilaricide that kills the adults worm is developed. In the meanwhile, people are far healthier, their sight has been preserved, and they are farming fertile land that might otherwise have been unavailable to them and to the development of their society (Hotez 2007; WHO 2003).

Other chronic, global causes of blindness

A number of major blinding diseases are not readily responsive to present treatment or prevention modalities. Chief among them is Age-Related Macular Degeneration (AMD), a disease that generally causes severe visual impairment and blindness in middle and old age. As such, it is already the leading cause of irreversible blindness in high-income countries, which are aging, and where 'avoidable' causes of blindness, like unoperated cataract, have largely been dealt with. AMD will soon pose a major problem for the already overburdened developing world as their population ages. A great deal of research is being directed at the cause(s) of AMD, but existing treatments remain relatively ineffective and expensive, and little is known about causative factors that might suggest effective means of prevention.

Glaucoma is claimed to be the second most prevalent cause of blindness globally. Primary Open Angle Glaucoma (POAG), prevalent in Caucasian and many Asian populations, but most commonly among Africans and those of African descent, is difficult to identify early in the course of the disease, before 'elevated' intraocular pressure results in blindness from destruction of the optic nerve. Effective 'screening' requires regular, repeated evaluation of the status of the optic nerve, a cumbersome and costly practice. Treatment, whether medical or surgical (commonly both), is also costly and requires careful, long-term monitoring. It may also have only modest efficacy, particularly where patients cannot be monitored frequently and are unable to afford expensive interventions. The costs and infrastructure needed for identifying and treating POAG is beyond the means of most low-, or even some middle-income countries. It is not yet clear that the benefits of screening and treatment in high-income countries are particularly impressive or cost-effective.

Primary Angle Closure Glaucoma (PACG), most common among some Asian populations, is amenable to early therapy, but the ability to identify cases early through large-scale screening programmes is limited by the accuracy of the available techniques, the need for trained personnel to interpret them, and the natural impediments to examining those at greatest risk.

Diabetic retinopathy, common among patients with both type one and type two disease, is likely to become far more prevalent as the obesity epidemic spreads around the globe, fuelling a secondary epidemic of type two diabetes and its accompanying retinopathy. Modestly effective interventions exist, from tackling obesity in the first place, to tight control of diabetes and laser therapy of the retinal abnormalities. Unfortunately, each of these has their limitations, though there is little doubt that the need for laser and related treatment of retinopathy is going to increase dramatically. As with other ophthalmic disorders, particularly those requiring regular examination and sophisticated intervention, poorer, less developed countries will find it more challenging to mount an appropriate response.

Conclusion

Visual impairment and economic development are tightly intertwined. Many poor countries do not have the resources to adequately prevent and treat blinding disorders, with the result that large numbers of individuals who might otherwise contribute to the development of their societies are, instead, disabled and require societal resources to survive. The WHO and the International Agency for the Prevention of Blindness (IAPB) have launched an ambitious, highly coordinated and regionally based programme to more effectively protect vision, and prevent blindness around the globe (Vision 2020, http://www.v2020.org). The World Health Assembly has recognised the need for this initiative and has encouraged the development of strong regional and national programmes with specific goals and clearly delineated approaches for meeting them.

References

Foster, A. (2001) 'Cataract and "Vision 2020: The Right to Sight" Initiative', *British Journal of Ophthalmology*, 85: 635–9.

Frick, K. and Foster, A. (2003) 'The Magnitude and Cost of Global Blindness: An Increasing Problem that can be Alleviated', *American Journal of Ophthalmology*, 135(4): 471–6.

Ho, V. and Schwab, I. (2001) 'Social Economic Development in the Prevention of Global Blindness', *British Journal of Ophthalmology*, 85: 653–7.

Hotez, P. (2007) 'Control of Onchocerciasis: The Next Generation', *The Lancet*, 369: 1,979–80.

Javitt, J., Sommer, A., and Venkataswamy, G. (1983) 'The Economic and Social Impact of Restoring Sight', in P. Henkind (ed.) *Acta: XXIV International Congress of Ophthalmology*, Philadelphia, PA: Lippincott Co.: 1,308–12.

Resnikoff, S., Pascolini, D., Etya'ale, D., Kocur, I., Pararajasegaram, R., Pokharel, G., and Mariotti, S.P. (2004) 'Global Data on Visual Impairment in the Year 2002', *Bulletin of the World Health Organization*, 82(11): 844–51.

Schachter, J., West, S.K., Mabey, D., Dawson, C., Bobo, L., Bailey, R., Vitale, S., Quinn, T.C., Sheta, A., Sallam, S., Mkocha, H., Mabey, D., and Faal, H. (1999) 'Azithromycin in Control of Trachoma', *The Lancet*, 354: 630–35.

Sommer, A. and West, K.P. (1996) *Vitamin A Deficiency*, Oxford: Oxford University Press.

Taylor, H., Velasco, F.M., and Sommer, A. (1985) 'The Ecology of Trachoma: An Epidemiological Study in Southern Mexico', *Bulletin of the World Health Organization*, 63: 559–67.

Taylor, H.R. (2008) *Trachoma: A Blinding Scourge from the Bronze Age to the Twenty-first Century*, Victoria, Australia: Haddington Press.

West, C., Eilander, A., and van Lieshout, M. (2002) 'Consequences of Revised Estimates of Carotenoid Bioefficacy for Dietary Control of Vitamin A Deficiency in Developing Countries', *Journal of Nutrition*, 132: 2920S–2926S.

West, K.P. (2002) 'Extent of Vitamin A Deficiency among Preschool Children and Women of Reproductive Age', *Journal of Nutrition*, 132: 2857S–2866S.

West, S., Muñoz, B., Lynch, M., Kayongoya, A., Chilangwa, Z., Mmbaga, B.B., and Taylor, H.R. (1995) 'Impact of Face-washing on Trachoma in Kongwa, Tanzania', *The Lancet*, 345: 155–8.

West, S.K., Muñoz, B., Lynch, M., Kayongoya, A., Mmbaga, B., and Taylor, H. (1996) 'Risk Factors for Constant, Severe Trachoma among Preschool Children in Kongwa, Tanzania', *American Journal of Epidemiology*, 143: 73–8.

WHO (World Health Organization) (2003) '28-year River Blindness Campaign Celebrates Completion', *Bulletin of the World Health Organization*, 81(1): 75.

34

Improving Maternal and Newborn Survival through Community Intervention

Tanja A. J. Houweling, Anthony Costello, and David Osrin

This chapter discusses maternal and newborn mortality as key population health issues for the twenty-first century. The challenges and contentions illustrate major themes in global public health: measuring and addressing socio-economic inequalities, the balance between top-down and bottom-up approaches, the need for better data, and the importance of monitoring.

The importance of maternal and newborn survival to population health

The targets associated with Millennium Development Goals 4 and 5 were to reduce under-five mortality by two-thirds and maternal mortality by three-quarters in every country, taking 1990 as a baseline and 2015 as the endline (United Nations 2000). In 2008, only 15 of 68 priority countries with high under-five mortality rates were on track towards the target, 28 had made insufficient progress, and 25 had made no progress at all. In 12 countries, under-five mortality had actually increased (Bryce *et al.* 2008). Reliable figures for trends in newborn mortality were not available, and this information gap needs urgent attention. As under-five mortality rates fall, the proportion of deaths occurring in the neonatal period (up to 28 days after birth) rises (Black *et al.* 2003). Neonatal mortality now accounts for about half of under-five deaths in South Asia. Added to this are a global 3–4 million annual stillbirths which do not appear in official statistics (Lawn *et al.* 2009).

Trends in maternal survival are equally distressing. The global maternal mortality ratio (MMR: deaths during pregnancy or up to 42 days postpartum) was recently estimated at 402 per 100,000 live births (uncertainty bounds 216–654) (Hill *et al.* 2007). Two points are worth noting. First, the countries that lacked tracking data were the 61 poorest, representing 25 per cent of global births and most maternal deaths. Second, there was little change in MMR in sub-Saharan Africa between 1990 and 2005 (921 and 905, respectively). In South Asia and sub-Saharan Africa, improvements in routine and emergency obstetric care in hospitals, health centres, and midwifery services have not been achieved at scale, which means that we must renew our efforts to understand why policies have not been successful, and whether new approaches are needed.

Box 34.1 Funding for maternal and child health

How can we address the shortfall of investment in mother and child health in the poorest countries? Greco and colleagues estimate that donor disbursements increased from US $2,119 million in 2003 to $3,482 million in 2006 (Greco *et al.* 2008). Funding for child health increased by 63 per cent and for maternal and newborn health by 66 per cent. In the 68 priority countries, child-related disbursements increased from a mean $4 to $7 per child between 2003 and 2006, and disbursements for maternal and neonatal health increased from $7 to $12 per live birth. Nonetheless, disbursements fell in some countries, much of the spending on maternal and child survival was directed at routine immunisation programmes, and aid specifically for maternal and newborn health did not seem to be well targeted towards countries with the greatest needs. A critical issue is the lack of a coordinating mechanism for aid investment, specifically for maternal and newborn health. We called previously for a global fund for mothers and children, but the question has turned towards the possibility of broadening the remit of the existing Global Fund for health, which currently focuses on AIDS, tuberculosis, and malaria. Whatever mechanism is used, the total aid directed to maternal and newborn health (about $1,172 million in 2006) is pitifully low compared with the sudden commitment of trillions of dollars to rescue the global financial system. Health and development professionals need to pressurise their governments to be more generous in assisting this effort.

Global concern about maternal and newborn survival has developed piecemeal. To some degree this reflects epidemiology. Child health has always been a priority for public health, and was the objective of the 'child survival revolution' which began in the 1970s (Schuftan 1990). The global tragedy of maternal mortality only became widely appreciated in the 1980s, and newborn survival joined the agenda even later, because of the relative invisibility of perinatal deaths and because earlier priorities mandated reductions in post-neonatal mortality from conditions such as vaccine-preventable disease, diarrhoea, and acute respiratory infection. Global concern equates with funding (Box 34.1), and developments since the 1990s have involved advocacy for maternal and newborn health issues at the same time as accretion of experience with model programmes. Initiatives have coalesced around key events (for example, a 1987 conference in Nairobi, Kenya, which launched the Safe Motherhood Initiative), alliances (for example, the White Ribbon Alliance for Safe Motherhood and the Partnership for Maternal, Newborn and Child Health), and literature reviews (Kidney *et al.* 2009). A current consensus is that the need is more for an understanding of how to deliver existing interventions than for new clinical approaches and technologies.

Socio-economic inequalities in maternal and newborn mortality

One particular concern is how to reduce socio-economic health inequalities. Average mortality rates at a country level hide as much as they reveal. The inverse care law – those who need interventions most get them least, and those who need them least get them most – applies dramatically in low- and middle-income countries (LMICs) (Tudor Hart 1971). Maternal, newborn, and childhood mortality rates are systematically and substantially higher in lower socio-economic groups. In India, for example, neonatal mortality is 56 per 1,000 in the poorest quintile, but 25 in the wealthiest (Macro International Inc. 2009). Mortality inequalities are found along many dimensions of social stratification, including household wealth, parental education, ethnic group, religion, caste, migration status, and occupation. In most countries there is a social gradient in mortality: for each step down in the social hierarchy, mortality rises. This means that inequalities are not limited to the most deprived, but pervade entire societies (Houweling and Kunst, 2010).

Socio-economic inequalities in newborn, child, and maternal mortality are found in almost every LMIC with available data. Yet their magnitude varies between countries and over time, suggesting that they are amenable to policy intervention (Houweling and Kunst, 2010). Huge population health gains would be made if inequalities were addressed. If the mortality rate for the richest 40 per cent of people in each country was extended to everyone, one-third of under-five deaths in the year 2000 would have been avoided (3.5 of 10.8 million) (Houweling and Kunst, 2010).

Socio-economic inequalities in infant and under-five mortality have, until now, received more research attention than inequalities in newborn mortality. This is partly due to sample size requirements for stratified analyses and other data-related problems, and partly because post-neonatal and child mortality are still important problems in many LMICs and tend to over-shadow attention to neonates. A more refined understanding is required, and sources such as the Demographic and Health Surveys and sentinel surveillance sites can be used to produce summaries such as Figure 34.1, which shows absolute poor–rich inequalities in under-five mortality in

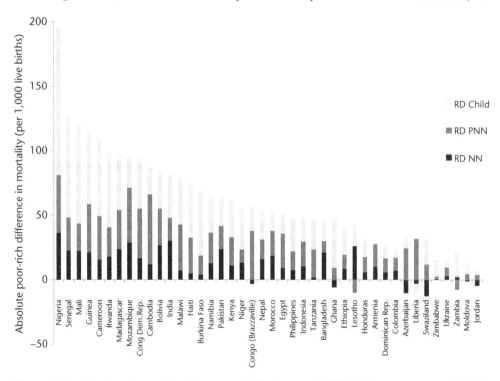

Figure 34.1 Absolute inequalities in neonatal (0–1 month) (RD NN), post-neonatal (1–12 months) (RD PNN), and child (1–5 years) mortality (RD child) between the poorest and richest quintiles for 43 low- and middle-income countries, using the most recent Demographic and Health Surveys data. The sum of inequalities in neonatal, post-neonatal and child mortality equals the poor-rich rate difference in under-five mortality

43 LMICs, and their decomposition into neonatal (0–1 month), post-neonatal (1–12 months), and child (1–5 years) categories. While these results should be interpreted with some caution because of problems such as age heaping (a tendency to report ages with easy estimates such as 7 days, 1 month, 1 year), some general conclusions can be drawn. Twenty to 25 per cent of under-five mortality inequalities are seen in the neonatal period. This contribution varies, and seems to be higher in countries with lower under-five mortality rates. Absolute poor–rich inequalities in neonatal mortality are substantial in many LMICs, reaching differences of 15–30 per 1,000 live births.

Socio-economic inequalities in maternal mortality have received even less attention. Data availability and reliability are, as above, critical obstacles. Inequalities in childhood mortality can be estimated by interviewing mothers to obtain full birth histories and socio-economic information, or through demographic surveillance. Similar approaches can be used to measure maternal mortality, but large surveillance populations are needed to allow for stratified analysis. Household surveys sometimes use the sisterhood method, in which adults are interviewed about the survival of their sisters, and particularly about the relationship of deaths with pregnancy. Combined with the familial technique, in which women are assigned the same socio-economic position as their sibling respondent, substantial inequalities in maternal mortality have been demonstrated (Graham *et al.* 2004).

Socio-economic inequalities in maternal, newborn, and child mortality are caused by factors within and outside the health care sector. Health care sector inequalities are huge in LMICs: use of maternity and child care services is much lower among lower socio-economic groups (Figure 34.2). Socio-economic position and health care use are linked across the entire social

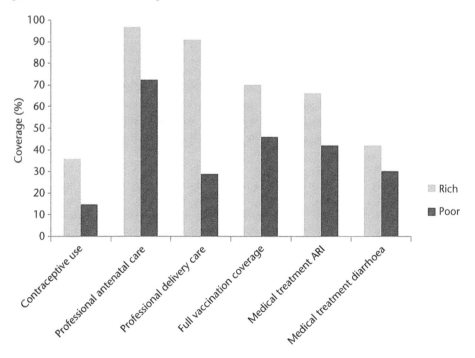

Figure 34.2 Median levels of health care use across 45 low- and middle-income countries, among the poorest 20 per cent and among the richest 20 per cent population groups, using the most recent Demographic and Health Surveys data (number of countries included varies from 36 to 45 depending on data availability)

hierarchy within countries, with each progressively more deprived group having progressively lower use (Houweling and Kunst, 2010). Even within urban slums, and in seemingly homogeneously poor rural areas, inequalities in health care use have been reported (More *et al.* 2009; Schellenberg *et al.* 2003). Inequalities in delivery care are particularly large. In most LMICs, most of the better-off receive professional delivery care, in contrast with only a minority of poor women. Some of this inequality is explained by private sector care, but much of it applies to public sector deliveries, by nurses as well as by doctors (Houweling and Kunst, 2010). These inequalities in health care use reflect inequalities in availability, accessibility, affordability, and acceptability of services between socio-economic groups and regions within countries.

Factors outside the health care sector are also important determinants of inequality. Lower socio-economic groups have, for example, less opportunity for healthy home care practices, such as hand-washing with soap, increasing the risk of illnesses such as diarrhoea (Houweling and Kunst, 2010). Community-level determinants include service provision such as piped water supply, influencing exposure to infections. More distally, social structural realities such as gender inequalities, food and economic security, limited transport and communication systems, and priorities in public policy-making unfavourable to low-income populations, are likely to be important determinants of inequality (CSDH 2008).

Community intervention to improve maternal and newborn survival

While there is a history of descriptive and explanatory research on socio-economic inequalities in health, particularly in high-income countries, and more recently in LMICs, intervention research still tends to focus on how to improve average maternal and newborn survival. If equitable improvements in maternal and newborn health are the goal, should the means be the provision of clinical care through health systems (which some refer to as supply-side), or alternatively, the mobilisation of communities to ensure the health of women and children (which some would call demand-side)? Figure 34.3 is an attempt to simplify the types of interventions that have been contemplated, tested, or introduced to improve maternal and newborn survival. The journey from home to health facility is represented as an uphill struggle, and its slope is both literal and metaphorical. Access to healthcare may involve travel across difficult terrain, but it is also undertaken against a gradient of disincentives. Poorer people live at the bottom of the slope, and the disincentives decline as socio-economic position rises. Physical distance and cost are the most familiar obstacles, and among the most common that programmes have addressed; but healthcare may not be sought because it is not usual for a family or community to do so, because it is known or presumed to be substandard, because of previous experiences with health workers, and because of a narrative of negativity about healthcare quality, costs, and outcomes.

Figure 34.3 identifies ten approaches which, though not necessarily exclusive, do tend to fall into groups. Interventions to address newborn mortality have tended to cluster towards the left-hand side of the diagram ('down the slope'), and strategies to increase maternal survival towards the right ('up the slope'). This reflects some differences in perspective. On one hand, it is argued that substantial reductions in maternal mortality will not be brought about by community-based interventions – what we require are skilled birth attendance and care for obstetric emergencies. On the other, it is argued that skilled attendance is uncommon in many places and the idea of achieving universal coverage is ambitious in the short or medium term. At current rates and without extra financial resources, coverage in Africa will still be below 50 per cent by 2015 (Knippenberg *et al.* 2005). Could maternal and newborn survival be improved through simultaneous interventions in health services and communities?

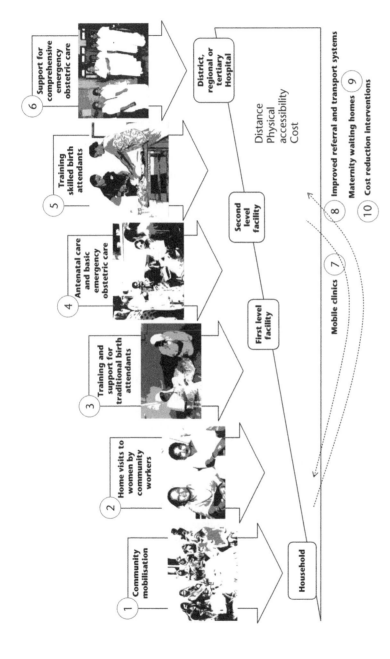

1 Community mobilisation

2 Home visits to women by community workers

3 Training and support for traditional birth attendants

4 Antenatal care and basic emergency obstetric care

5 Training skilled birth attendants

6 Support for comprehensive emergency obstetric care

Household

First level facility

Second level facility

District, regional or tertiary Hospital

Distance
Physical accessibility
Cost

7 Mobile clinics

8 Improved referral and transport systems

9 Maternity waiting homes

10 Cost reduction interventions

Figure 34.3 Types of interventions to improve average maternal and newborn survival

This is not an either-or choice; it is a decision about the balance of inputs (Kerber *et al.* 2007), but the point of balance (for which read 'investment') is uncertain (Haws *et al.* 2007). Of course, healthcare institutions are located within communities, and health workers are community members. This means that local antenatal care can, for example, be seen as a community-based intervention (Kidney *et al.* 2009), especially if reducing it to a minimum number of visits and goal-directed activities does not seem to compromise maternity outcomes (Carroli *et al.* 2001). Likewise, although the aim of training cadres of skilled birth attendants is primarily to increase institutional deliveries and improve their outcomes, these same skilled attendants may deliver babies at home. By this argument, an excellent 'community' strategy to improve maternal and newborn survival would be to improve maternity care services so that high-quality antenatal care, institutional delivery, and emergency obstetric and paediatric services are available to all. This is what we should be working towards (Campbell and Graham 2006).

A continuum of activity is required: between maternal and newborn care, between community and health systems, and between informal and formal sectors. Precisely what this would look like at district level is hazy. Moving 'down the slope' in Figure 34.3, there has been limited success with mobile clinics, but coverage is difficult and life-threatening events are unpredictable, and they have not captured the imagination in many countries. Moving up the slope, transport systems have been introduced in several vulnerable settings. Another option (again, one that seems to have translated poorly from theory to practice, despite having been successful in Cuba) is to move women closer to obstetric care services at the time of delivery by creating maternity waiting homes (Lee *et al.* 2009). Expense, either predicted or actual, is an important barrier to care. The remainder of this chapter discusses community interventions towards the left of Figure 34.3.

Community mobilisation

The mobilisation of communities, or groups within them, for change has a long history. This history is political as well as social, calling on Latin American liberation theology and the growth of community action for health. It seems that substantial improvements in health can be achieved without recourse to clinical inputs or technology. The Warmi programme worked successfully with Aymara women's groups in rural Bolivia to understand maternity in their communities, identify opportunities to improve maternal and newborn health, and design and implement local strategies to do so (Howard-Grabman *et al.* 2002). The model was adapted and tested in rural Nepal, where a cluster randomised trial suggested that women's groups facilitated by a local community worker could reduce neonatal mortality rates by about 30 per cent, without extensive inputs on the supply side (Manandhar *et al.* 2004). There were also unexpected reductions in maternal mortality, and this observation raises questions about the resilience of maternal complications to intervention. The model is being tested with rural groups in Bangladesh, India, and Malawi, and in urban slums in India.

Home visits to women by community workers

Several programmes, all from rural South Asia so far, have shown that adequately trained and supported community workers, making repeated home visits, can reduce newborn mortality. It is not clear how far this extends to maternal survival. The seminal work was done in rural Maharashtra, India, where a non-government organisation trained community health workers to conduct group health education, identify pregnant women and make antenatal care visits to their homes, attend delivery, give vitamin K injections, make several further postnatal home visits, identify and manage infants at risk from birth asphyxia, low birth weight, and sepsis, and encourage appropriate referral (Bang *et al.* 1999). This model reduced neonatal mortality by 62 per cent and has since been adapted and tested in other situations, including north India, Bangladesh, and Pakistan. Important questions are whether the model could be less intensive, whether it could be run through existing government health systems, and how it will fare when subjected to the diluting effects of scale-up.

Training and support for traditional birth attendants

The question of whether traditional birth attendants can be agents for maternal and newborn survival, once embraced by health services and trained and supported, is a vexed one (Sibley and Sipe 2006). At a policy level, their popularity has waxed and waned on the basis of patchy evidence, but ground-level programmes continue to involve them. For example, a programme in rural Pakistan sought to connect traditional birth attendants with government community health workers, by recommending antenatal home visits, registration of pregnancies, and the use of delivery kits. Newborn mortality fell by 30 per cent (Jokhio *et al.* 2005).

We have, then, reasonable evidence that community interventions can improve newborn survival. Maternal mortality, though catastrophic, is less common. The evidence for its tractability to non-specialist community interventions is limited, but there may be a place for community interventions in situations where mortality ratios are high (Kidney *et al.* 2009). None of the programmes mentioned above worked exclusively on community mobilisation. All made some effort to improve health service delivery, and programmes based on individual home visits also conducted community group events.

Can community interventions also reduce inequalities in newborn and perhaps even maternal mortality? Research on this is still underdeveloped, and fairly little is known about how to reach lower socio-economic groups, particularly since there is some evidence that health interventions in general tend to reach higher socio-economic groups first, increasing inequalities in the short term (Victora *et al.* 2000). Community mobilisation initiatives have successfully reached lower socio-economic groups in urban slums and tribal areas in India, and in remote communities in Nepal. To what extent they reduce inequalities within these marginalised communities is a topic of ongoing research. Conversely, while community-based skilled birth attendant programmes seem to be able to improve overall use of professional delivery care, inequalities in uptake remain. This might be due in part to reliance on private fees, which may deter the poor: the implementation and financing details of community-based interventions matter.

Challenges for research and intervention

Addressing the gradient in mortality, rather than only reaching the most marginalised, may require a combination of bottom-up and more universal top-down approaches (CSDH 2008). This is a challenge for research and implementation in the next decade. The existing portfolio of interventions with proven efficacy for maternal and child survival is large (Campbell and Graham 2006). The challenge is to translate efficacy into community effectiveness for either prevention or management of illness. In part, this will depend upon the reach and quality of the primary health care system, which in turn depends upon political will, adequate financing, district-level management, and community involvement. The Integrated Management of Childhood Illness strategy (IMCI) has recognised that increasing child survival requires interventions to improve health worker skills, to address health system issues (especially in relation to drug supply), to stimulate community awareness of maternal and child health problems and care, and to hold local health services accountable. Coverage of the population in need is the key indicator for health-related service and community interventions. Recent community effectiveness trials of interventions based on health worker home visits or participatory women's groups share a common challenge: how to ensure adequate coverage at scale. There is good evidence that the diagnostic skills of health workers are often weak, although IMCI training can bring about rapid improvements (Chowdhury et al. 2008). The reality, however, is that many of the most vulnerable women and children do not have access to essential care. In Bangladesh, the increase in caesarean sections in a rural population was almost wholly confined to the richest 40 per cent (Anwar et al. 2008). In Tanzania, evaluation of an IMCI programme in one district revealed that none of the children with pneumonia in the poorest quintile received an antibiotic (Victora et al. 2006).

These problems are an argument for a stronger focus on implementation in global health, for research addressing the need for better data, for statistical power to monitor time trends in inequalities in mortality, and for the development of innovative methods to allow systematic monitoring and policymaking. More evidence is needed on what works to reduce inequalities, and on the differential impact of interventions across socio-economic groups. Downstream, there are research questions around the most effective ways to achieve community mobilisation. We also need to look upstream at interventions to improve district management, collection, and analysis of key coverage indicators, and timely disbursement of funds to allow programmes to run effectively year round. Finally – but crucially – more understanding is needed of the social determinants of inequalities in maternal and newborn mortality, such as gender inequity, food and economic insecurity, and lack of water, sanitation, and transport infrastructure.

Conclusion

While the second half of the last century witnessed substantial improvements in child survival, good maternal, newborn, and child health are far from a reality in many populations. There has been a striking lack of progress in reducing maternal mortality, declines in child mortality have stagnated or even reversed in several countries, and while the relative importance of newborn mortality increases, there is a gap in epidemiological information. The technical solutions are by and large available; the social solutions require more systematic attention. Improving global health in the twenty-first century requires us to address key implementation issues: how to achieve effective coverage, how to balance community-based and health systems-based approaches, how to address health inequalities in addition to improving averages, and how to monitor progress, even in the poorest settings.

References

Anwar, I., Sami M., Akhtar N., Chowdhury M.E., Salma, U., Rahman, M., and Koblinsky, M. (2008) 'Inequity in Maternal Health-care Services: Evidence from Home-based Skilled-Birth-Attendant Programmes in Bangladesh', *Bulletin of the World Health Organization*, 86: 252–9.

Bang, A.T., Bang, R.A., Baitule, S.B., Reddy, M.H., and Deshmukh, M.D. (1999) 'Effect of Home-based Neonatal Care and Management of Sepsis on Neonatal Mortality: Field Trial in Rural India', *The Lancet*, 354: 1,955–61.

Black, R.E., Morris, S.S., and Bryce, J. (2003) 'Where and Why are 10 Million Children Dying Every Year?', *The Lancet*, 361: 2,226–34.

Bryce, J., Daelmans, B., Dwivedi, A., Fauveau, V., Lawn, J.E., Mason, E., Newby, H., Shankar, A., Starrs, A., and Wardlaw, T. (2008) 'Countdown to 2015 for Maternal, Newborn, and Child Survival: The 2008 Report on Tracking Coverage of Interventions', *The Lancet*, 371: 1,247–58.

Campbell, O.M.R. and Graham, W. (2006) 'Strategies for Reducing Maternal Mortality: Getting on with What Works', *The Lancet*, 368: 1,284–99.

Carroli, G., Villar, J., Piaggio, G., Khan-Neelofur, D., Gulmezoglu, M., Mugford, M., Lumbiganon, P., Farnot, U., and Bersgjo, P. (2001) 'WHO Systematic Review of Randomised Controlled Trials of Routine Antenatal Care', *The Lancet*, 357: 1,565–70.

Chowdhury, E.K., El Arifeen, S., Rahman, M., Hoque, D.E., Hossain, M.A., Begum, K., Siddik, A., Begum, N., Sadeq-ur Rahman, Q., Akter, T., Haque, T.M., Al-Helal, Z.M., Baqui, A.H., Bryce, J., and Black, R.E. (2008) 'Care at First-level Facilities for Children with Severe Pneumonia in Bangladesh: A Cohort Study', *The Lancet*, 372: 822–30.

CSDH (Center on Social Disparities in Health) (2008) *Closing the Gap in a Generation: Health Equity through Action on the Social Determinants of Health. Final Report of the Commission on Social Determinants of Health*', Geneva: World Health Organization, available at http://www.who.int/social_determinants/final_report/en/ (accessed 10 March 2010).

Graham, W.J., Fitzmaurice, A.E., Bell, J.S., and Cairns, J.A. (2004) 'The Familial Technique for Linking Maternal Death with Poverty', *The Lancet*, 363: 23–7.

Greco, G., Powell-Jackson, T., Borghi, J., and Mills, A. (2008) 'Countdown to 2015: Assessment of Donor Assistance to Maternal, Newborn, and Child Health between 2003 and 2006', *The Lancet*, 371: 1,268–75.

Haws, R.A., Thomas, A.L., Bhutta, Z.A., and Darmstadt, G.L. (2007) 'Impact of Packaged Interventions on Neonatal Health: A Review of the Evidence', *Health Policy and Planning*, 22: 193–215.

Hill, K., Thomas, K., AbouZahr, C., Walker, N., Say, L., Inoue, M., and Suzuki, E. (2007) 'Estimates of Maternal Mortality Worldwide between 1990 and 2005: An Assessment of Available Data', *The Lancet*, 370: 1,311–19.

Houweling, T.A.J. and Kunst, A.E. (2010) 'Socio-economic Inequalities in Childhood Mortality in Low and Middle Income Countries: A Review of the International Evidence', *British Medical Bulletin*, 93(1): 7–26.

Howard-Grabman, L., Seoane, G., Davenport, C.A., Mothercare, and Save the Children (2002) *The Warmi Project: A Participatory Approach to Improve Maternal and Neonatal Health, An Implementor's Manual*, Westport, CT: John Snow International, Mothercare Project, Save the Children.

Jokhio, A.H., Winter, H.R., and Cheng, K.K. (2005) 'An Intervention Involving Traditional Birth Attendants and Perinatal and Maternal Mortality in Pakistan', *New England Journal of Medicine*, 352: 2,091–9.

Kerber, K.J., de Graft-Johnson, J.E., Bhutta, Z.A., Okong, P., Starrs, A., and Lawn, J.E. (2007) 'Continuum of Care for Maternal, Newborn, and Child Health: From Slogan to Service Delivery', *The Lancet*, 370: 1,358–69.

Kidney, E., Winter, H.R., Khan, K.S., Gulmezoglu, A.M., Meads, C.A., Deeks, J.J., and Macarthur, C. (2009) 'Systematic Review of Effect of Community-level Interventions to Reduce Maternal Mortality', *BioMed Central Pregnancy and Childbirth*, 9: 2.

Knippenberg, R., Lawn, J.E., Darmstadt, G.L., Begkoyian, G., Fogstad, H., Walelign, N., Paul, V.K., and the Lancet Neonatal Survival Steering Team (2005) 'Systematic Scaling Up of Neonatal Care in Countries', *The Lancet*, 365: 1,087–98.

Lawn, J.E., Yakoob, M.Y., Haws, R.A., Soomro, T., Darmstadt, G.L., and Bhutta, Z.A. (2009) '3.2 Million Stillbirths: Epidemiology and Overview of the Evidence Review', *BioMed Central Pregnancy and Childbirth*, 9(Supplement 1): S2.

Lee, A.C.C., Lawn, J., Cousens, S., Kumar, V., Osrin, D., Bhutta, Z.A., Wall, S.N., Nandakumar, A.K., Syed, U., and Darmstadt, G. (2009) 'Linking Families and Facilities for Care at Birth: What Works to Avert Intrapartum-related Deaths', *International Journal of Gynecology and Obstetrics*, 107: S65–S88.

Macro International Inc. (2009) *Demographic and Health Surveys: STAT Compiler*, available at http://www.statcompiler.com/ (accessed 6 August 2009).

Manandhar, D.S., Osrin, D., Shrestha, B.P., Mesko, N., Morrison, J., Tumbahangphe, K.M., Tamang, S., Thapa, D., Shrestha, B., Thapa, J.R., Shrestha, A., Wade, Borghi, J., Standing, H., Manandhar, M. and Costello, A.M.L. (2004). 'Effect of a Participatory Intervention with Women's Groups on Birth Outcomes in Nepal: Cluster Randomized Controlled Trial', *The Lancet*, 364: 970–79.

More, N.S., Bapat, U., Das, S., Barnett, S., Costello, A., Fernandez, A., and Osrin, D. (2009) 'Inequalities in Maternity Care and Newborn Outcomes: One-year Surveillance of Births in Vulnerable Slum Communities in Mumbai', *International Journal of Health Equity*, 8: 21.

Schellenberg, J.A., Victora, C.G., Mushi, A., de Savigny, D., Schellenberg, D., Mshinda, H., and Bryce, J. (2003) 'Inequities among the Very Poor: Health Care for Children in Rural Southern Tanzania', *The Lancet*, 361: 561–6.

Schuftan, C. (1990) 'The Child Survival Revolution: A Critique', *Family Practice*, 7: 329–32.

Sibley, L.M. and Sipe, T.A. (2006) 'Transition to Skilled Birth Attendance: Is There a Future Role for Trained Traditional Birth Attendants?', *Journal of Health, Population, and Nutrition*, 24: 472–8.

Tudor Hart, J. (1971) 'The Inverse Care Law', *The Lancet*, 1: 405–12.

UN (United Nations) (2000) *Millennium Development Goals*, New York: United Nations.

Victora, C.G., Huicho, L., Amaral, J.J., Armstrong-Schellenberg, J., Manzi, F., Mason, E., and Scherpbier, R. (2006) 'Are Health Interventions Implemented Where they are Most Needed? District Uptake of the Integrated Management of Childhood Illness Strategy in Brazil, Peru and the United Republic of Tanzania', *Bulletin of the World Health Organization*, 84: 792–801.

Victora, C.G., Vaughan, J.P., Barros, F.C., Silva, A.C., and Tomasi, E. (2000) 'Explaining Trends in Inequities: Evidence from Brazilian Child Health Studies', *The Lancet*, 356: 1,093–8.

35

Chronic Diseases

The Urgent Need for Action

Henry Greenberg, Susan Raymond, Angela Beaton,
Ruth Colagiuri, and Stephen Leeder

The overarching problems of chronic disease

Chronic diseases, including CVDs such as coronary heart disease, stroke, and hypertension, as well as cancer, lung disease, and diabetes mellitus, account for most deaths in nearly all regions of the world except sub-Saharan Africa. The peak mortality from CVD occurred in the 1960s in the United States, in the 1970s in Western Europe, and in the 1980s and 1990s in Eastern Europe. While infectious diseases, lack of nutrition, and poor childbearing practices are claiming fewer lives in developing countries, deaths attributable to chronic diseases are rising (Levenson *et al.* 2002; Yusuf *et al.* 2001). This current epidemiologic transition in developing countries, a collision of emerging epidemics of non-communicable diseases and injury, with existing epidemics of infectious diseases, malnutrition, and complications of childbirth, creates complexity in countries where health infrastructure is often inadequate to deal with already existing health challenges and needs, and where health systems are often not agile enough to respond with the development of preventive and cost-effective interventions. This chapter provides an overview of the problem of chronic disease, and the urgent need for action globally, with a specific focus on CVD, a term we will use to encompass coronary artery disease, hypertension, stroke, and diabetes.

The steady global rise of non-communicable disease has occurred in parallel with changing social and economic circumstances. A massive migratory movement is occurring with the shift of populations from rural settings to cities. The movement is complicated because many cities are not citadels of shining affluence, and contain pockets of poverty, especially around the edges. Likewise, the features of city living that create the greatest cause for concern when it comes to contributing to chronic disease, such as easy availability of cheap, processed, high-fat, high-salt, and calorie-dense foods and beverages, including alcohol, and the loss of opportunities for incidental physical activity, are realities that are also beginning to permeate rural life.

These changes in the environment in which hundreds of millions of people live, combined with a simultaneously relentless effort by the tobacco industry to recruit smokers among people in developing economies as industry markets shrivel in more developed, health-conscious countries, suggest the need for preventive programmes aimed not only at high-risk individuals, but at entire populations who stand at heightened risk of chronic disease, especially diabetes mellitus and cardiovascular disorders (CVD).

The subsequent economic effects of non-communicable chronic disease are especially damaging in developing countries, in large part because many of the chronically ill are of working age. For instance, it is estimated that globally the greatest cumulative proportion of CVD deaths in the next 20 years will occur in those 65 years and over (Leeder *et al.* 2004). However, what is perhaps more striking is that the comparative cumulative CVD death percentage for those between 35 and 64 will increase dramatically. This will affect the economic 'bottom line' at both a macro- and micro- level, decreasing the national productivity of affected countries, while also bankrupting individuals and their families because they cannot work and are unable to afford their out-of-pocket health care expenses (Leeder *et al.* 2004).

Four decades of focus on reproductive maternal health have tightly bound the concept of 'women's health' to that of childbearing and motherhood. These remain, of course, important dimensions, but they are no longer (if they ever were), the only ones critical for addressing women's health needs in emerging economies, especially during the years of family formation. In fact, chronic diseases like CVD exact a much higher mortality toll among women in their reproductive and motherhood years than reproductive-related causes that receive the largest share of research, funding, and policy attention.

Chronic disease is often thought of as a disease of the elderly. For women in particular, it is not that simple. In Latin America, for women aged 35 to 44, an estimated 40 to 55 per cent of mortality is attributable to non-communicable chronic diseases (such as CVD), compared to less than 10 per cent of mortality attributable to causes associated with childbearing and HIV/AIDS combined (Raymond *et al.* 2005). In South Africa and China, non-communicable chronic diseases account for a much higher proportion of deaths among women of late child-bearing or early motherhood ages, compared to mortality attributable to causes associated with childbearing (Raymond *et al.* 2005).

The burden of non-communicable chronic diseases is matched by highly prevalent ante-cedents such as obesity. While the impact of low-cost, high-fat, high-salt, calorie-dense food and reduced physical activity are first manifest among the newly affluent in developing economies, this group can alter its lifestyle. The educated and well-to-do in developing countries are likely to be the first to realise the need for behavioural and other changes to reverse their risk, based on the experiences from high-income countries. Those who are less educated and less wealthy will be more likely to keep smoking, eat high-fat food, and not act to protect their health. The less affluent or overtly poor acquire these behaviours, but lack the education and affluence to get rid of them. The ongoing burden of death and disability from chronic disease is likely, therefore, to fall on the poorer (although possibly not the very poorest) sections of society, as it continues to do in more-developed countries (Leeder *et al.* 2004).

Obesity is also a phenomenon that must be disaggregated by gender. In the Middle East, the proportion of women who are obese far exceeds that of men in all countries. This is exemplified by Egypt, where 45 per cent of women are obese (BMI $\geq$ 30kg/m^2), and Kuwait and Bahrain, where 30 per cent of women are obese (WHO 2010a). Also in Egypt, deaths from CVD and/or diabetes are 15 times more common than deaths from reproductive health causes in women aged 35–44. Illustrating a health differential across the globe, CVD death rates for women aged 55 in Egypt are ten times those in the US (WHO 2010b). Living in low-income countries certainly does not immunise women against non-communicable chronic disease mortality at relatively young ages. In fact, the exact opposite has shown to be true.

The narrow definition of 'women's health' in global public health that has long focused on reproductive conditions and diseases needs to reflect this changed epidemiology. Likewise, with rising levels of obesity among children and adolescents, non-communicable chronic diseases must become part of a global definition of women's and children's health that matches a changing epidemiological reality.

Responses to non-communicable chronic disease

To combat non-communicable chronic disease in vulnerable populations requires a focus on prevention at the level of the population, supplemented by efforts to detect and treat early those at special risk, including children (Leeder *et al.* 2004). The potential benefits associated with this course of action, such as helping those with pre-diabetes to reduce their risk of developing diabetes and CVD, and reducing children's exposure to tobacco advertising, are not yet fully appreciated, especially in low- and middle-income countries.

When we consider the implementation of population-based approaches to prevention, it is easy to see why spirits fail and enthusiasm evaporates given the magnitude of the challenge – not unlike that of addressing climate change. First, there is the likely extended future duration of required action to effect change. Second, the necessary strategies, learned from efforts over the last few decades in developed countries – inter-sectoral action, political persuasion, battle with vested commercial interests and greed, social marketing of uncomfortable messages about what we eat and how much exercise we take – are also daunting. Third, and crucial to the success of any social change that might diminish the risk of chronic disease, is recruitment of the population to healthier lifestyles. Fourth – and this should never be discounted – the experience of many millions of people is that trade and commerce, and the move to the cities that economic progress has enabled, have made a massive, positive contribution to their quality of life and to chances of their children surviving, receiving an education, and progressing to a better life. The cards, therefore, are stacked against those favouring, as the late Professor Geoffrey Rose put it so memorably, 'sick population' approaches to prevention (Rose 1985: 1).

Unfortunately, the population-based prevention strategies, such as immunisation and attempts to change lifestyle characteristics, of enormous potential importance to the population as a whole, offer only a small benefit to each individual, since most of them were going to be all right anyway, at least for many years (Rose 1985).

Therefore, it would seem preferable to just seek out the high-risk individuals and treat them. Help them to quit smoking, to treat their elevated blood pressure and cholesterol, maybe even help them to change their diet. Combine this approach with an endorsement of the recommendations contained in the Framework Convention on Tobacco Control (WHO 2010c), such as price and tax measures to reduce the demand for tobacco, and non-price measures to reduce the demand for tobacco (namely, protection from exposure to tobacco smoke, packaging and labelling of tobacco products, and education, communication, training, and public awareness), and you may be doing the best that is possible in a near-impossible setting.

In the short term, as Rose (1985) acknowledged, an approach to 'sick individuals' may be the best tactic. There is no future, however, in restricting our strategies to the detection and treatment of sick individuals – we will be treating high-risk people for as long as the social and economic conditions that create their problems are not dealt with. Realistically, many chronic diseases will require that we take both approaches – that we use case-centred epidemiology to identify susceptible individuals (the 'high-risk strategy') and, at the same time, attempt to control the determinants of incidence (the 'population strategy'). The Finnish North Karelia project documents the benefits attainable in a 'sick population' approach that focused on community risk rather than individual risk (Vartiainen *et al.* 2000).

All of these concerns do not mean that the task at hand is impossible. Social movements do not owe all their origin and power to carefully considered and organised programmes designed by experts. To believe that the affected communities are not concerned by the problems they are experiencing is naïve. For instance, many economically advanced societies have witnessed a downturn in CVD mortality and morbidity of massive proportion since the mid-1960s, with this owing as much to community modification of lifestyle, as to complex, dazzling, and frequently highly expensive medical and surgical interventions. Where descriptive analytical work has looked back over the change in CVD rates, about 50 per cent on average (perhaps less lately) settles on actions that the populations have taken to reduce their exposure to risk factors. The other half can be credited to improved care (Vartiainen *et al.* 2000).

Encouragingly, if implemented, the positive impact of prevention and early treatment would manifest mostly in younger adults in their economically productive years, thereby mitigating the macro- and micro-economic implications of CVD already mentioned (Leeder *et al.* 2004). Visible results in the relatively short term, such as stroke reduction in treated hypertensives or diminished pneumonia admissions in reformed smokers, would be necessary to sustain investment in prevention programmes by non-health bureaucracies. But, as argued above, prevention programmes must be locally sustainable for an indefinite future, pending environmental change that reduces or eliminates risk. For this reason, developing countries must be encouraged to take the first step themselves, now, as a prelude to recruiting assistance from elsewhere, and as a reflection of genuine concern among the members of their communities.

Taking action on chronic diseases

The link between environmental changes associated with economic growth, urbanisation, and improvements in personal financial status, and the evolution of chronic disease that has been observed in many nations, lumbers the poor with the highest CVD risk profiles today. The social determinants of health, the conditions in which people are born, grow, live, work, and age, including the health system, are shaped by the distribution of power, resources, money, and policy at all levels – global, national, and local. The social determinants of health are mostly responsible for health inequities – the unfair and avoidable differences in health status seen within and between countries. They contextualise the origin of the disease, and make it less likely that the affected individuals will have the efficacy and money to seek treatment and change their lifestyles. Chronic disease is one of the biggest land masses on the map of inequality and inequity today.

Cultural and critical barriers to chronic disease management

In order to deal effectively with chronic diseases, the context in which they are addressed is extraordinarily important. On one level, the goal is quite straightforward. If one simply tells the patient (and also the seemingly disease-free population) to eat well and wisely, stop smoking, exercise, and maintain a normal weight, the chronic diseases that have become scourges of the modern age would almost disappear. The problem would be solved. As we all know, though, that advice is simple to give and accurate, but its implementation is extraordinarily difficult in any society and in any social strata, although more so for those in lower socio-economic classes for whom healthy and affordable foods, and safe neighbourhoods in which to exercise, may not be accessible.

Let us look at several examples of this complexity. First, take the need to swallow pills every day for an asymptomatic disease, such as when a person is found to have elevated blood pressure or cholesterol. In the United States and other high-income countries, this has been done for 60 years for hypertension and other conditions. This approach gained enormous publicity after the death of former president, Franklin Roosevelt, in the 1940s from high blood pressure. Yet, in spite of this robust history and widespread publicity, only 30 per cent of hypertensive patients in the US and other high-income countries today achieve the therapeutic goal of normal blood pressure. Nonetheless, because the response curve is continuous, this graded outcome has had a profound impact on CVD endpoints, with strokes falling by more than 75 per cent since 1940, and heart disease by more than 56 per cent from 1965 at its peak, until 2000 (CDC 1999).

If we then take the need for chronic disease management, and think about applying it to the nomadic herdsmen on the Mongolian steppes, to the favelas of Rio de Janeiro, or to the new urban areas of Mumbai, the magnitude of the response required is obviously amplified and the barrier seems even more formidable.

The second example comes from the political arena. The world is awash in empty, high-calorie, high-salt-containing fast foods. These foods are adored by billions, consumed in large amounts, and play an important role in the obesity, hypertensive, and diabetes epidemics currently in progress. These foods are available for several reasons. Most countries offer a variety of agricultural subsidies that are deeply embedded in the political and entrepreneurial fabric of the country. They are also supported by global trade agreements, the most obvious of which are the World Trade Organization (WTO) agreements, negotiated and signed by the bulk of the world's trading nations and ratified in their parliaments. However, there are also many other smaller bilateral treaty obligations based in agriculture. Changing this political reality is extraordinarily difficult, if not impossible.

While the World Health Organization (WHO), as a representative and protector of global public health interests, has observership status at WTO meetings, there is no obligation on the part of the negotiators at WTO meetings to pay any heed to the WHO. Since the WTO meetings go on for months, and are often in remote parts of the world, the expense is great for the WHO to maintain observers. Hence, there is virtually no input from the public health arena to the WTO. At some point, if we are to confront the mentioned global epidemics, this dynamic has to change.

The third example of the complexity of CVD control in particular comes from the fast food revolution that is supported by robust advertising campaigns. The retail companies that market these foods are extremely successful, enjoy the backing of the financial community, are supported enthusiastically by their customers, and have very little incentive to change a successful formula. There have, however, been some dents made in this armour.

In the United States, the main purveyors of soft drinks were persuaded to take sweetened drinks out of vending machine in schools (Burros and Warner 2006). They did this and deservedly got credit for doing it, but it is telling to examine the background to that decision.

A large effort has been directed by schools, parents, and non-governmental organisations to inhibit the abusive marketing and sales of energy-dense, low-nutrient foods. The food companies, given their acutely tuned political antennae, recognised this shift in public opinion, and broadened their portfolios to include juice and water companies. When the companies were finally ready to change, they simply altered the mix of drinks that they put in the vending machine. This, then, was a win-win operation; schools now have an environment with more healthy foods, and the companies have the capacity to continue marketing to a group that spends a great deal on what it drinks.

Essential strategies for prevention and management of chronic disease

Chronic disease management (and indeed prevention) requires continuity, trust, access, and supplies. The environment in which this kind of health care delivery system can thrive requires a civil society that is active on its own behalf in seeking support for such services. In wartime, prevention and management of chronic disease is not a priority and probably will not be done, during periods of social upheaval it cannot be done, and in an environment where the population has reason to dread its own government it will not happen unless somehow it can be seen as a movement independent of government. For effective prevention and management to occur, citizens must interact with the health care system, be open about their issues and problems, and have access to, and know that the personnel and supplies required for ongoing care are going to be there (Raymond *et al.* 2004).

If these social conditions exist, then action can follow. First, the Ministry of Health in a country needs, through mechanisms such as social marketing and education, to create a receptive environment for implementing the required changes, especially if chronic disease and their treatment and prevention are unknown entities to the local culture. Embarking on a new treatment programme for a chronic disease within a country's health system, and its clinical risk precursors in which medicines are offered for both symptomatic and asymptomatic disease, requires an informed population. A detailed publicity campaign, with structured public relations programmes and advocacy pronouncements by leading public figures, as well as health leadership, could be used to good effect to launch such a programme. This is not an easy sell and will require both health care delivery and public health leadership to collaborate and cooperate for common goals, and there may be a long lag time while such a programme is inaugurated before actual implementation occurs.

The second necessary strategic step is that the government agencies beyond those specifically devoted to health need to buy into this programme. This was argued persuasively by the WHO Macroeconomic Commission on Health (WHO 2001). All government ministries need to acknowledge that health is a part of its portfolio; that they must give health more than token attention; and that they must incorporate health issues into their policies, particularly those policies that relate to the food supply, the physical environment, and tobacco, all of which impinge on health. The broad government writ large needs to understand that it is important to have healthy workers, healthy soldiers, and healthy retirees. Without those, running a government becomes difficult, expensive, and politically risky in today's volatile world.

The third strategy relates to very new technologies. Remote medical monitoring offers the opportunity for patients with chronic disease to be followed where they live (Coye *et al.* 2009). Patients with hypertension, congestive heart failure, diabetes, asthma, and obesity can be followed from afar by mobile communication technology (Vital Wave Consulting 2009). For example, if mobile phones are used, patients can weigh themselves, document what they have been eating, confirm they have taken pills, even check their blood pressure or blood sugar – having been taught in the clinic – and report this in to the medical centre by phone. When they do this, they can be given extra telephone subscription minutes for that month or for that week. This saves the patient the need to make long trips, giving up work, and spending money to get to the clinic simply to have their blood pressure or blood sugar checked. The implementation of this technology is in its infancy but has great promise for the developing world, especially given the high levels of mobile phone ownership throughout Africa, India, and China, for example.

These strategies and no doubt others all need to be blended together to make a chronic disease prevention programme work. Clearly, the effort has to be broad-based throughout the government and society. It will require the input and cooperation of the corporate world, the national and international trading communities, military, labour and management, and the educational communities.

All relevant actors do not have to begin at a level of 100 per cent effort simultaneously, but ultimately, each of these groups and agencies will need to be engaged. The initiating leadership, whether the health advice comes from afar or from within their country or ministries, needs to recognise that this is a long-term strategy that needs to be built piece by piece, engaging the support and cooperation of multiple players.

Engaging the private sector, civil society and international organisations

Effective chronic disease prevention cannot be simply a matter of public health policy. Risk factors are embedded in all manner of social and economic structures and institutions. To implement policy effectively requires coalitions among a variety of institutions and interests of which public health will be one, and only one, part. Who else must be part of that coalition? The list is long. Employers, because the CVD threat occurs in the workforce, and reaching that workforce at work is most efficient; civil society organisations, because public communication and policy advocacy rests within their sphere of influence; educators, because risk behaviour is learned and needs to be un-learned; central banks, because investments in health infrastructure will be required; food companies, because nutrition inputs are critical to consumer food behaviour; and communications companies, because messaging about behaviour change is fraught with difficulty. To achieve this outcome, two changes of heart in public health are essential.

First, public health must see itself as one of many sectors needing to be mobilised. Only appreciating the need for coalitions, however, will be insufficient.

Second, related to the above, public health must see these other participants as its equal if policy is to be crafted and enthusiastically executed. Many seats at the coalition table must be filled, and they must be filled willingly and actively. Public health must see its peers in business, commerce, finance, communications, and the like, not as followers who are present to do the will of public health, but as leaders whose own interests must be accommodated in a jointly perceived priority. Effective coalitions are comprised of multiple gears that turn on their own separate axes for their own self-interest, but mesh to move a policy forward. It is the separateness that makes the movement possible.

This is by far the most difficult challenge for global public health. It cannot dominate chronic disease control strategy because the risk factors, behaviours, and institutional pathways are not within its grasp or power. Building coalitions of the willing and relevant is the way forward.

References

Burros, M. and Warner, M. (2006) 'Bottlers Agree to a School Ban on Sweet Drinks', *New York Times*, 4 May.
CDC (Centers for Disease Control and Prevention) (1999) 'Achievements in Public Health, 1900–1999: Decline in Deaths from Heart Disease and Stroke–United States, 1900–1999', *MMWR Morbidity and Mortality Weekly Report*, 48(30): 649–56.
Coye, M.J., Haselkorn, A., and DeMello, S. (2009) 'Remote Patient Management: Technology-enabled Innovation and Evolving Business Models for Chronic Disease Care', *Health Affairs*, 28(1): 126–35.
Leeder, S., Raymond, S., Greenberg, H., Liu, H., and Esson, K. (2004) *A Race Against Time: The Challenge of Cardiovascular Disease in Developing Countries*, available at http://www.earth.columbia.edu/news/2004/images/raceagainsttime_FINAL_051104.pdf (accessed 7 September 2009).

Levenson, J.W., Skerrett, P.J., and Gaziano, J.M. (2002) 'Reducing the Global Burden of Cardiovascular Disease: The Role of Risk Factors', *Preventive Cardiology*, 5: 188–99.

Raymond, S., Greenberg, H.M., Liu, H., and Leeder, S.R. (2004) 'Civil Society Confronts the Challenge of Chronic Illness', *Development*, 47: 97–103.

Raymond S.U., Greenberg, H.M., and Leeder, S.R. (2005) 'Beyond Reproduction: Women's Health in Today's Developing World', *International Journal of Epidemiology*, 34(5): 1,144–8.

Rose, G. (1985) 'Sick Individuals and Sick Populations', *International Journal of Epidemiology*, 14(1): 32–8.

Vartiainen, E., Jousilahti, P., Alfthan, G., Sundvall, J., Pietinen, P., and Puska, P. (2000) 'Cardiovascular Risk Factor Changes in Finland, 1972–1997', *International Journal of Epidemiology*, 29: 49–56.

Vital Wave Consulting (2009) *mHealth for Development: The Opportunity of Mobile Technology for Healthcare in the Developing World*, Washington, DC and Berkshire: UN Foundation-Vodafone Foundation Partnership, available at http://www.unfoundation.org/global-issues/technology/mhealth-report.html (accessed 7 August 2009).

WHO (World Health Organization) (2001) *WHO: Report of the Commission on Macroeconomics and Health: Investment in Health for Economic Development*, Geneva: WHO.

WHO (World Health Organization) (2010a) *WHO Global Database on Body Mass Index*, available at http://apps.who.int/bmi/index.jsp (accessed 27 January 2010).

WHO (World Health Organization) (2010b) *WHO Mortality Database*, available at http://www.who.int/whosis (accessed 27 January 2010).

WHO (World Health Organization) (2010c) *WHO Framework Convention on Tobacco Control*, available at http://www.who.int/fctc/en/ (accessed 27 January 2010).

Yusuf, S., Reddy, S., Ôunpuu, S., and Anand, S. (2001) 'Global Burden of Cardiovascular Diseases: Part I: General Considerations, the Epidemiologic Transition, Risk Factors, and Impact of Urbanization', *Circulation*, 104: 2,746–53.

36

Creating Access to Health Technologies in Poor Countries[1]

Laura J. Frost and Michael R. Reich

Many people in developing countries lack access to health technologies, even basic ones. These technologies include life-saving medicines, such as antiretrovirals for HIV/AIDS, as well as life-enhancing medicines, such as medications that help stop asthma attacks and improve breathing. Limited access is also a problem with many other health products, such as vaccines that can prevent debilitating diseases, diagnostics for infectious and chronic diseases, preventive technologies such as insecticide-treated bed nets, and various kinds of contraceptives. In 1999 the World Health Organization (WHO) estimated that since the mid-1980s, around 1.7 billion people – approximately one-third of the world's population in 1999 – did not have regular access to essential medicines and vaccines.

In recent years, the issue of access to medicines and other health technologies has risen on the global policy agenda. The most contentious debates about inadequate access in poor countries have focused on drugs and vaccines, but similar problems exist for other health technologies. Access to diagnostics, for example, has been relatively unexplored in policy debates. And the focus on certain types of access barriers (especially pricing and patents) has tended to obscure other important obstacles to access such as distribution, delivery, and adoption problems.

To provide a more comprehensive view of creating access, we explored the histories of six health technologies: praziquantel to treat schistosomiasis (a parasitic worm disease), hepatitis B vaccine, the Norplant contraceptive, malaria rapid diagnostic tests, vaccine vial monitors, and the female condom. A full description of each case study, along with a more complete analysis of the issues related to access, can be found in our book on this topic (Frost and Reich 2008). Due to space limitations, this chapter only provides an overview of access and the lessons from the case studies.

Four criteria guided our selection of case studies. We chose cases that: (1) included different types of health technologies; (2) reflected a range of health problems; (3) spanned different phases of access; and (4) included examples that have been successful, as well as those that have encountered obstacles and faltered. Our approach in these case studies draws from anthropological research that traces the 'life-cycles' or 'biographies' of medicines from production to end-user

(Van der Geest *et al.* 1996; Reynolds *et al.* 2002), and from public health case study research on barriers to technology access (Sevene *et al.* 2005). For each case study, we analysed the social, economic, political, and cultural processes that shaped access to the health technology in developing countries. We followed the technology's flow through different phases of access, identified barriers, and looked for measures that create access (Frost and Reich 2008).

Our findings have important implications for initiatives to develop global health products. These organisations are seeking to introduce new health products for poor countries (such as the Global Alliance for TB Drug Development, the Foundation for Innovative New Diagnostics, the International AIDS Vaccine Initiative, and OneWorld Health). Once developers demonstrate that a product can improve the health of poor people in poor countries, they confront a series of new problems related to creating access. This chapter presents seven lessons about the bottlenecks to access and the strategies to overcome them.

What do we mean by access?

Stated simply, *access* refers to people's ability to obtain and use good quality health technologies when they are needed. Access is not just a technical issue involving the logistics of transporting a technology from the manufacturer to the end-user. Access also involves social values, economic interests, and political processes. Access requires a product, as well as services, and depends on how health systems perform in practice. We think of access not as a single event but as a continuous process involving a series of activities and actors over time.

Access framework

Our conception of access is based on four As: architecture, availability, affordability, and adoption (Figure 36.1). These four As are activity streams that occur simultaneously. Our framework provides more complexity than the conventional view of a linear 'value chain' based on, for example, the stages of discovery, development, and delivery (IBM Institute for Business Value 2004). Our approach builds on previous research on barriers to access (Andersen and Andersen 1974; Hanson *et al.* 2003). It adapts the approach developed by the Global Alliance for TB Drug Development called the AAA strategy (Global Alliance for TB Drug Development 2009). We have changed some terms and added some ideas to improve both the clarity and comprehensiveness of the analysis. Our framework explicitly recognises the organisational dimension of access, or architecture. The second stream concerns the availability of health technologies. The third stream concerns the affordability of technologies for developing-country governments, non-governmental agencies, and individual end-users. The final stream involves the adoption of health technologies.

Access activities

Our framework uses a comprehensive approach to access and maps activities from the global level to the end-user. In the case studies in our book (Frost and Reich 2008), we broke down the process into access activities, which were defined by specific events and which must occur for access to achieve its potential health benefits. In the framework, we viewed access as beginning in the product development stage and concluding when end-users (including both providers and patients) were using the technology appropriately. Importantly, we have extended our view of access beyond simply reaching the end-user

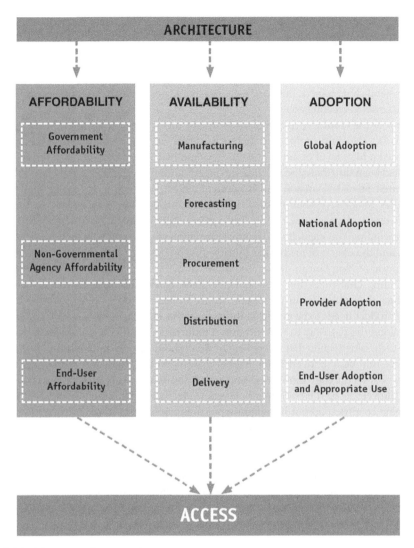

Figure 36.1   The access framework
Source: Frost and Reich 2008.

because we recognise that how people use the technology plays a major role in the ultimate effects produced. Thus, our concept of access includes ideas about both appropriate and inappropriate use of technology.

Findings for product development initiatives

Getting the four activity streams right can produce successful access for health technologies. But doing so is not easy. Based on the case histories, we reached the following findings about the process of creating access.

Finding 1: Developing a safe and effective technology is necessary but not sufficient for ensuring technology access and health improvement

Showing that a new technology is safe and efficacious in clinical trials represents an exciting and important result. Working through the regulatory process to licence the new technology also constitutes significant progress. But these measures should not be viewed as endpoints; they are only midway successes in creating access.

The case of the contraceptive implant Norplant nicely illustrates this point. Norplant was developed by the non-profit Population Council in New York City. Clinical trials demonstrated a high level of safety and efficacy, and by the end of 1996, more than 5 million implants had been distributed worldwide (about 3.6 million in Indonesia and close to a million in the United States) (Harrison and Rosenfield 1998). But Norplant's use in the field faced many hurdles. Major access barriers arose in many countries related to affordability, the training and competence of providers, the health infrastructure's capability to deliver high-quality services (including the capacity to remove the implant), adoption of new technologies by end-users, and the effects of media and litigation on product reputation. These problems led to the withdrawal of Norplant in the United States in 2002.

This finding challenges the view held by some product developers that 'if we make a good product that addresses an important health problem in developing countries, it will be used'. The product needs to be managed throughout the access process to address the numerous obstacles along the pathway to the end-user. Products do not fly off the shelf on their own – especially technologies aimed at improving health conditions in poor countries, because these products do not fit a conventional market-driven model. Many problems exist between the processes of technology innovation and actual diffusion and appropriate use in developing countries (Juma et al. 2001). Some technology developers do not know or understand the markets in developing countries, do not have existing organisational bases in those markets, and do not know how to enter those markets. For example, Temptime Corporation, the developer of vaccine vial monitors (VVMs), had not previously worked in global health and needed help from the Program for Appropriate Technology in Health (PATH) in entering this market, negotiating with international agencies, and redesigning its product for end-users. On the other side, developing-country governments often lack the financial capacity to purchase new technologies, and adequate purchasing mechanisms to push down prices for innovative products or to assure good quality. For these and other reasons, creating access for good health technologies requires concerted efforts.

Finding 2: Creating access depends on effective product advocacy by a product champion to construct and manage the architecture of access

Product champions in global health are people or organisations that believe in new technologies and are committed to developing products with wide access in poor countries. Product champions also take a major role in constructing and managing the architecture of access, especially the relationships among different organisations. Champions are found in many types of organisations working in global health (including technical agencies, non-profit organisations, academic institutions, and manufacturers). In the case of VVMs, staff from PATH collaborated closely with WHO staff to ensure the introduction and scale-up of the technology on all Expanded Programme on Immunization (EPI) vaccines. For Norplant, Population Council staff developed the product, introduced it, and acted as product champion. The main product champion for the female condom has been the manufacturer, the Female Health Company, and its foundation. Funding is key to the effectiveness of product champions. The product champion's role can range from stimulating awareness of the technology to more strategic activities of overcoming difficult development or access barriers.

One example of an effective product champion is the work of PATH in guiding the development of VVMs. The VVM is a miniature time-temperature indicator printed onto the label of a vaccine vial during the labelling process of vaccine production that aims to reduce vaccine wastage. At a critical point during product development in 1989, when Temptime had decided to give up on the project after months of failing to achieve technical success, representatives from PATH visited the company, explained the global significance of VVMs, and convinced Temptime to continue its work (without additional funding) (PATH 2005). PATH staff members continued to guide the access process for VVMs and provided crucial support to WHO staff through mentoring, technical assistance, and project documentation. By the end of 2005, close to 100 per cent of WHO-pre-qualified vaccine producers used the technology on their vaccine labels. Major challenges, however, still remain in expanding VVM access in the Pan American Health Organization (PAHO) region and in developing-country vaccine markets (Frost and Reich 2008: 158).

Effective product advocacy depends on an access plan that frames the work activities of champions and partners and takes into account the perspectives of different actors. Product champions and their partners need to develop an access plan to assess potential barriers and opportunities at the global and national levels and identify strategies to navigate and shape the complex terrain of access. In constructing relationships among different groups and individuals, advocates work with actors who may have widely divergent views of new health technologies. In the case of VVMs, WHO staff and health workers viewed the technology as key to improving the cold chain (the process of keeping a vaccine at a safely cold temperature throughout production and transportation) and decreasing vaccine wastage. For the UNICEF Supply Division, VVMs challenged the UNICEF policy on sole suppliers and created stress in relationships with vaccine producers. For vaccine producers, attaching VVMs to their vaccines sold to UNICEF meant a number of legal, logistical, and commercial challenges to their business. Providing VVMs required a concerted effort – and a significant amount of time – to bring these diverse groups together and address their different perspectives on the technology. Product champions and their partners can use an access plan to frame their activities, map the position and power of these diverse actors, identify obstacles and opportunities, and prepare concrete strategies that promote access.

The female condom case shows what can happen when there is no access plan. In the product introduction phase, individuals and organisations promoting the female condom identified next steps for access in global meetings. However, the steps were not prioritised or written into a plan; as a result, the next steps were never systematically implemented. This meant that advocates had no clear guide for moving access efforts forward.

Finding 3: Product champions need to create expert consensus about their health technology in international technical agencies and global health policy communities

Our case studies highlight the importance of creating 'expert consensus' on a new technology, within both the international health technical agencies and the broader international public health community. This role for expert consensus is emphasised by other public health analysts (Levine 2004). Product champions need to design strategies for producing expert consensus as one of their first tasks. The key question is: Whose consensus needs to be gained at the global level? The answer differs by technology because the specific actors vary. For most technologies, approval by the relevant international technical agency is required to move forward on other areas of adoption for the product. Agencies signal their adoption with official decisions about the technology and the related disease or health condition. This approval process often occurs through WHO expert groups, which can challenge or confirm the conventional wisdom.

One good example is the resolution adopted at the World Health Assembly in May 2001 on treatment for schistosomiasis and soil-transmitted helminths (intestinal worms that include ascaris and hookworm). This official statement helped promote new efforts to make praziquantel (the drug to treat schistosomiasis) more widely available in Africa. In the case of Norplant, the WHO conducted a technical evaluation and stated that the contraceptive was 'particularly advantageous to women who wish an extended period of contraceptive protection' (WHO 1985: 491). These official announcements by an international agency, however, are not simply the result of technical consultations and decisions. They often depend on highly political negotiations among actors with different interests in the technology. Product champions would be helped in these tasks by conducting an analysis of the key players involved and designing explicit political strategies for managing the stakeholders and the process of producing expert consensus to support their technology (Reich 2002).

Finding 4: End-user adoption of a technology is an essential but often overlooked component of the entire process of creating access

Adoption of a technology by the end-user is vital to ensuring access – whether the end-user is a patient, a consumer, or a provider. Adoption by end-users is influenced by the characteristics of the technology and the health problem it addresses, and by the social, political, and historical contexts.

The female condom demonstrates how a technology's characteristics can make adoption difficult for end-users in some contexts. Some women, for example, consider the female condom to be extremely large and bulky, aesthetically unappealing, prone to slippage and twisting during sexual intercourse, and stiff in its internal rings (AIDSCAP 1997). Developers of the first generation of female condoms did not adequately take into account the perspective of end-users. These negative impressions can be addressed and the chances of long-term use can be increased through extended and supportive counselling by providers (Telles Dias et al. 2006). Some women, however, do not have access to counselling, while others are unwilling to endure a series of awkward 'practice sessions' in order to get the female condom 'right'. Sales of the female condom have remained low since its introduction in the early 1990s. By 2004, approximately 12.2 million units were sold per year, representing only 0.1–0.2 per cent of the number of male condoms sold worldwide (The Female Health Company 2005). New female condom designs in development are seeking to address the adoption issues of end-users by changing these negative technology characteristics, making female condoms more user-friendly, and using less expensive material to make the technology more affordable.

Our cases show that paying attention to adoption by end-users must begin early. This attention starts during product development when technical characteristics of a new technology are first under consideration. It continues in field trials and pilot projects, when end-user views of a new technology can be assessed and addressed through technical changes. Attention is also important in later phases, when managing the perceptions of the technology is central to creating access. Strategies to help developers understand the perspectives of end-users include conducting early research on their perceptions, applying research findings to product development and programme design, hiring local project managers, and creating strategies for national and local ownership in programme implementation.

Finding 5: The cost of health technologies and related services is a key barrier to access: strategies to expand access must address affordability

The literature on access highlights cost to governments and individuals as a major obstacle, and our findings support this. Decreasing product costs for governments can involve a range of strategies. For example, in seeking to lower the price of praziquantel, the Schistosomiasis Control Initiative (SCI) has used a bulk purchasing approach and has sought to expand competition by assisting manufacturers with registration and stimulating local formulation in Africa. By increasing the number of registered suppliers in Burkina Faso, for example, the SCI helped to create a more competitive bidding process for government purchases, reducing the price per tablet for praziquantel from US $0.14 to $0.09 (Frost and Reich 2008). Other strategies to address government affordability are tiered pricing (used by the Population Council for Norplant) and threats of compulsory licensing (used by Brazil for antiretroviral products for HIV/AIDS) (Reich and Bery 2005).

Another measure to address high costs is external funding for government procurement. For example, the Bill & Melinda Gates Foundation supports SCI to finance praziquantel purchases for six African countries. The biggest problem with the external financing approach concerns its sustainability over the medium and long term, because donors persistently seek to limit the timeframe of funding commitments. Although affordability is essential, our cases show that making a technology more affordable is rarely sufficient on its own to create access. Availability constraints as well as factors related to adoption and architecture all need to be considered and addressed.

Finding 6: Supply-side strategies that ensure the availability of a technology are needed to help expand access for health technologies in developing countries

Two supply-side strategies to assure availability are of particular importance. The first relates to information failures. Suppliers often lack good or complete information about product demand in developing countries. These information problems affect supply, since manufacturers may underestimate the potential market in a poor country or region and may not take the necessary steps to enter the market (such as registering the product with the government). Strategies to address these problems include disseminating information to manufacturers about demand and assisting companies in product registration. A Global Health Forecasting Working Group, convened by the Washington-based Center for Global Development in 2006, provides recommendations to the global health community for improving demand forecasting.

Another information barrier is that government procurement agencies in poor countries often have incomplete information about the availability and quality of products and suppliers for a particular health technology. For example, although many government procurement agencies have financing from the Global Fund to Fight AIDS, TB and Malaria to procure malaria rapid diagnostic tests, they confront a rapidly changing range of available products and suppliers, making the purchase of diagnostics extremely difficult. One simple strategy that the WHO has used is to give countries regularly updated information about rapid diagnostic products and suppliers on its website (http://www.wpro.who.int/rdt) and in a 'Sources and Prices' document for malaria products (http://www.who.int/medicines/areas/access/AntiMalariaSourcesPricesEnglish.pdf).

A second important supply-side strategy relates to the difficulty of finding commercial partners willing to develop or manufacture a technology for use in poor countries. Such challenges are a major access barrier, particularly for lower-profit technologies (relative to, for instance, drugs and vaccines for sale in rich countries). Our study found that suitable private partners for low-profit technologies may be located among small- to mid-size companies that have existing commercial products, are already generating revenues from these products, and have experience in working with regulatory authorities (such as the US Food and Drug Administration). This finding concurs with a 2005 study on neglected disease drug development that urged policymakers to target commercial incentives for research and development to smaller companies that have a good chance of becoming engaged with neglected disease markets (Moran 2005).

One example of a technology that was produced by a small- to mid-size company is the case of a rapid diagnostic test for malaria. In this instance, when the Walter Reed Army Institute (WRAI) looked for a commercial partner to manufacture its malaria diagnostic, it encountered many barriers. Because the diagnostic would be used for US soldiers, WRAI needed a company that could take the product through the FDA regulatory process. After years of seeking a partner, WRAI found Binax Inc., a mid-size company. In this search, WRAI learned that most diagnostic companies are small 'mom-and-pop' businesses that do not possess the resources, know-how, experience, or willingness to navigate the FDA process. It also discovered that the large companies with these features were not interested in partnering because the technologies were not profitable enough.

Product developers and champions therefore need to expand their search for partners to small- and mid-size companies willing to take on niche products, and also high-quality manufacturing firms in emerging markets (such as China and India). The challenges of finding good partners in emerging markets should not be underestimated, especially given the problematic regulatory environments in those countries (Yardley and Barboza 2008). It is worth noting, however, that a number of groups have found good manufacturing partners in these countries, as shown by the success of the SCI in working with praziquantel producers in both China and India.

Finding 7: Limited health infrastructure in many developing countries impedes technology access, making it important to invest in health-system strengthening to ensure sustained access

The successful delivery of technologies to patients and consumers depends in large part on the capacity of the health sector's human resources, network of public and private providers, and availability of functioning equipment – in short, how the health system performs on a daily basis (Roberts *et al.* 2004). Health-system strengthening is especially important for new technologies (because many require the development of new systems and skills) and provider-dependent technologies. But it is also necessary for products designed for use in areas with limited health infrastructure – such as poor countries.

The Norplant case study demonstrates how the failure to invest in health systems can impede access. Norplant required both insertion and removal by a trained provider. In the rapid scale-up of Norplant in countries such as Indonesia and the United States, many providers received training (particularly on insertion techniques), but the instruction was not comprehensive enough. As a result, many health professionals were not well-trained on removal techniques, and these training shortfalls led to later difficulties with implant removals. Other health system problems that emerged globally included the lack of sufficient information and counselling about the method for end-users and concerns about informed choice, particularly whether uneducated, poor women were targeted for Norplant or steered to that method over other contraceptives. Overall, our study shows that strategies for health-system strengthening are product- and context-specific, but they all require sufficient funding, attention, and time to adequately address health system barriers if access is to be produced and sustained.

Concluding remarks

Access to health technologies in poor countries is hindered by multiple obstacles. Inadequate access is rarely a single-failure problem. Access problems typically result from a combination of market failures, government failures, and NGO failures. The problems often affect all four dimensions of access – architecture, availability, affordability, and adoption – although the patterns differ by specific technology. Addressing the multiple failures requires many steps directed at global-, national-, and local-level actors and depends on various kinds of expertise. The solutions often require strategies involving economics, politics, and perceptions – efforts to shape how people perceive different technologies, and how they perceive both the illness and the treatment.

Our case studies show that one of the most challenging obstacles is to design political strategies that produce consensus for a technology at the national or global level; these are time-consuming and difficult, and they are often underestimated by product champions. Rarely can access problems be solved simply by providing more money.

But access to health technologies in poor countries can be achieved. Creating access requires that individuals and organisations devote time, passion, and resources to a new technology and carefully craft strategies for addressing the multiple barriers along the pathways to access. The seven lessons presented above can help advance the complex process of creating access and help assure that new, safe, and effective health technologies reach the hands of people in poor countries who need them most.

Note

1 The authors thank the Bill & Melinda Gates Foundation for providing support for this work. They also appreciate the assistance of experts who were interviewed for the studies of the individual technologies and reviewed the full case studies, and the helpful comments of Philip Musgrove and two reviewers on the initial draft. Figure 36.1 was designed by Carol Maglitta. A previous version of this chapter was published in *Health Affairs* July/August 2009, 28(4): 962–73; it is adapted here with permission.

References

AIDSCAP Women's Initiative (1997) *The Female Condom: From Research to the Marketplace*, Arlington, VA: Family Health International/AIDSCAP.

Andersen, L.A. and Andersen, R. (1974) 'A Framework for the Study of Access to Medical Care', *Health Services Research*, 9: 208–20.

The Female Health Company (2005) *No More Excuses: The Female Health Company 2005 Annual Report*, Chicago: The Female Health Company.

Frost, L.J. and Reich, M.R. (2008) *Access: How Do Good Health Technologies Get to Poor People in Poor Countries?* Cambridge, MA: Harvard Center for Population and Development Studies, distributed by Harvard University Press.

Global Alliance for TB Drug Development (2009) *Our AAA Strategy*, available at http://www.tballiance.org/aaa/mandate.php (accessed 19 September 2009).

Hanson, K., Ranson, M.K., Oliveira-Cruz, V., and Mills, A. (2003) 'Expanding Access to Priority Health Interventions: A Framework for Understanding the Constraints to Scaling-up', *Journal of International Development*, 15: 1–14.

Harrison, P.E. and Rosenfield, A. (eds) (1998) *Contraceptive Research, Introduction, and Use: Lessons from Norplant*, New York: National Academy Press.

IBM Institute for Business Value (2004) *Pharma 2010: Silicon Reality*, Somers, NY: IBM Global services, available at http://www-935.ibm.com/services/us/index.wss/ibvstudy/imc/a1002316?cntxtId=a1000060 (accessed 28 April 2009).

Juma, C., Fang, K., Horca, D., Huete-Perez, J., Konde, V., Lee, S.H., Arenas, J., Ivinson, A., Robinson. H., and Singh, S. (2001) 'Global Governance of Technology: Meeting the Needs of Developing Countries', *International Journal of Technology Management*, 22: 629–55.

Levine, R. (2004) *Millions Saved: Proven Successes in Global Health*, Washington, DC: Center for Global Development.

Moran, M. (2005) 'A Breakthrough in R&D for Neglected Diseases: New Ways to Get the Drugs we Need', *PLoS Medicine*, 2: e302.

PATH (Program for Appropriate Technology in Health) (2005) *HealthTech Historical Profile: Vaccine Vial Monitors*, Seattle: PATH.

Reich, M.R. (2002) 'The Politics of Reforming Health Policies', *Promotion & Education*, 9: 138–42.

Reich, M.R. and Bery, P. (2005) 'Expanding Global Access to ARVs: The Challenges of Prices and Patents', in K.H. Mayer and H.F. Pizer (eds) *The AIDS Pandemic: Impact on Science and Society*, San Diego, CA: Elsevier Academic Press.

Reynolds Whyte, S., Van der Geest, S., and Hardon, A. (2002) *Social Lives of Medicines*, Cambridge: Cambridge University Press.

Roberts, M.J., Hsiao, W.C., Berman, P., and Reich, M.R. (2004) *Getting Health Reform Right: A Guide to Improving Performance and Equity*, New York: Oxford University Press.

Sevene, E., Lewin, S., Mariano, A., Woelk, G., Oxman, A.D., Matinhure, S., Cliff, J., Fernandes, B., and Daniels, K. (2005) 'System and Market Failures: The Unavailability of Magnesium Sulphate for the Treatment of Eclampsia and Pre-eclampsia in Mozambique and Zimbabwe', *British Medical Journal*, 331: 765–9.

Telles Dias, P.R., Souto, K. and Page-Shafer, K. (2006) 'Long-term Female Condom Use among Vulnerable Populations in Brazil', *AIDS Behavior*, 10: S67–75.

Van der Geest, S., Reynolds Whyte, S., and Hardon, A. (1996) 'The Anthropology of Pharmaceuticals: A Biographical Approach', *Annual Review of Anthropology*, 25: 153–79.

WHO (World Health Organization), Special Programme of Research, Development and Research Training in Human Reproduction (1985) 'Facts about an implantable contraceptive', memorandum from a WHO meeting, *Bulletin of the World Health Organization*, 63: 485–94.

Yardley, J. and Barboza, D. (2008) 'Despite Warnings, China's Regulators Failed to Stop Tainted Milk', *The New York Times*, 27 September, A1.

Part VIII
Global Mental Health

37

Closing the Treatment Gap for Mental Disorders[1]

Vikram Patel, Mirja Koschorke, and Martin Prince

Introduction

An analysis of the treatment gaps for mental disorders must begin with an acknowledgement that mental disorders cover a wide range of conditions affecting people across the life course and that the distinctions between psychiatric and neurological disorders, widely ingrained in specialist medical contexts, have little relevance in the global health context (Table 37.1).

A core concern of global mental health is the care and treatment of people with mental disorders. While most people with mental disorders live in low- and middle-income countries (LMIC), these countries enjoy only a tiny fraction of the available global resources for mental health. Global mental health is a relatively young discipline. Its growth has been fuelled by a series of influential publications from the past two decades. The *World Mental Health* report (1995) emphasised the robust relationship between mental health and social factors such as violence and poverty, contextual realities which have a higher prevalence in LMIC (Desjarlais *et al.* 1995). The 2001 *World Health Report* was devoted to mental health, indicating the priority given to this important issue (WHO 2001). The World Health Organization's Commission on Social Determinants of Health reported robust evidence demonstrating the strong bi-directional relationship between social disadvantage and the two mental disorders reviewed: depression in adults and ADHD in children, yet another indication of the social contexts of mental disorders in LMIC (Patel *et al.* 2009b). In spite of these initiatives and the substantial evidence of the large global burden of mental disorders, recent estimates suggest that between 50 to 90 per cent of people with severe mental disorders fail to receive even basic treatment, with treatment gaps evident in all countries, particularly in LMIC (Wang *et al.* 2007). Even the few who do access treatment do not receive appropriate care; appalling neglect of human rights, often under the guise of hospital care, continue to blot the mental health care landscape in many countries. This astonishing 'treatment gap', in spite of the growing evidence of cost-effective interventions for many mental disorders (Patel *et al.* 2007), is one of the greatest public health scandals of our times.

This chapter presents a review of the evidence on the global burden of mental disorders, and the interaction between mental health and other health conditions, in order to make the case that 'there is no health without mental health' (Prince *et al.* 2007). We describe the impact of

Table 37.1 Major mental disorders across the life course

Childhood	Mental retardation
	Conduct and behaviour disorders (e.g. ADHD)
	Other neurodevelopmental disabilities (e.g. autism)
Adolescence	Mood disorders (e.g. depression)
	Substance use disorders (e.g. alcohol abuse)
Adult	Mood disorders
	Psychotic disorders (e.g. schizophrenia)
	Substance use disorders
Older people	Dementia
	Mood disorders

mental disorders on the lived experiences of those affected and their families, demonstrating the enormous burden of stigma and discrimination that exists across all countries. We report on the barriers to scaling up services for people with mental disorders, challenges that remain despite the substantial evidence on the cost-effectiveness of treatments, and new evidence on the feasibility and effectiveness of task-shifting in mental health care (Patel *et al.* 2007). Finally, we describe new global initiatives which seek to use this evidence to scale up services and close the treatment gap for mental disorders.

Burden and impact of mental disorders

Globally, the absolute health burden of mental disorders does not vary much between world regions. However, proportionately, mental disorders account for 9 per cent of the burden in low-income countries (LIC), 18 per cent in middle-income (MIC), and 27 per cent in high-income countries (HIC) (Murray and Lopez 1996). The proportional differences are due to the burden of other health conditions being much greater in LICs, thus swelling the denominator. It has been suggested that the burden of mental disorders is in fact underestimated in reports of the global burden of disease (GBD) (Prince *et al.* 2007). First, according to the GBD, mental disorders account for 31.7 per cent of all years lived with disability, but only 1.4 per cent of years of life lost through premature mortality (WHO 2008a). However, each year, at least 800,000 people commit suicide, 86 per cent in LMIC, and over half involving young people. Mental disorder is overwhelmingly the most important preventable factor of this cause of premature mortality. Non-suicide mortality is also elevated in psychosis, depression, and dementia. Thus, the poor quality of general health care received by those in LMIC with mental disorders may explain some of the excess mortality. Second, much of the burden of mental ill health may be mediated through complex interactions with other health conditions, including infectious disease, reproductive, and maternal and child health, thus hiding the true burden of mental disorders.

The relationships between physical and mental disorder are complex. First, primary care personnel in LMIC commonly encounter symptoms that are medically unexplained. Such somatic symptoms, coupled with psychological distress and help-seeking, is present in around 15 per cent of patients seen in primary care (Gureje *et al.* 1997). Those affected are chronically disabled, consult frequently, and account for a high proportion of healthcare costs (Escobar *et al.* 1998).

Second, mental disorders are risk factors for the development of communicable and non-communicable diseases, and many physical health conditions increase the risk for mental disorder. For example, in population-based studies, depression is a prospective risk factor for cardiovascular diseases (CVD) including angina, myocardial infarction (Hemingway and Marmot 1999), and stroke (Larson *et al.* 2001). These associations are largely independent of CVD risk factors, despite the high incidence of hypertension (Jonas *et al.* 1997), obesity (Simon *et al.* 2006), and smoking (Patel *et al.* 2006) among those with mood disorders. Around 15 per cent of people with schizophrenia have type 2 diabetes, as a consequence of lifestyle factors, the metabolic effects of antipsychotic medication, and possible underlying disease-specific mechanisms (Holt *et al.* 2005). Tuberculosis (TB) is also more common among people with serious mental illness (McQuistion *et al.* 1997). Up to 10 per cent of HIV cases worldwide are attributable to injection-drug use (Chander *et al.* 2006). In the US, those with chronic severe mental illness have a high seroprevalence of HIV (5–7 per cent) (Cournos *et al.* 2005). Living with a communicable disease increases the risk for mental disorder, through a variety of mechanisms. Infection with HIV is consistently associated with a high prevalence of affective disorder (Maj *et al.* 1994). Apart from the psychological trauma of the diagnosis, HIV infection (Dube *et al.* 2005) and HAART treatment (Cournos *et al.* 2005) have direct central nervous system (CNS) effects. MDR-TB is associated with particularly poor mental health attributed to loss of work and social roles, feelings of hopelessness, and stigma (Sweetland *et al.* 2002). In Peru, the prevalence of mood disorders at diagnosis was 52 per cent with a further substantial incidence of mood disorders and psychosis during MDR-TB treatment (Vega *et al.* 2004). In an in-patient study in Turkey, the prevalence of mood disorder was 19 per cent for recently diagnosed TB, 22 per cent for defaulted TB, and 26 per cent for MDR-TB (Aydin and Ulusahin 2001).

Third, co-morbidity complicates help-seeking, diagnosis, and treatment, and affects outcomes of treatment for physical conditions, including disease-related mortality. Co-morbid depression predicts re-infarction and death after myocardial infarction (Hemingway and Marmot 1999). Post-stroke depression is associated with a 3.4 times higher mortality over ten years (Morris *et al.* 1993). In diabetes, depression is associated with poor glycaemic control (Lustman *et al.* 2000), complications (de Groot *et al.* 2001), and death (Katon *et al.* 2005). In the US, chronic depressive symptoms were associated with increased AIDS-related mortality (Cook *et al.* 2004; Ickovics *et al.* 2001) and more rapid disease progression (Ickovics *et al.* 2001) independent of receipt of treatment. There is consistent evidence from developed countries that adherence to HAART is adversely affected by depression (Ammassari *et al.* 2004), cognitive impairment (Hinkin *et al.* 2004), and alcohol and substance use (Chander *et al.* 2006). There are fewer studies from LMIC (Collins *et al.* 2006), but depression was associated with impaired adherence in Ethiopia (Tadios and Davey 2006).

Fourth, there may be a particular salience of mental disorders for women, given important associations between mental disorders and reproductive, maternal, and child health. Women are at heightened risk for mood disorders, with a typical female to male gender ratio of 1.5 to 2.0 (Patel *et al.* 2009b). Mood and substance use disorders are all robustly associated with dys menorrhoea, dyspareunia, and pelvic pain. Maternal mental health may also have important implications for infant growth and survival, with maternal schizophrenia consistently associated with pre-term delivery, low birth-weight, still birth, and infant mortality (Patel *et al.* 2004). Post-partum depression affects 10 to 15 per cent of women, and in developed countries there are adverse consequences for the early mother–infant relationship and for the child's psychological development (Patel *et al.* 2004). In Asia, where physical development of infants is a particular problem, studies suggest an independent association between antenatal mood disorder and low birth weight, and associations between perinatal mood disorder and infant undernutrition at six months (Rahman *et al.* 2004).

Stigma and discrimination

The stigma associated with mental illness contributes significantly to the burden of mental illness; in fact, subjective accounts of persons affected by mental illness testify that the effects of stigma and discrimination are often perceived as more burdensome and distressing than the primary condition itself (Thornicroft 2006). Stigma can be conceptualised as consisting of problems of ignorance, prejudice, and discrimination (Thornicroft 2006). Discrimination, the behavioural consequence of stigma, contributes to the disability of persons with mental illness and leads to disadvantages in many aspects of life including personal relationships, education, work, housing, parenting, childcare, and access to physical healthcare.

Paradoxically, mental health institutions and staff themselves often act as a source of discrimination. People with mental illness frequently report feeling patronised or humiliated by contact with mental health services, with stigmatising views often held by mental health staff themselves. Human rights violations are also often pervasive within mental health services. Some people with mental illness accept the negative beliefs and prejudices and lose self-esteem, resulting in self-stigmatisation, and in turn, feelings of shame, hopelessness, a sense of being separate from society, and social withdrawal (Thornicroft 2006). People with mental illness frequently expect to be treated in a discriminatory way and may therefore try to hide their illness, be reluctant to seek help, or stop themselves from applying for a job, thereby reinforcing the cycle of dependency and disability.

Research on stigma has been carried out in many parts of the world (Thornicroft 2006), with the evidence suggesting that 'there is no known country, society or culture where people with mental illness are considered to have the same value or be as acceptable as people who do not have mental illness' (180). Stigma and discrimination associated with mental illness are important both as a cause and as a consequence of the treatment gap for mental disorders. Stigma triggers a vicious cycle that leads to disadvantages in many aspects of life, and increased levels of disability. Stigma may lead health decision-makers to allocate a lower priority to the needs of people with mental illness, and may influence the efforts and resources spent for the treatment of mental disorders. For a stigmatised individual, feelings of shame and low self-esteem may reduce self-efficacy and act as a barrier to recovery. Stigma may influence access to and utilisation of health care as people may fear being identified and labelled, therefore delaying or avoiding seeking help for their condition. Undesirable and often dehumanising conditions in many mental health institutions may contribute further to decisions by persons with mental disorders not to take up available treatments. All these factors, both within the individual and the programme and policymakers, adversely influence adherence to and the effectiveness of existing treatments for mental disorders, leading to poor recovery rates, continued disability, and further reinforcing negative attitudes and discrimination about mental disorders.

The stigma attached to mental illness has been identified as 'the main obstacle to the provision of care for people with mental disorders' (Sartorius 2007: 810), and the need to tackle this important issue has been emphasised as a key intervention to closing the treatment gap. While there are promising initiatives to combat stigma both at the local and international level, much remains to be done to better understand and effectively address this complex phenomenon.

Treatments of mental disorders

A substantial evidence base testifies to the efficacy and cost-effectiveness of treatments for mental disorders, though much of this evidence is derived from HIC. Fortunately, there is a growing evidence base from LMIC (Patel *et al.* 2007) which shows that for most mental disorders, a combination of pharmacological and psychological treatments is the most appropriate and cost-effective package of care. Among the existing pharmacological treatments, older, generic medications are often as effective as newer drugs, and are more cost-effective. In addition, for many disorders, pharmacological treatments are indicated only for the most serious cases (for example, mood disorders). Among the available and recommended approaches, brief structured treatments such as cognitive-behavioural or interpersonal therapies are the most effective. There is ample evidence that treatment of co-morbid mental disorder (with a physical disorder) is highly effective in improving mental health and quality of life across a range of disorders, including cancer, diabetes, heart disease, and HIV/AIDS. Structured treatment recommendations, antidepressants, and cognitive behavioural therapy (CBT) can reduce 'medically unexplained' somatic complaints, and costs.

The evidence base on whether mental health interventions can improve physical disease outcomes is more mixed. Psychological interventions have been shown to improve diabetic control in Type 1 and Type 2 diabetes (Ismail *et al.* 2004; Winkley *et al.* 2006), while antidepressants and CBT are safe and moderately effective treatments for depression post-myocardial infarction, but do not reduce re-infarction rates or overall mortality (Berkman *et al.* 2003). The evidence base for the effectiveness of antidepressants post-stroke is weak, both for prevention and treatment. In terms of maternal and child health, a randomised clinical trial of a CBT-based intervention for depressed mothers integrated into the routine work of community-based primary health workers in rural Pakistan was effective in increasing immunisation rates, reducing diarrhoeal episodes in their infants, and improving the mental health outcome of mothers (Rahman *et al.* 2008).

Barriers to scaling up evidence-based services

In spite of the evidence and many previous initiatives to highlight the crisis in global mental health care, the unmet need for care for people with mental disorders remains astonishingly large. Even where treatments are available, these tend to focus on pharmacological interventions and on care within mental hospitals (rather than primary and community care models). There are several barriers to scaling up evidence-based services (Saraceno *et al.* 2007), which operate in varying degrees in all countries of the world. First, lack of resources is a major barrier; in Africa, for example, 80 per cent of countries spend less than 1 per cent of their national health budget on mental health. The small overall size of health budgets makes the absolute figures even less adequate in the poorest countries. Although tax and insurance-based systems are all more appropriate than out-of-pocket payment, the latter are most commonly used in LMIC. A relatively modest investment of US $2–3 per capita is all that is needed to provide a basic package of mental health services (focusing on schizophrenia, bipolar disorder, and depression) in many of the poorest LMIC (Lancet Global Mental Health Group 2007).

Second, a great scarcity of psychiatrists and other mental health specialists exists in most countries. Mental health specialists are also very inequitably distributed between and within countries (Saxena *et al.* 2007). This scarcity and inequity is further exacerbated by the migration of specialists, both internationally from poorer to richer countries, and within nations, from poorer to richer regions, and from public to private services. Third, there are issues of inefficiency: most mental health specialists work in similar ways, regardless of the resource contexts in which they work. Thus, face-to-face clinical work remains their predominant approach, one which is incompatible with scaling up services to increase the pitiful coverage rates for basic mental health care across countries. Furthermore, the concentration of scarce resources in many countries in large mental hospitals, with little or no investment in community or primary mental health care services, is another example of inefficient use of scarce resources. Finally, additional barriers include the prevailing public health priority agenda and its impact on funding, the complexity of and resistance to decentralising mental health services, challenges in implementing mental health care in primary care settings, and the lack of public health perspectives in mental health leadership (Saraceno *et al.* 2007).

Closing the treatment gap

One of the most important advances in mental health care in recent years has been the demonstration of the safety and effectiveness of task shifting in the delivery of efficacious treatments. This evidence provides the key to overcoming the huge barrier posed by the scarcity of specialist mental health human resources. *Task shifting* refers to the strategy of rational redistribution of tasks among the health workforce team: specific tasks are moved, where appropriate, from highly qualified health workers to health workers with shorter training and fewer qualifications in order to make more efficient use of the available human resources for health. In recent years, a series of controlled evaluations have shown that psychological treatments, or complex packages of care, can be delivered by low-cost health professionals (lay people or community health workers), who are appropriately trained and supervised for treating depression, schizophrenia, and dementia (Patel *et al.* 2007).

Mental health remains a low priority in most LMIC. When mental disorders are seen as a distinct health domain, with separate services and budgets, then investing in mental health is perceived as having an unaffordable opportunity cost. The ideal setting of care should be within the primary health care model using strategies which are common to all chronic diseases: (1) opportunistic case finding for early detection; (2) a combination of pharmacological and psychosocial interventions, often in a stepped care fashion; and (3) long-term follow-up with regular monitoring and promotion of adherence to treatment. A recent WHO-WONCA (World Association of Family Doctors) report reviewed the key strategies and successful models for integration in primary care (WHO 2008b), and supports this approach.

Modern classifications of mental and neurological disorders (MND), such as the International Classification of Diseases (ICD), have more than a hundred diagnostic categories. However, there also exist shorter, pragmatic classifications, many of which can be merged for the delivery of effective health service interventions (Patel *et al.* 2009a). One such model categorises MND into two broad groups: the common MNDs comprising mood and substance use disorders; and severe MNDs comprising the psychoses, epilepsy, strokes, and dementia. This classification is the basis for designing the intervention framework of the District Mental Health Programme (DMHP) in India (Patel *et al.* 2009a), with services delivered at the primary health care level. Thus, the management of common MND relies principally on early detection through routine or high-risk group screening of general or primary health care attendees. The management of severe MND relies principally on active case-finding and follow-up in the community, and adequate provision for inpatient care for severe presentations.

Scaling up services: a call to action for global health

The sheer scale of unmet need for care was the key motivation for the publication, in 2007, of the landmark *Lancet* series on global mental health, a six-article series produced independently by a group of global mental health leaders. The articles argued for scientific evidence to be used as the basis for global advocacy (Lancet Global Mental Health Group 2007), and ended with a call to action for the scaling up of evidence-based mental health services throughout the world, and the implementation of policies protecting the rights of mentally ill people. These messages are relevant in all countries, not just in LMIC. The principles set out in the *Lancet* series do not necessarily find expression in the developed world, for example, in the non-parity in mental health care compared to general medical care in most developed countries. Fortunately, local, regional, and international initiatives have begun to materialise in response to this call to action. A prominent example is the WHO's Mental Health Gap Action Programme (mhGAP) (http://www.who.int/mental_health/mhGAP/en/index.html) (WHO 2008c), which aims to identify and scale up cost-effective packages of care for eight priority mental health conditions.

The *Movement for Global Mental Health*, launched on 10 October 2008, aims to build a coalition of individuals and institutions committed to improving the health care of people with mental disorders anywhere in the world. The ultimate aim is straightforward: *the provision of basic, affordable, care comprising generic medications, brief psychological treatments and attention to the social needs and human rights of people with mental disorders and their families.* The Movement embodies the hope that 'the substantial progress in scaling up of services for people with mental disorders will take its place alongside progress in HIV/AIDS treatment and maternal and child survival as one of the great public health successes of our times' (www.globalmentalhealth.org). It is only when the treatment gaps for people with mental disorders are systematically addressed on the basis of evidence derived both from bio-medical disciplines, and the lived experiences of people with mental disorders, that the rights and entitlements of the mentally ill will be realised at the standards which we should expect and demand.

Note

1 A longer version of this chapter with a full list of references is in press in a forthcoming textbook *Mental Health in Public Health*, Oxford University Press (2011).

References

Ammassari, A., Antinori, A., Aloisi, M.S., Trotta, M.P., Murri, R., Bartoli, L., Monforte, A.D., Wu, A.W., and Starace, F. (2004) 'Depressive Symptoms, Neurocognitive Impairment, and Adherence to Highly Active Antiretroviral Therapy among HIV-infected Persons', *Psychosomatics*, 45: 394–402.

Aydin, I.O. and Ulusahin, A. (2001) 'Depression, Anxiety, Comorbidity, and Disability in Tuberculosis and Chronic Obstructive Pulmonary Disease Patients: Applicability of GHQ-12', *General Hospital Psychiatry*, 23: 77–83.

Berkman, L.F., Blumenthal, J., Burg, M., Carney, R.M., Catellier, D., Cowan, M.J., Czajkowski, S.M., Debusk, R., Hosking, J., Jaffe, A., Kaufmann, P.G., Mitchell, P., Norman, J., Powell, L.H., Raczynski, J.M., and Schneiderman, N. (2003) 'Effects of Treating Depression and Low Perceived Social Support on Clinical Events after Myocardial Infarction: The Enhancing Recovery in Coronary Heart Disease Patients (ENRICHD) Randomized Trial', *JAMA*, 289: 3: 106–16.

Chander, G., Himelhoch, S., and Moore, R.D. (2006) 'Substance Abuse and Psychiatric Disorders in HIV-positive Patients: Epidemiology and Impact on Antiretroviral Therapy', *Drugs*, 66: 769–89.

Collins, P.Y., Holman, A.R., Freeman, M., and Patel, V. (2006) 'What is the Relevance of Mental Health to HIV/AIDS Care and Treatment Programs in Developing Countries? A Systematic Review', *AIDS*, 20: 1,571–82.

Cook, J.A., Grey, D., Burke, J., Cohen, M.H., Gurtman, A.C., Richardson, J.L., Wilson, T.E., Young, M.A., and Hessol, N.A. (2004) 'Depressive Symptoms and AIDS-related Mortality among a Multisite Cohort of HIV-positive Women', *American Journal of Public Health*, 94: 1,133–40.

Cournos, F., McKinnon, K., and Sullivan, G. (2005) 'Schizophrenia and Comorbid Human Immunodeficiency Virus or Hepatitis C Virus', *Journal of Clinical Psychiatry*, 66(Supplement 6): 27–33.

De Groot, M., Anderson, R., Freedland, K.E., Clouse, R.E., and Lustman, P.J. (2001) 'Association of Depression and Diabetes Complications: A Meta-analysis', *Psychosomatic Medicine*, 63: 619–30.

Desjarlais, R., Eisenberg, L., Good, B., and Kleinman, A. (1995) *World Mental Health: Problems and Priorities in Low-Income Countries*, Oxford: Oxford University Press.

Dube, B., Benton, T., Cruess, D.G., and Evans, D.L. (2005) 'Neuropsychiatric Manifestations of HIV Infection and AIDS', *Journal of Psychiatry and Neuroscience*, 30: 237–46.

Escobar, J.I., Waitzkin, H., Silver, R.C., Gara, M., and Holman, A. (1998) 'Abridged Somatization: A Study in Primary Care', *Psychosomatic Medicine*, 60: 466–72.

Gureje, O., Simon, G.E., Ustun, T.B., and Goldberg, D.P. (1997) 'Somatization in Cross-cultural Perspective: A World Health Organization Study in Primary Care', *American Journal of Psychiatry*, 154: 989–95.

Hemingway, H. and Marmot, M. (1999) 'Evidence Based Cardiology: Psychosocial Factors in the Aetiology and Prognosis of Coronary Heart Disease. Systematic Review of Prospective Cohort Studies', *British Medical Journal*, 318: 1,460–67.

Hinkin, C.H., Hardy, D.J., Mason, K.I., Castellon, S.A., Durvasula, R.S., Lam, M.N., and Stefanik, M. (2004) 'Medication Adherence in HIV-infected Adults: Effect of Patient Age, Cognitive Status, and Substance Abuse', *AIDS*, 18(Supplement 1): S19–S25.

Holt, R.I., Bushe, C., and Citrome, L. (2005) 'Diabetes and Schizophrenia 2005: Are We Any Closer to Understanding the Link?', *Journal of Psychopharmacology*, 19: 56–65.

Ickovics, J.R., Hamburger, M.E., Vlahov, D., Schoenbaum, E.E., Schuman, P., Boland, R.J., and Moore, J. (2001) 'Mortality, CD4 Cell Count Decline, and Depressive Symptoms among HIV-seropositive Women: Longitudinal Analysis from the HIV Epidemiology Research Study', *JAMA*, 285: 1,466–74.

Ismail, K., Winkley, K., and Rabe-Hesketh, S. (2004) 'Systematic Review and Meta-analysis of Randomised Controlled Trials of Psychological Interventions to Improve Glycaemic Control in Patients with Type 2 Diabetes', *The Lancet*, 363: 1,589–97.

Jonas, B.S., Franks, P., and Ingram, D.D. (1997) 'Are Symptoms of Anxiety and Depression Risk Factors for Hypertension? Longitudinal Evidence from the National Health and Nutrition Examination Survey I Epidemiologic Follow-up Study', *Archives of Family Medicine*, 6: 43–9.

Katon, W.J., Rutter, C., Simon, G., Lin, E.H., Ludman, E., Ciechanowski, P., Kinder, L., Young, B., and Von, K.M. (2005) 'The Association of Comorbid Depression with Mortality in Patients with Type 2 Diabetes', *Diabetes Care*, 28: 2,668–72.

Lancet Global Mental Health Group (2007) 'Scaling Up Services for Mental Disorders – a Call for Action', *The Lancet*, 370: 1,241–52.

Larson, S.L., Owens, P.L., Ford, D., and Eaton, W. (2001) 'Depressive Disorder, Dysthymia, and Risk of Stroke: Thirteen-year Follow-up from the Baltimore Epidemiologic Catchment Area Study', *Stroke*, 32: 1,979–83.

Lustman, P.J., Anderson, R.J., Freedland, K.E., De, G.M., Carney, R.M., and Clouse, R.E. (2000) 'Depression and Poor Glycemic Control: A Meta-analytic Review of the Literature', *Diabetes Care*, 23: 934–42.

McQuistion, H.L., Colson, P., Yankowitz, R., and Susser, E. (1997) 'Tuberculosis Infection among People with Severe Mental Illness', *Psychiatric Services*, 48: 833–5.

Maj, M., Satz, P., Janssen, R., Zaudig, M., Starace, F., D'Elia, L., Sughondhabirom, B., Mussa, M., Naber, D., and Ndetei, D. (1994) 'WHO Neuropsychiatric AIDS Study, Cross-sectional Phase II. Neuropsychological and Neurological Findings', *Archives of General Psychiatry*, 51: 51–61.

Morris, P.L., Robinson, R.G., Andrzejewski, P., Samuels, J., and Price, T.R. (1993) 'Association of Depression with 10-year Poststroke Mortality', *American Journal of Psychiatry*, 150: 124–9.

Murray, C. and Lopez, A. (1996) *The Global Burden of Disease*, Boston, MA: Harvard School of Public Health, WHO, and World Bank.

Patel, V., Rahman, A., Jacob, K.S., and Hughes, M. (2004) 'Effect of Maternal Mental Health on Infant Growth in Low Income Countries: New Evidence from South Asia', *British Medical Journal*, 328: 820–23.

Patel, V., Kirkwood, B.R., Pednekar, S., Weiss, H., and Mabey, D. (2006) 'Risk Factors for Common Mental Disorders in Women: Population-based Longitudinal Study', *British Journal of Psychiatry*, 189: 547–55.

Patel, V., Araya, R., Chatterjee, S., Chisholm, D., Cohen, A., De Silva, M., Hosman, C., McGuire, H., Rojas, G., and Van Ommeren, M. (2007) 'Treatment and Prevention of Mental Disorders in Low-income and Middle-income Countries', *The Lancet*, 370: 991–1,005.

Patel, V., Goel, D., and Desai, R. (2009a) 'Scaling Up Services for Mental and Neurological Disorders', *International Health*, 1: 37–44.

Patel, V., Lund, C., Heathrill, S., Plagerson, S., Corrigal, J., Funk, M., and Flisher, A. (2009b) 'Social Determinants of Mental Disorders', in E. Blas and A. Sivasankara Kurup, (eds) *Priority Public Health Conditions: From Learning to Action on Social Determinants of Health*, Geneva: World Health Organization: 115–34.

Patel, V., Koschorke, M., Prince, M., and Cottler, L. (2011) 'Closing the Treatment Gap for Mental Disorders', in L.B. Cottler (ed.) *Mental Health and Public Health – The Next 100 Years*, Oxford: Oxford University Press.

Prince, M., Patel, V., Saxena, S., Maj, M., Maselko, J., Phillips, M.R., and Rahman, A. (2007) 'No Health without Mental Health', *The Lancet*, 370: 859–77.

Rahman, A., Iqbal, Z., Bunn, J., Lovel, H., and Harringon, R. (2004) 'Impact of Maternal Depression on Infant Nutritional Status and Illness: A Cohort Study', *Archives of General Psychiatry*, 61: 946–52.

Rahman, A., Malik, A., Sikander, S., Roberts, C., and Creed, F. (2008) 'Cognitive Behaviour Therapy-based Intervention by Community Health Workers for Mothers with Depression and their Infants in Rural Pakistan: A Cluster-randomised Controlled Trial', *The Lancet*, 372: 902–909.

Saraceno, B., Van Ommeren, M., Batniji, R., Cohen, A., Gureje, O., Mahoney, J., Sridhar, D., and Underhill, C. (2007) 'Barriers to Improvement of Mental Health Services in Low-income and Middle-income Countries', *The Lancet*, 370: 1,164–74.

Sartorius, N. (2007) 'Stigma and Mental Health', *The Lancet*, 370: 810–11.

Saxena, S., Thornicroft, G., Knapp, M., and Whiteford, H. (2007) 'Resources for Mental Health: Scarcity, Inequity, and Inefficiency', *The Lancet*, 370: 878–89.

Simon, G.E., Von, K.M., Saunders, K., Miglioretti, D.L., Crane, P.K., Van, B.G., and Kessler, R.C. (2006) 'Association between Obesity and Psychiatric Disorders in the US Adult Population', *Archives of General Psychiatry*, 63: 824–30.

Sweetland, J., Guerra, D., Kleiman, A., and Saraceno B. (2002) 'Enhancing Adherence: The Role of Group Psychotherapy in the Treatment of MDR-TB in Urban Peru', in A. Cohen, A. Kleinman, and B. Saraceno (eds) *World Mental Health Casebook: Social and Mental Health Programmes in Low-Income Countries*, Kluwer: Academic/Plenum Press: 51–80.

Tadios, Y. and Davey, G. (2006) 'Antiretroviral Treatment Adherence and its Correlates in Addis Ababa, Ethiopia', *Ethiopian Medical Journal*, 44: 237–44.

Thornicroft, G. (2006) *Shunned: Discrimination against People with Mental Illness*, Oxford: Oxford University Press.

Vega, P., Sweetland, A., Acha, J., Castillo, H., Guerra, D., Smith Fawzi, M.C., and Shin, S. (2004) 'Psychiatric Issues in the Management of Patients with Multidrug-resistant Tuberculosis', *International Journal of Tuberculosis and Lung Disease*, 8: 749–59.

Wang, P.S., Aguilar-Gaxiola, S., Alonso, J., Angermeyer, M.C., Borges, G., Bromet, E.J., Bruffaerts, R., de Girolamo, G., de Graaf, R., Gureje, O., Haro, J.M., Karam, E.G., Kessler, R.C., Kovess, V., Lane, M.C., Lee, S., Levinson, D., Ono, Y., Petukhova, M., Posada-Villa, J., Seedat, S., and Wells, J.E. (2007) 'Use of Mental Health Services for Anxiety, Mood, and Substance Disorders in 17 Countries in the WHO World Mental Health Surveys', *The Lancet*, 370: 841–50.

Winkley, K., Ismail, K., Landau, S., and Eisler, I. (2006) 'Psychological Interventions to Improve Glycaemic Control in Patients with Type 1 Diabetes: Systematic Review and Meta-analysis of Randomised Controlled Trials', *British Medical Journal*, 333: 65.

WHO (World Health Organization) (2001) *The World Health Report 2001: Mental Health: New Understanding, New Hope*, Geneva: WHO.

WHO (World Health Organization) (2008a) *The Global Burden of Disease: 2004 Update*, Geneva: WHO.

WHO (World Health Organization) (2008b) *Integrating Mental Health into Primary Care: A Global Perspective*, Geneva: WHO and World Organization of Family Doctors (WONCA).

WHO (World Health Organization) (2008c) *Mental Health Gap Action Programme (mhGAP): Scaling Up Care for Mental, Neurological and Substance Abuse Disorders*, Geneva: WHO.

38

Stigma, Discrimination, Social Exclusion, and Mental Health

A Public Health Perspective

Nicolas Rüsch, Sara Evans-Lacko, Sarah Clement, and
Graham Thornicroft

Introduction

People with mental illness face a twofold problem. In addition to experiencing symptoms such as mood swings, hallucinations, or anxiety, they often encounter stigma and discrimination, which can present a greater burden than the illness itself. Mental illness stigma is pervasive in developing and developed countries alike (Thornicroft *et al.* 2009), and typically leads to social exclusion in various life domains such as personal relationships, work, housing, or access to care. Given that stigma affects all areas of life, it is a major public health concern. There is a rich and growing literature on mental illness stigma in particular (Corrigan 2005; Hinshaw 2007; Thornicroft 2006), and on the concepts of stigma and discrimination in general (Link and Phelan 2001; Major and O'Brien 2005; Nelson 2009). In this chapter, we will first briefly define three domains in which stigma and discrimination can operate: public stigma, self-stigma, and structural discrimination. We will then discuss the daily life consequences of these three types of stigma for people with mental illness. Finally, we will outline some ongoing initiatives, for example from Scotland and New Zealand, meant to reduce stigma and discrimination.

Types of stigma and terminology

Public stigma and discrimination

Public stigma comprises reactions of the general public towards a group based on preconceptions about that group. For example, if members of the public consider people with mental illness dangerous, they will be more likely to avoid individuals with mental illness. Stigma is a broad term that is linked to the seminal work of Erving Goffman, who defined it as a discrediting attribute that reduces the stigmatised person 'from a whole and usual person to a tainted, discounted one' (Goffman 1963: 3). Modern social-psychological and sociological conceptualisations of stigma distinguish several interrelated components of stigma (Corrigan 2005; Link and Phelan 2001). First, in order to become the source of stigma, a characteristic, such as skin colour or mental illness, must be used to label individuals. There is no clear boundary between mental illness and mental health, and across cultures perceptions of mental illness and health vary. Therefore, the label of 'mental illness' is a social construct that changes over time. For example, dissociative states or hallucinations are mostly considered pathological in Western societies, but may be considered normal, for example as part of religious practices, in other societies. Second, stereotypes are associated with the labelled characteristic. Stereotypes are knowledge structures known to most members of a social group. They are often based, however, on ignorance or misinformation, and therefore ignorance is another way of thinking about stereotypes (Thornicroft 2006). Typical stereotypes about people with mental illness are that they are violent and dangerous, are to blame for their condition, cannot live independently, are rebellious free spirits, or have childlike perceptions of the world (Wahl 1995). Third, prejudice occurs if members of the public are both familiar with negative stereotypes, and also agree with them, and have negative emotional reactions as a consequence ('That's right! All people with mental illness are violent and they all scare me'). Fourth, prejudice leads to discrimination as a behavioural reaction. Anger-related prejudice may lead to withholding help or replacing health care with the criminal justice system. As mentioned above, fear leads to avoidant behaviour. For example, employers often do not want persons with mental illness around them for reasons based on fear, so they do not hire them. As a final component of stigma and discrimination, social, economic, and political power is necessary to effectively discriminate against a stigmatised group.

Self-stigma

Self-stigma or internalised stigma refers to the reactions of individuals who belong to a stigmatised group and turn the stigmatising attitudes against themselves (Corrigan 2005). It is a process parallel to public stigma, starting with (negative) self-labelling and stereotypes, and finally affects the behaviour of the stigmatised individuals. Persons with mental illness are usually well aware of negative stereotypes against their group. If they agree with the stereotypes, and apply them to themselves, this results in decreased self-esteem and self-efficacy ('I have a mental illness and therefore I do not deserve good treatment and am not capable to work'). Self-stigma is associated with shame as an emotional correlate (Rüsch *et al.* 2006), and with reduced empowerment, seriously undermining the quality of life of people with mental illness, and their subsequent motivation to pursue life goals such as work or independent living.

Structural discrimination

Discrimination does not only result from individual attitudes or intentions. Societal rules and regulations may systematically disadvantage people with mental illness, something which is referred to as *structural discrimination*. Examples include legislation, funding decisions about research and mental health services, or health insurance policies that exclude people with mental illness from insurance coverage. For example, when making decisions about health insurance coverage, an insurance employee may discriminate against applicants with schizophrenia unintentionally, just by following the insurance company's rules of handling applications.

Consequences of stigma

Public stigma, discrimination, and social exclusion

Stigma and *discrimination* can lead to social exclusion of people with mental illness. People with mental illness indicate that discrimination most typically occurs in relationships with friends and families, in intimate relationships, and at work or school (Thornicroft *et al.* 2009). Unfortunately, recent evidence suggests that the stigma of mental illness may have increased rather than decreased over the last decades in Western countries (Angermeyer and Matschinger 2005; Phelan *et al.* 2000).

In terms of global patterns, we know very little about levels of public stigma across different countries. In a recent survey of over 700 people with schizophrenia in 27 countries (Thornicroft *et al.* 2009), nearly half of the participants reported being discriminated against in making or keeping friends, and in contact with family members. Over a quarter experienced discrimination finding or keeping a job, as well as in intimate relationships or contact with their neighbours. Rates of anticipated discrimination were even higher. These data underline the pervasiveness of mental illness stigma and the potential for experiencing multiple threats in different areas of life. Rates of experienced and anticipated discrimination were similar across countries, suggesting that stigma and discrimination are a global phenomenon.

The results of assessing stigma in Africa, Asia, the Americas, in Islamic countries of North Africa and the Near East, and in Europe have produced generally consistent findings (Sartorius and Schulze 2005). First, there are few countries, societies, or cultures in which people with mental illness are considered to have the same value as people who do not have mental illness, as shown, for example, in lower rates of financial investment in mental health services. Second, the quality of information that we have is relatively poor, with few comparative studies having been conducted between countries or over time. Third, there are clear links between popular understandings of mental illness, and whether or not people in mental distress seek help or feel able to disclose their problems. The core experiences of shame (to oneself or to one's family) and blame (from others) are common, although they vary to some extent between cultures. Where comparisons with other conditions, such as physical illnesses, have been made, mental illnesses are usually more stigmatised. Finally, the behavioural consequences of stigma (rejection and avoidance) by others to the stigmatised individual appear to be universal phenomena (Sartorius and Schulze 2005).

Self-stigma: secrecy, withdrawal, avoidance of treatment

Many people with mental illness try to avoid the negative consequences of labelling, stigma, and discrimination by keeping their mental illness a secret. Unlike many other stigmatised characteristics such as ethnicity, mental illness is usually not visible. Depending on the severity and course of their disorder, people with mental illness can therefore often decide whether or not to disclose, and secrecy is a common reaction to the threat of stigma. As noted above, discrimination is anticipated so widely that it may lead to social withdrawal when persons with mental illness avoid other people who are perceived to be potentially stigmatising. While these coping reactions may help to avoid some experiences of discrimination, unfortunately they are also associated with negative outcomes, such as demoralisation and unemployment (Link *et al.* 1991; Rüsch *et al.* 2009b).

A second common consequence of secrecy and label avoidance is that individuals with mental illness may opt not to seek care because they fear being labelled as a consequence of entering treatment. There is mounting evidence that high levels of perceived stigma and low resilience to stigma (Rüsch *et al.* 2009a) are associated with low levels of care-seeking. Stigma, therefore, contributes to poor treatment participation worldwide (Schomerus and Angermeyer 2008; Thornicroft 2008), which is a major public health concern (Wang *et al.* 2007). Stigma-related barriers to treatment-seeking are a burden that compounds the effects of mental health services that are often of poor quality or even entirely absent.

Structural discrimination: consequences for funding and other policies

Discrimination is not necessarily deliberate (Corrigan *et al.* 2004). Legal or cultural rules and regulations can profoundly disadvantage minorities, intentionally or unintentionally. One example of structural discrimination is legislation that restricts the rights of people with mental illness in areas such as voting or parenting (Corrigan *et al.* 2005). It is important to note here that some restrictions may be justified because of an individual's current psychiatric symptoms or disabilities, and therefore do not necessarily constitute discrimination. For example, it can be appropriate and necessary to preclude a person with a current and serious thought disorder from driving buses. However, a mental illness per se does not justify the restriction of rights if no current disability is present that specifically impairs performance of the activity in question. Mental health funding is another example of structural discrimination. A German study found that the public had a strong preference to cut funding for mental rather than physical illnesses, thus facilitating structural discrimination (Schomerus *et al.* 2007). Underfunding of mental health services is a global problem. According to the World Health Organization (WHO), mental illnesses cause about 12 per cent of all illness-related disability (Disability Adjusted Life Years); however only about 2 per cent of overall health care budgets are allocated for mental health services, indicating a dramatic lack of resources (Saxena *et al.* 2007). This is reflected in the view of service users in Hong Kong, who saw poor quality and accessibility of mental health services as a major source of structural discrimination (Lee *et al.* 2006). However, there is a scarcity of research on international aspects of structural discrimination, especially for developing countries.

Interventions to reduce stigma and discrimination

We now discuss strategies and some ongoing initiatives to fight the three main types of stigma and discrimination: public, self-stigma, and structural discrimination.

Public stigma

Three main strategies have been used to reduce public stigma: protest, education, and contact (Corrigan and Penn 1999). Protest, by stigmatised individuals or members of the public who support them, is often applied against stigmatising public statements, such as media reports and advertisements. Many protest interventions, for example against stigmatising advertisements or soap operas, have successfully suppressed negative public statements, and for this purpose they are clearly very useful (Wahl 1995). However, it has been argued (Corrigan and Penn 1999) that protest is not effective for improving attitudes towards people with mental illness. Education interventions aim to diminish stigma by replacing myths and negative stereotypes with facts, and have reduced stigmatising attitudes among members of the public. However, research on educational campaigns suggests that behaviour changes are often not evaluated, and the degree of change achieved is both limited and may fade quickly. The third strategy is personal contact with persons with mental illness. In a number of interventions in secondary schools, education and personal contact have been combined (Pinfold *et al.* 2003). Contact appears to be the more efficacious part of the intervention. Factors that create an advantageous environment for interpersonal contact and stigma reduction include equal status among participants, a cooperative interaction, and institutional support for the contact initiative.

For both education and contact, the content of anti-stigma programmes matters. Biogenetic models of mental illness are often highlighted because viewing mental illness as a biological, mainly inherited problem, may reduce shame and blame associated with it. Evidence supports this optimistic expectation (i.e. that a biogenetic causal model of mental illness will reduce stigma) in terms of reduced blame. However, focusing on biogenetic factors may increase the perception that people with mental illness are fundamentally different, and thus biogenetic interpretations have been associated with increased social distance, perceptions of mental illness as more persistent, serious, and dangerous, and with more pessimistic views about treatment outcomes (Phelan *et al.* 2006). Therefore, a message of mental illness as being 'genetic' or 'neurological' may be overly simplistic and unhelpful for reducing stigma.

Anti-stigma initiatives can take place nationally, as well as locally. National campaigns often adopt a social marketing approach, whereas local initiatives usually focus on target groups. An example of a large multifaceted national campaign is 'Time To Change' in England (Henderson and Thornicroft 2009). It combines mass-media advertising and local initiatives. The latter try to facilitate social contact between members of the general public and mental health service users, as well as target specific groups such as medical students and teachers. The programme is evaluated by public surveys assessing knowledge, attitudes, and behaviour, and by measuring the amount of experienced discrimination reported by people with mental illness. Similar initiatives in other countries, for example 'See Me' in Scotland (Dunion and Gordon 2005), 'Like Minds, Like Mine' in New Zealand (Vaughan and Hansen 2004), or the World Psychiatric Association anti-stigma initiative (Sartorius and Schulze 2005) in, among many other countries, Japan, Brazil, Egypt, have reported positive outcomes.

In summary, there is evidence for the effectiveness of anti-stigma initiatives. On a more cautious note, individual discrimination, structural discrimination, and self-stigma lead to innumerable mechanisms of stigmatisation. If one mechanism of discrimination is blocked or diminished through successful initiatives, other ways to discriminate may emerge (Link and Phelan 2001). Therefore, to substantially reduce discrimination, stigmatising attitudes and behaviours of influential stakeholders need to change fundamentally.

Efforts to reduce self-stigma and to increase empowerment

Before discussing more specific interventions to tackle self-stigma and to increase empowerment, we need to make it clear that we do not see self-stigma as a clinical problem or somehow the fault of the person with mental illness. On the contrary, it is a consequence of unfair public discrimination. However, as long as public stigma continues, many people with mental illness will internalise stigma, and therefore, strategies to reduce self-stigma matter. One way to reduce self-stigma is to discuss and refute negative stereotypes in groups of people with mental illness that are run by professionals or peers, using paradigms of cognitive therapy. Research suggests that to accept stigma as fair and to hold the group of people with mental illness in low regard is associated with more negative reactions to stigma (Rüsch *et al.* 2009c). Therefore, efforts to reduce self-stigma should enable people with mental illness to reject stigma as unfair and to think better of themselves and their group. Psycho-education and empowerment interventions can facilitate informed choices and shared decision-making. Further, mutual-help/peer-support groups can be a source of support and empowerment, thus decreasing self-stigma. Another approach is to promote active participation in mental illness service provision, either through consumer-operated services, or through using advance statements that give service users more control over their treatment.

Fighting structural discrimination

Improving public attitudes and behaviours is not sufficient to fight stigma, because discrimination can persist in long-lived social and cultural rules and regulations despite the best intentions of individuals. Comprehensive anti-stigma efforts can effect structural discrimination by specifically addressing legislation, mental health care funding, or health insurance policies which disadvantage people with mental illness. Differences between developing and developed countries should be taken into account (Rosen 2006) because structural discrimination, and initiatives to fight it, depend on legal and cultural local factors.

Conclusions

We outlined forms and consequences of mental illness stigma and discrimination and discussed anti-stigma initiatives. There is growing interest in stigma research among service users, clinicians, and researchers, and work from different disciplines such as psychology, sociology, and public health has increased our understanding over the last decades. Still, there is much to be done.

Research in this field would, in our view, benefit from addressing the following topics. First, while surveys of attitudes and intentions have been helpful, it is now time to focus on discriminatory behaviour. Behaviour of, for example, a stigmatising employer, is an outcome that seriously affects people with mental illness. Second, future studies should be more theory-driven instead of merely offering descriptive reports. For example, applying social-psychological models derived from other stigmatised groups to mental illness stigma may be promising (Rüsch *et al.* 2009b, 2009c). Third, emotional aspects of both stigmatisers (e.g. disgust) and their targets (e.g. shame) have been neglected in previous work (Link *et al.* 2004). Fourth, future studies should rigorously test the effectiveness of anti-stigma interventions, especially in terms of long-term behaviour change (Thornicroft *et al.* 2008). Fifth, the voice of service users has been under-represented, and more qualitative and quantitative work is needed to fill this gap (Rose 2001). Sixth, investigations of mental illness stigma have largely neglected the impact of structural discrimination on stigmatised individuals (Corrigan *et al.* 2004). Finally, to gain a global perspective, we need studies that assess cultural factors and international similarities and differences (Thornicroft *et al.* 2009).

Future anti-stigma initiatives should take comprehensive steps to address different aspects of stigma and discrimination simultaneously. In particular, they should measure success in terms of reduced discrimination as experienced by people with mental illness, which in our view is the most relevant outcome. This is not an easy task, but recent anti-stigma initiatives provide reason for cautious optimism. Success will depend on the continuing collaboration of many groups in society, involving people with mental illness as well as key stakeholders such as teachers, mental health professionals, faith leaders, employers, police officers, and legislators. Judging from the history of the civil rights movement, a long-term collaborative effort is needed to achieve profound social change and substantially reduce mental illness stigma.

References

Angermeyer, M.C. and Matschinger, H. (2005) Causal Beliefs and Attitudes to People with Schizophrenia: Trend Analysis Based on Data from Two Population Surveys in Germany', *British Journal of Psychiatry*, 186: 331–4.

Corrigan, P.W. (ed.) (2005) *On the Stigma of Mental Illness: Practical Strategies for Research and Social Change*, Washington, DC: American Psychological Association.

Corrigan, P.W. and Penn, D.L. (1999) 'Lessons from Social Psychology on Discrediting Psychiatric Stigma', *American Psychologist*, 54(9): 765–76.

Corrigan, P.W., Markowitz, F.E., and Watson, A.C. (2004) 'Structural Levels of Mental Illness Stigma and Discrimination', *Schizophrenia Bulletin*, 30(3): 481–91.

Corrigan, P.W., Watson, A.C., Heyrman, M.L., Warpinski, A., Gracia, G., Slopen, N., and Hall, L.L. (2005) 'Structural Stigma in State Legislation', *Psychiatric Services*, 56(5): 557–63.

Dunion, L. and Gordon, L. (2005) 'Tackling the Attitude Problem: The Achievements to Date of Scotland's See Me Anti-stigma Campaign', *Mental Health Today*, March: 22–5.

Goffman, E. (1963) *Stigma: Notes on the Management of Spoiled Identity*, Englewood Cliffs, NJ: Prentice Hall.

Henderson, C. and Thornicroft, G. (2009) 'Stigma and Discrimination in Mental Illness: Time to Change', *The Lancet*, 373(6): 1,930–32.

Hinshaw, S.P. (2007) *The Mark of Shame: Stigma of Mental Illness and an Agenda for Change*, Oxford: Oxford University Press.

Lee, S., Chiu, M.Y., Tsang, A., Chui, H., and Kleinman, A. (2006) 'Stigmatizing Experience and Structural Discrimination Associated with the Treatment of Schizophrenia in Hong Kong', *Social Science & Medicine*, 62(7): 1,685–96.

Link, B.G. and Phelan, J.C. (2001) 'Conceptualizing Stigma', *Annual Review of Sociology*, 27: 363–85.

Link, B.G., Mirotznik, J., and Cullen, F.T. (1991) 'The Effectiveness of Stigma Coping Orientations: Can Negative Consequences of Mental Illness Labeling be Avoided?', *Journal of Health & Social Behavior*, 32(3): 302–20.

Link, B.G., Yang, L.H., Phelan, J.C., and Collins, P.Y. (2004) 'Measuring Mental Illness Stigma', *Schizophrenia Bulletin*, 30(3): 511–41.

Major, B. and O'Brien, L.T. (2005) 'The Social Psychology of Stigma', *Annual Review of Psychology*, 56: 393–421.

Nelson, T.D. (ed.) (2009) *Handbook of Prejudice, Stereotyping, and Discrimination*, New York: Psychology Press.

Phelan, J.C., Link, B.G., Stueve, A., and Pescosolido, B.A. (2000) 'Public Conceptions of Mental Illness in 1950 and 1996: What is Mental Illness and is it to be Feared?', *Journal of Health & Social Behavior*, 41(2): 188–207.

Phelan, J.C., Yang, L.H., and Cruz-Rojas, R. (2006) 'Effects of Attributing Serious Mental Illnesses to Genetic Causes on Orientations to Treatment', *Psychiatric Services*, 57(3): 382–7.

Pinfold, V., Toulmin, H., Thornicroft, G., Huxley, P., Farmer, P., and Graham, T. (2003) 'Reducing Psychiatric Stigma and Discrimination: Evaluation of Educational Interventions in UK Secondary Schools', *British Journal of Psychiatry*, 182(4): 342–6.

Rose, D. (2001) *Users' Voices: The Perspectives of Mental Health Service Users on Community and Hospital Care*, London: The Sainsbury Centre.

Rosen, A. (2006) 'Destigmatizing Day-to-Day Practices: What Developed Countries can Learn from Developing Countries', *World Psychiatry*, 5(1): 21–4.

Rüsch, N., Hölzer, A., Hermann, C., Schramm, E., Jacob, G.A., Bohus, M., Lieb, K., and Corrigan, P.W. (2006) 'Self-stigma in Women with Borderline Personality Disorder and Women with Social Phobia', *Journal of Nervous and Mental Disease*, 194(10): 766–73.

Rüsch, N., Corrigan, P.W., Wassel, A., Michaels, P., Larson, J.E., Olschewski, M., Wilkniss, S., and Batia, K. (2009a) 'Self-stigma, Group Identification, Perceived Legitimacy of Discrimination and Mental Health Service Use', *British Journal of Psychiatry*, 195: 551–2.

Rüsch, N., Corrigan, P.W., Powell, K., Rajah, A., Olschewski, M., Wilkniss, S., and Batia, K. (2009b) 'A Stress-coping Model of Mental Illness Stigma: II. Emotional Stress Responses, Coping Behavior and Outcome', *Schizophrenia Research*, 110: 65–71.

Rüsch, N., Corrigan, P.W., Wassel, A., Michaels, P., Olschewski, M., Wilkniss, S., and Batia, K. (2009c) 'Ingroup Perception and Responses to Stigma among Persons with Mental Illness', *Acta Psychiatrica Scandinavica*, 120: 320–28.

Sartorius, N. and Schulze, H. (2005) *Reducing the Stigma of Mental Illness: A Report from a Global Association*, Cambridge: Cambridge University Press.

Saxena, S., Thornicroft, G., Knapp, M., and Whiteford, H. (2007) 'Resources for Mental Health: Scarcity, Inequity, and Inefficiency', *The Lancet*, 370(9,590): 878–89.

Schomerus, G. and Angermeyer, M.C. (2008) 'Stigma and its Impact on Help-seeking for Mental Disorders: What do We Know?', *Epidemiologia e Psichiatria Sociale*, 17(1): 31–7.

Schomerus, G., Matschinger, H., and Angermeyer, M.C. (2007) 'Familiarity with Mental Illness and Approval of Structural Discrimination against Psychiatric Patients in Germany', *Journal of Nervous and Mental Disease*, 195(1): 89–92.

Thornicroft, G. (2006) *Shunned: Discrimination against People with Mental Illness*, Oxford: Oxford University Press.

Thornicroft, G. (2008) 'Stigma and Discrimination Limit Access to Mental Health Care', *Epidemiologia e Psichiatria Sociale*, 17(1): 14–19.

Thornicroft, G., Brohan, E., Kassam, A., and Lewis-Holmes, E. (2008) 'Reducing Stigma and Discrimination: Candidate Interventions', *International Journal of Mental Health Systems*, 2: 3.

Thornicroft, G., Brohan, E., Rose, D., Sartorius, N., and Leese, M. (2009) 'Global Pattern of Experienced and Anticipated Discrimination against People with Schizophrenia: A Cross-sectional Survey', *The Lancet*, 373(9,661): 408–15.

Vaughan, G. and Hansen, C. (2004) 'Like Minds, Like Mine: A New Zealand Project to Counter the Stigma and Discrimination Associated with Mental Illness', *Australasian Psychiatry*, 12(2): 113–17.

Wahl, O.F. (1995) *Media Madness: Public Images of Mental Illness*, New Brunswick, NY: Rutgers University Press.

Wang, P.S., Aguilar-Gaxiola, S., Alonso, J., Angermeyer, M.C., Borges, G., Bromet, E.J., Bruffaerts, R., de Girolamo, G., de Graaf, R., Gureje, O., Haro, J.M, Karam, E.G., Kessler, R.C., Kovess, V., Lane, M.C., Lee, S., Levinson, D., Ono, Y., Petukhova, M., Posada-Villa, J., Seedat, S., and Wells, J.E. (2007) 'Use of Mental Health Services for Anxiety, Mood, and Substance Disorders in 17 Countries in the WHO World Mental Health Surveys', *The Lancet*, 370(9,590): 841–50.

39

Developing Mental Health Programmes in Low- and Middle-Income Countries

Florence Baingana

Introduction

This chapter begins with a discussion of the context of low- and middle-income countries (LMIC), including health systems and their relevance to mental health programming. The chapter then outlines key steps to take in developing a mental health programme and concludes with a discussion of gender, HIV and AIDS, children's mental health, and conflicts. Uganda is used as a case study quite frequently throughout the chapter, simply because that is where the author has most experience.

The context of low- and middle-income countries

In order to understand the current status of mental health programmes in LMIC, it is essential to first explain the present social, economic, and political context of these country groupings. LMIC are not just characterised by poverty as measured by income or consumption, but also include 'social exclusion, social vulnerability and denial of opportunities and choice' for their populations (Saxena *et al.* 2007: 883). In addition, many LMIC have a high incidence and prevalence of HIV and AIDS. According to the 2008 Report of the Global AIDS Epidemic, 67 per cent of all people living with HIV, and 72 per cent of AIDS deaths in 2007, were in sub-Saharan Africa (SSA). An estimated 90 per cent of the 2 million children below 15 years living with HIV are in SSA (UNAIDS 2008). Lastly, LMIC are disproportionately affected by violence as compared to high-income countries (HIC); whereas conflict-related deaths per 100,000 are 0 in HIC, the rate of conflict-related deaths in low income countries (LIC) are 6.2 per 100,000. This overall figure is misleading, however, as in the World Health Organization (WHO) Africa Region, there were 32 per 100,000 conflict-related deaths; 8.1 per 100,000 in the WHO Eastern Mediterranean Region; and 4.2 per 100,000 for the WHO European Region (the latter has mainly HIC but also middle-income countries (MIC)) (WHO 2002a).

Currently, LMIC are going through a demographic transition, with a simultaneously increasing ageing population, and the biggest cohort of children and adolescents below 18 years of age thus far in existence. Globally, there are 1.2 billion youth aged 15 to 24 years, 90 per cent of whom are in developing countries (or LMIC), and 80 per cent living in SSA and Asia. Due to HIV and AIDS, and conflicts and complex emergencies, the population of children and youth growing up today has the lowest human capital levels in the history of the world (World Bank 2006). In many countries, young people have not gone to school or have had a very poor education, the existence of poor health services implies poor health status and premature mortality for many of them, and the continued presence of early marriage implies high rates of teenage pregnancies. All of these factors add up to a poorly educated, low-skilled potential workforce, unlikely to contribute substantially to the development efforts of these countries (Desjarlais *et al.* 1995; World Bank 2006).

Health systems and mental disorders in LMIC

Of particular importance to the delivery of mental health care in these contexts is the current status of overall health care systems, and in particular, the *human resources for health crisis* that is global in nature. In LMIC this crisis is characterised by shortages of all cadres of health care-related personnel, both specialised and non-specialised; a mal-distribution of the few existing health care professionals, both within and between countries; and poor working conditions for those health workers who do exist (Pick 2008; Pillay and Mahlati 2008).

Set against this health system background is the growing burden of mental and neurological disorders. Such disorders have an increasing prevalence not only in HIC, but also across LMIC. According to the 2005 Burden of Disease data, neuropsychiatric disorders contribute 14 per cent to the global burden of disease (Prince *et al.* 2007). Important to note is the likelihood that the existing data on mental disorders captured within LMIC is in fact greatly underestimated, due to the limited research conducted on mental disorders in these countries. A survey carried out in general outpatient clinics in 15 districts of Uganda found rates of depression ranging from 8 to 50 per cent (Kinyanda 2004). Other studies have reported consistently higher rates of anxiety, depression, and post-traumatic stress disorder (PTSD) in the Africa Region (Baingana *et al.* 2006; Kinyanda 2004).

Along with increasing the burden of mental health morbidity in LMIC, mental disorders also make a significant contribution to mortality, accounting for 1.2 million deaths every year in the region. Annually, an estimated 800,000 people commit suicide in LMIC. This figure, though significant, is likely to be an underestimate given the continued stigma that exists around suicide, the likelihood that suicide is frequently not reported, and the poor status of birth and death records in this part of world. Suicide deaths are generally categorised by the WHO as injuries, yet it is estimated that up to 91 per cent of people who commit suicide have an underlying mental disorder. An estimated 86 per cent of all global suicides occur in LMIC (Prince *et al.* 2007).

The huge morbidity and mortality burden of mental disorders is important, but is insufficient in itself to make a case for investment in mental health. Mental disorders within a population are also costly; they impact productivity at the individual, household, and institution levels. There is therefore a significant cost to be borne by countries not adequately investing in mental health care (World Bank 2003; Hyman *et al.* 2006; Saxena *et al.* 2007).

It is in this context that the challenges of developing a mental health programme in LMIC are going to be discussed.

How best can quality mental health services be provided in LMIC, taking into account the limited existing human and financial resources?

Since the Alma-Ata Declaration of Health for All of 1978, WHO has recommended the integration of mental health into primary health care. This was reiterated in the 1990s with the Nations for Mental Health programme (WHO 2002b). In 1995, the seminal work by Desjarlais and others made three far-reaching recommendations on addressing the challenges facing mental programmes. The recommendations are: (1) investing in strengthening of mental health integrated into a strengthened health care system; (2) a new approach to public health that takes into account mental health; and (3) integration of mental health into relevant national and international development policies (Desjarlais *et al.* 1995). In 2001, almost identical recommendations were made in the World Health Report with the theme 'Mental Health: New Understanding New Hope' (WHO 2001), which suggested integration of mental health into primary health and provided three scenarios for doing this, for low-, middle-, and high-income countries. Finally, in 2007, *The Lancet* ran a series of articles on mental health that culminated with a Call for Action, which reinforced the recommendation of integrating mental health into primary health care (Chisholm *et al.* 2007).

What is meant by integration of mental health into primary health care, and how does this differ from community-based mental health care, which is also recommended? WHO defines *primary health care* as:

> ... providing 'essential health care' which is universally accessible ... and provided as close as possible to where people live and work. It refers to care which is based on the needs of the population. It is decentralized and requires the active participation of the community and family.
>
> (WHO, 1978: Declaration of Alma-Ata)

> Providing mental health services in primary health care involves diagnosing and treating people with mental disorders; putting in place strategies to prevent mental disorders and ensuring that primary heath care workers are able to apply key psychosocial and behavioral science skills, for example, interviewing, counselling and interpersonal skills, in their day to day work in order to improve overall health outcomes in primary health care.
>
> (WHO, 2003)

In responding to the numerous recommendations for the integration of mental health into primary health care, there are key areas that are important to consider, and a step-wise approach that is essential. The steps to be followed by individual LMIC countries include the following.

First, determine a set of mental disorders that can be managed by all health care workers, especially those at the lower levels of care. This is frequently determined based on the categorisation of the severity and disease burden of the disorder. Uganda represents a useful case study: schizophrenia and manic depressive illness were included in the set based on severity, and depression, anxiety disorders, alcohol, and drug abuse were included based on disease burden. Also included were disorders that pertain to children. Although minimal research has been carried out on child-specific mental disorders, the widespread existence of conflicts and HIV in Uganda, and the related high numbers of orphans and vulnerable children, would suggest that the need is likely to be large. Lastly, epilepsy, although a neurological disorder, was added to the priority set, as an estimated 60 to 70 per cent of patients who attend regularly at mental health outpatient clinics are people with epilepsy. In the lay thinking/understanding of the community, these are all 'disorders of the brain/head'.

Second, a country should develop standards and guidelines for the management of these common or essential mental health problems at the three levels of care (primary, secondary, and tertiary).

Third, required cadres of health care workers should be trained at all three levels. This includes training all primary-level health care workers to recognise and manage the identified priority mental health disorders. The types of primary health workers in the countries and regions of the world are different. For example, in SSA and some parts of South Asia, primary health care workers are likely to be low-level nurses or nursing assistants, while in MIC, like the former Soviet Union countries, they will be physicians. Prior training is important to consider when adding mental health training to workers' existing portfolios. The secondary level of the health care system will often have specialised mental health workers, such as psychiatric nurses or psychiatric clinical officers in LIC, and psychiatrists in MIC. Finally, the tertiary level will often have higher-level specialised mental health personnel, such as psychiatrists, psychologists, and psychiatric social workers, working together as a team in the management of patients, and in the training of health workers in mental health.

Fourth, a list should be compiled of essential mental health drugs that are required to manage the priority mental disorders, and integrate them into the national essential drugs list (EDL). An EDL includes all those drugs that are purchased by the Ministry of Health, and that can be ordered by districts through a credit line system, or through the PHC (Primary Health Care) Fund for the HIPC (Highly Indebted Poor Countries). Fifth, a linkage should be established between the health care system and any existing psycho-social care systems within a country, especially in those countries affected by conflicts and/or by HIV and AIDS. This step is especially important, since the psycho-social sector within many LMIC is provided by non-governmental organisations (NGOs), with government-level responsibility lying within the Ministry of Social Affairs (Gender and Social Affairs, Family and Social Affairs, etc.), as opposed to governmental responsibility for mental health, which lies with the Ministry of Health. Unfortunately in many countries there exist two parallel systems, mental health and psycho-social, providing services to the same populations without ever meeting. This can result in wastage of scarce resources, replication of services, and confusion for the clients (Baingana et al. 2004).

Sixth, mental disorders should be integrated into a country's Health Management Information System (HMIS). Each country must determine which disorders will be specifically counted and which will be lumped under 'other'. The disorders to be included in the HMIS also depend on the ability of lower-level cadres to make correct diagnoses.

Management and infrastructure for mental health

Critical to the successful integration of mental health into primary health care is ensuring that support supervision (higher-level workers travelling regularly to lower levels of care to provide support) exists, and that functioning referral systems (in both directions, higher to lower and lower to higher levels of care) are in place (WHO 2001). Five key areas that determine a fully integrated mental health care system include: (1) outpatient clinics, whether mobile or static; (2) community mental health teams that carry out regular outreach; (3) availability of beds for acute in-patient care; (4) long-term rehabilitation based in the community, including drop-in centres; and (5) home visiting or residential care and rehabilitation, occupation, and work. To have an effective mental health system integrated into primary health care requires collaboration with the social welfare sector, housing, and employment/labour; not an easy feat in many LMIC. For further information, read WHO's *Integrating Mental Health into Primary Health Care* (WHO and Wonca 2008).

The issue of mental health facilities, and specifically beds, is an important one for implementing a successful national mental health system. Countries must determine the optimum number of beds per population, and optimum distribution of beds across the country. Many countries have too few beds, with these beds located in one large central institution. Overall, Africa has a median of 0.34 beds per 10,000 population, with 73 per cent in hospitals; and Southeastern Asia has 0.33 beds per 10,000 population, with 83 per cent located in hospitals (Saxena *et al.* 2007). The challenge is to increase available beds for mental health, based on need, at the primary level, with a few designated beds in general medical wards at district hospitals, and a stand-alone mental health unit with separate male and female wards at the regional referral level. In comparison, in LMIC within Eastern Europe, there are an estimated eight beds per 10,000 population, but 80 per cent are located in large institutions (Saxena *et al.* 2007). The challenge in Eastern European LMIC is to decrease the overall bed numbers, along with moving the existing beds from large institutions into lower levels of care and the community. It is essential that there also be beds in the community-based health care system.

In recommending examples of countries who have undertaken such efforts, Byaruhanga *et al.* (2008) describe in further detail the mental health system of Uganda. In addition, the 'Mental Health at a Glance Factsheet' contains a short synopsis of where to start, objectives, key activities, and beneficiaries/target groups, as well as indicators and some important do's and don'ts for implementing or improving mental health services (World Bank 2003). Lastly, Jenkins *et al.* (2002) provide a comprehensive text on developing a national mental health policy; and a recent WHO publication brings the state of the knowledge together as well as providing ten case studies (WHO and Wonca 2008).

What is the difference between community-based mental health care and integration of mental health into primary care?

The previous section elaborated on the elements for integrating mental health into primary health care. At the same time, it is important to develop and/or strengthen community-based mental health programmes. Community-based mental health is defined as 'any type of care, supervision and rehabilitation of patients with mental illness outside the hospital by health and social workers based in the community' (Saxena *et al.* 2007: 879). Only half the countries in Africa, the eastern Mediterranean, and southeastern Asia provide such care. And in many countries, community-based mental health care may be available in some areas of the country but not in others, such as in China, India, Paraguay, and Zambia (Saxena *et al.* 2007).

What are the different dimensions that must be considered in developing a national mental health programme?

There are additional critical dimensions to be considered during a country's planning phase for developing a mental health programme. Although these will not be discussed in depth, these dimensions include the following:

- *Planning mental health services across the lifespan.* Very often, mental health services are planned for the adult population; however, there remains a dire shortage of services for children. In most countries even information on what is available for children is lacking, due to there being no focal person for child and adolescent mental health, no system for gathering data on children's mental disorders, and the difficulty of making a diagnosis with a scarcity of specialists for child and adolescent psychiatry. Existing data suggest that whereas most LIC have non-existent child and adolescent mental health programmes, an estimated 78 per cent of HIC have programmes. The regions with the lowest numbers of child and adolescent mental health programmes are Africa, with 6.3 per cent, eastern Mediterranean with 33.3 per cent, and the Americas with 45 per cent.

- The other dimension is that of *prevention, promotion, treatment,* and *care,* as well as *rehabilitation.* Many mental disorders can be prevented, especially those related to lifestyle, such as alcohol and drug abuse. Mental health promotion involves integrating mental health into public health action (Desjarlais *et al.* 1995; Herrman and Swartz 2007), and can be promoted alongside population-based public health measures, such as universal immunisation, iodinisation of salt, de-worming of children, and encouraging pregnant women to attend antenatal clinics. Rehabilitation may involve reintegration of people with mental disorders back into their families and communities, re-socialising them, providing sheltered workshops, day drop-in centres, vocational skills training, and job placements.

What are the human resources of the country in general, and of mental health personnel in particular?

As mentioned, there is a *human resources for health crisis.* This is of particular importance to mental health since provision of services requires that personnel be available, and be trained in the right skills (Saxena *et al.* 2007). Human resources are in even shorter supply in conflict-affected countries (Doull and Campbell 2008). Proposed solutions to this problem include creating incentives to get health personnel to work in rural and hard-to-reach areas of the country; and specific to mental health, implementing task-shifting. The latter has been utilised since the 1970s, when paramedical personnel such as nurses, physician assistants, and clinical officers were trained to manage people with mental disorders (Ghebrehiwet and Barret 2008). In Uganda, all nurses now receive training in the recognition and management of common mental disorders during their basic training, as well as getting in-service refresher courses. One challenge is that the overall shortage of nurses and other paramedical health workers in the country means that those to be re-trained in mental health are in short supply. Studies also suggest that, as lower-level health workers are trained to take on more tasks, the quality of care deteriorates, mainly due to the huge patient loads they then must handle. These workers often do not receive increased remuneration for the added workload (Philips *et al.* 2008).

What are the present financing mechanisms for health care and which are best suited to mental health financing in LMIC?

It is futile to plan a state-of-the-art mental health programme without taking into account how it will be financed. Unfortunately, almost one-third of countries globally do not have a designated budget line for mental health, and of those that do – 21 out of 101 countries – most of them in Africa and southeastern Asia, spend less than 1 per cent of the health budget on mental health (Saxena *et al.* 2007).

The manner in which available financial resources are used is also important. Prepayment mechanisms, such as social insurance, voluntary health insurance, and tax-based schemes would be best suited to assisting poor individuals; however, these are not widely used in LMIC. Poorer countries, and the poor within countries, tend to pay out-of-pocket. More than one-third of LIC rely on out-of-pocket payments as the main mode of financing mental health care, compared to only 3 per cent of HIC (Saxena *et al.* 2007). It is important to consider equity (equal access for equal need); allocative efficiency (whether the distribution of resources best meets a society's needs); as well as technical efficiency; and whether health improvements and quality of life gains match the resources committed to treatment and support for people with mental illness (Saxena *et al.* 2007).

What related issues must be considered as relevant to mental health, such as gender, conflicts and complex emergencies, and HIV/AIDS?

Lastly, there are some critical cross-cutting issues that have particular relevance to mental disorders and mental health delivery services. These will not be explored in depth, but they include the following.

Gender and mental health

First, more women than men, especially women with little education and low social class, suffer from depression and anxiety, the most common mental disorders (Saxena *et al.* 2007). Second is the prevalence of violence against women and its consequences for women's mental and physical health (Garcia-Moreno 2002). Third, women's needs are often not addressed, possibly due to stigma, in relation to alcohol and drug abuse treatment. Women abuse alcohol and drugs; however, units that provide care for alcohol and drug abuse often do not have facilities for women, and shelters for abused or homeless women may not include alcohol and drug treatment as part of the care package (Baingana 2009). In planning mental health services, care must be taken to ensure that women have equal access to care as men. Fourth is the excess mortality of males in the former Soviet Union countries. In this region, men die at much higher rates than women, as well as men living in western Europe. It is postulated that the stress linked to the recent economic and political transition has led men to take on unhealthy lifestyles, like excessive consumption of alcohol and drugs, which has contributed to excess mortality. In the former Soviet Union countries, males are also more likely to die of injures and to commit suicide (Paci 2002). It is therefore important to look at mental health from a gendered view, taking into account differential expression in males and in females.

Interrelationship between conflicts and other complex emergencies and mental and neurological disorders

There is an interrelationship between conflicts and other complex emergencies and mental and neurological disorders, with NGOs and UN agencies having specific programmes to address mental health and psychosocial disorders in conflict and complex emergencies. These include the WHO, United Nations Development Programme (UNDP), United Nations Children's Fund (UNICEF), United Nations Population Fund (UNFPA), and the Inter-Agency Standing Committee (IASC) Guidelines Working Group. Critical areas in programming for mental health and psycho-social interventions in conflict and complex emergency situations include the integration of psycho-social and mental health activities, so there are not two parallel silos of work. It is also important to plan for the post-emergency phase, ensuring that there is an exit plan for NGOs whose mandate for the provision of mental health services may only pertain to emergency activities. Very often, an emergency mental health and psycho-social programme can be the beginning of mental health reforms in the post-conflict and the development period, as was the case in Rwanda, Sri Lanka, and Afghanistan.

Mental health and psycho-social issues are closely interrelated to HIV and AIDS

Both HIV and mental disorders are associated with high levels of stigma. The impending death associated with HIV and AIDS, as well as opportunistic infections, such as cryptococcal meningitis, TB meningitis, and AIDS Dementia Complex, may present as organic mental disorders (Baingana *et al.* 2005). There is also the challenge of orphans and vulnerable children, some of whom are born with HIV, and many of whom are now living up to young adulthood. These young people living with HIV have been counselled as if they will not live long, yet many now have to decide whether to have relationships, whether to have relationships with HIV-positive people or HIV-negative ones, whether to marry, or even to have a child. These are all critical issues for mental health (Baingana *et al.* 2008).

Finally, prevention of mother-to-child transmission of HIV programmes previously counselled pregnant women and encouraged them to test for HIV. Those who were found positive were provided with a single pill during delivery, with the baby put on an antiretroviral therapy (ART) regimen. The sole aim was to prevent transmission of HIV to the child, but often no further counselling or drug treatment was provided to the mother, not even support on how to disclose her status to her husband. It was only after HIV-negative children of HIV-positive mothers started to die at a rate much higher than anticipated was it realised that the mental health status of the mother, and the care and support provided to the mother, is probably as much, if not more important, to the health and well-being of the baby than just the ARTs alone. It is therefore essential for country health systems to collaborate with HIV programmes in order to ensure that the mental health issues are addressed in treatment and care programmes.

Conclusion

Mental health programming is a complex process that takes into account the context of the country, including the present status of mental health services, available resources, the burden of mental health disorders in that country, and available health personnel, both in general and specifically in mental health care. Programming is not done once. A strategic plan must be drawn up within each LIMC, with the involvement of all key stakeholders, including people with mental disorders. Once resources are mobilised, the plan should be implemented, monitored, and evaluated, and then reviewed, with a new strategy developed as population and resource changes occur. Even with limited resources, it is possible to develop and implement a quality mental health programme that is accessible to as much of the population as possible.

References

Baingana, F., Bannon, I., and Thomas, R. (2004) 'Mental Health and Conflicts: Conceptual Framework and Approaches', Health, Nutrition and Population (HNP) Discussion Paper, Washington, DC: World Bank.

Baingana, F., Thomas, R., and Comblain, C. (2005) *Mental Health and HIV/AIDS*, Washington, DC: World Bank.

Baingana F., Alem, A., and Jenkins, R. (2006) 'Mental Health and the Abuse of Alcohol and Controlled Substances', in D. T. Jamison, R. G. Feachem, M. W. Makgoba, E. R. Bos, F. K. Baingana, K. J. Hofman, and K. O. Rogo (eds) *Disease and Mortality in Sub-Saharan Africa*, 2nd edn, Washington, DC: World Bank.

Baingana, F., Fuller, F., Levy Guyer, A., Holman, S. R., Kim, J. Y., Li, M., McKeever, J., Mungherera, L., Psaki, S., Sematimba, B., Serukka, D., Smith Fawzi, M. C., and Zaeh, S. (2008) *The Implementation Gap in Services for Children Affected by HIV and AIDS*, Boston, MA: François Xavier Bagnoud Center for Health and Human Rights, Harvard School of Public Health.

Baingana, F. (2009) 'Alcohol and Substance Abuse', in P.S. Chandra, H. Herrman, J. Fisher, M. Kastrup, U. Niaz, M.B. Rondon, and A. Okasha (eds) *Contemporary Topics in Women's Mental Health: Global Perspectives in a Changing Society*, West Sussex: John Wiley & Sons, pp. 139–48.

Byaruhanga, E., Cantor-Graae, E., Maling, S., Kabakyenga, J. (2008) 'Pioneering Work in Mental Health Outreach in Rural South Western Uganda', *Interventions*, 6(2): 117–31.

Chisholm, D., Flisher, A.J., Lund, C., Patel, V., Saxena, S., Thornicroft, G., Tomlinson, M. (2007) 'Scale Up Services for Mental Disorders: A Call to Action', *The Lancet*, 370(9,594): 1,241–52.

Desjarlais, R., Eisenberg, L., Good, B., and Kleinman, A. (1995) *World Mental Health*, New York: Oxford University Press.

Doull, L. and Campbell, F. (2008) 'Human Resources for Health in Fragile States', *The Lancet*, 371(9,613): 626–7.

Garcia-Moreno, C. (2002) 'Violence against Women: Consolidating a Public Health Agenda', in G. Sen, A. George, P. Ostin (eds) *Engendering International Health: The Challenge of Equity*, Cambridge, MA: The MIT Press, pp. 111–141.

Ghebrehiwet, T. and Barret, T. (2008) 'Nurses and Mental Health Services in Developing Countries', *The Lancet*, 370(9,592): 1,016–17.

Herrman, H. and Swartz, L. (2007) 'Promotion of Mental Health in Poorly Resourced Countries', *The Lancet*, 370:(9,594): 1,195–7.

Hyman, S., Chisholm, D., Kessler, R., Patel, V., and Whiteford, H. (2006) 'Mental Disorders', in World Health Organization and Disease Control Priorities Project, *Disease Control Priorities Related to Mental, Neurological, Developmental and Substance Abuse Disorders*, Geneva: World Health Organization.

Jenkins, R., McCulloch, A., Friedli, L., and Parker, C. (2002) *Developing a National Mental Health Policy*, Maudsley Monograph No. 43, East Sussex: Psychology Press.

Kinyanda, E. (2004) 'Mental Health', in Information Discovery and Solutions Limited (eds), *The Support to the Health Sector Strategic Plan Project, Results of the Baseline Survey Report to Provide Basic Data for the Development of the National Communication Strategy, for the Promotion of the National Minimum Health Care Package (NMHCP)*, Kampala, Uganda: Ministry of Health.

Paci, P. (2002) *Gender in Transition*, Washington, DC: World Bank.

Philips, M., Zachariah, R., and Venis, S. (2008) 'Task-shifting for Antiretroviral Treatment Delivery in Sub-Saharan Africa: Not a Panacea', *The Lancet*, 371(9,613): 682–4.

Pick, W. (2008) 'Lack of Evidence Hampers Human-resources Policy Making', *The Lancet*, 371(9,613): 629–30.

Pillay, Y. and Mahlati, P. (2008) 'Health-worker Salaries and Incomes in Sub-Saharan Africa', *The Lancet*, 371(9,613): 632–4.

Prince, M., Patel, V., Saxena, S., Maj, M., Maselko, J., Phillips, M.R., and Tahman, A. (2007) 'No Health without Mental Health', *The Lancet*, 370(9,590): 859–77.

Saxena, S., Thornicroft, G., Knapp, M., and Whiteford, H. (2007) 'Resources for Mental Health: Scarcity, Inequity, and Inefficiency', *The Lancet*, 370 (9,590): 878–89.

UNAIDS (Joint United Nations Programme on HIV/AIDS) (2008) *2008 Report on the Global AIDS Epidemic*, Geneva: UNAIDS.

World Bank (2003) *Mental Health at a Glance*, Washington, DC: World Bank, available at http://siteresources.worldbank.org/INTPHAAG/Resources/AAGMentalHealth110703.pdf (accessed 15 September 2010).

World Bank (2006) *World Development Report 2007: Development and the Next Generation*, Washington, DC: World Bank.

WHO (World Health Organization) (2001) *The World Health Report 2001: Mental Health: NewUnderstanding, New Hope*, Geneva: WHO.

WHO (World Health Organization) (2002a) *World Report on Violence and Health*, Geneva: WHO.

WHO (World Health Organization) (2002b) *Nationals for Mental Health: Final Report*, Geneva: WHO.

WHO (World Health Organization) and Wonca (2008) *Integrating Mental Health into Primary Care: A Global Perspective*, Geneva: WHO.

40

Sexual Violence

A Priority Research Area for Women's Mental Health

Jill Astbury and Rachel Jewkes

Sexual violence is a violation of human rights and a serious global public health problem. To date, the challenge of sexual violence has been massively neglected by researchers, policy-makers, and programme designers. Yet the problem is widespread, occurs in all countries, and mars the lives of over one in three female children and at least one in four women globally (Jewkes *et al.* 2002). Rape is carried out, often with impunity, in peace as well as in conflict situations, and results in a wide range of mental and physical health problems. Significantly, the use of sexual violence against women as a military tactic during war has been described by the United Nations (UN) Security Council in resolution 1820 as a 'threat to global security'.

Sexual violence is a broad notion that was defined in the *World Report on Violence and Health* as:

> any sexual act, attempts to obtain a sexual act, or acts to traffic for sexual purposes, directed against a person using coercion, and unwanted sexual comments, harassment or advances made by any person regardless of their relationship to the victim, in any setting, including but not limited to home and work.

> (Jewkes *et al.* 2002: 149)

The most common severe forms of sexual violence perpetrated are rape and attempted rape, but the notion also includes acts of trafficking for sex, female genital mutilation, all forms of unwanted sexual touching, and sexual harassment. In this chapter, we chiefly focus on the severest forms of sexual violence as related to global health, those of rape and attempted rape. Sexual violence is a deeply gendered health and social issue that serves to perpetuate gender inequality, reinforce the social subordination of girls and women, and repudiate their human rights, including their right to dignity, security, and health. Mostly perpetrated by men, rape predominantly affects girls and women. This chapter examines how rape violates victims' fundamental right to health, especially mental health. The social power dynamics and psychological consequences of rape against boys and men need to be addressed as a topic in its own right.

Social dynamics

Globally, the prevalence of rape varies widely, reflecting the role of gendered cultural attitudes in facilitating or preventing sexual violence in particular settings. The most important social dynamic influencing risk of rape is the extent of the subordination of women within a society, which relates to dominant ideals of masculinity, including expectations of male control over women (Seedat *et al.* 2009). Other factors that are important in the perpetration of rape include poverty, unemployment, and limited educational opportunities, all of which influence the risk of rape due to the challenges they present to fulfilling local ideals of masculinity. In addition, the childhood contexts within various societies, including parental absence and exposure to bullying and violence, all influence boys' development and their socialisation in ways that impact on the risk of perpetrating rape. Finally, social attitudes and responses towards rape influence its prevalence through the rigour and efficiency of law enforcement in responding to claims of rape, and the treatment of victims of violence. In settings where both adequate law enforcement and sensitive treatment of victims are absent, a powerful message about the seriousness of rape is conveyed.

Risk of being a victim is obviously influenced by these broader dimensions of context. While rape occurs, and recurs, across the life course, female sex is the most obvious risk factor, with teenagers and young women most at risk. Children everywhere are disproportionately targeted by those they know, including the members of their own families (Astbury 1996).

The context of rape varies considerably between settings. While in many countries the highest rates of sexual violence have been reported for rape by intimate partners, in South Africa, men are more likely to report having raped a woman who is not an intimate partner (Jewkes *et al.* 2009). The World Health Organization's (WHO) *Multi-country Study on Women's Health and Domestic Violence* reported the prevalence of rape by an intimate partner varied from 6 per cent in Japan, Serbia, and Montenegro, to 59 per cent in rural Ethiopia. Rape by a man who was not a partner varied from less than 1 per cent in rural Ethiopia and Bangladesh, to over 10 per cent in Peru, Samoa, and urban Tanzania (Garcia-Moreno *et al.* 2005). While women report marital rape in surveys, social and legal recognition that rape can and does occur within marriage is far from universal. For women in 53 nations, rape in marriage remains a legal impossibility (BBC 2008). Social and gender mores continue, in many settings, to privilege the 'rights' of husbands and instruct women that their marital obligation is to have sex whenever their partners want it. One participant in a study in Zimbabwe observed, 'You as the woman will not have sex only if he does not feel like it' (Watts *et al.* 1998).

In South Africa, many young women feel unclear about the boundary between the uses versus abuses of their bodies by male partners, and make a distinction between 'unwanted sex' and 'rape' (Jewkes *et al.* 2001). 'Rape' is a concept often reserved for acts of sexual aggression by strangers, a term made familiar to girls and women in the abounding rape myths, and entails adoption of a devalued identity as a woman who has 'been raped' (discussed below). Yet epidemiological research, which measures experience of acts of unwanted sex, rather than using the more subjective notion of 'rape', suggests that the physical and psychological consequences of rape are not avoided by attempts by victims, or others, to minimise their experiences (and label them as other than rape). Research highlights the wide range of physical health consequences which stem from acts of rape, including injuries, unwanted pregnancy, unsafe abortion, and sexually transmitted infections, including HIV (Jewkes *et al.* 2002).

Serious as these physical consequences are, the psychological harms caused by rape are widespread, cause severe morbidity and mortality, and reverberate across the lives of the children and women affected. Harm is manifested in the unrealised human potential, multiple psychological disorders, impugnment of human dignity, and difficulties in interpersonal relationships, social, and occupational functioning. Sexual abuse in childhood significantly increases the risk of subsequent sexual victimisation (Dunkle *et al.* 2004) and intimate partner violence (Coid *et al.* 1998). Negative consequences are increased and compounded by re-victimisation, delay in disclosure, and the absence of appropriate psychosocial support (Ruggiero *et al.* 2004).

Sexual violence predicts precisely those psychological disorders in which women predominate, such as depression, anxiety, and post-traumatic stress disorder. These in turn make a large contribution to the global burden of disease (Vos *et al.* 2006). Consequently, improved understanding of the psychological impact of sexual violence may offer a unique insight into the characteristics of situations that underpin gender disparities in rates of psychological disorders. Psychological health and well-being are intensely important to victim/survivors of sexual violence, and play a critical role in their recovery. Health services need to be reoriented to better address the psychological concerns of victim/survivors both in the aftermath of rape, and as part of their health care in other contexts. Post-rape care rarely offers mental health services beyond the immediate containment of acute psychological distress, and psychological support for court preparation. This chapter thus focuses on the psychological impact of sexual violence.

Psychological responses to sexual violence

Immediate effects of sexual assault include shock, fear, and feelings of helplessness, with many survivors meeting the criteria for Acute Traumatic Stress Disorder. High levels of physical and psychological co-morbidity that frequently define the acute aftermath of rape, may continue over the medium and long term. Symptoms of depression, anxiety, and traumatic stress are the most common forms of psychological distress reported, all of which result in poor self-rated health (Cloutier *et al.* 2002). Physical manifestations of traumatic stress are also seen in reported gastrointestinal, sexual and reproductive health problems, pain syndromes including chronic pelvic pain, eating disorders, and chronic sleep problems (Jewkes *et al.* 2002; Krakow *et al.* 2002). Rates of deliberate self-harm and suicidality are significantly higher, and women raped before the age of 16 are three to four times more likely to attempt suicide than those assaulted at older ages (Davidson *et al.* 1996). Also important, high-risk behaviours such as alcohol, tobacco, and illicit and licit drug use, may add to the complex mix of adverse psychological and physical health problems experienced by victims, exacerbating the original risk, as well as frequently being employed as a means of coping with rape-related distress.

In general, sexually victimised women are more likely to use medical services than non-victimised women, but are less likely to utilise preventive health services (Springs and Friedrich 1992). They report finding Pap test screenings traumatic because it reminds them of sexual assault, which may contribute to their lower rates of participation (Farley *et al.* 2002). Survivors are also less likely to use mental health services despite having high rates of psychological disorder (Resnick *et al.* 1997).

Post-traumatic stress disorder (PTSD)

Three different sets of symptoms define PTSD. Briefly, these include recurrent and intrusive distressing recollections of the event, persistent avoidance of stimuli associated with the trauma, and numbing of general responsiveness not present before the trauma and persistent symptoms of increased arousal. All three sets of symptoms must persist for more than one month, and significantly affect functioning, before the diagnosis is made according to the DSM-IV criteria. Of all the traumatic stressors, rape most strongly predicts PTSD (Kessler *et al.* 1995). It also predicts depression. In the US Co-Morbidity Survey, 49 per cent of women with PTSD also had a lifetime history of depression (Kessler *et al.* 1995). Women who experience sexual violence are six times more likely to develop PTSD than non-abused women (Kilpatrick *et al.* 1992).

Psychological distress after rape is very acute in the first week, may increase in intensity over the next couple of weeks, and then is often sustained at high levels for one to two months. Typically, levels of distress begin to decline at two to three months after the incident of assault. Darves-Bornoz's (1997) research with sexual abuse survivors in France found that at one month post-assault, 87 per cent had PTSD, decreasing to 70 per cent three months post-assault, and 65 per cent at six months post-assault. Mathews *et al.* (2008) studied PTSD in South African girls, and found that two-thirds of those who developed PTSD had symptoms persisting three months after the rape.

Frequently, symptoms of intrusive thoughts and distressing recollections, or symptoms of avoidance and dissociation, interfere with the social and occupational functioning of victim/survivors during the day. At night, getting a good night's sleep may prove impossible due to ongoing nightmares and sleep-related breathing and movement disorders (Krakow *et al.* 2002). Incorrect diagnosis of sleep problems, and their relationship to sexual trauma, can result in the prescription of unsuitable medications and may add to survivors' psychological burden. One study of 187 sexual assault survivors with post-traumatic stress symptoms found sleep problems including sleep-disordered breathing and nightmares had lasted for an average of 20 years and had not responded to repeated use of psychotropic medications or psychotherapy (Krakow *et al.* 2002).

Mediating factors

PTSD is more likely if the rape is more violent or a weapon used (Dutton *et al.* 2006). Levels of psychological distress during the attack significantly predict increased levels of fear and anxiety at 3–12 months post-rape (Girelli *et al.* 1986). Some evidence suggests that women raped in locations rated as 'safe' develop more symptoms (Cascardi *et al.* 1996). Survivors who are less educated and have greater self-blame post-assault have more psychological symptoms (Frazier and Borgida 1997), as do those who are more blamed and stigmatised (Ullman and Filipas 2001). Conversely, being believed, disclosing soon after the rape has taken place, and being offered empathy and access to effective psychological interventions result in better psychosocial outcomes for victims. Meta-analysis has revealed that tangible and other forms of social support are very strongly protective against developing PTSD (Brewin *et al.* 2000).

Much of the research into sexual assault has focused on a single event. The assumption that trauma has terminated, implicit in the diagnosis of 'post-traumatic stress disorder', is inaccurate when considering the repetitive sexual trauma over an extended period of time experienced by children and women who cannot escape their perpetrator/s. A diagnosis of complex PTSD (cPTSD) recognises the loss of a coherent sense of self and pervasive insecure attachment following chronic repetitive trauma (Herman 1992). However, trauma-focused cognitive-behavioural therapy appears to be effective in treating both PTSD and cPTSD in child sexual-abuse survivors (Resick *et al.* 2003).

Health services interventions

High-quality, appropriate health services can reduce all forms of violence-related harms, and meet survivors' needs for assistance in dealing with the impact of sexual violence on their lives (WHO 2004). The majority of services provided globally focus on the immediate post-rape period, and their quality is highly variable. In some northern countries, post-rape care professionals have been specifically trained, such as the sexual assault nurses of Canada, and often work from dedicated post-rape facilities. In many other countries, however, health professionals consulted after rape have no specific training, conduct examinations in general facilities, and often lack basic equipment and medication (Christofides *et al.* 2005; Claramunt and Cortes 2003). In one hospital in Karachi, Pakistani, women who had been raped were examined by a forensic examiner on a table used for post-mortems (Aahung 2007). South African research shows that even where staff generally lack training in post-rape care (75 per cent of service providers at the time had no training), better care was provided by staff who were specifically motivated to engage in the work and saw rape as a serious problem for women (Christofides *et al.* 2005).

In the absence of a specialised rape-care health service, the widespread social judgement that 'victims are responsible for rape' pervades care for rape victims, and deters them from coming forward for assistance. Research in the Dominican Republic, Peru, and Venezuela showed many service providers held survivors, not perpetrators, responsible for rape (Guedes *et al.* 2002). Victims of rape and child abuse often remain symptomatic for PSTD many years after the assault in the absence of treatment. Even if they do not disclose to services at the time of the assault, they may continue to manifest problems from the rape, and can still benefit from treatment. Health providers remain a potent gateway into care, having a unique opportunity to identify a history of sexual violence, diagnose psychological disorders, and provide effective responses to survivors' mental health needs and concerns.

In countries and settings where there have been strenuous efforts to improve post-rape care, essential features of successful efforts have included: (1) selecting people for the work who choose the area, (2) deepening their understanding of the social context of rape, and (3) exploring their values more generally in an effort to provide an empathetic and non-judgmental service. In a good service, efforts should seek to start the process of psychological healing from the moment rape victims enter the safety of the facility, through a supportive and caring response from health workers. In very low-resource settings, this may be as much as can be provided, alongside emergency contraception and treatment for sexually transmitted infections, and documentation of findings from a basic examination. The importance of this affirmation for rape victims should not be undervalued.

Basic mental health interventions in post-rape care require training, but are not essentially complex interventions to deliver. For example, survivors find it very helpful to be told about the common psychological reactions to rape. It is much easier to cope with nightmares, flashbacks, feelings of panic, sleep disorders, overwhelming desire for flight, anorexia, memory loss, and so forth if they are explained as 'normal' after rape rather than a sign of 'going mad'.

In South Africa, the obligation to meet mental health needs of rape survivors has been written into the national Sexual Assault Care Policy of the Department of Health (2005). Two days of training are included as part of the national curriculum for training professionals in post-rape care (Jina *et al.* 2008), spanning from basic counselling methods to trauma-focused cognitive behavioural therapy. This model of mental health care includes immediate support and containment, with discussion over the early follow-up visits of psychological reactions to rape, supported by a brochure for survivors. Two effective techniques used in trauma-focused cognitive behavioural therapy, *in vivo* exposure and imaginal exposure, are also taught (Foa and Rothbaum 1998). While in well-resourced settings trained clinical psychologists would provide such interventions, in a country with one psychologist for 100,000 population, there is a need to identify techniques that reduce the symptoms of PTSD in the short and long term, and that can be delivered by sensitive trained professionals from a broader range of backgrounds. *In vivo* exposure is of great value in helping survivors overcome powerful feelings of avoidance of circumstances related to the rape that they often have afterwards. Such feelings can be extremely socially debilitating if they result in a survivor feeling, for example, she cannot leave her house, or cannot use public transport because of fear of being raped again. Imaginal exposure is valuable in helping survivors process the rape, through revisiting the events in a safe environment. PTSD symptoms, including the pervasive sense of fear engendered by thinking of the trauma, are believed to stem from a failure of processing of the rape. Revisiting events through verbal and written descriptions can lead to new and important insights being developed related to possibilities of avoidance of the rape, culpability, and so forth, which are essential for recovery.

The South African model of training doctors and nurses needs to be evaluated properly and tested in other settings. One of the biggest threats to its utilisation is the time needed for the training, time often being a scarce commodity in the public health sector. Yet early feedback from staff who have been trained suggests they have enormously valued being given some resources to utilise, essentially being empowered to help victims deal with highly distressing mental health problems.

Conclusions

The high prevalence and serious health and human rights consequences of sexual violence are at odds with its neglect as an international health issue. The Sexual Violence Research Initiative, an initiative of the Global Forum for Health Research, was set up in 2004 to address this disparity, and respond to the urgent need for high-quality evidence on all health-related aspects of sexual violence, including its profound mental health consequences (for further information, see www.svri.org).

PTSD is more common after rape than after any other traumatic event, and a substantial proportion of affected survivors remain symptomatic months and years after the rape in the absence of treatment. The global neglect of mental health services is compounded within post-rape care, where, historically, services have also been neglected. When initiatives have occurred, these have often been driven by a desire to improve the quality of evidence available for the criminal justice system. Little wonder that mental health services for rape survivors are all but non-existent globally. There are signs of this beginning to change. The South African post-rape care curriculum is an exciting example of an effort to put mental health service provision in a more prominent place within post-rape care. The essential challenge is to create a global impetus to move thinking after post-rape care from a medico-legal framework to one which centres on the needs of victims, among which mental health needs predominate. Critical questions remain about what capacity services in developing countries have for delivering such care, how and which cadres of health professional are best equipped to do this, and what modalities of care provision offer the most meaningful assistance to survivors. A lengthy journey lies ahead, but the most important first steps have been taken.

References

Aahung (2007) A Research Study on the Medico-legal Sector in Karachi, Karachi: Aahung.
Astbury, J. (1996) Crazy for You: The Making of Women's Madness, Melbourne: Oxford University Press.
Breslau, N., Kessler, R.C., Chilcoat, H.D., Schultz, L.R., Davis, G.C., and Andreski, P. (1998) 'Traumatic and Posttraumatic Stress Disorder in the Community: The 1996 Detroit Area Survey of Trauma', Archives of General Psychiatry, 55: 626–32.
Brewin, C.R., Andrews, B., and Valentine, J.D. (2000) 'Meta-analysis of Risk Factors for Posttraumatic Stress Disorder in Trauma-exposed Adults', Journal of Consulting and Clinical Psychology, 68: 748–66.
BBC (British Broadcasting Corporation) (2008) Women Face Bias Worldwide – UN, British Broadcasting Corporation News, 5 April, available at http://news.bbc.co.uk/go/pr/fr/-/2/hi/europe/7331813.stm (accessed 10 August 2008).

Cascardi, M., Riggs, D.S., Hearst-Ikeda, D., and Foa, E.B. (1996) 'Objective Ratings of Assault Safety as Predictors of PTSD', *Journal of Interpersonal Violence*, 11(1): 65–78.

Christofides, N., Jewkes, R., Webster, N., Penn-Kekana, L., Abrahams, N., and Martin, L. (2005) '"Other Patients are Really in Need of Medical Attention" – The Quality of Sexual Assault Services in South Africa', *Bulletin of the World Health Organization*, 83: 495–502.

Claramunt, M.C. and Cortes, M.V. (2003) *Situation Analysis of Medico-legal and Health Services for Victims of Sexual Violence in Central America, Subregional Report: Belice, Costa Rica, El Salvador, Guatemala, Honduras, y Nicaragua*, San Jose: Pan American Health Organization.

Cloutier, S., Martin, S., and Poole, C. (2002) 'Sexual Assault among North Carolina Women: Prevalence and Health Risk Factors', *Journal of Epidemiology and Community Health*, 56: 265–71.

Coid, J., Petruckevitch, A., Feder, G., Chung, W., Richardson, J., and Moorey, S. (1998) 'Relation between Childhood Sexual Abuse and Physical Abuse and Risk of Revictimisation in Women: A Cross Sectional Study', *The Lancet*, 358: 450–54.

Darves-Bornoz, M. (1997) 'Rape-related Pscyhotraumatic Syndromes', *European Journal of Obstetrics and Gynecology*, 71: 59–65.

Davidson, J.R.T., Hughes, D.C., George, L.K., and Blazer, D.G. (1996) 'The Association of Sexual Assault and Attempted Suicide within the Community', *Archives of General Psychiatry*, 53: 550–55.

Dunkle, K.L., Jewkes, R.K., Brown, H.C., Yoshihama, M., Gray, G.E., McIntyre, J.A., and Harlow, S.D. (2004) 'Prevalence and Patterns of Gender-based Violence and Revictimization among Women Attending Antenatal Clinics in Soweto, South Africa', *American Journal of Epidemiology*, 160: 230–39.

Dutton, M.A., Green, B.L., Kaltman, S.I., Roesch, D.M., Zeffiro, T.A., and Krause, E.D. (2006) 'Intimate Partner Violence, PTSD and Adverse Health Outcomes', *Journal of Interpersonal Violence*, 21(7): 955–68.

Farley, M., Golding, J., and Minkoff, J. (2002) 'Is a History of Trauma Associated with a Reduced Likelihood of Cervical Cancer Screening?', *Journal of Family Practice*, 51: 827–31.

Foa, E.B. and Rothbaum, B.O. (1998) *Treating the Trauma of Rape: Cognitive Behavioural Therapy for PTSD*, Guildford: Guildford Press.

Frazier, P.A. and Borgida, E. (1997) 'The Scientific Status of Research on Rape Trauma Syndrome' in D. Faigman, D. Kaye, M. Saks, and J. Saunders (eds) *Modern Scientific Evidence: The Law and Science in Expert Testimony*, St Paul, MN: West Group Publishing.

Garcia-Moreno, C., Hansen, H.A., Ellsberg, M., Heise, L., and Watts, C. (2005) *WHO Multi-country Study on Women's Health and Domestic Violence against Women*, Geneva: World Health Organization.

Girelli, S.A., Resnick, P.A., Marhoefer-Dvorak, S., and Hutter, C.K. (1986) 'Subjective Distress and Violence during Rape: Their Effects on Long Term Fear', *Violence and Victims*, 1: 35–45.

Guedes, A., Bott, S., and Cuca, Y. (2002) 'Integrating Systematic Screening for Gender-based Violence into Sexual and Reproductive Health Services: Results of a Baseline Study by the International Planned Parenthood Federation, Western Hemisphere Region', *International Journal of Gynecology and Obstetrics*, 78: 557–63.

Herman, J.L. (1992) *Trauma and Recovery*, New York: Basic Books.

Jewkes, R., Vundule, C., Maforah, F., and Jordaan, E. (2001) 'Relationship Dynamics and Adolescent Pregnancy in South Africa', *Social Science & Medicine*, 52(5): 733–44.

Jewkes, R., Sen, P., and Garcia-Moreno, C. (2002) 'Sexual Violence' in E. Krug, J. Mercy, A. Zwi, and R. Lozano (eds) *World Report on Violence and Health*, Geneva: World Health Organization: 147–81.

Jewkes, R., Sikweyiya, Y., Morrell, R., and Dunkle, K. (2009) *Understanding Men's Health and Use of Violence: Interface of Rape and HIV in South Africa*, Pretoria: Technical Report, Medical Research Council.

Jina, R., Jewkes, R., Christofides, N., and Loots, L. (eds) (2008) *Caring for Survivors of Sexual Assault: A Training Programme for Health Care Providers in South Africa*, Pretoria: Department of Health.

Kessler, R.C., Sonnega, A., Bromet, E., Hughes, M., and Nelson, C. (1995) 'Posttraumatic Stress Disorder in the National Comorbidity Survey', *Archives of General Psychiatry*, 52: 1,048–60.

Kilpatrick, D.G., Edmonds, C.N., and Seymour, A.K. (1992) *Rape in America: A Report to the Nation*, Arlington, VA: National Victim Center.

Krakow, B., Melendrez, D., Johnston, L., Warner, T.D., Clark, J.O., Pacheco, M., Pedersen, B., Koss, M., Hollipfield, M., and Schrader, R. (2002) 'Sleep-disordered Breathing, Psychiatric Distress and Quality of Life Impairment in Sexual Assault Survivors', *Journal of Nervous and Mental Disease*, 190: 442–52.

Mathews, S. and Abrahams, N. (2008) *Child Sexual Assault: Exploring the Psychosocial Needs of the Girl Child and their Carer Post-Rape*, Gender and Health Research Unit, South Africa: South African Medical Research Council.

Resnick, H.S., Acierno, R., and Kilpatrick, D.G. (1997) 'Health Impact of Interpersonal Violence. 2. Medical and Mental Health Outcomes', *Behavioral Medicine*, 23: 65–78.

Resick, P.A., Nishith, P., and Griffin, M.G. (2003) 'How Well does Cognitive-behavioral Therapy Treat Symptoms of Complex PTSD? An Examination of Child Sexual Abuse Survivors within a Clinical Trial', *CNS Spectrums*, 8: 340–55.

Ruggiero, K.J., Smith, D.W., Hanson, R.F., Resnick, H.S., Saunders, B.E., Kilpatrick, D.G., and Best, C.L. (2004) 'Is Disclosure of Childhood Rape associated with Mental Health Outcome? Results from the National Women's Study', *Child Maltreatment*, 9: 62–77.

Seedat, M., Van Niekerk, A., Jewkes, R., Suffla, S., and Ratele, K. (2009) 'Violence and Injuries in South Africa: Prioritising an Agenda for Prevention', *The Lancet*, 374: 1,011–22.

Springs, F.E. and Friedrich, W.N. (1992) 'Health Risk Behaviours and Medical Sequelae of Childhood Sexual Abuse', *Mayo Clinic Proceedings*, 67: 527–32.

Ullman, S. and Filipas, H. (2001) 'Predictors of PTSD Symptom Severity and Social Reactions in Sexual Assault Victims', *Journal of Traumatic Stress*, 14: 369–89.

Vos, T., Astbury, J., Piers, S., Magnus, A., Heenan, M., Walker, L., and Webster, K. (2006) 'Measuring the Health Impact of Intimate Partner Violence on the Health of Women in Victoria, Australia', *Bulletin of the World Health Organization*, 84: 739–44.

Watts, C., Keogh, E., Ndlovu, M., and Kwaramba, R. (1998) 'Withholding of Sex and Forced Sex: Dimensions of Violence against Zimbabwean Women', *Reproductive Health Matters*, 6: 57–65.

WHO (World Health Organisation) (2004) *Preventing Violence: A Guide to Implementing the Recommendations of the World Report on Violence and Health*, Geneva: WHO.

Part IX
Global Access to Essential Medicines

41

Global Access to Essential Medicines

Past, Present, and Future

Jonathan D. Quick and Eric Olawolu Moore

Introduction

Access to essential medicines has led to dramatic health impacts, saving lives and improving health. Each year an estimated 10 million men, women, and children – nearly all in low- and middle-income countries (LMIC) – die from conditions for which safe, effective, affordable prevention or treatment exists through medicines, vaccines, and improved health habits. Medicines also have a huge financial impact on individuals, families, communities, and governments.

This chapter briefly describes the rapid emergence of modern pharmaceuticals in the last century. It reviews the two 'eras' in access to medicines: the development of the essential medicines concept from the mid-1970s, and the access to medicines campaign from the late 1990s. It then uses the lens of access to AIDS medicines to illustrate core essential medicines concepts and the success of the access to medicines campaign. The concluding section looks at some of the opportunities and challenges for essential medicines in the twenty-first century.

The century of the modern pharmaceutical

Cave paintings discovered in Lascaux, France, tell us that humankind has used herbal and other traditional medicines since at least 12000 BC. Yet by 1900, there were no mass-produced, widely available medicines or vaccines. It was only in 1928 that Alexander Fleming discovered penicillin, and not until the mid-1940s that the world saw the first clinical use of modern pharmaceuticals when antibiotics, anti-malarials, tuberculosis medicines, smallpox vaccine, tetanus toxoid, and other vaccines were used for large military populations during the Second World War. The 1950s, 1960s, and 1970s saw an explosion of development and marketing of antibiotics, mental health medicines, oral contraceptives, cardiovascular medicines, and many other medicines and vaccines. By the year 2000, over 7,000 unique pharmaceutical compounds had been discovered, and tens of thousands of different individual products were on the market in countries around the globe. In less than 100 years, the lives of literally billions of people had been transformed by the widespread availability of medicines and vaccines, contributing to greater productivity, increased well-being, and the near doubling of average life expectancy in high-income countries.

Two eras in access to essential medicines

The twentieth century truly was the century of the modern pharmaceutical. By the mid-1970s, the world had developed vaccines and medicines for prevention or treatment for the majority of known major killers. Yet an estimated 2 billion people – half the world's population at that time – lacked regular access to essential medicines (WHO 2004a). Mostly living in Africa, Asia, and Latin America, these people might as well have been living in the year 1900 – or the year 12,000 bc.

This 'fatal gap' between those with access to medicines in the world's richest countries and those without access led in the mid-1970s to the first era in access to medicines, which focused on the World Health Organization's (WHO) 'essential drugs concept'. Then, in the late 1990s, the stark gap in access to AIDS medicines and to new medicines for tropical diseases led to an 'access to medicines campaign', driven initially by advocacy organisations. These two eras have defined the access to medicine landscape over the last 30 years.

Rise of the essential medicines concept

Building on successful experiences in countries as diverse as Norway, Sri Lanka, Bangladesh, and Papua New Guinea, the WHO in 1975 formally adopted the concepts of 'essential medicines' and 'national drug policies' aimed at ensuring the availability, safety, and rational use of medicines. Two years later, WHO produced the first 'model list of essential drugs', which contained 224 medicines and vaccines. The list has been updated nearly every two years by a WHO committee on essential medicines, consisting of relevant experts from around the globe. In 2001, WHO fundamentally revised the entire process for selecting essential medicines to make it more evidence-based, transparent, responsive, and timely (WHO 2001). According to WHO:

> essential medicines are those that satisfy the priority health care needs of the population. Essential medicines are selected with due regard to disease prevalence, evidence on efficacy and safety, and comparative cost-effectiveness. Essential medicines are intended to be available within the context of functioning health systems at all times in adequate amounts, in the appropriate dosage forms, with assured quality, and at a price the individual and the community can afford.
>
> (WHO 2009a)

> A national drug policy is a commitment to a goal and a guide for action. It expresses and prioritises the medium- to long-term goals set by the government for the pharmaceutical sector, and identifies the main strategies for attaining them. It provides a framework within which the activities of the pharmaceutical sector can be coordinated. It covers both the public and the private sectors, and involves all the main actors in the pharmaceutical field.
>
> (WHO 2001)

Within 25 years of the first model list, nearly 160 countries had developed national or local essential medicines lists; over 130 countries had developed independent treatment guidelines and/or formulary manuals; over 100 countries had national medicines policies to guide public and private action in the field; and numerous countries had established programmes to assure medicines' quality, implement generic competition, provide public price information, and incorporate essential medicines into their training. Most heartening for public health was the fact that over 25 years of community, national, and international action by public, private, and civil society actors had expanded the number of people estimated to have regular access to essential medicines from 2.1 billion in 1977 to over 4 billion in 2003 – roughly increasing from one-half to two-thirds of the world's population (Quick 2003a).

Access to medicines campaign

During the late 1990s, three new challenges in access to medicines began to command the world's attention: (1) the 'fatal gap' in access to AIDS treatments in resource-poor countries, (2) the dearth of research and development for malaria and other tropical diseases, and (3) the potential impact of new international patent and other intellectual property requirements on access to medicines.

In many ways, each of these three challenges had its own driving forces and public health implications. Yet across individual issues, the era of the 'access to medicines campaign' has been characterised by new dynamics of engagement by political leaders, public health leaders, advocacy groups, international organisations, superstars, the general public, and communities of affected people. Of the three challenges, measureable progress has been greatest in reducing the gap in access to AIDS medicines. In many respects, this reflects the combined effect of applying both the 'classic' essential medicines concept and this 'modern' campaign dynamic. Lessons from this approach are described in the following section.

Access through the lens of AIDS medicines

The dramatic increase in AIDS treatment medicines between 2002 and 2007 represents the largest access to medicines scale-up in public health history. In just five years, the estimated number of HIV-positive people on antiretroviral (ARV) medicines in Africa increased 40-fold, from roughly 50,000 to over 2 million. For all LMIC combined, the total number on treatment reached nearly 3 million people – 30 per cent of the estimated number of people needing treatment (WHO et al. 2008). As recently as 2001, however, ARV prices remained unafford-able, the quality of generic ARVs was unproven, views varied widely on treatment regimens and monitoring requirements, funding for large-scale ARV treatment programmes was non-existent, and few supply systems were up to handling the projected volume of ARVs.

In its framework for access to essential medicines, WHO defines four critical factors, each of which must be in place to ensure access: rational selection and use, affordable prices, sustainable financing, and reliable supply and quality assurance systems (Quick 2003b; WHO 2004a). The role of each of these factors is well-illustrated by the scale-up in access to AIDS medicines.

Selection and rational use

The WHO list of essential medicines has no direct authority over the production, procurement, distribution, or use of medicines in any major health system in the world. Similarly, WHO treatment guidelines have no inherent authority over diagnosis, treatment, clinical monitoring, or patient care. As expert guidance, however, such tools provide essential information and send important signals to public health officials, donors, the generic and brand-name pharmaceutical industry, low-cost essential medicines suppliers such as the United Nations Children's Fund (UNICEF) and the International Development Association (IDA), and many others. As a result, the addition of 12 ARVs to the WHO model list and the publication of WHO guidelines for scaling up antiretroviral treatment (ART) in resource-limited settings – both in 2002 – represented significant steps forward in scaling up AIDS treatment.

The guidelines for scaling up ART provided health officials, clinicians, and others with much needed and heartily welcomed advice on when and how to start ART; recommended first-line and second-line treatments; ART in pregnancy, adolescents, children, and infants; adherence to treatment; and monitoring of ART (WHO 2002). A key principle underlying these guidelines was that the inability of an AIDS treatment programme to provide optimal laboratory monitoring did not justify withholding treatment, as long as the basic recommended or absolute minimum testing could be provided. The addition of selected ARVs to the WHO model list included the most comprehensive publicly available analysis of ART effectiveness and safety to date, authoritative formulary information on ARV use, quality assurance standards for ARVs, and additional reference information. For the treatment advocates, such information may have seemed like academic footnotes to a foregone conclusion. But for Ministry of Health officials, donors, international agencies, and many in the public health community, such definitive guidance from the world's leading health authority helped to convince the undecided and counter the sceptics (of which there were still many).

Scaling up ART has contributed to a range of efforts to promote rational use. Programmes to strengthen adherence counselling skills in Kenya and Ethiopia have improved communication skills to the benefit of all patients (MSH 2009a). In Namibia and other countries, AIDS treatment has increased attention on pharmacovigilance (monitoring drug effectiveness and safety) to inform patient and provider decisions, improve treatment results, and minimise adverse effects (MSH 2009b; Sagwa et al. 2009).

Affordable prices

The prices of medicines matters a lot, especially for low-income countries and poor households. Getting to the best achievable price for pharmaceuticals requires a combination of strategies. Patients in low-income countries pay as much as 25 times the international reference price for the lowest-costing essential medicines (Cameron et al. 2009). Whereas in high-income countries the cost of supply chain, dispensing, and taxes rarely adds more than 20 per cent to a manufacturer's price, in developing countries such intermediary costs can double, triple, or in some cases even quintuple the final cost to the patient.

Affordability strategies, therefore, must target the full range of factors that determine the final cost of a medicine. Effective strategies include use of price information; competition among qualified suppliers; bulk procurement; generic substitution; differential pricing for newer essential medicines; elimination of duties, tariffs and taxes on essential medicines; more efficient distribution and dispensing systems; local production of quality essential medicines where feasible and financially competitive; and appropriate use of compatible safeguards such as compulsory licensing and price negotiation (see Figure 41.1).

In the case of ART, a stunning and unprecedented 98 per cent price reduction (from over US $10,000 to less than $200 per person per year) was achieved over just six years through a combination of negotiation and competition. In 1997, the UNAIDS Drug Access Initiative negotiated the price to between $7,000 to $8,000; by 1999, competition within Brazil's AIDS programme lowered the price to $5,000; in May 2000, five pharmaceutical companies offered UN agencies prices of less than $2,000; in 2001, the Indian manufacturer, Cipla, offered competitive pricing of $360 ($1 per patient per day); and finally, in 2003, the Clinton Foundation announced that it had negotiated with manufacturers a price of less than $140

Rational selection and use of essential medicines

- Develop national treatment guidelines based on the best available evidence concerning efficacy, safety, quality, and cost-effectiveness
- Develop a national list of essential medicines based on national treatment guidelines
- Use a national list of essential medicines for procurement, reimbursement, training, donations and supervision

Affordable prices

- Use available and impartial price information
- Allow price competition in the local market
- Promote bulk procurement
- Implement generics policies
- Negotiate equitable pricing for newer essential medicines for priority diseases
- Undertake price negotiation for newly registered essential medicines
- Eliminate duties, tariffs, and taxes on essential medicines
- Reduce mark-ups through more efficient distribution and dispensing systems
- Encourage local production of essential medicines of assured quality when appropriate and feasible
- Include WTO/TRIPS compatible safeguards into national legislation and apply

Sustainable financing

- Increase public funding for health, including for essential medicines
- Reduce out-of-pocket spending, especially by the poor
- Expand health insurance through national, local, and employer schemes
- Target external funding – grants, loans, donations – at specific diseases with high public health impact
- Explore other financing mechanisms, such as debt-relief and solidarity funds.

Reliable supply systems

- Integrate medicines in health sector development
- Create efficient public-private-NGO mix approaches in supply delivery
- Assure quality of medicines through regulatory control
- Explore various purchasing schemes: procurement cooperatives
- Include traditional medicines in the health care provision

Figure 41.1 WHO Framework for Equitable Access to Essential Medicines
Source: Management Sciences for Health/WHO 1997.

per person per year for one of the most commonly used triple combinations (Kapstein and Busby 2009).

Sustainable financing

With the feasibility of treatment demonstrated through thousands of patients in over half a dozen developing countries, expert support available for treatment protocols, and falling ARV prices, the question of funding became predominant. Following an intensive two-year effort by AIDS activists, politicians, governments north and south, multilateral organisations such as the UN and WHO, outspoken academics, and high-profile rock stars, the Global Fund to Fight AIDS, Tuberculosis and Malaria (GFATM) opened its doors in January 2002. Within three months, the GFATM had approved initial grants to 36 countries. The GFATM has since approved grants for over $15.5 billion – almost 60 per cent allocated to HIV response, and nearly 50 per cent allocated for medicines and commodities (GFATM 2009).

The launch of the Global Fund was followed by the five-year US President's Emergency Plan for AIDS Relief (PEPFAR) in 2003, the US President's Malaria Initiative (PMI) in 2004, the French-initiated UNITAID in 2006, and re-authorisation of PEPFAR in 2008. Together, this explosion of 'mega-funds' has resulted in the commitment of over $80 billion to global health, the largest share to HIV and AIDS, and a sizable share of this to AIDS treatment.

Reliable supply and quality assurance systems

Responding to the AIDS epidemic has provided developing country pharmaceutical supply and quality assurance systems with huge challenges. At the same time, there are a growing number of examples of the positive effects of AIDS funding on pharmaceutical systems. In Rwanda, the stakeholder Coordinated Procurement and Distribution System helped to standardise ART and commodity selection across all external donors; simplify pharmaceutical management; enable CAMERWA, the national procurement agency, to access pooled donor basket funding; and optimise use of donor resources. In a growing number of countries, new pharmaceutical supply and dispensing information systems help reduce stock-outs, quantify ART use, calculate inventory requirements, report patient care statistics, and reduce staff needs through automated labelling. In Namibia and South Africa, task-shifting for ART has led to increased production of pharmacy assistants (Embrey *et al.* 2009; Walkowiak and Keene 2009).

The desire to address HIV scale-up challenges helped bring together the 14 member countries of the East, Central and Southern Africa Health Community (ECSA HC) to create the Regional Pharmaceutical Forum to provide technical leadership, enable national policy environments, share best practices, and exchange price and supplier information. Supply of HIV-related pharmaceuticals and commodities has increasingly been integrated into the essential medicines supply system, thereby strengthening existing systems (Oomman *et al.* 2008).

Increasingly, large-scale public health programmes are looking at options for integrated systems that use an appropriate mix of public, private, and non-governmental capacity. Alternatives to the classic central medicines stores include autonomous supply agencies, direct delivery, and the primary distributor model (MSH 1997). Innovative public–private arrangements such as these have been tested in several African countries, including Zambia, parts of South Africa, Tanzania, Kenya, and Uganda (Quick *et al.* 2005). The success of such efforts depends on reliable private sector partners, capable public oversight, and accountable governance.

Faith-based organisations provide a large share of health care services, especially in rural Africa, and have played a vital role in the AIDS response. A WHO study of 15 faith-based medicines supply organisations in ten countries found that these organisations served 25 to 60 per cent of the population. Though performance varied, these organisations were generally performing well, had transparent procurement procedures, competitive prices, and highly motivated staff; maintained strong relationships with their customers, Ministries of Health, and founding church bodies; and operated like small business entities, with boards or committees to oversee their work (Banda *et al.* 2006).

In the face of rapidly falling pharmaceutical prices and uncertainty about the quality of generic ARVs and other AIDS medicines, in 2001 WHO, with other UN partners, set up the Prequalification Programme for Medicines (PQP). The programme has since been expanded to cover malaria, tuberculosis, and reproductive health. Initially focused on products ready for patient use ('finished dosage forms'), the programme has been broadened to manufacturing sites for active pharmaceutical ingredients, research organisations involved in bioequivalence and other testing, prequalification of pharmaceutical quality control laboratories (QCLs), advocacy for medicines quality, and capacity-building drug regulatory authorities (WHO 2009b).

The WHO PQP and US Food and Drug Administration (USFDA) Fast Track Approval Process have facilitated generic procurement, with literally billions of dollars being spent by PEPFAR, the GFATM, and others. The USAID-funded Supply Chain Management System (SCMS), for example, during its first three years of operation, saved an estimated $364 million (compared to the purchase of equivalent branded products) by purchasing 90 per cent of its ARVs as generic products (SCMS 2009).

Global access opportunities and challenges in the twenty-first century

Since the first widespread use of essential medicines and vaccines barely 70 years ago, tremendous progress has been achieved in creating access to these life-saving products. The effectiveness of the essential medicines public health concepts for access, quality, and rational use of medicines have been proven by the test of time. Yet millions of people still lack regular access, needed new medicines are slow in coming, and vast amounts of resources are wasted through mismanagement. The following section addresses a few of the many global access opportunities and challenges which face us in the twenty-first century.

Access to essential medicines as human right

The International Covenant of Economic, Social and Cultural Rights (ICESCR) forms the reference text in international treaties regarding the right to health. The ICESCR explicitly recognises that not all rights can be realised immediately. Thus, the right to health is a 'progressive right'. The right to health includes a right to health care and a right to healthy conditions, but not the right to be healthy, as such, since this reflects individuals' genetic make-up, socio-economic conditions, and the resources of the state (WHO 2009c). As a result of WHO's joint effort with the United Nations Committee on Economic, Social and Cultural Rights, in 2000, access to essential medicines was explicitly incorporated into the right to health (Seuba 2006).

The power of rights-based social mobilisation in securing access to medicines is vividly illustrated by the 1996 victory by AIDS activists in the legal battle for universal access to ARV treatment in Brazil. This groundbreaking action provided the critical catalyst for Brazil to build its successful national AIDS treatment programme and become the inspiration for scaling up AIDS treatment throughout the world. The growing international recognition of health as a human right, and the now explicit recognition of access to essential medicines as part of that right, is becoming an increasingly potent tool in expanding access to medicines. This is especially true in pursing the rights of the vulnerable and underserved in areas such as child, reproductive, and maternal health. One caveat, however, is that misapplication of this right can, and has, led to legal action forcing health care programmes to provide access to medicines which are unproven or of marginal value.

Essential medicines for priority needs

Keeping the essential medicines relevant and dynamic is both a challenge and an opportunity for the twenty-first century. Two recent examples illustrate how the essential medicines approach continues to catalyse action by the international health community to address priority health needs. The first addresses access to medicines for children, and the second to medicines for reproductive health.

Most of the 9 million annual deaths of children under five years are preventable with adequate access to essential medicines and vaccines for children. The WHO and other international partner agencies have launched several initiatives to address the global need for safe, effective, and accessible medicines for children through the 'Better Medicines for Children' and 'Make Medicines Children Size' campaigns. Some of the issues surrounding access to medicines for children include the absence of children's medicines on essential medicines lists, inadequate development and production of children's medicines, availability and regulation of dosage forms for children, and unclear ethical guidelines for clinical trials in children (WHO 2009d). Progress is currently being made with funding research and development, and forming ethical guidelines for drug trials in children.

Reproductive health covers a range of conditions that include healthy sexual development, reproductive and fertility regulation, prevention of STIs and HIV/AIDS, and safe motherhood. Reproductive health problems account for up to 18 per cent of the global burden of disease and 32 per cent of the total burden of disease for women of reproductive age (AGI and UNFPA 2004). A 2006 review of national health policies and essential medicines lists found that inclusion of reproductive health medicines to be absent or inadequate in the majority of cases (PATH *et al.* 2006). Without question, the addition of needed reproductive health medicines to essential medicines, and action to ensure access, quality, and appropriate use is essential for the reproductive and overall health of women and their families.

Global access to new medicines

The stunning gap in research and development of drugs for neglected diseases such as malaria, sleeping sickness, and other tropical diseases was incisively documented by Médecins sans Frontières/Doctors without Borders (Trouiller *et al.* 1999), which launched the Drugs for Neglected Diseases Initiative that same year with the funds from winning the Nobel Peace Prize.

Since 1999, there has been series of promising new initiatives aimed at developing new medicines, vaccines, and other technologies for global health, including the Bill & Melinda Gates Foundation Grand Challenges in Global Health initiative, the Medicines for Malaria Venture, the Global Alliance for TB Drug Development, the International AIDS Vaccine Initiative, and the Malaria Vaccine Initiative. In addition to these initiatives for tropical and other neglected diseases of developing countries, it must be borne in mind that developing and developed countries alike face significant 'pharmaceutical gaps' in areas of chronic disease, children's medicines, reproductive health, and other areas of public health importance for which pharmaceutical treatments either do not exist or are inadequate (Kaplan 2004).

Long delays in the adoption of community-based treatment of childhood pneumonia and in expanding access to artemisinin-based combination therapies (ACTs) attest to the challenge of ensuring rapid, widespread global access to new medicines. Initiatives involved in developing these products must from the outset work together with the full range of public health, pharmaceutical, regulatory, financial, and other expertise to ensure rapid widespread adoption.

Drug financing through health insurance

Community financing broadly describes a wide variety of health financing arrangements, some of which include community cost-sharing, community prepayment, micro-insurance, community health funds, rural health insurance, revolving drug funds, and community involvement in user-fee management (Ekman 2004). In low-income countries, community health insurance (CHI) has been introduced in different forms to pool risks and reduce the economic burden of out-of-pocket spending on health. Out-of-pocket payments account for 85 per cent of private health care expenditures, and over 50 per cent of total health care expenditures in these countries (Vialle-Valentin et al. 2008). Medicines were also found to constitute the largest reported component of out-of-pocket payments for health care ranging from 11.1 per cent of health expenditures in Chad to 68.8 per cent in Nepal.

Drug benefits are thus an integral part of community health insurance. There is a paucity of detailed information on the extent to which medicines are covered in CHI in low-income countries. A 2008 study identified CHI plans in only one-third (19 out of 54) low-income countries (Vialle-Valentin et al. 2008). Several medicine coverage forms include medicine co-payment, in-patient and outpatient medicine benefits, and essential medicines and generic policies. Some of the challenges of medicines coverage in CHI include weak drug supply systems, low enrolment and 'access' among the poor, insufficient political support, low voluntary enrolment and diversity of communities, and lack of infrastructure and technical capacity. If scaled up adequately to include medicines coverage, CHI can improve access to and use of essential medicines in low-income countries.

Quality assurance in a global market

Pharmaceutical quality cannot be 'tested into a product' – it must be built in by its manufacturer through the formulation, production, and packaging processes. Effective medicines regulation by an established government authority provides the needed oversight to ensure that quality is created by manufacturers, and preserved at each step in the supply chain from producer to patient (WHO 2003). The effects of counterfeit and substandard medicines are seen around the world, from the consumption of harmful ingredients in fake medicines, to the promotion of drug-resistant microbial strains of diseases, drug resistance in individuals and populations, intellectual property theft, loss of productivity, loss of confidence in health-delivery systems, and death. Estimates of the prevalence of counterfeit medicines range from less than 1 per cent of market value in most industrialised countries, to 50 per cent in parts of Africa, Asia, and Latin America (WHO 2009e; Newton et al. 2006).

Factors encouraging counterfeiting of medicines include lack of regulation and enforcement in many developing countries, greed, relative high costs of genuine medicines, and light penalties for producers and traffickers (Newton et al. 2006). Several interlinked strategies are required to effectively combat the problem of counterfeit medicines. Greater intergovernmental collaboration, stricter penalties at points of source, and increased diplomatic pressure are needed to minimise the production, trading, and selling of fake medicines around the globe.

Good governance for medicines

The World Bank has described corruption as the 'greatest obstacle to economic and social development', and Transparency International (TI) has estimated that 10 to 25 per cent of global public health procurement spending is stolen or otherwise misused. Corruption in the pharmaceutical sector can occur through bribery of procurement official; theft in the distribution chain; falsification of data on quality, efficacy, or safety; or any of a number of other ways (Vian 2002).

Though spoken of quietly for decades, corruption and other failures in good governance for medicines has only received systematic visible attention by the international community since the early 2000s. TI, the leading global civil society organisation committed to fighting corruption, has taken as one of its global priorities corruption in the health sector, including in health services, the pharmaceutical industry, and in the procurement of medicines and equipment (TI 2009). The WHO Good Governance for Medicines (GGM) programme, started in 2004, works with governments and other stakeholders to reduce corruption in the pharmaceutical sector (WHO 2009f). Lastly, a comprehensive initiative of the UK Department for International Development (DFID), the Medicines Transparency Alliance (MeTA), brings together governments, pharmaceutical companies, civil societies, and other stakeholders aimed at promoting access to essential medicines in developing countries (MeTA 2009). The effects of a more transparent and accountable pharmaceutical system has seen the reduction in pricing of medicines in several countries including Tanzania, Jordan, and Zambia (MeTA 2009).

Anti-microbial resistance

The world has been experiencing a steady increase in microbial resistance to traditional first-line medicines for malaria, tuberculosis, HIV, and other diseases. Anti-microbial resistance (AMR) has severe consequences, some of which include treatment failure, prolonged illnesses, avoidable death, and the higher cost and often toxicity of second- and third-line medicines. It is estimated that more than half of all medicines are prescribed, dispensed, or sold inappropriately. Achieving rational use of medicines is dependent on the whole health system, health practitioners, and consumers (WHO 2009g). Active local coalitions can do a great deal to contain AMR (MSH 2008).

Conclusion

It is sobering to note that modern medicines and vaccines have been available to the world for barely 70 years, and that for the first half of this period, access to these magic bullets was quite limited in most LMIC. Yet over the last 30 years, tremendous progress has been achieved in access to essential medicines, and the last ten years has seen stunning progress in access to AIDS medicines.

Amid this progress, serious challenges remain. The dearth of research and development for malaria and other tropical diseases, unreliable supply systems in many places, the high prevalence of counterfeit and substandard medicines in several parts of the world, slow uptake of new medicines, unaffordable medicine pricing, and AMR are but a few of the challenges which remain unresolved.

At the same time, there are promising efforts and some notable progress in areas such as development of needed new medicines for children, neglected diseases and other unmet needs; expanded financing of essential medicines through health insurance; and innovative efforts to improve governance for medicines. Ultimately, the success of twenty-first century medicines programmes will be determined by the accessibility of medicines to the populations and regions where they are needed most.

References

AGI (Alan Guttmacher Institute), UNFPA (United Nations Population Fund) (2004) *Adding It Up: The Benefits of Investing in Sexual and Reproductive Health Care*, New York: AGI, UNFPA, available at http://www.guttmacher.org/pubs/covers/addingitup.html (accessed 10 August 2009).

Banda, M., Everard, M., Logez, S., and Ombaka, E. (2006) *Multi-Country Study of Medicine Supply and Distribution Activities of Faith-Based Organizations in Sub-Saharan African Countries*, Geneva: World Health Organization and Ecumenical Pharmaceutical Network.

Cameron, A., Ewen, M., Ross-Degnan, D., Ball, D., and Laing, R. (2009) 'Medicine Prices, Availability, and Affordability in 36 Developing and Middle-income Countries: A Secondary Analysis', *The Lancet*, 373: 240–49.

Ekman, B. (2004) 'Community-based Health Insurance in Low-income Countries: A Systematic Review of the Evidence', *Health Policy Planning*, 19(5): 249–70.

Embrey, M., Hoos, D., and Quick, J.D. (2009) 'How AIDS Funding Strengthens Health Systems: Progress in Pharmaceutical Management', *Journal of Acquired Immune Deficiency Syndromes*, 52: S34–S37.

GFATM (Global Fund to Fight AIDS, Tuberculosis and Malaria) (2009) *Distribution of Funding after 7 Rounds*, available at http://www.theglobalfund.org/en/distributionfunding/?lang=en (accessed 10 October 2009).

Kaplan, W. and Laing, R. (2004) *World Health Organisation: Priority medicines for Europe and the World*, Geneva: World Health Organization.

Kapstein, E. and Busby, J. (2009) 'Making Markets for Merit Goods: The Political Economy of Antiretrovirals', Center for Global Development, Working Paper 179, Washington, DC: Center for Global Development.

MSH (Management Sciences for Health) (1997) 'Drug supply strategies', in MSH and World Health Organization (eds), *Managing Drug Supply*, 2nd edn, Bloomfield, CT: Kumarian Press.

MSH (Management Sciences for Health) (2008) *Building Local Coalitions for Containing Drug Resistance: A Guide*, submitted to the US Agency for International Development by the Rational Pharmaceutical Management Plus Program, Arlington, VA: Management Sciences for Health.

MSH (Management Sciences for Health) (2009a) *Pharmaceutical Management Interventions that Improve Country Health Systems: The Strengthening Pharmaceutical Systems Program*, Arlington, VA: Management Sciences for Health.

MSH (Management Sciences for Health) (2009b) *Strengthening Pharmaceutical Systems (SPS). Supporting Pharmacovigilance in Developing Countries: The Systems Perspective*, submitted to the US Agency for International Development by the SPS Program, Arlington, VA: MSH.

MeTA (Medicines Transparency Alliance) (2009) *MeTA: Medicines Transparency Alliance*, available at http://www.medicinestransparency.org/ (accessed 8 October 2009).

Newton, P.N., Green, M.D., Fernandez, F.M., Day, N.P., and White, N.J. (2006) 'Counterfeit Anti-infective Drugs', *Lancet Infectious Diseases*, 6: 602–13.

Oomman, N., Bernstein, M., and Rosenzweig S. (2008) *Seizing the Opportunity on AIDS and Health Systems*, Washington, DC: Center for Global Development.

PATH (Program for Appropriate Technology in Health), WHO (World Health Organization), UNFPA (United Nations Population Fund) (2006) *Essential Medicines for Reproductive Health: Guiding Principles for their Inclusion on National Medicines Lists*, Seattle, WA: PATH.

Quick, J.D. (2003a) 'Essential Medicines Twenty-five Years On: Closing the Access Gap', *Health Policy and Planning*, 18(1): 1–3.

Quick, J.D. (2003b) 'Ensuring Access to Essential Medicines in the Developing Countries: A Framework for Action', *Clinical Pharmacology and Therapeutics*, 73(4): 279–83.

Quick, J.D., Boohene, N.A., Rankin, J., and Mbwasi, R.J. (2005) 'Medicines Supply in Africa', *British Medical Journal*, 331: 709–10.

Sagwa, E., Nwokike, J., Mabirizi, D., Lates, J., Gaeseb, J., and Mengistu, A. (2009) *The Therapeutics Information and Pharmacovigilance Centre: Namibia's Approach to Monitoring Medicine Safety*, presented at the HIV Implementers Meeting, Winhoek, Namibia, available at http://www.hivimplementers.com/pdfs/Session%2057/57_2078_Nwokike.pdf (accessed 10 October 2009).

Seuba, X. (2006) 'A Human Rights Approach to the WHO Model List of Essential Medicines', *Bulletin of the World Health Organization*, 84: 405–407.

SCMS (Supply Chain Management System) (2009) *Three Years of Saving Lives through Stronger HIV/AIDS Supply Chains: A Report on the Global Impact of SCMS*, available at http://scms.pfscm.org/scms/resources/other/three%20year%20report.pdf (accessed 4 March 2010).

TI (Transparency International) (n.d.) *Corruption and Health*, available at http://www.transparency.org/global_priorities/other_thematic_issues/health (accessed 8 October 2009).

Trouiller, P., Battistella, C., Pinel, J., and Pecoul, B. (1999) 'Is Orphan Drug Status Beneficial to Tropical Disease Control? Comparison of the American and Future European Orphan Drug Acts', *Tropical Medicine & International Health*, 4(6): 412–20.

Vialle-Valentin, C.E., Ross-Degnan, D., Ntaganira, J., and Wagner, A.K. (2008) 'Medicines Coverage and Community-based Health Insurance in Low-income Countries', *Health Research Policy and Systems*, 6: 11.

Vian, T. (2002) *Corruption and the Health Sector*, Washington, DC: Management Systems International and Joint United Nations Programme on HIV/AIDS.

Walkowiak, H. and Keene, D. (2009) 'Managing Medicines and Supplies for HIV/AIDS Program Scale-Up', in R.G. Marlink and S.J. Teitelman (eds) *From the Ground Up: Building Comprehensive HIV/AIDS Care Programs in Resource-Limited Settings*, Washington, DC: Elizabeth Glaser Pediatric AIDS Foundation.

WHO (World Health Organization) (2001) *How to Develop and Implement a National Drug Policy*, 2nd edn, available at http://apps.who.int/medicinedocs/en/d/Js2283e/4.1.2.html (accessed 10 October 2009).

WHO (World Health Organization) (2002) *Scaling Up Antiretroviral Therapy in Resource-Limited Setting: Guidelines for a Public Health Approach*, Geneva: WHO.

WHO (World Health Organization) (2003) *Effective Medicines Regulation: Ensuring Safety, Efficacy and Quality*, WHO Policy Perspectives on Medicines Number 7, Geneva: WHO.

WHO (World Health Organization) (2004a) *Equitable Access to Essential Medicines: A Framework for Collective Action*, WHO Policy Perspectives on Medicines Number 8, Geneva: WHO.

WHO (World Health Organization) (2004b) *Scaling Up Antiretroviral Therapy in Resource-Limited Setting: Guidelines for a Public Health Approach, 2003 Revision*, Geneva: WHO.

WHO (World Health Organization) (2009a) *Essential Medicines*, available at http://www.who.int/medicines/services/essmedicines_def/en/index.html (accessed 2 September 2009).

WHO (World Health Organization) (2009b) 'WHO medicines prequalification: Progress in 2008', *WHO Drug Information*, 23(1): 3–7.

WHO (World Health Organization) (2009c) *Health and Human Rights*, available at http://www.who.int/hhr/Economic_social_cultural.pdf (accessed 11 August 2009).

WHO (World Health Organization) (2009d) *Report on Country Support and Interventions to Improve Use of Medicines in Children*, Geneva: WHO, available at http://www.who.int/childmedicines/progress/Country_Meeting_June2009.pdf (accessed 10 August 2009).

WHO (World Health Organization) (2009e) *Fact Sheet on Counterfeit Medicines*, available at http://www.who.int/medicines/services/counterfeit/CfeitsFactSheetJuly09.pdf (accessed 7 September 2009).

WHO (World Health Organization) (2009f) *Good Governance for Medicines*, available at http://www.who.int/medicines/ggm/en/index.html (accessed on 8 October 2009).

WHO (World Health Organization) (2009g) *Rational Use of Medicines*, available at http://www.who.int/medicines/areas/rational_use/en/ (accessed 5 September 2009).

WHO, UNAIDS, and UNICEF (World Health Organization, Joint United Nations Programme on HIV/AIDS, and United Nations Children's Fund) (2008) *Towards Universal Access: Scaling Up Priority HIV/AIDS Interventions in the Health Sector. Progress Report 2008*, available at http://www.who.int/hiv/pub/2008progressreport/en/ (accessed 10 October 2009).

42

Challenges of Local Production of Pharmaceuticals in Improving Access to Medicines

David Ofori-Adjei and Paul Lartey

Access to medicines (ATM) is sometimes loosely taken to imply the medicines in hand for the use of particular patients. In recent times, ATM approaches have focused on medicines for the treatment of malaria, tuberculosis, and HIV-opportunistic infections and AIDS, with particular attention on low-income countries (LICs), especially in sub-Saharan Africa. Fortunately, there exist some therapeutic options for these three large-scale health problems, and providing patients access to these medicines is important. However, there also exist health problems posing major public health challenges for which effective treatment is neither readily available nor being developed. The diseases in this category include African sleeping sickness, leishmaniasis, Buruli ulcer, and other diseases categorised as 'neglected diseases'. In this chapter, we will look broadly at the current situation regarding access to medicines and its determinants in the context of the low-income country's perspective. We will look at the production capacities and share of the pharmaceutical market, using examples mainly from Ghana. Problems faced by local pharmaceutical industries, including the acquisition of active pharmaceutical ingredients, production costs, generic manufacturing, patents/intellectual property, fake and/or substandard medications, competition, and public sector procurement penetration will also be addressed.

Perceived threats to local manufacturers by the Global Fund to Fight AIDS, TB and Malaria (GFATM), including the Affordable Medicines Facility – malaria (AMF-m), the World Health Organization (WHO) certification scheme, and other donor-supported activities in the pharmaceutical sector will also be addressed. The virtual absence of research and development (R&D) investment in LIC, and the high expectations that exist for herbal products in LIC will be covered. Lastly, suggestions for encouraging the participation of local LIC manufacturers in improving access to pharmaceutical products within their respective countries will be discussed.[1]

Background: measuring the availability of medicines

In order to address the lack of systematic measurement of access to medicines across countries, an international conference was organised by Management Sciences for Health (MSH) and WHO in December 2000. The aim of the conference was to draw up measurement indicators for the purpose of better assessing national and global availability of essential medicines. These indicators focused on availability, geographic accessibility, affordability, and acceptability of medicines around the world. The indicators also covered the cross-cutting issue of quality for both services and products. These indicators became part of the Gates Foundation-supported Strategies to Enhance Access to Medicines (SEAM) project run by MSH.

At the core of the concept of access to medicines is the provision of safe, efficacious, cost-effective, and good quality medicines to satisfy the health problems of populations. The challenges of poverty, weak health care systems, and social upheavals have focused the agenda of ATM on LICs. These LICs must deal with the double burden of persistent communicable diseases, as well as emerging non-communicable and chronic diseases. Despite the disease-specific focus of recent global funding mechanisms, the scope of medicines required to respond to the health problems of LICs extends far beyond anti-malarials, anti-mycobacterials, and antiretrovirals. While it is well recognised that malaria, tuberculosis, and HIV/AIDS cause high morbidity and mortality in LICs and affect primarily the young, women, and the poor, there are equally prevalent conditions that are silent killers. For example, schistosomiasis constitutes a major disease burden in LICs, but its related morbidity and mortality does not inspire the same level of global support despite the existence of effective treatment. Similarly, respiratory tract infections and cerebro/cardiovascular diseases also disproportionately cause mortality in LICs, again in spite of the availability of (but lack of access to) effective existing medicines.

In 1999, WHO estimated that nearly 80 per cent of the world's population without access to essential medicines lived in LICs, a disproportionate share considering that 60 per cent of the global population currently lives in LICs, while only 0.3 per cent of those populations without access to essential medicines live in high-income countries (HIC) (UN Millennium Project 2005). A decade later, the disparity has not significantly changed despite the implementation of various initiatives and strategies to improve access (for example, the WHO Access to Medicines initiative and the Rational Pharmaceutical Management programme of MSH). The WHO estimates that nearly half the population of Africa has no access to the most essential medicines, including anti-malarials like the artemisinin combination therapies (ACT), antiretroviral medicines, and medicines for non-communicable diseases like hypertension and diabetes (WHO 2004a).

The access gap and development of new medicines

Three out of eight Millennium Development Goals (MDGs), eight of the 16 MDG targets, and 18 of 48 MDG indicators are health-related. Medicines are necessary for the achievement of most of the MDGs' health-related targets, with access to essential medicines as a target unto itself: 'Proportion of population with access to affordable essential drugs on a sustainable basis' (MDG Target 8E and Indicator 8.13).[2]

Before discussing the issue of local production of medicines, it is essential to understand the nature of the access gap. There are four medicine-specific factors required to ensure that medicines are available wherever and whenever they are needed: (1) affordable prices, (2) sustainable financing, (3) rational selection, and (4) reliable health care supply system. In general, access to medicines has been described in the context of availability, affordability, geographic access, and acceptability (quality) (WHO 2007).

Overall, product (medicines) availability is a good measure of supply chain performance in any particular country. Using product availability as a measure of supply chain performance in HICs, it is estimated that availability at most retail pharmacies is over 95 per cent and 90 per cent for Organisation for Economic Co-operation and Development (OECD) and European

Table 42.1 Comparison of availability and price in private, public, and faith-based sectors in urban and rural communities in Ghana

	Public		Private		Faith-inspired	
	Availability	MPR	Availability	MPR	Availability	MPR
Urban	80% (n = 15)	3.44 (n = 15)	91% (n = 18)	3.04 (n = 18)	62.5% (n = 4)	3.19 (n = 4)
Rural	40% (n = 15)	3.07 (n = 15)	39.3% (n = 14)	3.13 (n = 14)	54.2% (n = 12)	3.26 (n = 12)

Source: Ghana MoH/WHO/HAI Collaboration Ghana – Medicine Price and Availability Monitor, September 2007–March 2008, sponsored by HAI Africa.
MPR – The MPR is a ratio of the local price divided by an international reference price converted into the same currency. An MPR of 1 means the local price is equivalent to the reference price, whereas an MPR of 2 means the local price is twice the reference price. The MPR results in this survey were based on the 2006 MSH International Drug Price Indicator guide (http://erc.msh.org/).

Union countries, respectively (Dalberg Global Development Advisors and MIT-Zaragoza International Logistics Program 2008). In contrast, in most low- and middle-income countries (LMIC), public health facilities are reported on average to have a product availability of 38 per cent, with less than 60 per cent availability reported in private outlets (WHO/HAI 2008). As shown in Table 42.1 through the case study of Ghana (an LIC), the availability of medicines within a country can also differ significantly between urban and rural communities, and between the type of health facility/institution (e.g. public, private, and faith-inspired organisations).

These differences in availability occur with both generic and branded medicine products (HAI, n.d.). Figure 42.1 shows the differences that exist in various economic groups.

The lack of access to medicines and its associated impact on increased morbidity, mortality, and national economies has been of concern to leaders of LICs. These concerns have been expressed at various forums and reflected in statements and international position papers and initiatives. Regional economic groupings in Africa and Asia have also addressed these concerns. At the 2006 World Health Assembly (WHA), member states established an Intergovernmental Working Group on Public Health, Innovation, and Intellectual Property to address the issue of

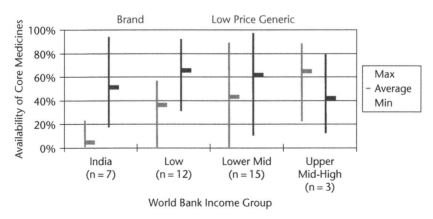

Figure 42.1 Availability of medicines in private retail outlets by country income groups
Source: Ross-Degnan 2007.

better access to health care products for poor populations and to address conditions dispropor-tionately affecting developing countries. The report[3] recommends, inter alia, prioritising research and development needs, technology transfer, and improving delivery and access to health products.

At the Bamako Ministerial Forum on Research for Health, ministers of health, education, science and technology, and finance (or their representatives) also emphasised the need for research and development for solving local health problems. The Call to Action, among others, requested promoting and sharing 'the discovery and development of, and access to, products and technologies addressing neglected and emerging diseases which disproportionately affect low- and middle-income countries (LMIC)' (Global Ministerial Forum on Research for Health 2008: 3). The need to work in partnership with the private sector requires important attention, as most of the investments in developing new medicine products for health come from that sector. Indeed, the cost of health technology development is such that most national budgets of developing (or LIC) countries cannot support it.

The development of new medicines and local production

It is in the area of new drug discoveries for 'emerging' diseases that perhaps the major or multinational pharmaceutical companies take on unfair criticism. The 'emerging' health care problems of the HICs link to lifestyle and related social and environmental issues within HICs, such as the need for more effective cholesterol-lowering drugs, and safer anti-anxiety medicines. Given the reality of the international (based on HICs) pharmaceutical industry's focus on HICs' health-related priorities, a logical sequence of events is for local pharmaceutical manufacturers within LICs to discover and develop medicines for diseases that disproportionately affect the populations of LICs. Unfortunately, there is little or no research or a development agenda involving innovation in current local LIC industries. We will next explore some of the reasons for the present gap in local development and production.

First, although some academic and publicly funded research facilities in LICs, such as the Centre for Scientific Research into Plant Medicine, Mampong-Akwapim, Ghana and the National Institute for Pharmaceutical Research and Development, Federal Ministry of Health, Abuja, Nigeria, have some existing capacity for drug discovery research, these facilities generally lack development capabilities and experience, and are in no position to commercialise bona fide discoveries. However, there is potential here that can be harnessed. Technology transfers and collaborations within the global private sector, between the manufacturers in HICs, and those in LICs, should be encouraged and facilitated. Genuine assistance from major international pharmaceutical manufacturers to help build research and development (R&D) capacities in LICs will empower local manufacturers to tackle emerging local health care problems, and will help to stem the current global perception of the international manufacturers as uncaring entities with only profit as their motivation.

Second, mechanisms should be developed within LICs to foster public–private partnerships for collaborative research toward the development of new medicines against emerging diseases, and for the commercialisation of health care innovations. For example, recent efforts by the McLaughlin-Rotman Centre for Global Health (University of Toronto) in Ghana and Tanzania are laudable. In an initiative termed 'Life Sciences Commercialization and Convergence', the McLaughlin-Rotman Centre is challenging government, academic, research, and financial institutions in both countries, in collaboration with private sector pharmaceutical manufacturers, to come up with practical approaches towards commercialising healthcare innovations in their resource-constrained environments. Such initiatives can lead to creative approaches in the development of new medicines.

Third, the lack of access to medicines in LICs has mostly been viewed in terms of regulation, manufacturing, procurement, and distribution. These issues all relate, albeit some indirectly, to the lack of existing incentives to develop new medicines that target diseases disproportionately affecting poor countries, and to the inadequate existing local pharmaceutical manufacturing capacity.

Local development and production in low-income countries

There have been several initiatives, mainly sponsored by international health partners such as WHO, UNICEF, and MSH, that have sought to address the question of access to medicines. However, the focus has generally been on models that address issues of supply chain management and the rational use of drugs. The local manufacture of medicines has not been a significant component of these interventions. In general, LICs are not major players in the pharmaceutical manufacturing arena, and most local manufacturing companies focus on a limited number of generic medicines.

In Ghana, for example, the local pharmaceutical industry started in earnest at the time of independence in 1957. Currently, there are 35 companies registered with the Pharmaceutical Manufacturers Association of Ghana, and they supply less than 30 per cent of the country's needs. The companies' portfolios include analgesics, haematinics, and anti-malarial medicines. There is only one manufacturer of antiretrovirals, and only three manufacturers of anti-malarial medicines in Ghana. The majority of medicines are imported, with an estimated 60 per cent coming from Asia and 10 per cent from the United States and Europe (Harper and Gyansa-Lutterodt 2007).

The import versus local manufacturing situation is no different in many other LICs. The WHO (2004a) indicates that HIC dominate in pharmaceutical production (by value), with a share of production of 89.1 per cent in 1985, which increased to 92.9 per cent in 1999. The combined manufacturing share of LMIC decreased from 10.9 per cent to 7.1 per cent over the same period. In general, local manufacturers in LICs are reproducer firms which manufacture medicines that are not protected by patent (unless under licence). These firms may be publicly or privately owned, and are typically small to medium-sized.

Local pharmaceutical manufacture occurs mainly in the private sector in LICs. Government involvement in local pharmaceutical manufacture has been found to be inefficient and subject to political interference (Bate 2008). Therefore, an increased public sector role in local manufacturing has not been encouraged.

Among the numerous challenges faced by private sector companies are insufficient financing, the high cost of utilities, the availability of cheaper imports, and the absence of needed economies of scale within the population. Increasing the challenge is the poor economic performance of many LICs, which bring high inflation and base lending rates, which in turn contribute to local manufacturers' difficulty in accessing affordable financing. Irregular supply and the high cost of local utilities, such as electricity and water, contribute substantially to the cost of production. Finally, many of the inputs for pharmaceutical manufacture, such as active pharmaceutical ingredients (APIs), excipients, and packaging materials, have to be imported and are not only costly inputs, but also subject to exchange rate fluctuations.

The challenge of medicine quality and counterfeits

The circulation of fake medicines appears to be increasing in many LICs, and also in LMICs (Cockburn *et al.* 2005). Alternatively, it may be that fake medicines are simply increasingly recognised as a result of improved surveillance activities using local minilabs and through collaboration with established laboratories such as the United States Pharmacopoeia (USP) Convention. The increased awareness of the health, economic, and social consequences of fake medicines has also promoted the interest of civil society organisations and the general public. A recent posting on E-drug,[4] the USP Drug Quality and Information Program, reported in a press release the discovery of quantities of a prescribed anti-malarial medication that did not contain any active ingredient in Ghana. The discovery was made by a vigilant citizen who contacted the Medicines Quality Monitoring programme set up by the US Agency for International Development (USAID)-supported Drug Quality and Information (DQI) Program,[5] implemented by the US Pharmacopeial (USP) Convention (USP Convention 2009).

In Ghana, the drug regulatory agency, the Food and Drugs Board (FDB), and the Catholic Health Services, have installed minilabs to monitor the quality of selected medicines being circulated in the country. The Medicines Transparency Alliance (MeTA), supported by the UK's Department for International Development (DFID), the WHO, and the World Bank, works with Ghana as one of its pilot countries. One of the issues of interest to MeTA in Ghana is the question of fake and substandard drugs. Through the concerted effort of these three agencies, MeTA-Ghana should provide a systematic basis for monitoring medicines in general use throughout the country. The role of civil society organisations and citizens is an important factor in abating the risk of existing fake medicines. The promotion of transparency and accountability in the pharmaceutical sector involving medicines procurement, distribution, pricing, and utilisation is one of the ways in which LICs can be adequately informed to make decisions on the efficient use of resources.

In many LICs, the quality of locally produced medicines is perceived to be poorer than those imported from HICs. This is not entirely unjustified, as poor regulatory control and enforcement, as well as failure to adhere to industry standards of Good Manufacturing Practices (GMP),[6] can result in the production and distribution of substandard medicines. The problem in the marketplace has been affected by open market policies, originally sponsored by the World Bank (for example, Ghana's Structural Adjustment Programme of the early 1980s), which resulted in the influx of a range of poor and satisfactory quality medicines to Ghana from other LICs (mainly India, Southeast Asia, and China). Thus, the question as to whether to import medicines or procure them from local manufacturers is confounded by the poor quality of some imported medicines.

Organisations such as MeTA have a role to play in this regard. A systematic study of issues surrounding medicines in each country, such as procurement, quality, availability, and distribution, has the potential of revealing the source of poor quality drugs, and how such drugs manage to reach the local market. Such empirical studies may help reveal the truth about locally manufactured medicines, and in particular reduce the perceptions that locally manufactured medicines are substandard. It would be a credit to the local industry if systematic studies showed that the quality of locally manufactured medicines is on par with imported ones from HICs when stringent drug regulatory authorities exist. If, on the other hand, perceptions of poor quality are confirmed as fact, then the industry, as well as their regulators, must be taken to task and mandated to improve the quality of their production, or be sidelined.

The role of external funders

In most LICs, key essential medicines for the predominant health problems (HIV and AIDS, malaria, and tuberculosis) are purchased primarily through the GFATM and other bilateral arrangements. The supply of these medicines requires pharmaceutical companies to satisfy WHO pre-qualification. The WHO pre-qualification scheme is designed to provide a rigorous but efficient assessment of products and manufacturing site inspection (Foster *et al.* 2006; WHO 2004b). Manufacturers must apply to be pre-qualified. Very few pharmaceutical companies in LICs have been pre-qualified. The pre-qualification exercise has been criticised by activists as confusing GMP standards with actual drug quality (Bate 2008). To clarify, GMP certification provides an assurance that a particular manufacturing plant is capable of producing products in a consistent manner that ensures quality. GMP certification does not cover content, quality, and effectiveness of specific medicines. The GFATM, for example, requires recipients of its grants to use WHO-prequalified products.

Anti-malarial medicines, analgesics, and anti-helminthics are some of the major medicines produced by local manufacturers, as most of the patents on these medicines have long expired or the existing patent holder has granted permission to a manufacturer to produce those products. Use of donor funds to procure or subsidise the purchase of these medicines poses a perceived threat to the local industry. The GFATM initiative, the AMF-m, for example, has been perceived as a major threat to local manufacturers of anti-malaria medicines. The AMF-m initiative, in its simplistic interpretation, seeks to make anti-malarial drugs affordable in LICs by reimbursing countries fully for their manufacture and offering them to distributors at a fraction of their normal wholesale cost. This approach, it is hypothesised, should translate into very low and affordable retail prices for such medicines. As there is a paucity of manufacturers in LICs that qualify to participate in this programme because of the requirement for WHO pre-qualification, such medicines would by necessity be imported and 'unfairly' compete with similar products from local manufacturers. Thus, the threat may not be in terms of volumes but rather price competition.

The reliance of most LICs on donor support for the procurement of pharmaceutical products is a major contributor to the stunted development of local pharmaceutical production. Using international competitive bidding, LIC governments are able to greatly increase the size of their drug imports, as opposed to procuring locally, given that local prices tend to be higher than those of imported medicines. In the absence of an effective pricing policy, private and public sector price mark-ups are arbitrarily determined. These mark-ups can sometimes push up retail prices by as much as 300 per cent (Cameron *et al.* 2009). In a recent study using the WHO/Health Action International methodology in Ghana, where sources of drugs were from a range of public, private, and faith-inspired organisations, price differences existed across these different sectors, and also between urban and rural communities.

Barriers to enhancing local production

The lack of financing, absence of technologies, lack of innovations, small market sizes, and weak regulatory systems constitute continuing barriers to enhancing local pharmaceutical manufacture. However, opportunities do exist for local pharmaceutical production to respond to national and regional demand in the supply of essential medicines. One major step in addressing such available opportunities is the role being played by regional super-bodies like the African Union (AU). The AU has convened several meetings seeking to address the issues surrounding the Agreement on Trade-Related Aspects of Intellectual Property Rights (TRIPS), which grants certain flexibilities meant 'to promote access to medicines for all'. These meetings have resulted in a call for the streamlining of patent regimes in order to take advantage of the TRIPS flexibilities.[7] A report by the WHO (Musungu and Oh 2005) found that many developing countries have not incorporated TRIPS flexibilities into their legislation. It remains up to governments to implement the necessary frameworks to take advantage of parallel imports, government use, and compulsory licensing. The fact still remains, however, that unless they advance from their current levels of technological know-how, pharmaceutical manufacturers in LICs will still not be able to take advantage of TRIPS flexibilities.

One idea is the approach taken by the German enterprise for sustainable development (GTZ) and the United Nations Industrial Development Organization (UNIDO), which is to consider capacity building in the local industry as a necessary step towards taking advantage of the TRIPS flexibilities (Harper and Gyansa-Lutterodt 2007). Realising that local industry not only contributes to health care, but can also contribute to industrial development and poverty alleviation, the two organisations conducted a comprehensive analysis of the industry in West and Central Africa. The outcome of the study was that in certain countries, such as Ghana, it may be possible to provide technical and related assistance that could help some companies to satisfy the conditions needed for WHO pre-qualification. Such an eventuality will enable the local industry to participate in donor-funded medicine supply, thereby boosting capacity utilisation, improving access, and contributing to industrial and technological growth. This could, in turn, position the industry to take advantage of the flexibilities. There is good potential for this approach, as the industry in Ghana benefits from relatively more stringent regulation by the Ghana FDB, and has a utilisation capacity of about 40 per cent, three facilities preparing for WHO pre-qualification, and is technologically more advanced (being the only one in the region with some capacity for the production of active pharmaceutical ingredients) (Harper and Gyansa-Lutterodt 2007).

Also of interest, regional groupings such as the Economic Community of West African States (ECOWAS), the East and Central African groupings, and the southern African group-ings are all focusing attention on the issue of improving access to medicines. It will be important for these economic groupings to pursue standardisation of regulatory policies and their harmo-nisation in order to encourage legitimate cross-border trade in pharmaceuticals. An important consequence of the harmonisation of regional regulatory rules is the opportunity to do pooled procurement (which would bring down prices), thereby helping with capacity utilisation, and hence growth of the local pharmaceutical industry.

In recent times, there have been several funding opportunities for capacity building in research directed at the health needs and diseases of LICs. A recent mapping exercise carried out by the WHO/TDR programme called the African Network for Drugs and Diagnostics Initiative (ANDI) paints a good picture of the potential of African countries to undertake research for new drugs and diagnostics (TDR 2008). What is missing from the existing initiative is a commercialisation component, which would enable local manufacture of the innovations and products. It is this component that needs to be simultaneously addressed at the onset of such a project, and linked to local manufacturing. Unless this is incorporated into the agenda, the status quo will continue, and scientific institutions in LICs will remain testers of products for HIC pharmaceutical concerns.

One of the final key challenges of R&D activities in LICs is the critical protection of intellectual property. This challenge is not limited to academic research institutions, but also to indigenous knowledge. The cost of patenting an invention internationally can be prohibi-tive. Having patented the invention, scientists are also faced with finding investors willing to proceed with further development. There have been several attempts to improve the lot of LICs scientists in this regard, but national governments should focus on assisting such industries with the filing of patents. The practice of 'evergreening' and extended data exclusivity limit LIC pharmaceutical companies from taking advantage of expired patents to manufacture generic versions of the off-patent product. 'Evergreening' is a procedure by which originator manufacturers (product patent holders) hold on to patent protection through obtaining separate patents for multiple attributes of a single product (read more at http://www.egagenerics.com/gen-evergrn.htm). Extended data exclusivity is another strategy used by originator manufacturers to protect their products from generic manufacturers. Unlike evergreening, extended data exclusivity prevents local health authorities from accepting applications for generic medicine during the period of exclusivity (additional information available at http://www.egagenerics.com/gen-dataex.htm).

Conclusion

In conclusion, it is in the interest of the governments of LICs to pursue policies that will enable local pharmaceutical companies to close the gap between external and domestic supplies of essential medicines. Efforts at enhancing plant utilisation capacities, acquisition of APIs, fair trade (including management of the issues surrounding TRIPS flexibilities), equitable financing systems, and intellectual property must be pursued at continental, regional, and national levels. The LICs must also make a special effort to deal with the challenges they face in the provision of essential medicines for child survival, reproductive health, HIV/AIDS, malaria, tuberculosis, and neglected diseases.

Notes

1 Further reading: (a) World Health Organization (2004) *The World Medicines Situation*, Geneva: WHO, available at http://apps.who.int/medicinedocs/en/d/Js6160e/3.html (accessed 25 June 2009).
(b) Foster, S., Laing, R., Melgaard, B., and Zaffran, M. (2006) 'Ensuring Supplies of Appropriate Drugs and Vaccines', in D. T. Jamison, J. G. Breman, A. R. Measham, *et al.* (eds) *Disease Control Priorities in Developing Countries*, 2nd edn, New York: Oxford University Press, available at http://www.dcp2.org/pubs/DCP/72/Section/10392 (accessed 23 December 2009).
2 *The Millennium Development Goal Indicators*, available at http://unstats.un.org/unsd/mdg/Hostaspx?Content=Indicators/OfficialList.htm (accessed 23 December 2009).
3 http://apps.who.int/gb/ebwha/pdf_files/WHA59/A59_R24-en.pdf.
4 'E-DRUG is the English version of SATELLIFE's electronic discussion groups on essential drugs. E-DRUG is used by health care professionals, researchers, and policymakers to obtain and discuss current information on essential drugs, policy, programme activities, education, and training. Members also use E-DRUG to announce and learn of upcoming conferences or courses in their field'. For more information, visit http://www.essentialdrugs.org/edrug/.
5 The USP DQI Program is a cooperative agreement first awarded to USP by USAID in 2000 and renewed in 2005. Through the programme, USP works in countries throughout Asia, Eastern Europe, Latin America, and sub-Saharan Africa. For more information, visit http://www.uspdqi.org/.
6 Good manufacturing practice (GMP) is the part of quality assurance which ensures that products are consistently produced and controlled to the quality standards appropriate for their intended use and as required by the marketing authorisation. For more information, visit http://www.who.int/medicines/areas/quality_safety/quality_assurance/production/en/index.html.
7 The TRIPS flexibilities include compulsory licensing, parallel importation, limits on data protection, and other exceptions to patentability. These provisions are meant for incorporation into national legal frameworks in order to improve access to medicines.

References

Bate, R. (2008) *Local Pharmaceutical Production in Developing Countries*, London: International Policy Network.
Cameron, A., Ewen, M., Ross-Degnan, D., Ball, D., and Laing, R. (2009) 'Medicine Prices, Availability and Affordability in 36 Developing and Middle-income Countries: A Secondary Analysis', *The Lancet*, 373(9,659): 240–9.

Cockburn, R., Newton, P.N., Agyarko, E.K., Akunyili, D., and White, N.J. (2005) 'The Global Threat of Counterfeit Drugs: Why Industry and Governments Must Communicate the Dangers', *PLoS Medicine*, 2(4): e100.

Dalberg Global Development Advisors and MIT-Zaragoza International Logistics Program (2008) *Private Sector Role in Health Supply Chains: Review of the Role and Potential for Private Sector Engagement in Developing Country Health Supply Chains*, New York: Rockefeller Foundation.

Foster, S., Laing, R., Melgaard, B., and Zaffran, M. (2006) 'Ensuring Supplies of Appropriate Drugs and Vaccines', in D.T. Jamison, J.G. Breman, A.R. Measham, G. Alleyne, M. Claeson, D.B. Evans, P. Jha, A. Mills, and P. Musgrove (eds) *Disease Control Priorities in Developing Countries*, 2nd edn, New York: Oxford University Press, pp. 1328–33, available at http://www.dcp2.org/pubs/DCP/72/Section/10392 (accessed 23 December 2009).

Global Ministerial Forum on Research for Health (2008) *The Bamako Call To Action on Research For Health: Strengthening Research For Health, Development, And Equity*, Bamako, Mali, 17–19 November, available at http://www.tropika.net/svc/specials/bamako2008/call-for-action/call (accessed 10 February 2010).

Harper, J. and Gyansa-Lutterodt, M. (2007) *The Viability of Pharmaceutical Manufacturing in Ghana to Address Priority Endemic Diseases in the West Africa Sub-Region*, Eschborn: Deutsche Gesellschaft für Technische Zusammenarbeit (GTZ) GmbH.

HAI (Health Action International) (n.d.) *Medicine Prices, Availability, Affordability, and Price Components*, available at http://www.haiweb.org/medicineprices/ (accessed 6 August 2009).

Musungu, S.F. and Oh, C. (2005) *The Use of Flexibilities in TRIPS by Developing Countries: Can They Promote Access to Medicines?* Commission on Intellectual Property Rights, Innovation and Public Health, Geneva: World Health Organization and the South Centre.

Ross-Degnan, D. (2007) *Toward a Medicines Transparency Alliance (MeTA) Issues for Consumers and Civil Society*, available at http://www.dfidhealthrc.org/meta/documents/MeTA%20demand-side%20framework%20(13%20Mar% 202007)%20-%20for%20participants.ppt (accessed 30 June 2009).

TDR (2008) 'African Network for Drugs and Diagnostics Innovation (ANDI): New Network Launched in Abuja, Nigeria', *TDRnews*, available at http://apps.who.int/tdr/svc/publications/tdrnews/issue-81/african-network (accessed 11 February 2010).

UN (United Nations) Millennium Project (2005) *Prescription for Healthy Development: Increasing Access to Medicines, Report of the Task Force on HIV/AIDS, Malaria, TB, and Access to Essential Medicines*, Working Group on Access to Essential Medicines, Sterling, VA: Earthscan.

USP (US Pharmacopeial) Convention (2009) *Counterfeit Antimalarial Drug Discovered in Ghana with Aid of USP Drug Quality and Information Program*, available at http://vocuspr.vocus.com/vocuspr30/ViewAttachment.aspx?EID=RSVIlQYucB5oeaAqQ%2beRWsGX7Qy88vEXkpB6QDmSuOM%3d (accessed 28 April 2010).

WHO (World Health Organization) (2004a) *The World Medicines Situation*, Geneva: WHO, available at http://apps.who.int/medicinedocs/en/d/Js6160e/3.html (accessed 27 December 2009).

WHO (World Health Organization) (2004b) *The WHO Prequalification Project*, Geneva: WHO, available at http://mednet3.who.int/prequal/ (accessed 11 February 2010).

WHO (World Health Organization) (2007) *Measuring Availability, Affordability, and Appropriate Use of Medicines: Use of the WHO Pharmaceutical Sector Level II Monitoring Tools*, Geneva: WHO, available at http://apps.who.int/medicinedocs/documents/s14877e/s14877e.pdf (accessed 11 February 2010).

WHO/HAI (World Health Organization/Health Action International, Africa) (2008) *Medicine Prices in Ghana Summary Report*, Nairobi: Health Action International, Africa.

43

Medicine Safety and Safe Access to Essential Medicines

Time for Renewed Attention and Innovation

Malebona Precious Matsoso, Ushma Mehta, and Fatima Suleman

Introduction

Medicines play a critical role in the prevention, cure, and alleviation of suffering from diseases for billions of people around the globe. They continue to be the mainstay of managing the infectious diseases that continue to devastate low- and middle-income countries (LMIC) while preventing and managing complications associated with chronic diseases that predominate in high-income countries. It cannot be disputed that medicines, as well as vaccines, have made a significant contribution to public health and have changed the course of modern medicine.

Despite these public health gains, problems associated with the appropriate use of and inadequate access to medicines by communities and individuals most in need of them prevent the full potential of these gains from being realised. Where reasonable access to medicines exists, system-related problems, costs, and inappropriate use continue to undermine the benefits that are possible with these treatments. In addition, the risks associated with adverse reactions are under-appreciated even in the most well-resourced settings.

Adverse drug reactions[1] *(ADRs)* have been shown to contribute substantially to morbidity and mortality, but continue to be a relatively neglected area of research and policy (Nebeker *et al.* 2004). Medawar (1992) contends that the risks and levels of drug injury are much higher than they should be. Although the true extent of the problem at the global level is unknown, studies and analyses conducted in various regions of the world unanimously suggest that the problem of ADRs is significant. A meta-analysis of 69 prospective and retrospective studies conducted in various regions of the world involving 419,000 patients found that approximately 6.7 per cent of all hospitalisations were drug-related (Wiffen *et al.* 2002). A report by the US Institute of Medicine (IOM) estimated that between 44,000 and 98,000 people in US hospitals die each year because of medical errors, especially medication errors (Kohn *et al.* 1999). Similarly, Runciman (2003) reports from Australia that medication errors are a major contributor to medical errors, with 26 per cent of 27,000 hospital-related incidents being medication-related, along with 36 per cent of 2,000 anaesthesia-related incidents, and 50 per cent of 2,500 general practice incidents. Needless to say, several studies have also indicated that the cost of managing ADRs places a significant burden on health care budgets (Lundkvist and Jonsson 2004).

Unfortunately, data on the nature and extent of medication-related injury in low-income countries (LIC) is scarce. In a study conducted in South Africa in the medical unit of a secondary level hospital, ADRs with treatment of HIV/AIDS and TB in the population were noted. This study highlighted the need for caution in extrapolating the results of data derived from a particular country or region to other countries where the burden of disease, access to medicines, and health care system may differ.

There is a need for global research into the burden of ADRs on public health and patient care, and to ensure that access to, and use of, essential medicines is as safe as possible. Innovative approaches need to be developed and assessed to ensure that the burden of preventable adverse reactions, medication errors, and drug-related problems are minimised, while optimising the considerable benefits of essential medicines to those individuals and communities most in need.

Understanding the scope of pharmacovigilance

The WHO (2002) defines *pharmacovigilance* as the science and activities related to the detection, assessment, understanding, and prevention of ADRs and drug-related problems. This definition encompasses the traditional practices of spontaneous reporting, and includes all activities relating to medicines safety, such as those that are aimed at collecting information on ADRs, and events and activities that aim to prevent and manage the burden of ADRs in individuals and populations.

In this chapter, we emphasise the importance of medicines safety as a public health priority within an integrated approach to medicines selection, procurement, distribution, and use as a part of public health programmes. We also consider this to be an imperative for those who have regulatory oversight.

Pharmacovigilance should not just be given attention when the products are marketed or clinical trials are conducted, but well-conceived even at the time when drugs are designed. Novel approaches are needed on how safety concerns can be mitigated through innovation from the early phases of drug development throughout the life cycle of medicines.

Pharmacovigilance is a responsibility shared by manufacturers, drug regulators, public health programmes, clinical institutions, academic researchers, health care workers, the media, and consumers alike. This area of public health can be approached from a variety of perspectives, including programmatic, legal, regulatory, and institutional frameworks, and will be discussed further in this chapter.

Drug development and pharmacovigilance

The pharmaceutical landscape has changed over the years, influenced mainly by disease burdens, particularly in developing countries, epidemiological transitions, and the international flow of funds. Drug development has also undergone significant shifts, with more attention given to optimising the characteristics of novel chemical entities to improve their potential toxicity profiles.

One of the key objectives of preclinical studies and pre-marketing clinical trials is to ensure that medicines intended for the global market are safe. Within this context, a *safe medicine* is one in which the nature, severity, and frequency of adverse effects (i.e. risk of harm) are outweighed by the benefits demonstrated by the medicine under controlled circumstances. However, this measure of safety is based on data derived from controlled clinical trial settings where the sample size, duration of exposure, and population of subjects exposed are not a good reflection of the way these medicines will be used by the global population after licensing. Pregnant women, children, the elderly, and patients who are particularly ill or affected by co-morbid conditions are often systematically excluded from such studies. Furthermore, studies have consistently shown that safety monitoring procedures during clinical trials are far from adequate despite the dissemination of international guidelines for safety monitoring during clinical trials (Ioannidis 2009; Ioannidis *et al.* 2004).

In recent years, there have been increased efforts to develop medicines for tropical neglected diseases, and diseases almost exclusively endemic to the developing world. Novel drugs, drug combinations, and vaccines have been introduced on a large scale to communities where the context of use varies considerably from the conditions in the developed world.

In some developing countries, regulatory control is weak, and medicines requiring a prescription are often dispensed by retail vendors with no medical training (Whitty *et al.* 2008). Furthermore, the significant barriers to accessing care faced by impoverished communities make the detection and management of ADRs extremely challenging. Several novel drugs and vaccines are being introduced into countries in large populations concurrently. In such situations, it can be argued that the standards of safety monitoring during clinical trials and the threshold of acceptable risk of harm for such medicines needs to be particularly high. A key challenge facing drug developers is that of maintaining a balance between ensuring that novel essential medicines are safe prior to marketing, without compromising the access of these medicines to those most in need, in as inexpensive and timely a manner as possible (Craft 2008).

Post-marketing pharmacovigilance

Regulatory pharmacovigilance

When medicines are used in health care facilities by medical doctors, nurses, or pharmacists, little is known about whether a new medicine interacts with other medicines the patient may be taking, or whether it will be as safe and effective in a population of a particular ethnicity or with a high prevalence of other concurrent diseases not included in the clinical trial population. Within this uncontrolled setting, some medicines continue to demonstrate a favourable risk-benefit profile, while others pose a risk of harm that overwhelms any benefit the medicine may provide. Swayzey (1991: 291) describes this more succinctly: 'they are unavoidably unsafe but can also not be viewed as unreasonably dangerous'. It must be remembered that the merit or value of a medicine may evolve with changes in the epidemiology of the disease being treated, and the availability of safer or more effective alternatives.

It is for these reasons that the manner in which medicines are selected and used is regulated beyond the time of initial licensing, and the information that is provided to both health professionals and patients is continually reassessed and updated throughout the life cycle of the medicine. To maximise the overall effectiveness of medicines in society, it is important to have functional systems of selection and procurement at the national and subnational levels, as well as an effective and responsive regulatory system with institutional capacity to react and respond to real or suspected drug safety concerns.

Regulatory pharmacovigilance focuses on developing a greater understanding of the risk-benefit profile of licensed medicines. Regulatory authorities employ various measures to address new safety concerns. These include product withdrawals, restrictions in use, amendments to package inserts (by including warnings and precautions), and the dissemination of alerts via the media. A number of countries have introduced measures that are aimed at improving medicines safety. To date, there are 96 countries that serve as full members of the World Health Organization's (WHO) International Drug Monitoring Programme. In all of these countries, an operational spontaneous reporting system for suspected ADRs exists. An additional 30 countries are associate members of the programme, and are in the process of developing their pharmacovigilance systems to a point where they will be able to pool and share their safety data with other countries.

The field of drug regulation is changing globally, with more onus being placed on LMIC to rely less on the regulatory decisions made in the developed world for medicines, which target neglected diseases and diseases not prevalent in the developed world. The fight against counterfeits and illegal trade in medicines is an important issue that requires urgent attention. Supporting and strengthening regulatory systems in these countries is being recognised as a high priority for safeguarding the public.

Institutional pharmacovigilance

In resource-limited countries in particular, the selection of suitable drugs as part of an essential drugs list (EDL) to meet the needs of the population is an important component of health policy, and provides the rational basis for determining a country's essential drug needs, and for guiding procurement at the national level in order to meet the requirements of different levels of the health sector. This selection should consider the efficacy, safety, quality, and cost of these medicines, identifying issues such as systems of health practice, diagnostic capacity at various levels of the health care system, and human resources available for the optimal provision of these medicines. The process of drug selection not only considers whether or not a medicine should be used within a particular country or setting, but also what health systems and policy changes are needed to ensure that the benefits of these medicines are optimised, and the potential risk of harm minimised. The EDL approach has been successful in improving the rational and safe use of medicines by health workers in many countries. Health workers become more familiar and confident in using the medicines on the list, thus further reducing the possibility of inappropriate or irrational use.

Institutional pharmacovigilance relates to activities occurring within health facilities such as clinics, hospitals, and pharmacies. These activities are usually coordinated by a pharmacy and therapeutics committee, pharmacists, and a quality assurance department. The focus of pharmacovigilance within these institutions is to minimise the potential for preventable ADRs and drug-drug or drug-disease interactions. This is likely to reduce hospital costs, the duration of hospitalisation in patients, and liability to the institution. Activities such as therapeutic drug monitoring, formulary management, and specific monitoring of high-risk medicines are some examples of programmes within institutions that can have a positive impact on patient safety.

Some countries have addressed drug safety broadly as part of patient safety campaigns, while others have specifically targeted medicine safety as a priority in itself.

Public health pharmacovigilance

Over the years, novel medicinal products with limited clinical experience have been introduced as a critical part of vertical public health programmes (e.g. antiretrovirals (ARVs), antimalarials, novel vaccines, antibiotics). Public health programmes have a responsibility for ensuring that these medicines enjoy the public's confidence, and that the use of these medicines within the public health programme occurs as safely as possible.

For instance, national immunisation programmes are being encouraged to introduce surveillance systems for adverse events following immunisation. These systems are designed to ensure that preventable 'programme errors' and serious adverse events that have the potential to cause community concerns, are detected and reported as soon as possible. In-depth investigations into these concerns are immediately initiated, and any shortcomings addressed in order to minimise any further problems.

Access to safe medicines vs. safe access to medicines

In recent years, global access programmes have evolved to provide essential medicines to those most in need. Programmes such as the Affordable Medicines Facility – malaria (AMF-m) managed by the Global Fund, the President's Malarial Initiative (PMI), President's Emergency Plan For AIDS Relief (PEPFAR), Global Alliance Vaccine Initiative (GAVI) and more recently UNITAID (international facility for the purchase of drugs against HIV/AIDS, Malaria and Tuberculosis), are examples of funding programmes that have facilitated widescale access of vaccines, ARVs, and artemisinin-based combination treatments for malaria in LMIC at practically every level of health care.

Thus, medicines are likely to be used by health workers and vendors in the private sector, who have limited access to drug information and limited training in the principles of pharmacology and therapeutics. Misuse and overprescribing of these medicines are likely to occur in these settings of limited diagnostic capacity and expertise. Clinical suspicion that adverse experiences in patients could be drug-related is low in settings with poor reporting cultures and poor awareness of the safety profile of these medicines. Drug interactions, shared toxicities, and medication errors are likely to occur when patients are exposed concurrently to more than one essential medicine.

As mentioned earlier, *safe medicines* are medicines with an inherently favourable risk-benefit profile based on data from clinical trials, and that may or may not include data from the post-licensing period. These represent the inherent pharmacological profile of the medicines, and also include a medicine's potential to cause toxicities and significant drug interactions, the risk in specific vulnerable populations, and potential for abuse/misuse and toxicity as a result of a narrow therapeutic window (the range of dosage of a drug or of its concentration in a bodily system that provides safe effective therapy) or pharmacokinetic profile (the absorption, distribution, metabolism, and excretion of drugs in the body).

Safe access to medicines refers to the extrinsic conditions under which the medicine in question is likely to be used, and whether these conditions support the safe use of the medicine. For example, if a medicine has a narrow therapeutic window and therefore requires careful clinical or laboratory monitoring, safe access would imply the concurrent provision of such laboratory tests, and relevant training of healthcare workers, to ensure that appropriate monitoring of patients is possible at institutions where the medicine is likely to be used or prescribed.

Of course, safe medicines and safe access are linked, although one is more inherent to the properties of the medicine itself, while the latter is a function of the health care system, environment, and conditions of use of the medicine.

Pharmaceutical assessments in some countries have revealed that ineffective drug supply management, inappropriate medicines use, and weak medicines regulation are barriers to sustainable availability and safe access to quality medicines. One of the key factors that make access safe is the provision of drug information to users and consumers of these medicines. Additionally, safe access is the provision of a consistent supply of safe, effective, and good quality medicines, where it is most needed. These are discussed in more detail below.

Access to drug information

The provision of useful, unbiased, and evidence-based drug information to consumers, health professionals, and the public is fundamental to ensuring that access to medicines occurs as safely as possible. In this context, drug information does not only relate to the characteristics of the medicine in question, but also to training around when the medicine can and cannot be used, how it should be used, what alternatives exist, and how they compare to each other. The provision of drug information also relates to providing users with guidance on how to manage situations of adverse events and failed treatment.

Drug information is made available in legally mandated expressions in the form of package inserts and patient information leaflets. In addition, drug information centres based within regulatory authorities, Ministries of Health, hospitals, pharmaceutical companies, and non-governmental organisations (NGOs) have played a role in providing information primarily to health professionals who prescribe and dispense medicines. In most developed countries, manufacturers have a legal duty and responsibility to monitor their products, and to ensure that prescribers and patients have the most up-to-date information on cautions and contra-indications. Most legal provisions in consumer protection laws hold companies responsible for failure to warn. However, in countries with poorly evolved regulatory mechanisms, relevant legislation and such enforcement powers are lacking.

In addition, the efforts to ensure that these medicines are used correctly are derailed by aggressive marketing practices that create confusion and misunderstanding among users of this information. Uncontrolled access to misinformation, particularly via the internet, has added to the complexity of access to drug information. Conversely, in resource-limited settings, access to even basic drug information is rare, and medicines are often prescribed or dispensed by unskilled individuals with no knowledge about the risk and benefits of these products. A key challenge facing policymakers today is how to counteract the effects of misinformation and aggressive marketing practices, while still ensuring that reliable, user-friendly, evidence-based drug information is consistently available to health care workers and consumers. Drug information needs to be made available at all levels of health care, including at the community level, and delivered in a manner that is suitable for the intended audience and purpose. This calls for innovation and investment in appropriate resources, and partnership between the various stakeholders, including drug regulators, policymakers, academics, essential drug programmes, health care providers, and consumers.

Perhaps one of the most fundamental, but most neglected functions of drug information systems is the provision of feedback to health staff and communities. While performing their daily health care activities, care providers within the health unit record data for patient/client and health unit management. Routine health unit-based data can also be aggregated to generate information on services provided to the population, for disease surveillance, and for pharmacovigilance. However, these professionals are poorly motivated to produce quality data, because most data collected are irrelevant to their own information needs. They rarely receive feedback on the data reported at higher levels, so they have little incentive to ensure the quality of the collected data, and comply with reporting requirements. The provision of drug information has been shown to be a powerful incentive to supporting pharmacovigilance surveillance systems (Bukirwa *et al.* 2008).

Safeguarding the drug delivery chain

Safe access to medicines also refers to careful planning and forecasting by national procurement agencies in order to ensure that adequate quantities of essential medicines are available at the relevant levels of health care over time. This is a critical activity that has a significant impact on reducing the potential for waste and critical drug shortages, which could have a devastating impact on public health programmes and clinical care. However, in many countries, public health officials have limited experience in designing an optimal procurement system to fit their market context.

Drug shortages are a challenge for the health care community, particularly since they typically appear with little or no warning, and significant resources may be needed to manage patients when a particular therapy is in short supply. Health workers at the facility level are then left to deal with the problems this creates. Which drug should the patient be switched to in the absence of the prescribed drug? How do health workers emphasise adherence to therapy if drugs are not supplied consistently? In the cases of countries facing epidemics of HIV/AIDS, TB, and malaria, shortages of these drugs can be disastrous. Failure to strictly adhere to TB/HIV medication increases the likelihood that a patient will develop resistant strains of the disease and may become unresponsive to treatment once drug supply is re-established. It also adversely impacts patients with chronic conditions who are controlled on their current therapy, and may be the difference between life and death in the case of acute, life-threatening conditions.

Changes in drug supply can alter the way drugs are prepared in the pharmacy, the way they are administered to patients, and, in some cases, whether patients receive drugs at all. Aside from managing the drug supply cycle more diligently, health policymakers and managers need to be more proactive. To encourage greater transparency and accountability around the procurement, supply, and use of medicines, information should be made available as soon as a shortage is detected. Prescribers are more constructive and cooperative if they are involved in the process, and information regarding the shortage needs to be disseminated to those who will be impacted by it as soon as possible (Tyler and Mark 2002).

Key elements to a successful programme for managing supply and procurement problems include analysis of the root causes of inadequate drug supply; a tested system for involving the entire health care organisation quickly; and clear channels for communicating information and plans with all those involved, especially patients, when necessary (Neame and Boelen 1993).

Conclusion

Access to essential medicines that are safe, effective, and meet quality standards for those most in need still remains a challenge. A growing body of research indicates that ADRs, medication errors, and other drug-related problems are a major cause of hospitalisation in the developed and possibly developing world. The need for prioritising the safe access to medicines is becoming internationally recognised by donors and governments alike. The elements of safe, reliable access of essential medicines include: (1) the creation of pharmacovigilance systems from the earliest point of drug development throughout the life cycle of the medicine. This includes regulatory, institutional, and programmatic pharmacovigilance systems; (2) the provision of reliable and useful drug information to policymakers, prescribers, dispensers, and users of medicines; and (3) the development and maintenance of a reliable drug supply chain at national and international levels.

However, in most countries, ensuring safe access to essential medicines remains a major and under-appreciated challenge. In order to meet this challenge, the size and severity of the problem must be acknowledged by policymakers and society alike, and an ethos of safety awareness cultivated among users of medicines. Within this culture of awareness, innovation at all levels of health care and drug development is likely to arise. Strategies that are locally responsive, cost-effective, and meaningfully improve the level of health care offered to patients and the public can be developed to minimise the risk of harm and optimise the benefits of medicines.

Note

1 An adverse drug reaction is defined by the World Health Organization as 'any response to a drug which is noxious and unintended, and which occurs at doses normally used in man for prophylaxis, diagnosis or therapy of disease, or for the modification of physiological function' (World Health Organization (2002) *The Importance of Pharmacovigilance: Safety Monitoring of Medicinal Products*, Geneva: WHO).

References

Bukirwa, H., Nayiga, S., Lubanga, R., Mwebaza, N., Chandler, C., Hopkins, H., Talisuna, A.O., and Staedke, S.G. (2008) 'Pharmacovigilance of antimalarial treatment in Uganda: community perceptions and suggestions for reporting adverse events', *Tropical Medicine and International Health*, 13(9): 1,143–52.

Craft, J.C. (2008) 'Challenges facing drug development for malaria', *Current Opinion in Microbiology*, 11: 428–33.

Ioannidis, J.P. (2009) 'Adverse events in randomized trials: neglected, restricted, distorted and silenced', *Archives of Internal Medicine*, 169(19): 1,737–9.

Ioannidis, J.P., Evans, S.J., Gotzsche, P.C., O'Neill, R.T., Altman, D.G., Schulz, K., Moher, D., and CONSORT Group (2004) 'Better reporting of harms in randomized trials: An extension of the CONSORT statement', *Annals of Internal Medicine*, 141(10): 781–8.

Kohn, L.T., Corrigan, J.M., and Donaldson, M.S. (eds) (1999) *To Err is Human: Building a Safer Health System*, Washington, DC: National Academy Press, available at http://books.nap.edu/openbook.php?record_id=9728andpage=R1 (accessed 13 November 2009).

Lundkvist, J. and Jonsson, B. (2004) 'Pharmacoeconomics of adverse drug reactions', *Fundamental and Clinical Pharmacology*, 18: 275–80.

Medawar, C. (1992) *Power and Dependence: Social Audit on the Safety of Medicines*, London: Social Audit.

Neame, R. and Boelen, C. (1993) *Information Management for Improving Relevance and Efficiency in the Health Sector: A Framework for the Development of Health Information Systems*, Geneva: World Health Organization.

Nebeker, J.R., Barach, P., and Samore, M.H. (2004) 'Clarifying adverse drug events: a clinician's guide to terminology, documentation, and reporting', *Annals of Internal Medicine*, 140: 795–801.

Runciman, W.B., Roughead, E.E., Semple, S.J., Adams, R.J. (2003) 'Adverse drug events and medication errors in Australia', *International Journal for Quality in Health Care*, 15(suppl 1): i49–59.

Swayzey, J.P. (1991) 'Prescription Drug Safety and Product Liability', in P.W. Huber and R.E. Litan (eds) *The Liability Maze: The Impact of Liability Law on Safety and Innovation*, Washington, DC: Brookings Institution Press: 291–333.

Tyler, L.S., and Mark, S.M. (2002) 'Understanding and Managing Drug Shortages', in the American Society of Health-System Pharmacists, Midyear Clinical Meeting, Atlanta, GA, 9 December.

Whitty, C.J.M., Chandler, C., Ansah, E., Leslie, T., and Staedke, S.G. (2008) 'Deployment of ACT antimalarials for treatment of malaria: challenges and opportunities', *Malaria Journal*, 7(Supplement 1): S7.

Wiffen, P., Gill, M., Edwards, J., Moore, A. (2002) 'Adverse drug reactions in hospital settings: A systematic review of the prospective and retrospective studies', *Bandolier Extra*, available at http://www.medicine.ox.ac.uk/bandolier/extra.html (accessed 13 November 2009).

WHO (World Health Organization) (2002) *The Importance of Pharmacovigilance*, available at http://www.who.int/medicinedocs/en/d/Js4893e/ (accessed 13 November 2009).

44

Saving the Lives of Children by Improving Access to Essential Medicines in the Community

Martha Embrey, Jane Briggs, and Grace Adeya

Global financial resources for health

A number of global initiatives, such as the President's Emergency Plan for AIDS Relief (PEPFAR) and UNITAID, have resulted in a quadrupling of health resources for poorer countries between 1990 and 2007, mostly for HIV/AIDS, but also with increases for malaria and tuberculosis (Ravishankar *et al.* 2009). For example, the Global Fund to Fight AIDS, Tuberculosis and Malaria (GFATM) alone has approved grants for over $15.5 billion – nearly 50 per cent of which is allocated for medicines and commodities.[1] These new pharmaceutical funding sources have greatly affected medicine and commodity procurement, distribution, and pharmacy management systems, especially in countries heavily affected by HIV. Although the largest initiatives have focused on particular diseases and not specifically on child health, there has been leveraging, especially in malaria activities that focus on community medicine distribution and generally target vulnerable children under five years of age.

Pushing a global agenda to improve child health

Aside from the global focus on AIDS, tuberculosis, and malaria, child mortality is still a huge problem. Fortunately, the increased attention and resources for international health have also produced several global initiatives to improve the state of children's health. Many of these initiatives support the Millennium Development Goals (MDGs) by promoting the Integrated Management of Childhood Illness (IMCI) strategy and addressing widespread recommendations to increase community-based access to medicines. MDG 4 is to reduce the under-five mortality rate by two-thirds between 1990 and 2015. To achieve this goal, the global recommendations include preventing and providing effective treatment of childhood illnesses and promoting universal coverage of primary health care through community health workers (UN 2008; WHO/UNICEF 2004a, 2004b). These objectives rely on the availability of quality-assured and appropriate medicines, but planners of community health care interventions often forget about the importance of managing medicines.

The IMCI strategy, developed by the World Health Organization (WHO) and the United Nations Children's Fund (UNICEF), targets the leading causes of childhood mortality: acute respiratory infection, diarrhoea, malaria, malnutrition, and measles (WHO/UNICEF 1999). The strategy involves three components: (1) improving the case management skills of health care providers, (2) improving the health system needed to manage childhood illness, and (3) improving family and community health practices.

Most affected countries started implementing IMCI between 1996–2001, which helped reduce under-five mortality (Murray *et al.* 2007). However, an evaluation of IMCI implementation showed that countries need to concentrate more on improving how childhood illness is managed within the community (Bryce *et al.* 2005).

In 2003, the *Lancet* published a series of articles on child survival that combined evidence, analysis, and advocacy related to decreasing the estimated 10.8 million annual deaths of children under five years of age. One article concluded that low-cost interventions, such as the use of oral rehydration therapy for diarrhoea, were already available to reduce child deaths by two-thirds, but that widespread coverage across countries was lacking (Jones *et al.* 2003). In fact, recent data show that across 68 countries, a median of 38 per cent of children with diarrhoea receive oral rehydration therapy, while only 32 per cent receive antibiotics for pneumonia (Countdown to 2015, 2008).

Jones and colleagues concluded that 'There is no need to wait for new vaccines, new drugs, or new technology. … The main challenge today is to transfer what we already know into action …' (2003: 70). This series served as an effective call-to-action as child health advocates mobilised to expand the reach of existing interventions and to leverage resources from other organisations receiving global health funding. For example, the Partnership for Maternal, Newborn and Child Health was launched in 2005 to bring together the maternal, newborn, and child health communities to support the work underway to achieve related MDGs. One of the Partnership's six priority areas is *essential commodities* (e.g. medicines and health supplies needed to treat the main causes of morbidity and mortality in children), and the Partnership strives to have members harmonise their commodity management and supply strategies to maximise resources.

Health-seeking and medicine use practices in the community

People's care-seeking patterns differ according to geography, wealth, and health condition, and on factors such as availability of medicines and comfort with the care provider. Although children are more likely than adults to receive formal health care, caretakers frequently treat children at home for common illnesses, such as malaria and diarrhoea, and often with medicines obtained from a community source, such as a drug shop (Goodman *et al.* 2007). The inefficient and even unsafe treatment of illnesses through inappropriate medicine use is a problem in many settings. These problems can be caused by inappropriate or irrational practices on the part of providers, such as dispensing an unsuitable medicine, or poor treatment adherence on the part of caregivers. Therefore, improving child health means ensuring that the correct treatment is available at the community level and that families seek, obtain, and appropriately use the right medicines.

What is community case management?

Community case management (CCM) is a strategy responding to international recommendations to deliver community-level treatment for common, serious childhood infections (CORE Group *et al.* 2010). CCM relies on trained, supervised community members to provide interventions, such as antibiotics, oral rehydration therapy, anti-malarials, zinc, and vitamin A. These community-based providers can be in the public or private sectors, and can include traditional healers and pharmacists (Box 44.1).

Box 44.1 Community health care providers

- Health facilities (e.g. government, private, or mission facilities)
- Licensed retail medicine sales outlets (e.g. pharmacies, chemists, drug shops)
- Other retail outlets selling medicines (e.g. general stores, kiosks)
- Licensed individuals dispensing medicines (e.g. community health workers (CHWs), health huts)
- Other individuals dispensing medicines (e.g. traditional healers, street vendors)
- Child's caregiver in a household

Source: Nachbar *et al.* 2003.

Many countries have established CCM using networks of community health workers (CHWs), but other informal health care providers in the community can also provide curative services; for example, in many resource-limited countries, community members often first seek advice and medicines from retail drug sellers – especially in rural areas, where public facilities may not be easy to reach. Because many of these outlets are loosely regulated, the quality of the medicines and services they offer are suspect. Initiatives to improve service quality include training to improve drug sellers' case management skills, and franchising and accreditation models for drug shops. For example, in Kenya and Rwanda, the Child and Family Wellness Shops use a franchising model to assure quality pharmaceuticals and services in its network of small clinics and pharmacies, whereas the accredited drug dispensing outlet (ADDO) programme in Tanzania uses government accreditation and inspection to maintain quality standards as described below (see Box 44.2).

Box 44.2 Using the private sector to improve child health in Tanzania: the Accredited Drug Dispensing Programme

By applying the IMCI strategy in the public sector, Tanzania has improved case management and reduced child mortality. To fill the gap for the many who seek care in the private sector, the government endorsed incorporating a child health component based on IMCI methodology into services provided by ADDOs. The ADDO programme created retail medicine shops that must adhere to quality standards to achieve and maintain government accreditation. The ADDOs' package of child health interventions focuses on increasing the number of children correctly treated for malaria, acute respiratory infection, and diarrhoea, and improving community awareness of the importance of promptly attending to a sick child. A key objective is to promote ADDOs as a source of treatment and advice for child health in communities with poor access to health facilities.

Over 1,300 dispensers from four regions have been trained to deliver child health services. Supportive supervision is key to the success of the ADDO programme, and for the child health component, a district team initially visits stores every three months to review records, observe store operations, and discuss issues with the dispensers. Thousands of posters and flyers related to child health, family planning, and HIV/AIDS have been distributed to ADDOs, which help establish them as centres of community public health information. In addition, outreach meetings with almost 1,000 regional, district, and community leaders have garnered local support for delivering child health services through ADDOs.

Sources: RPM Plus, CEEMI, and BASICS 2007.

The role of managing medicines in community case management

As mentioned previously, community health care interventions often ignore the importance of managing medicines. For CCM to succeed, medicines and supplies need to be available, managed appropriately, and used rationally (according to standardised treatment guidelines). Even with the increased funding for pharmaceuticals in developing countries mentioned earlier, major challenges remain in assuring that children have access to essential medicines. For example, Robertson and colleagues (2009) found that on average, public and private outlets in 14 central African countries had only half the essential medicines on their shelf. Clearly, children cannot receive appropriate treatment if medicine shortages are common.

Pharmaceutical management involves four basic functions: selection, procurement, distribution, and use (Figure 44.1) (Management Sciences for Health/WHO 1997). In the CCM context, *selection* involves reviewing the community's health problems, identifying treatments that can be appropriately delivered at the community level, and deciding which medicines will be available in the CCM programme. *Procurement* for CCM includes determining what quantity and how medicines will be bought or obtained on a national level and how they will be financed. *Distribution* establishes how the CHWs or other community providers will receive and maintain the right amounts of the products needed. *Use* includes diagnosing, prescribing, and dispensing by the provider plus proper usage by the patient.

In the pharmaceutical management framework, each major function builds on the previous function and leads logically to the next – all dependent on information systems, management support, and a policy and legal framework. For example, medicines and supplies used in CCM programmes should be consistent with the national child health programme's recommendations and other pharmaceutical regulations.

Many factors influence whether medicines are available and used appropriately, and ultimately, whether young children recover from potentially life-threatening illnesses. The diagram in Figure 44.2 details the framework for the availability and appropriate use of medicines for childhood illnesses at the community level.

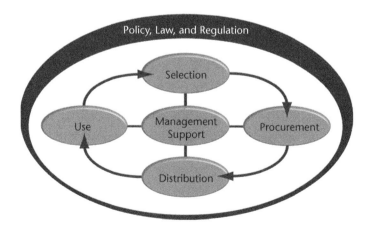

Figure 44.1   Pharmaceutical management
Source: Management Sciences for Health/WHO 1997.

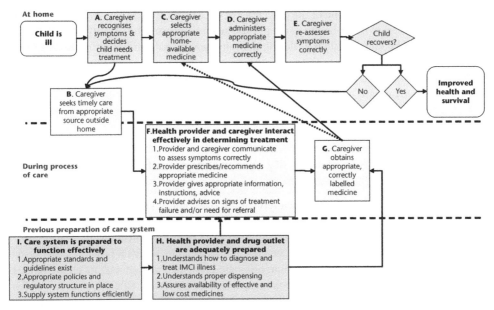

Figure 44.2 Framework for appropriate community drug management for childhood illness
Source: Ross-Degnan *et al.* 2008.

Barriers to initiating community case management

Although many experts, organisations, and initiatives support CCM as a feasible strategy to improve child health and reduce deaths, barriers often stand in the way of initiating large-scale programmes that feature community-based treatment. For example, many countries have policies that limit medicine dispensing, especially antibiotics, by non-medical providers. In addition, getting CCM onto a national health care agenda can be difficult. In a recent survey, only 18 of 68 priority countries reported having CCM policies, with respondents' progress limited by decision-making about who would be permitted to administer antibiotics (Countdown to 2015, 2008).

A key component of the ADDO programme's success in Tanzania was the policy change allowing accredited dispensers to dispense select antibiotics, and showing that with proper training, they dispensed them appropriately; however, revising existing policies is often complicated. Sometimes, countries allow CCM only with special restrictions, such as in emergency settings or in sparsely populated states. Because CHWs in Tanzania are not allowed to dispense medicines, ADDO dispensers fill an important niche, especially in rural communities.

To get around policy limitations, many government and NGO programmes use a model in which CHWs promote healthy practices, assess sick children, and offer simple remedies, but then refer children who need antimicrobial treatment to primary health facilities. The problem, however, with a referral-based model is that caretakers often choose not to seek treatment in public facilities for reasons such as distance and long lines. In addition, community providers who cannot supply curative treatment lose credibility (Lehmann and Sanders 2007).

For those programmes that do allow community-based providers to dispense some medicines, finding a reliable source of medicines can be a challenge. CHWs usually rely on the nearest public health facility, but often those facilities have trouble keeping medicines in stock for their own use. And because one of the objectives of CCM is to provide care in places that may not have easy access to other health care options, such as a nearby clinic, getting medicines to these places can be difficult, such as during the rainy season, so distribution needs to be well planned.

Another medicine-related challenge for CCM is the lack of appropriate paediatric formulations, which simplify treatment administration and improve adherence. When available, paediatric formulations need to be in the national procurement and medicine supply system to assure that CHWs have them on hand.

Ongoing challenges in community case management

Established CCM programmes also face challenges, such as assuring that community providers receive continuous support, adding new interventions over time, and achieving and maintaining financial sustainability. In addition to the operational factors, the success of CCM ultimately relies on the providers' standing in their community and their relationship with its members.

Years of experience have shown that viable CCM programmes rely on providing supportive supervision and refresher training to community-based providers and enough incentive to keep them engaged. In some settings, face-to-face supervision may not be efficient or even possible because of the sheer number of workers, which requires more innovative supervisory mechanisms. For example, in Rwanda, CHWs are supervised by a peer who is selected based on performance or educational criteria (Manning *et al.* 2008). Incentives for community providers, either monetary or non-monetary, help prevent attrition and maintain motivation. Some compensation systems are based on a revolving fund, where in addition to medicines, providers sell products such as soap and toothpaste for a small profit. Incentive packages, however, will vary depending on the national policy and community context.

Additional ongoing issues include the temptation of programme planners to overload providers with conditions to treat and changing existing case management recommendations, which requires careful coordination. When zinc was recently added as a recommended diarrhoea treatment, countries needed to ensure that it was incorporated into the supply system and work with providers to assure its correct use by providing training and informational materials.

Finally, many government budgets do not include funding for CCM programmes, in the belief that such programmes are low-cost and self-sustainable. These issues may be easily addressed in a geographically restricted or pilot programme, but scaling up and ultimate integration into the country's health system results in logistical and financial challenges. Leveraging among different donor organisations can provide the resources to initiate and scale-up CCM, but financial sustainability may be more elusive.

Community case management successes

Countries with supportive policies and successful CCM programmes can provide technical support and exchange lessons learned with neighbouring countries. Examples of successful community case management follow.

Afghanistan

After decades of war, Afghanistan's child survival rates were close to the world's worst. Geographic isolation, culture, and security prevent many women and children from accessing care at public health facilities, so the Afghan government trained 20,000 CHWs – half of them women and most illiterate. Their jobs include providing IMCI and advice to mothers on child care and family planning. About half of all sick children are now seen by CHWs and increased access has contributed to the 25 per cent decline in child mortality seen over five years (Aitken *et al.* 2009).

Nepal

The Ministry of Health in Nepal trains female community health volunteers (FCHVs) to provide some health services in their community. When FCHVs were given responsibility for managing childhood pneumonia using co-trimoxazole, some questioned the cadre's ability to correctly diagnose and treat pneumonia, especially those who were semi-literate. These concerns were addressed by using pictorial training materials to facilitate understanding. The intervention also includes regular refresher training for the FCHVs and community orientation to the concept. In the programme's first decade, districts with FCHVs doubled the number of children who received treatment – saving an estimated 6,000 lives a year. The intervention now covers about 80 per cent of children, with plans for universal coverage in the next two years (Dawson *et al.* 2008; Global Health Council 2009).

Democratic Republic of Congo

Since 2005, the CCM programme in DRC has trained hundreds of CHWs to manage uncomplicated childhood conditions. A key component of the CCM strategy was managing medicines, and training included how to track inventory and calculate medicine needs. Initial programme results showed that 90 per cent of 20 randomly sampled CHWs dispensed the correct quantity of medicine; all said the medicine name and formulation and how to administer it; 90 per cent asked the caregiver to repeat the instructions to assure understanding; and stock-outs were rare (Bukasa *et al.* 2008). Investing in pharmaceutical management from programme initiation has encouraged positive results including minimised stock-outs and appropriate dispensing practices.

Senegal

Based on evidence showing wide misuse of antibiotics, the Ministry of Health introduced a policy permitting CHWs with special training and close supervision to treat cases of childhood pneumonia with co-trimoxazole. Evaluation showed that nearly 90 per cent of workers correctly evaluated, classified, and treated acute respiratory illnesses, plus there were no co-trimoxazole stock-outs. In addition, nearly twice as many pneumonia cases were treated in intervention areas than in control districts. As a result, the Ministry of Health extended the community-based pneumonia treatment project nationwide (Senauer *et al.* 2008).

Detailing the experiences countries have had with community case management and community health workers to improve child health is beyond the scope of this chapter, however, Box 44.3 includes a number of resources to consult for further reference.

Tools

A variety of tools are available to help implement community case management programmes; for example, a useful programmatic guide is *Community Case Management Essentials: A Guide for*

Box 44.3 Additional resources on community health worker programmes

Community Health Workers: A Review of Concepts, Practice and Policy Concerns
(Prasad and Muraleedharan 2007)
Achieving Child Survival Goals: Potential Contribution of Community Health Workers
(Haines *et al.* 2007)
Community Health Workers: What do we know about them? The State of the Evidence on Programmes,
Activities, Costs and Impact on Health Outcomes of using Community Health Workers
(Lehmann and Sanders 2007)
Scaling up Health and Education Workers: Community Health Workers
(Abbatt 2005)
Do Lay Health Workers Improve Healthcare Delivery and Healthcare Outcomes? Evidence Update
(Effective Healthcare Alliance Programme 2006)

Program Managers. This resource provides guidance for the design, implementation, and monitoring of CCM. The book includes a chapter on managing medicines and supplies.

An example of a community assessment tool is *Community Drug Management for Childhood Illness: Assessment Manual*. This tool evaluates practices of use of medicines to treat childhood illnesses and malaria at two levels in the community – provider and household. The tool has been used in Cambodia, DRC, Peru, Mali, Zambia, and Senegal, and is available in English, French and Spanish.

Improving Community Use of Medicines in the Management of Child Illness: A Guide to Developing Interventions describes a series of steps for developing interventions to improve management of medicines for child illness in the community.

In addition to programmatic tools, CHWs need to have the proper training and tools on how to manage medicines appropriately. Such inventory tools can include stock cards, order forms, and monthly reports. Some training and reporting tools also need to be creatively adapted to account for semi- or non-literate CHWs. *Community Case Management Essentials: A Guide for Program Managers* lists examples of both inventory tools and picture-based tools for CHWs.

Conclusion

The growing international concern for high mortality rates in children under five years of age, as well as a global increase in funding and opportunities to improve health care delivery, has resulted in a surge of interest in using CCM to increase access to basic treatment in the community. Planners of community health care interventions, however, often forget about the importance of managing medicines. Experiences have shown that including pharmaceutical management early in CCM programmes produces positive results by equipping stakeholders with the necessary skills and tools to assure the availability and appropriate use of medicines.

Note

1 The Global Fund for AIDS, Tuberculosis and Malaria (no date) *Distribution of Funding after 7 Rounds*, available at http://www.theglobalfund.org/en/distributionfunding/?lang=en (accessed 16 June 2009).

References

Abbatt, F. (2005) *Scaling Up Health and Education Workers: Community Health Workers*, London: Department for International Development Health Resource Centre, available at http://www.dfidhealthrc.org/publications/health_service_delivery/05HRScalingUp03.pdf (accessed 18 August 2009).

Aitken, I., Omar, F., Raza, A., Noorzada, A., and Alawi, S.A. (2009) 'Pictorial C-IMCI Technology for Illiterate Community Health Workers in Afghanistan', in Global Health Council, The 36th Annual International Conference on Global Health, paper presented at the 36th Annual International Conference on Global Health, Washington, DC, 26–30 May.

Bryce, J., Victora, C.G., Habicht, J.P., Black, R.E., Scherpbier, R.W., and MCE-IMCI Technical Advisors (2005) 'Programmatic Pathways to Child Survival: Results of a Multi-country Evaluation of Integrated Management of Childhood Illness', *Health Policy and Planning*, 20(Supplement 1): i5–i17.

Bukasa, G., Senauer, K., Briggs, J., and Adeya, G. (2008) 'Don't Forget the Medicines: Community Case Management, DRC', in Global Health Council, The 35th Annual International Conference on Global Health, Washington, DC, 27–31 May.

CORE Group, Save the Children, and USAID (US Agency for International Development) (2010) 'What is CCM and Why Should it be Considered?' in *Community Case Management Essentials. Treating Common Childhood Illnesses in the Community: A Guide for Program Managers*, Washington, DC: CORE Group, Save the Children, and USAID.

Countdown to 2015, Maternal, Newborn, & Child Survival (2008) *Tracking Progress in Maternal, Newborn & Child Survival: The 2008 Report*, New York: United Nations Children's Fund.

Dawson, P., Pradhan, Y.V., Houston, R., Karki, S., Poudel, D., and Hodgins, S. (2008) 'From Research to National Expansion: 20 Years' Experience of Community-based Management of Childhood Pneumonia in Nepal', *Bulletin of the World Health Organization*, 86(5): 339–43.

Effective Healthcare Alliance Programme (2006) *Do Lay Health Workers Improve Healthcare Delivery and Healthcare Outcomes? Evidence Update*, Liverpool: Liverpool School of Tropical Medicine, available at http://www.liv.ac.uk/evidence/evidenceupdate/HSD_Health-workers_CD004015_MAR06.pdf (accessed 18 August 2009).

Global Health Council (2009) 'Female Community Volunteers Save Children from Pneumonia Deaths in Nepal', *Global Health*, available at http://www.globalhealthmagazine.com/field_notes/nepal_female_community_health_volunteers_saving_children_from_pneumonia-rel (accessed 18 August 2009).

Goodman, C., Brieger, W., Unwin, A., Mills, A., Meek, S., and Greer, G. (2007) 'Medicine Sellers and Malaria Treatment in Sub-Saharan Africa: What do They Do and How can Their Practice be Improved?', *American Journal of Tropical Medicine and Hygiene*, 77(Supplement 6): 203–18.

Haines, A., Sanders, D., Lehmann, U., Rowe, A.K., Lawn, J.E., Jan, S., Walker, D.G., and Bhutta, Z. (2007) 'Achieving Child Survival Goals: Potential Contribution of Community Health Workers', *The Lancet*, 369(9,579): 2121–31.

Jones, G., Steketee, R.W., Black, R.E., Bhutta, Z.A., Morris, S.S., and Bellagio Child Survival Study Group (2003) 'How Many Child Deaths Can We Prevent this Year?', *The Lancet*, 362(9,377): 65–71.

Lehmann, U. and Sanders, D. (2007) *Community Health Workers: What do We Know About Them? The State of the Evidence on Programmes, Activities, Costs and Impact on Health Outcomes of Using Community Health Workers*, Geneva: World Health Organization, available at http://www.who.int/hrh/documents/community_health_workers.pdf (accessed 18 August 2009).

Management Sciences for Health and WHO (World Health Organization) (1997) *Managing Drug Supply: The Selection, Procurement, Distribution, and Use of Pharmaceuticals*, 2nd edn, West Hartford, CT: Kumarian Press.

Manning, J., Hoffmann, K., and Forrest, J. (2008) *Rwanda Community Health Needs Assessment*, Washington, DC: US Agency for International Development.

Murray, C.J.L., Laakso, T., Shibuya, K., Hill, K., and Lopez, A.D. (2007) 'Can We Achieve Millennium Development Goal 4? New Analysis of Country Trends and Forecasts for Under-5 Mortality to 2015', *The Lancet*, 370: 1,040–54.

Nachbar, N., Briggs, J., Aupont, O., Shafritz, L., Bongiovanni, A., Acharya, K., Zimicki, S., Holschneider, S., and Ross-Degnan, D. (2003) *Community Drug Management for Childhood Illness: Assessment Manual*, submitted to the U.S. Agency for International Development by the Rational Pharmaceutical Management Plus Program, Arlington, VA: Management Sciences for Health.

Prasad, B.M. and Muraleedharan, V.R. (2007) *Community Health Workers: A Review of Concepts, Practice and Policy Concerns. International Consortium for Research on Equitable Health Systems*, available at http://www.hrhresourcecenter.org/hosted_docs/CHW_Prasad_Muraleedharan.pdf (accessed 18 August 2009).

RPM Plus, CEEMI, and BASICS (Rational Pharmaceutical Management Plus Program, Centre for Enhancement of Effective Malaria Interventions and Basic Support for Institutionalizing Child Survival) (2007) *Improving Child Health through the Accredited Drug Dispensing Outlet Program: Baseline from Five Districts in Tanzania, September 2006*, Arlington, VA: Basic Support for Institutionalizing Child Survival and Rational Pharmaceutical Management Plus Program/ Management Sciences for Health.

Ravishankar, N., Gubbins, P., Cooley, R.J., Leach-Kemon, K., Michaud, C.M., Jamison, D.T., and Murray, C.J.L. (2009) 'Financing of Global Health: Tracking Development Assistance for Health from 1990 to 2007', *The Lancet*, 373: 2,113–24.

Robertson, J., Forte, G., Trapsidac, J-M., and Hill, S. (2009) 'What Essential Medicines for Children are on the Shelf?' *Bulletin of the World Health Organization*, 87: 231–7.

Ross-Degnan, D., Backes-Kozhimannil, K., Payson, A., Aupont, O., LeCates, R., Chalker, J., and Briggs, J. (2008) *Improving Community Use of Medicines in the Management of Child Illness: A Guide to Developing Interventions*, Arlington, VA: Rational Pharmaceutical Management Plus Program/Management Sciences for Health.

Senauer, K., Briggs, J., Saleeb, S., and Adeya, G. (2008) 'Improving Child Health through Informed Policy Decisions and Targeted Interventions to Strengthen Medicine Management in the Community: The Example of Senegal', in Global Health Council, The 35th Annual International Conference on Global Health, Washington, DC, 27–31 May.

UN (United Nations) (2008) *Goal 4: Reduce Child Mortality Fact Sheet, DPI/2517 J*, New York: UN.

WHO/UNICEF (World Health Organization and United Nations Children's Fund) (1999) 'Management of Childhood Illness in Developing Countries: Rationale for an Integrated Strategy', WHO/CHS/CAH/98.1A. REV.1 1999, Geneva: WHO.

WHO/UNICEF (World Health Organization and United Nations Children's Fund) (2004a) 'WHO/UNICEF Joint Statement: Management of Childhood Pneumonia in Community Settings', WHO/FCH/CAH/04.06, Geneva: WHO.

WHO/UNICEF (World Health Organization and United Nations Children's Fund) (2004b) 'WHO/UNICEF Joint Statement: Clinical Management of Acute Diarrhoea', WHO/FCH/CAH/04.7, Geneva: WHO.

45

Antiretrovirals as Merit Goods

Ethan B. Kapstein and Josh Busby

The scale-up of antiretroviral therapy is the most ambitious public health undertaking of our lifetimes. We are making history…

(Gonsalves 2008)

When antiretrovirals (ARVs) first came on the market in the 1990s, they were exceedingly expensive; the cost of treatment was upwards of US $10,000 per year.[1] These drugs were thus only accessible to those with high incomes or exceptionally good health insurance, and gay activist groups – notably the militant organisation ACT-UP – targeted pharmaceutical companies, insurance providers, and governments for changes in their home governments, rather than at the global level (d'Adesky 2004; Kramer 2003; Johnson and Murray 1988; Smith and Siplon 2006).

By the year 2006, however, the 'international community', meeting as a United Nations General Assembly Special Session (UNGASS), made an astonishing pledge to those who were infected with HIV. It declared that there should be *universal access to ARV treatment*. This UNGASS, following up on an earlier historic UN special session devoted entirely to AIDS in 2001, marks the first time in history that the international community has set a policy goal of chronic care for the ill – of establishing what Mead Over has labelled an international 'entitlement scheme' (Over 2008) – which in this specific case includes the approximately 30 million people around the world estimated to be HIV positive (UN General Assembly 2006). Political declarations have been backed by ample funding, as financial commitments to address the AIDS crisis in the developing world have grown from almost nothing in the 1990s to about US $8.7 billion in 2008 (Kates *et al.* 2009). While funds from the global community only put about 4 million HIV-positive individuals in middle- and low-income countries on ARV therapy by the end of 2008, this was up from 400,000 at the end of December 2003 (UNAIDS 2009; WHO 2008b).

How do we explain the transformation of ARVs from private goods, which only a very few of those infected with the HIV virus in developing countries could afford, into merit goods or entitlements, defined as goods that *should* be made available to everyone, irrespective of their ability to pay for them (Musgrave 1959)? In other words, how does a norm of 'universal access to treatment' – that no person should be denied life-extending drugs – become the ethical basis for global public policy with respect to pharmaceutical allocation?

Briefly, in this chapter we argue that the policy entrepreneurs and activists who promoted the creation of a universal access to treatment regime did so by using compelling moral arguments, while enjoying favourable material conditions or circumstances. From the ethical perspective, the task of these entrepreneurs was to convince political leaders and the broader public *that it was morally wrong to allocate antiretroviral drugs solely on the basis of an individual's ability to pay*. From a material standpoint, these arguments were greatly facilitated by the falling prices of ARVs after the turn of the millennium, coupled with increases in foreign aid spending devoted to HIV/AIDS and other diseases – changes that activists helped to bring about.

Making the market for ARVS

> 'You can't say to your patients, "sorry you are dying of market failure"'.
> (Zackie Achmat, Treatment Action Campaign
> quoted in d'Adesky 2005)

The AIDS crisis is a tragedy of epic proportions. By 2007, more than 25 million people had reportedly died from AIDS, 2 million of them in that year alone. Another 33 million were living with the virus. There were an estimated 2.7 million new infections in 2007, 1.9 million of them in sub-Saharan Africa, the epicentre of the pandemic (UNAIDS 2008). In 2004, AIDS was the leading cause of death worldwide for people aged 15–59 (Kaiser Family Foundation 2005). As AIDS worked its grim way around the world, leaving in its train a growing number of casualties, the United Nations Security Council in 2000 called it a threat to peace and security. Soon after, in July 2000, Durban hosted the first international conference on AIDS to be held in Africa. This gathering was widely regarded by the AIDS community as the decisive turning point at which the idea of extending treatment to the developing world was deemed both medically feasible and morally necessary, since many of the developing world success stories with respect to treatment were presented at this time (Garrett 2009).

With the idea of broader access to ARV treatment now advancing on the international agenda, policy entrepreneurs like Peter Piot, the director of UNAIDS, sought political support from the growing number of activist organisations such as Doctors without Borders, Oxfam, the Global AIDS Alliance and ACT-UP that were beginning to take up this global cause (Piot 2009). UN Secretary-General Kofi Annan picked up their call and sought donor approval for a new special fund to fight AIDS. In 2002, donors agreed that a new financing vehicle, the Global Fund to Fight AIDS, TB, and Malaria, should be created. Soon thereafter, President Bush announced the five-year, $15 billion President's Emergency Plan for AIDS Relief (PEPFAR), which would become the world's biggest vehicle for AIDS spending.

To understand the political economy of the universal access policy, we seek to conceptualise ARVs as a class of 'merit goods'. It is crucial to recognise that merit goods could be, and indeed often are, produced by the private sector in something akin to a 'free market' setting. Unlike classic public goods like clean air and national defence, which are non-rival and non-excludable, merit goods are more like club goods, exhibiting qualities of both scarcity and excludability.[2] *The significant ideational and material challenge facing activists and policy entrepreneurs who wish to promote universal access to a particular good, therefore, is to transform private goods into merit goods.*

Why doesn't society simply transfer income to the poor so that they can buy what they so desire? As James Tobin pointed out many years ago, the merit goods argument provides an example of what he calls 'specific egalitarianism', meaning that society is often willing to provide specific interventions (e.g. vouchers and food stamps) rather than general income support, since the recipients of the merit good might not choose to buy the desired goods on their own (Tobin 1970). Another way to phrase the merit goods argument is in terms of 'paternalism', meaning that some members of society (say, public officials or even activists) know better than other individuals what people really need in order to live a better life. In the global context, paternalism often takes the form of 'activists' or 'policy entrepreneurs' in wealthy societies deciding what it is that consumers in 'poor societies' *really* need, and providing funding for certain goods and services that effectively shape a given society's consumption in a way that might well be different from the consumption that would be generated by consumers who were instead given additional income directly. *In short, the production of merit goods generally requires some degree of interference in the marketplace in order to match supply and demand* (Musgrave 1959).

So what specific types of interference in markets might be required to match merit good production and consumption? On the supply side, it is apparent that several possible solutions present themselves, assuming for the moment that constrained demand or under-consumption is mainly a function of high prices or inadequate incomes. First, a given 'home' society can raise taxes and transfer income via foreign aid, enabling the 'foreign' society to buy more of the merit good at the home price. Second, the home society can induce donations from wealthy individuals (e.g. via tax breaks) to pay for the merit goods which are then transferred overseas. However, the funding from such organisations like the Gates Foundation is likely to be small compared to the level of global needs that exist. Third, the home society can induce its firms to donate the merit goods overseas; this approach will have similar shortcomings to those noted above with any philanthropy, and vary depending upon general market conditions. Fourth, the home society can produce the merit good in question and then donate it overseas, or it can encourage competition from other producers (e.g. generic manufacturers in the case of drugs) so that the monopoly price falls to the level of marginal cost, say by reducing the amount of intellectual property protection that the monopolist can claim on its products. Fifth and finally, the home society can encourage its firms to engage in 'differential pricing' of the merit goods such that prices in developing countries are lower than they are in the home market. It is the combination of solutions four and five – generic competition and differential pricing – that became the economic basis for ARV delivery in the developing world.

Why is that the case? The argument made by ARV activists at the turn of the millennium was that drug donation and charitable giving programmes were basically 'not sustainable' (CPT *et al.* 2001). Sustainability, the activists claimed, required a pricing scheme that reconciled the needs of the poor for cheap drugs, with incentives to induce the pharmaceutical companies to continue their investments in research and development (R&D). Differential pricing, with the price in developing countries equal to something like marginal cost, was touted as reconciling profits with the provision of merit goods (Kremer 2002). Health economists also made the analytical case that differential pricing, also known as Ramsey pricing, reconciled the needs of profit-seeking firms with the demands of the poor for low-cost drugs (Danzon and Towse 2003; Jack and Lanjouw 2005).

Ramsey pricing works as follows. We assume that the company produces everywhere at the same marginal cost, and the firm exercises monopoly power, say through a patent. If it exercises monopoly power it can therefore price differently in each market, *so long as it can effectively segment these markets*, setting high prices in wealthy countries and lower prices in developing countries. The multinational pharmaceutical companies had not engaged in Ramsey pricing up to this time because they doubted whether the developing world provided a large enough market for these drugs at any price. Furthermore, they were concerned whether they could enforce market segmentation and prevent the illicit re-exportation of low-cost drugs back to the industrial world.

On the demand side, poor countries had no interest in importing high-cost ARVs because the price was much more than they could afford. The absence or deficiencies in health infrastructure also meant that extending access entailed substantial costs beyond the purchase of drugs, placing a strain on stretched health budgets, and, in any event, it was unclear whether ARV purchases would be or even should be the first priority of developing world health ministries. Even if they were, procurement and delivery mechanisms would have to, in many cases, be created from scratch, delivering drugs to rural areas over poor roads, with irregular electricity to areas that needed clinics and storehouses and procedures to manage all of that activity (Kremer 2002, summarises market failures for pharmaceuticals in the developing world).

Essentially, policy entrepreneurs like Peter Piot of UNAIDS – along with activists based within such organisations as Doctors without Borders, Partners in Health, Oxfam, and later the Clinton Foundation – brought together the pharmaceutical manufacturers with developing world governments by negotiating the lower prices at which demand would kick in and by showing through 'proof of concept' demonstration efforts that ARV uptake was medically feasible in poor country settings. In 1997, Brazil began to provide ARV therapy to people with HIV, including locally manufactured generic drugs, while in Haiti, Partners in Health, led by Dr Paul Farmer, extended treatment to another resource-poor setting. Among the other significant programmes in this respect was the UN's Drug Access Initiative of 1997–1998, which used Cote D'Ivoire, Vietnam, Thailand, and Chile as pilot countries for exploring the feasibility of universal access to treatment (UNAIDS 1998). So long as the prices paid by governments or philanthropies covered production costs, at least some firms would be prepared to increase output; and so long as prices were low enough the countries (perhaps using foreign aid funds) would be able to buy the drugs. *Again, the role of the activists was to construct the market for merit goods by matching demand and supply. On the supply side, drug companies were encouraged to lower the prices on their patented ARVs, while generic drug suppliers were encouraged to enter developing world markets. On the demand side, activists won substantially higher amounts of foreign aid funding from the US and other industrial world governments, specifically targeted at ARV purchases.*

Indeed, the activists' cause of advancing universal access was, paradoxically, assisted by ongoing developments regarding the Trade in Intellectual Property Rights (TRIPS) provisions of the Uruguay Round trade agreement of 1993 and its specific application to public health. These provisions required all members of the World Trade Organization (WTO), including developing countries, to put into place effective protections on intellectual property (IP), including patents on pharmaceutical products. The least developed countries, however, were given until 2006 (later extended to 2016) to create enforceable TRIPS mechanisms. The TRIPS agreement, reinforced by the Doha Declaration of 2001, allowed countries in principle to retain the possibility of issuing compulsory licences for drugs to generic manufacturers (Fink 2008).

In the meantime, as a Federal Reserve Bank of New York economist reported, competition from Indian and Brazilian generics producers put pressure on brand-name pharmaceuticals to lower the prices of ARVs in low- and medium-income countries. The average branded price of AIDS triple-combination drugs fell from nearly $10,500 per year to less than $1,000 per year in 2000. 'Indian and Brazilian generics companies' low prices began to put pressure on originator companies to reduce their prices in low- and medium-income countries. For example, competition from generics producers … forced the average branded price of an AIDS triple-combination therapy from $10,439 per year to less than $1,000 per year in 2000' (Hellerstein

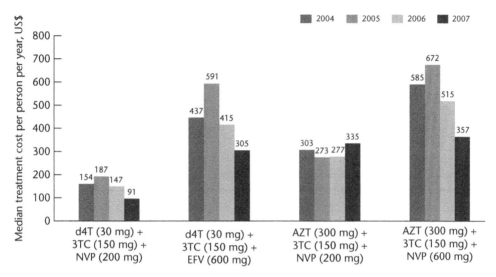

Figure 45.1 Median price (US$) of first-line antiretroviral drug regimens in low-income countries, 2004–07
Source: http://www.who.int/hiv/data/Universal_Access_Report_2008_Figures.ppt.

2004: 3). As Figure 45.1 suggests, the price of three out of four 'first-line' cocktails has fallen substantially since 2004 (and indeed, since 2001) thanks to pressure from generic competition, coupled with bulk purchases made possible by such organisations as the Clinton Foundation.

As prices fell, activists moved to increase public (and charitable) spending to buy ARVs for those with AIDS in the developing world, and the Global Fund and PEPFAR were soon launched. To explain the successful creation of these multi-billion dollar procurement vehicles, we must take a closer look at how activists were able to build a coalition of political interests that bridged AIDS activists and development campaigners on the left with the evangelical community on the right.

Why the AIDS treatment campaign succeeded

The success of the AIDS advocacy movement in generating a massive scale-up of ARV treatment naturally leads to the question, why was this particular campaign successful while many others both within and outside global health policy (e.g. the elimination of small arms, the reduction of carbon emissions, the Save Darfur Coalition) have failed or enjoyed much less success? This question is of intense interest for other campaigns for global public health and international development that are seeking to emulate the success of the AIDS campaign.

Permissive material conditions

While moral and ideational motivations may sometimes convince policymakers to embrace costly commitments (Busby 2007), campaigners must also often make utilitarian or cost-benefit arguments that they are not throwing taxpayer funds down the proverbial rat-hole. To that end, even if HIV/AIDS did not exhibit the characteristics necessary for successful disease eradication, like smallpox or polio, the proof of concept demonstrations in Brazil, Haiti, and other countries succeeded in showing that treatment could be effective in the developing world. These early programmes were especially important in overturning the presumption that poor people would not adhere to the drug regimen as faithfully as those in the advanced welfare states. The dramatic decline in drug prices brought about by competition from generic ARV suppliers also persuaded policymakers that treatment was now within the realm of affordability. Furthermore, unlike prevention programmes, the number of ARV treatments being provided to patients could readily be counted; politicians could thus set numerical targets whose progress could easily be followed.

Still, despite the favourable circumstances fostered by the combination of successful demonstration projects, declining drug prices, and a healthy global economy, a permissive material context was not enough to build a broad political coalition in support of the campaigners' aims. Why did decision-makers decide to promote and fund AIDS programmes and not something else?

The politics of AIDS treatment

Potentially, there are a number of different answers to explain why AIDS treatment campaigners were able to convert permissive material conditions into widespread political support: the degree of policy consensus; the attributes and expertise of AIDS activists; and, related, their ability to win over potential opponents in building a big tent for their cause. None of these on their own is sufficient to explain the emergence of the access to treatment regime, instead AIDS activists relied on each factor as they worked to forge a broad political coalition.

Degree of policy consensus

Other authors have highlighted that campaigns have failed due to their failure to forge a consensus on a policy prescription (Shiffman and Smith 2007; Youde 2008 discusses the failure of the universal primary health care norm). When too many ideas are at play, policy change is less likely. Thus, if this hypothesis is correct, the AIDS treatment campaign was ultimately successful because the movement coalesced towards a single consensus view of what was needed – greater access to ARVs – while other health concerns and other campaigns for maternal mortality, population control, or arguably the AIDS prevention agenda have lacked a single defining prescription.

Activist attributes and expertise

It is difficult to deny that much of the ARV treatment regime's relative success ultimately has to do with the quality of the individuals involved in this campaign, just as it would be hard to imagine modern Singapore without Lee Kuan Yew or South Africa without Nelson Mandela. One could argue that the characters involved in this story, such as Peter Piot, Bono, Franklin Graham, Paul Farmer, Jonathan Mann, and many others, had unusually strong persuasive skills. They combined substantive expertise with evangelical fervour, and they also exploited diffuse social networks that extended throughout the political and economic realms. Busby suggests that the personal attributes and expertise of advocates like the evangelist Franklin Graham and rock star Bono were persuasive because they shared a number of attributes (religion, ideology, gender, age) in common with key decision-makers like George W. Bush (Busby, ms). A different argument about advocate characteristics would focus on the shared scientific expertise of medical professionals (Haas 1992). As already noted, AIDS experts like Peter

Piot and Paul Farmer were converted early to the belief that ARV treatment should be extended globally, and they helped create an 'epistemic community' of like-minded advocates.

While the degree of policy cohesion and activist attributes are important and attractive in their simplicity, these alone cannot explain why policymakers were persuaded to support the demands of AIDS treatment activists, especially given the number of other health conditions in the developing world that are responsible for as many, if not more, premature deaths than AIDS, and whose solutions are relatively straightforward. For example, diarrhoeal disease – which can readily be reduced by access to clean water and better sanitation and for which effective treatments already exist – killed 1.81 million people in 2004 compared to 1.51 million who died from AIDS (WHO 2008a).

Building coalitions and overcoming opposition

In order to succeed politically, campaigns have to have broad support while overcoming the major sources of potential political opposition. One way they build political support for their cause is by framing the problem in ways that various groups find compelling. For example, HIV/AIDS has been framed as a public health issue, a human rights issue, a justice issue, a moral problem, an issue of intellectual property rights, and a security problem. The ethical/human rights-based argument was perhaps the most central frame that animated advocates' demands internationally, but there has been some local variation, with the moral frame having a decidedly more Christian religious flavour in the United States. While advocacy groups often adopt a dominant frame, they may also employ multiple messages to appeal to different groups, building political coalitions in the process.

From this perspective, the nature of the issue area can have a big effect on the relative success of different campaigns by changing the balance between coalitions and opponents. For example, advocates of climate change policy have sought to build a broad coalition drawn from both environmental and industrial groups, but they have confronted influential interest groups in the power generation sector. Who were the potential opponents of extending AIDS treatment programmes? These included pharmaceutical companies that were worried about profits, social conservatives who identified AIDS with a sinners' disease, and fiscal conservatives opposed to foreign aid spending. AIDS activists succeeded by reducing the political costs of supporting AIDS treatment. By creating a campaign with some cachet on both left and right, AIDS activists made their cause broadly attractive. Given that the potential opposition in the United States was concentrated on the political right, it was especially important to make inroads among evangelicals and social and fiscal conservatives who could vouch for the policy.

In sum, we would expect campaigns to be more successful when they (1) enjoy permissive materials conditions; (2) provide a coherent policy prescription; and (3) build a broad political coalition, on the one hand, while facing few influential political opponents on the other. With the AIDS case, activists were favoured in each of these three dimensions.

Conclusions

We have demonstrated the role of activists and policy entrepreneurs in building a market for ARVs in the developing world. By naming and shaming pharmaceutical companies and by promoting generics, the price of this treatment was greatly reduced, making the goal of universal access seemingly feasible. With lower prices, the activists pressured governments to provide more foreign assistance for the purchase of ARVs, bringing the supply and demand sides of the equation together. Activists thus succeeded in transforming ARVs from private goods into merit goods that everyone had the right to consume.

In thinking about the future, the AIDS treatment campaign raises several important questions for policymakers. First, can ARV treatment access continue to be extended? Second, can other campaigns (e.g. for universal access to education and clean water) replicate the success of the AIDS treatment campaign politically?

With respect to maintaining and extending ARV access, the answer is not a simple one. To the extent that the virus that causes AIDS will continue to mutate and generate drug resistance, branded pharmaceuticals companies are needed to develop new drug therapies for AIDS. These companies continue to press for maximal protection of intellectual property rights, and as drug resistance among first-line ARV drugs becomes more prevalent, it will become increasingly expensive to provide second-line drugs, since these are facing less competition from generic producers.

At the same time, the failure of AIDS prevention strategies is straining budgets at a time when governments are under unprecedented pressure to cut costs, especially given the 'Great Recession' that began in 2008, 'donor fatigue' with respect to AIDS, and the emergence of other priorities. For these reasons, a growing number of observers are expressing concern about the future sustainability of the global AIDS regime (Over 2008). Reneging on the commitments made to the more than 3 million people on ARV therapy would be morally indefensible. But advocates for AIDS broadly need to spur a renewed focus on prevention since the funds available for treatment will never be large enough to cover those in need, so long as the HIV-positive community continues to swell.

For other causes to replicate the AIDS campaign's success to date on treatment, activists must build broad coalitions of interests, including private sector generators (and copiers) of intellectual property. Mustering political support is likely to require very specific development programmes (like PEPFAR), which are much more politically popular than broad-based financial assistance to well-run governments to spend as they see fit (i.e. the Millennium Challenge Corporation). This coalition, in turn, must be joined by a convergent idea of what *can and should* be done. It is only through the fusion of a compelling set of ideas about how the world should work with favourable material conditions that activists will bring change to the global economy.

Notes

1 The authors would like to thank Matthew Flynn for his editorial support and research assistance. This piece is based on a longer working paper for the Center for Global Development and an academic journal article (Kapstein and Busby 2009, 2010).
2 Club goods are goods that are only provided to members of a particular group while others are excluded.

References

Busby, J. (2007) '"Bono Made Jesse Helms Cry": Debt Relief, Jubilee 2000, and Moral Action in International Politics', *International Studies Quarterly*, 51(2): 247–75.

Busby, J. (ms) 'From God's Mouth: Messenger Effects and the Politics of the Global AIDS Response in the United States', Austin, TX: University of Texas.

CPT, HAI, MSF, and TAG (Consumer Project on Technology, Health Action International, Médecins sans Frontières, and Oxfam and Treatment Action Group) (2001) *Joint Statement on Differential Pricing & Financing of Essential Drugs*, available at http://www.cptech.org/ip/wto/norwaystatement.html (accessed 22 January 2010).

d'Adesky, A.C. (2004) *Moving Mountains: The Race to Treat Global AIDS*, New York: Verso.

d'Adesky, A.C. (2005) *Pills Profits Protest - Voices of Global AIDS Activists*, New York: Outcast Films.

Danzon, P.M. and Towse, A. (2003) 'Differential Pricing for Pharmaceuticals: Reconciling Access, R&D and Patents', *International Journal of Health Care Finance and Economics*, 3: 183–205.

Fink, C. (2008) *Intellectual Property and Public Health: An Overview of the Debate with a Focus on US Policy*, Working Paper Number 146, Washington, DC: Center for Global Development, available at http://www.cgdev.org/content/publications/detail/16228/ (accessed 22 January 2010).

Garrett, L. (2009) Interview with Laurie Garrett, conducted by Ethan Kapstein, 31 January.

Gonsalves, G. (2008) *Scaling Up Antiretroviral Therapy and the Struggle for Health for All. AIDS and Rights Alliance for Southern Africa (ARASA)*, International Treatment Preparedness Coalition (ITPC), available at http://www.tac.org.za/community/node/2397 (accessed 22 January 2010).

Haas, P.M. (1992) 'Introduction: Epistemic Communities and International Policy Coordination', *International Organization*, 46(1): 1–35.

Hellerstein, R. (2004) *Do Pharmaceutical Firms Price Discriminate Across Rich and Poor Countries? Evidence from Antiretroviral Drug Prices. International Research, Federal Reserve Bank of New York*, available at http://www.ny.frb.org/research/economists/hellerstein/JDE2.pdf (accessed 22 January 2010).

Jack, W. and Lanjouw, J.O. (2005) 'Financing Pharmaceutical Innovation: How Much Should Poor Countries Contribute?', *The World Bank Economic Review*, 19(1): 45–67.

Johnson, D. and Murray, J.F. (1988) 'AIDS Without End', *New York Review of Books*, 35(13): 2–4.

Kaiser Family Foundation (2005) *The Global HIV/AIDS Epidemic*, available at http://www.kff.org/hivaids/upload/3030-06.pdf (accessed 22 January 2010).

Kapstein, E. and Busby, J. (2009) *Making Markets for Merit Goods: The Political Economy of Antiretrovirals*, Washington, DC: Center for Global Development, available at http://www.cgdev.org/content/publications/detail/1422655/ (accessed 22 January 2010).

Kapstein, E. and Busby, J. (2010) 'Making Markets for Merit Goods: The Political Economy of Antiretrovirals', *Global Policy*, 1(1): 75–90.

Kates, J., Lief, E, and Avila, C. (2009) *Financing the Response to AIDS in Low-and Middle-income Countries: International Assistance from the G8, European Commission and Other Donor Governments in 2008*, Washington, DC: Kaiser Family Foundation, available at http://www.kff.org/hivaids/7347.cfm (accessed 22 January 2010).

Kramer, L. (2003) *ACTUP Oral History Project: A Program of Mix – The New York Lesbian & Gay Experimental Film Festival*, available at http://www.actuporalhistory.org/interviews/images/kramer.pdf (accessed 22 January 2010).

Kremer, M. (2002) 'Pharmaceuticals and the Developing World', *Journal of Economic Perspectives*, 16(4): 67–90.

Musgrave, R.A. (1959) *The Theory of Public Finance*, New York: Mcgraw-Hill.

Over, M. (2008) *Prevention Failure: The Ballooning Entitlement Burden of US Global AIDS Treatment Spending and What to Do About It, Working Paper 144*, available from http://www.cgdev.org/content/publications/detail/15973/ (accessed 22 January 2010).

Piot, P. (2009) Interview with Peter Piot, conducted by Ethan Kapstein, 28 January.

Shiffman, J. and Smith, S. (2007) 'Generation of Political Priority for Global Health Initiatives: A Framework and Case Study of Maternal Mortality', *The Lancet*, 370(9,595): 1,370–79.

Smith, R.A. and Siplon, P.A. (2006) *Drugs into Bodies: Global AIDS Treatment Activism*, Westport, CT: Praeger.

Tobin, J. (1970) 'On Limiting the Domain of Inequality', *Journal of Law and Economics*, 13(2): 263–77.

UNAIDS (Joint United Nations Programme on HIV/AIDS) (1998) *UNAIDS HIV Drug Access Initiative - Providing Wider Access to HIV-related Drugs in Developing Countries, Pilot Phase Background Document*, Geneva: UNAIDS.

UNAIDS (Joint United Nations Programme on HIV/AIDS) (2008) *Global Facts and Figures*, available at http://data.unaids.org /pub/GlobalReport/2008/20080715_fs_global_en.pdf (accessed 22 January 2010).

UNAIDS (Joint United Nations Programme on HIV/AIDS) (2009) *More than Four Million HIV-positive People now Receiving Life-saving Treatment*, available at http://www.unaids.org/en/KnowledgeCentre/Resources/FeatureStories/archive/2009/20090930_access_treatment_4millions.asp (accessed 22 January 2010).

UN (United Nations) General Assembly (2006) *Resolution adopted by the General Assembly: 60/262. Political Declaration on HIV/AIDS*, available at http://data.unaids.org/pub/Report/2006/20060615_HLM_PoliticalDeclaration_ARES60262_en.pdf (accessed 22 January 2010).

WHO (World Health Organization) (2008a) *Fact Sheet: Top Ten Causes of Death*, available at http://www.who.int/mediacentre/factsheets/fs310/en/index.html (accessed 22 January 2010).

WHO (World Health Organization) (2008b) *Towards Universal Access: Scaling Up Priority HIV/AIDS Interventions in the Health Sector*, available at http://www.who.int/hiv/pub/2008progressreport/en/ (accessed 22 January 2010).

Youde, J. (2008) 'Is Universal Access to Antiretroviral Drugs an Emerging International Norm', *Journal of International Relations and Development*, 11(4): 415–40.

Part X
Health Systems, Health Capacity, and the Politics of Global Public Health

46

Health Systems Strengthening

Past, Present, and Future

Sara Bennett

Introduction

The national health systems of many European and some Latin American countries evolved in the post-war period. In many developing countries, the adoption of specific policies to strengthen national health systems is typically more recent, often dating back to independence in the 1960s or 1970s. It is perhaps not surprising, therefore, that the study of health systems, and how best to strengthen them, is also a relatively recent phenomenon.

This chapter documents how health systems strengthening has evolved over the past 40 years, what have been the major landmarks in this process, and how our understanding of health systems has also evolved. The discussion focuses on the health systems of low- and middle-income countries (LMIC). After a brief introduction of terms and definitions, the chapter provides an historical overview, discusses current debates regarding health systems, and finally looks to the future, and emerging challenges for health systems. Through this chronological approach, the chapter also seeks to give readers a grounding in the main debates concerning approaches to health systems strengthening, and to provide a language and terminology than can be used to describe and analyse health systems.

Thinking about health systems

Exactly what a health system is remains unclear to many: does it encompass solely the network of health care providers; does it include private as well as public sector actors; are interventions such as sanitation, health education, and food standard regulations that have little to do with health services but a lot to do with health, part of the health system or not? A system, a generic system, is often said to be a set of elements and interrelationships between those elements that exist to serve a specific goal. In the case of a health system, that goal is primarily to promote good health, although analysts have also suggested that offering financial protection (from the costs of ill health), and being responsive to patients' needs are other important goals (WHO 2000).

The World Health Organization (WHO) recently identified six elements of a health system: health financing, service delivery, drugs and supply systems, human resources for health, health information, and governance (WHO 2007). Other analysts have conceptualised the elements of a health system in different ways. Although there is a danger that different conceptual frameworks create confusion, in many respects they complement each other, offering different approaches to analysing health systems depending on the purpose and context.

Early efforts to strengthen health systems

Throughout the 1950s and 1960s, and extending into the 1970s, many efforts to improve health in developing countries took the form of mass campaigns or 'vertical programmes', focusing, for example, on the eradication of smallpox and polio (Mills *et al.* 2006). However, at independence, developing countries often embarked upon an era of health system strengthening, characterised in particular by efforts to expand their networks of basic health services through public sector investment. Public health centres were built in rural and remote areas, and schemes to develop cadres of largely unpaid community-level health workers were developed. Such efforts were often underpinned by new national policy documents such as the Bhore Report (1946) in India and the Titmuss Report (1964) in Tanganyika. In 1978, the Alma-Ata Declaration lent further support to this approach. Declaring health care a basic right, and embracing a broad definition of health, the Alma-Ata Declaration called for the launch and sustaining of primary health care 'as part of a comprehensive national health system' (WHO 1978).

The broader macro-economic context, however, was not supportive of health system development. The oil crisis and debt crisis of the late 1970s and early 1980s led to structural adjustment programmes in many developing country contexts that sought to rein in government spending. In this milieu, the concept of a comprehensive approach to primary health care was rapidly challenged. Walsh and Warren argued that in the context of limited resources, it was not feasible to provide comprehensive primary health care, and instead efforts should be focused on specific priority diseases. This approach, known as selective primary health care (Walsh and Warren 1979), represented the early salvos in a battle between broad approaches to systems strengthening versus more focused support to specific disease control interventions that has persisted to this day. Approaches that focus on specific diseases are often viewed to be better defined, more easily specified, shorter-term impacts, and hence more easily held accountable. In contrast, broader health systems strengthening approaches are viewed to be more likely to address the root causes of problems, and to be more sustainable, but are also likely to be more diffuse and their impacts longer term, making it harder to assess the impacts of investments. While these two approaches are probably best seen as complementary (Mills 2005), the practices of global health donors seem to swing backwards and forwards between one approach and the other, without finding a comfortable equilibrium.

A renewed focus on health systems was stimulated in the late 1980s through a World Bank publication, 'Financing Health Services in Developing Countries: An Agenda for Reform', that argued that 'continuing gains [in health outcomes] depend largely on the capacity of health systems to deliver' (Akin *et al.* 1987: 1). While 'An Agenda for Reform' stressed the importance of health systems, its line of argument was very different from previous documents. It proposed a series of market-oriented reforms – increasing user fees and expanding the role of the private sector, among others – with the aim of enhancing the efficiency of health systems. Several of the policy measures proposed were elaborated in the World Development Report of 1993, 'Investing in Health' (World Bank 1993), which also argued strongly for an 'essential package' of health services. These reports, which were particularly influential in developing country contexts as their recommendations were often reflected in World Bank lending conditionalities, were further supported by policy approaches fostered by some bilateral donors such as the United States Agency for International Development (USAID) and the United Kingdom Official Development Assistance (ODA) (now DfID). During the 1980s, policies adopted by these bilateral donors reflected contemporary thinking in their own countries about an appropriate role for government. The 'new public management' movement influenced the 1980s' 'health sector reform' movement in LMIC: policy reforms often included measures to separate the purchasers of health care from the providers of health care, in an effort to create greater transparency about which services were being purchased, and to engender higher levels of accountability and efficiency. For example, health reforms in Zambia espoused a contracting model whereby a new 'Central Board of Health' contracted with district health management teams to deliver health services. Similarly, in Colombia, reforms introduced under Law 100 in 1993 separated out functions of (1) policy and governance, (2) insurance, and (3) service delivery, and were intended to stimulate managed competition (Rosa and Alberto 2004).

Over time, however, many health sector reform policies became discredited, partly because of the negative consequences of some specific policies (such as user fees) on equity issues, and partly because of challenges in implementing these complex reforms. There was a lack of evidence that the policies had positive effects upon health outcomes. Later criticisms suggested that the end goal of health systems, that is improving the health of the population, was lost sight of in the eagerness to experiment with novel organisational arrangements. While WHO's World Health Report in 2000 (WHO 2000) sought to keep (or refocus) a spotlight on the health systems agenda, and the Report made considerable progress in terms of developing a clear analytical approach and strategies for measuring health system performance, the tide had already turned. Moreover, the Report's controversial application of measures to rank country health systems caused such a furore that it distracted from the ideas within the Report.

During the past decade, there has been dynamic growth in international investment in global health, but for the reasons described above, much of this has been channelled to tackle specific priority diseases. For example, the GAVI Alliance was established in 2000 to scale-up access to immunisation programmes in developing countries, and the Global Fund to Fight AIDS, TB and Malaria (GFATM) was established in 2002. Dramatic growth in spending by the Bill & Melinda Gates Foundation has further nurtured this focus on specific diseases and services. The Foundation has typically resisted investing in health system strengthening, instead favouring more vertically oriented approaches capable of delivering rapid results.

Current debates

The global growth in disease-specific financing, particularly for HIV/AIDs, translates into compelling statistics. In some heavily affected countries, external funding for HIV/AIDS grew from 500 to 1,000 per cent in a two-year period, with further external HIV/AIDS funding in high-prevalence countries often exceeding 150 per cent of government health budgets (Lewis 2005) . Such dramatic increases in funding have put pressure on already weak health systems. It has become apparent that, on the one hand, weak health systems are primary obstacles to the achievement of disease-specific targets and, on the other, that the scale and nature of some disease-specific funding, unless complemented by investments in health systems, might further distort and undermine health systems (Travis *et al.* 2004). For example, the '3 by 5' Initiative launched by the WHO in 2003 aimed to ensure that 3 million HIV-positive people in developing countries were receiving antiretroviral therapy by 2005. The Initiative fell far short of this ambitious target for multiple reasons, but the evaluation team identified weak health systems, and particularly health worker shortages, as a key constraint to achievement of the goal (Nemes *et al.* 2006).

Slowly, activists and analysts who do not typically concern themselves with health system issues have become concerned about the need for greater investment in and attention to health systems. Frequently, health worker shortages (particularly in sub-Saharan Africa), which are a very visible and emotive issue, have formed an entry point for such stakeholders. Both the Rockefeller-supported Joint Learning Initiative and a subsequent World Health Report highlighted shortages and the global imbalance in the distribution of health workers (Joint Learning Initiative 2004; WHO 2006). Increasingly, HIV/AIDS activists have taken up this cause, with some success, for example, in getting the US President's Emergency Plan for AIDS Relief (PEPFAR) to invest in this area.

In 2005, the GAVI Alliance Board launched a dedicated health systems window, and the GFATM first welcomed health systems strengthening proposals. More recently, the launch of the International Health Partnership in 2007 marked a renewed focus on health systems, with a call to 'action to scale-up coverage and use of health services, and deliver improved outcomes against the health-related MDGs and universal access commitments'.[1] So it appears that health systems strengthening is again back on the agenda.

One of the key challenges for the international development community in promoting health systems strengthening is the high degree of context-specificity, and often complexity, in terms of what needs to be done. Sometimes health system strengthening is viewed to be a black hole and a black box. While the goals of disease-specific programmes can sometimes be captured in simple and easily-specified targets (3 by 5, or universal child immunisation), the goals and strategies for health systems strengthening are rarely so simple to articulate. A recent evaluation of the World Bank's portfolio of health sector loans noted, for example, that:

> Health reforms promise to improve efficiency and governance but they are politically contentious, often complex and relatively risky.
>
> (World Bank, 2008: xviii)

While there is widespread agreement around the goals of health systems strengthening, there remains considerable dispute about how best to achieve these goals. At least four factors contribute to the difficulties of devising and implementing strategies for health systems strengthening:

- Health systems are inherently political and the selection of strategies for health systems strengthening depends as much on values and politics as it does on technical issues
- Appropriate policies for health systems strengthening are likely to be very context-specific, in particular, the nature of local institutions will influence the effectiveness of alternative approaches to systems strengthening
- Implementation processes can considerably influence the final effects of a health system strengthening strategy – the details of how the poor are identified in a targeting programme, or what incentives providers face to maintain quality of care, are often as important in determining impacts as the overall thrust of the reform
- Evidence about the effects of alternative health systems strengthening strategies is often lacking. Where evidence is available, it may be nuanced in terms of conclusions, and it may be very difficult to assess its transferability to different contexts.

Two policy examples, both first proposed by the World Bank in 1987 as part of 'The Agenda for Reform' report discussed above, serve to illustrate the complexities in determining appropriate strategies for health system strengthening. The two policy changes discussed are user fees and promoting service provision by the private health sector.

User fees were initially proposed as a policy option that would both raise extra revenue for health care services, and promote rational use of services. Early evidence from Malaysia and the Philippines suggested that imposing small fees at the point of service use would not discourage uptake of services and could critically improve quality of care, which would ultimately help increase use (Akin *et al.* 1986; Heller 1982). On this fairly slim evidence base, the World Bank supported the widespread implementation of user fees, particularly in sub-Saharan Africa, in the late 1980s and early 1990s. However, a growing body of research literature, largely but not exclusively from sub-Saharan Africa, demonstrated that in fact user fees frequently had negative effects, particularly for the poor (Lagarde and Palmer 2008). Further, mechanisms to protect the poor from their effects (such as exemption mechanisms) were often ineffective, as they were improperly implemented. Consequently, the World Bank, and some other donors such as the UK DFID, now have policies that support the abolition of user fees (in the case of the World Bank reversing a policy that they helped put in place many years ago). However, even for a relatively clearly defined policy issue such as this, there continues to be much debate about the relative merits and demerits of user fees when applied in different contexts.

The 'Agenda for Reform' report also highlighted the role of private health care providers in LMIC and argued that they should be encouraged to provide services for which people were willing to pay. Inevitably, this issue of the role of the private sector is very politically sensitive, and it has sometimes proved difficult to move beyond politicised positions and rhetoric to generate a deeper empirical understanding of the issues. Oxfam UK recently released a policy report, 'Blind Optimism', that urged caution in terms of promoting private sector channels as a means to scale-up health services (Oxfam International 2009). The report unleashed a furious debate online (Harding 2009) and on the pages of the *British Medical Journal*.[2] The broad thrust of critics' arguments was that the private sector is too big to be ignored, that lines between public and private sector activity in developing countries are often blurred, and that there is no evidence of the innate superiority of government health services over private services. While the evidence base regarding the private sector in developing countries has grown substantially during the past 20 years, it is still sufficiently fragile that different analysts can review the same body of evidence and come to quite different conclusions. The fragility of the evidence base is further exacerbated by the fact that the private sector looks very different in different country contexts – in some cases, private sector providers are largely for-profit hospitals and clinics, and in others contexts, they are largely traditional providers. Governments' regulatory powers and capacity also vary substantially.

In the face of complexities such as these, history tells us that there is a persistent tendency to retreat to the safe territory of single-disease or service programmes with discrete and easily quantifiable targets, and much shorter and more direct causal chains, where it is easier to see and assess the impacts of interventions. Encouragingly, however, there are signs that many stakeholders now recognise the symbiotic relationship between disease control programmes and health systems, and the need to act on both fronts simultaneously. Some analysts are talking of a 'diagonal approach' to health care that combines concerns with specific diseases with health systems strengthening (Ooms *et al.* 2008). The ongoing WHO initiative, 'Positive Synergies', claims that it is seeking to:

> ... finally put an end to the long-running debate about 'vertical versus horizontal' approaches to health, and to provide clear guidance to GHIs and country health systems so that each can support the other in the achievement of their shared goal: better health outcomes for more people.

> (WHO, 2009: 5)

However, for the global health community to be successful in this goal, much remains to be done. First, far greater conceptual clarity is required around what a 'diagonal approach' might look like: what actual behaviours and strategies are effective in both strengthening health systems and extending coverage of priority services, and conversely, which strategies may negatively affect one of the other. Second, major changes are required on the part of the international community in terms of the time frames for which they are willing to commit aid, the time frame over which they seek results, and the degree of attribution acceptable in accounting for the effects of their investments. While various international initiatives such as the Paris Declaration and the International Health Partnership have made significant progress in this direction, much remains to be done. Finally, the community of researchers and analysts engaged in health systems work, as well as funders of such research, need to redouble their efforts to strengthen the evidence base on which health systems strengthening rests.

Future challenges

While many of the 'old' problems of health systems in developing countries – ensuring adequate human resources, strategies to promote access for the poor, ways of working with the private sector – have not yet been resolved, a new series of challenges for health systems is already emerging. While attempting to forecast the future is always a risky act, this appears not to have deterred many from trying. Analysis of this nature consistently identifies a number of issues as presenting new challenges (as well as new opportunities) for health systems.

The rise of non-communicable disease

In many LMIC, the effects of the epidemiological transition are already being felt with rising morbidity and mortality due to non-communicable diseases such as heart disease, hypertension, and diabetes. Health systems in many developing countries have extremely poor patient records, fragmented health care systems, and weak referral systems, which means they are poorly prepared to deal with long-term patients requiring support in managing chronic conditions. One of the major challenges in scaling up antiretroviral therapy has been to strengthen patient record-keeping and referral channels so as to ensure continuity of care; lessons learnt in this process are likely to be relevant to the management of non-communicable disease. Furthermore, many of the underlying causes of non-communicable disease lie outside of the direct control of the health system. Obesity, alcohol and tobacco use, nutrition, and indoor smoke from fuels are all significant risk factors contributing to non-communicable disease. To tackle these risk factors requires multisectoral action, such as public education campaigns, changes to school curricula, clearer labelling of food products, regulation of food and beverage advertising, development of sports and leisure facilities, and redesign of the built environment to promote walking (Butland *et al.* 2007). Governments have historically been extremely weak at working across different sectors of government. Greater attention must be given to this aspect of governance in future health systems.

Globalisation

The governance function of a health system encompasses 'overseeing and guiding the whole health system, private as well as public, in order to protect the public interest' (WHO 2007: 23). Globalisation processes mean that national governments increasingly find that the key levers that influence population health lie outside of their direct national control, and instead depend upon global trade agreements, or policy lines pressed by influential external actors. The agreement of Trade-Related Aspects of Intellectual Property Rights (TRIPs) has already had significant effects on patterns of drug production and consumption in developing countries (Barton 2004). In addition to globalisation, the increasing number of NGOs, civil society organisations, and advocacy groups – both national and international – are also changing the way that ministries of health do business. Governments increasingly need to be adept at managing a diverse array of stakeholders, identifying who can support health systems changes, who might resist them, and creating coalitions and partnerships.

Information and communications technology (ICT)

It has been suggested that 'the impact of ICT on health systems will be substantial or even revolutionary. However, there is much less agreement as to the likely nature of that impact' (Lucas 2008: 2,129). In principle, ICT could dramatically change the way that health conditions are diagnosed and treated, facilitating access to scarce medical skills for those in remote and hitherto underserved areas. ICT could also dramatically change approaches to medical record-keeping, regulation of providers and insurers, and behaviour change communication. However, the successful application of ICT depends not only on appropriate technologies being available and funded, but also on significant changes in work processes, which would most likely affect power relations between government and private sector, physicians, and other cadres. Any fundamental changes in work practices (and power relations) are likely to be resisted and hence the feasibility of really benefiting from ICT to the full extent possible is still unclear.

Conclusions

As noted at the outset, the study of health systems is still a relatively new endeavour, so it is perhaps not surprising that the field continues to be plagued by a lack of shared understanding of key concepts, as well as a very weak evidence base. The level of interest in health systems in LMIC appears higher now than perhaps at any time previously. With many long-standing health system challenges remaining unaddressed, and new challenges rapidly emerging, it is imperative that the current interest in health systems is capitalised on. We need both to intensify the implementation of measures to strengthen health systems, and to learn from these efforts.

Notes

1 http://www.internationalhealthpartnership.net/ihp_plus_about.html
2 See http://www.bmj.com/cgi/eletters/339/jul06_1/b2737

References

Akin, J.S., Griffin, C., Guilkey, D.K., and Popkin, B.M. (1986) 'Demand for primary health care services in the Bicol region of the Philippines', *Economic Development and Cultural Change*, 34 (4): 755–82.
Akin, J.S., Birdsall, N., De Ferranti, D.M., and World Bank (1987) *Financing Health Services in Developing Countries: An Agenda for Reform*, Washington DC: World Bank.
Barton, J.H. (2004) 'TRIPS and the global pharmaceutical market', *Health Affairs*, 23(3): 146–54.
Butland, B., Jebb, S., Kopelman, P., McPherson, K., Thomas, S., Mardell, J., and Parry, V. (2007) *Tackling Obesity: Future Choices*, London: Department of Science and Technology.
Harding, A. (2009) 'Oxfam: this is not how to help the poor', *Global Health Policy*, Washington, DC: Center for Global Development.

Heller, P.S. (1982) 'A model of the demand for medical and health services in Peninsular Malaysia', *Social Science & Medicine*, 16(3): 267–84.

Joint Learning Initiative (2004) *Human Resources for Health: Overcoming the Crisis*, Cambridge, MA: Harvard University Press.

Lagarde, M. and Palmer, N. (2008) 'The impact of user fees on health service utilization in low- and middle-income countries: how strong is the evidence?', *Bulletin of the World Health Organization*, 86(11): 839–48.

Lewis, M. (2005) *Addressing the Challenge of HIV/AIDS: Macroeconomic, Fiscal and Institutional Issues*, Washington, DC: Center for Global Development.

Lucas, H. (2008) 'Information and communications technology for future health systems in developing countries', *Social Science & Medicine*, 66(10): 2,122–32.

Mills, A. (2005) 'Mass campaigns versus general health services: what have we learnt in 40 years about vertical versus horizontal approaches?', *Bulletin of the World Health Organization*, 83(4): 315–6.

Mills, A., Rasheed, F., and Tollman, S. (2006) 'Strengthening Health Systems', in D. Jamison, J. Bremen, and A. Meashamet (eds) *Disease Control Priorities in Developing Countries*, New York: Oxford University Press: 87–102.

Nemes, M.I., Beaudoin, J., Conway, S., Kivumbi, G.W., Skjelmerud, A., and Vogel, U. (2006) *Evaluation of WHO's Contribution to '3 by 5': Main Report*, Geneva: World Health Organization.

Ooms, G., Van Damme, W., Baker, B.K., Zeitz, P., and Schrecker, T. (2008) 'The 'diagonal' approach to Global Fund financing: a cure for the broader malaise of health systems?', *Global Health*, 4: 6.

Oxfam International (2009) *Blind Optimism: Challenging the Myth About Private Health Care in Poor Countries*, Oxford: Oxfam.

Rosa, R.-M. and Alberto, I.C. (2004) 'Universal health care for Colombians 10 years after Law 100: challenges and opportunities', *Health Policy*, 68: 129–42.

Travis, P., Bennett, S., Haines, A., Pang, T., Bhutta, Z., Hyder, A.A., Pielemeier, N.R., Mills, A., and Evans, T. (2004) 'Overcoming health-systems constraints to achieve the Millennium Development Goals', *The Lancet*, 364(9,437): 900–6.

Walsh, J.A. and Warren, K.S. (1979) 'Selective primary health care: an interim strategy for disease control in developing countries', *New England Journal of Medicine*, 301(18): 967–74.

World Bank (1993) *Investing in Health: World Development Report*, Washington DC: World Bank.

World Bank (2008) *Improving Effectiveness and Outcomes for the Poor in Health, Nutrition, and Population: An Evaluation of World Bank Group Support Since 1997*, Washington DC: World Bank.

WHO (World Health Organization) (1978) *Declaration of Alma-Ata, International Conference on Primary Health Care*, Geneva: WHO.

WHO (World Health Organization) (2000) *The World Health Report 2000: Health Systems: Improving Performance*, Geneva: WHO.

WHO (World Health Organization) (2006) *World Health Report 2006: Working Together for Health*, Geneva: WHO.

WHO (World Health Organization) (2007) *Everybody's Business: Strengthening Health Systems to Improve Health Outcomes: WHO's Framework for Action*, Geneva: WHO.

WHO (World Health Organization) (2009) *Initial Summary Conclusions: Maximizing Positive Synergies Between Health Systems and GHIs*, Geneva: WHO.

47

Politics of Global Health

Understanding the Politics of Aid[1]

Rebecca Dodd

Introduction

Health is a prominent political issue on the domestic agenda of most developed countries. At election time, voters show a keen interest in the health manifestos of political parties. The achievements or failures of national health systems are often centre-stage in debates. At the international level, too, health is frequently in the headlines: from the threat of a new infectious disease, to the resurgence of 'old' maladies such as tuberculosis or cholera; from the ethics of rich nations who recruit health workers from poor countries, to the price of medicines.

This chapter maps the various political forces affecting international health and provides a framework through which these can be understood. It focuses in particular on the politics of aid (development assistance), but looks also at the intersection of aid, foreign, and security policies. It attempts to answer four key questions: *why* do donors provide aid, *what* do they hope to achieve by doing so, *how* should aid be provided and managed, and does aid *achieve results*? The next section sets the context by discussing these questions in general terms and in relation to overall aid, while section three looks at the issue for health in particular.

What is aid?

The Development Assistance Committee (DAC) of the Organisation for Economic Co-operation and Development (OECD) calls aid Official Development Assistance (ODA) and defines it as 'grants or loans to countries and territories on the DAC list of ODA recipients (developing countries) and to multilateral agencies which are: (a) undertaken by the official sector; (b) with promotion of economic development and welfare as the main objective; (c) at concessional financial terms (if a loan, having a grant element of at least 25 per cent)' (OECD 2009).

Bilateral aid is provided directly by a donor country to an aid recipient country, while *multilateral* flows are channelled via an international organisation such as the World Bank or the United Nations. Multilateral aid represents about one-third of all ODA, and is seen as to have the advantage of being 'neutral' (because decisions about how it is spent are made on technical rather than political grounds) and 'knowledgeable' (as multilateral agencies develop expertise in particular areas of development). However, in recent years concerns have been raised about the increasing complexity of the multilateral aid architecture, with growing numbers of organisations and aid channels.

The politics of international development

Why do donors provide aid?

This is the quintessential political economy question in discussions of development aid. There are two perspectives:

- Aid is provided for moral, ethical, or altruistic reasons (Lumsdaine 1993). According to this perspective, aid contributes to the realisation of a shared international vision of a secure, prosperous world
- Aid is a tool of foreign policy, and therefore reflects the geopolitical and foreign policy priorities of donor countries (Lancaster 2007).

While scholars argue about the relative dominance of these different perspectives, they agree that aid decision-makers are influenced by both. Since the end of the Cold War, though, aid has been *less* influenced by geopolitics, and a consensus has emerged around the basic principles and attributes of aid: that is, it must be provided on concessional terms to developing countries, and its primary objectives must be developmental. This consensus is reflected in the OECD/DAC definition of aid provided above. Nevertheless, aid remains an instrument of international relations, and is therefore inevitably influenced by the ideological positions and persuasions of those who dominate international affairs. The role of the World Bank in responding to the international debt crisis of the 1980s and 1990s (see Box 47.1) is an illustration of this.

Box 47.1 The debt crisis, aid, and conditionality

Money lent by bilateral and multilateral creditors on non-concessional terms is called 'official development flows'. In the 1980s and 1990s, many developing countries began to default on their debt repayments to these creditors, creating a debt crisis. In response, further support – including concessional support and grants that qualified as aid – was often conditional upon recipient countries restructuring their economies and adopting Structural Adjustment Policies (SAPs). SAPs involved radical reductions in public sector spending, and came under criticism both for their impact on human development – as spending on health and education was slashed – and for effectively undermining the sovereign right of recipient countries to determine economic policy.

In the 2000s, various debt relief schemes were launched. These included the World Bank's Highly Indebted Poor Countries (HIPC) scheme, in which debt owed to the World Bank and IMF was cancelled if countries adopted Poverty Reduction Strategies. Again, these came to be criticised for promoting a particular model of economic development favoured by the World Bank.

It is not the role of this chapter to discuss the pros and cons of structural adjustment, poverty reduction strategies, or debt relief efforts. Rather, the point is to show that aid provision is inevitably influenced and inextricably linked to the politics, ideologies, and priorities that influence broader international relations. Recent efforts to de-politicise aid must be viewed in this light.

The altruism vs. self-interested dichotomy is most useful for analysing the motivations and actions of sovereign states. However, with globalisation, aid provision has become increasingly influenced by other actors such as civil society organisations (CSOs) and the private sector. As global communication becomes faster and cheaper and global networks easier to establish, non-state actors have emerged as a powerful force in the global arena, often with a greater influence than their size, resources, or mandate would warrant (Fidler 2007). Indeed, Northern lobby groups in rich countries often have better access to and influence over aid decision-makers than recipient countries. Research from the US suggests that, like nation states, these groups are motivated both by self-interest – for example, wanting aid to be used in ways that boost the domestic economy – and by altruism. When their focus is international rather than domestic, civil society groups often campaign on single issues – such as user fees and access to medicines – rather than overall health sector development.

Globalisation is also associated with the blurring of traditional distinctions between donors and recipients. China and Brazil are examples of countries that assume both roles. This evolution is reflected in the emergence of new political groupings such as the G20, which includes developed and developing countries, and which takes an interest in both economic issues and development policy. At the April 2009 meeting of the G20 in London, heads of state not only agreed on an economic strategy to address the global financial crisis, but also reiterated their commitment to supporting the world's poorest countries.

What *is the purpose of aid?*

What do those providing aid want to achieve? The answer is again multifaceted, an indication of the mix of influences that drive provision of aid in the first place. In the post-Cold War era, poverty reduction has provided the overarching framework for aid, as reflected by the Millennium Declaration and the subsequent agreement of the Millennium Development Goals (MDGs). This broad consensus on the purpose of aid is located within a more widely shared vision of development, as set out in the 2002 Monterrey Consensus (United Nations 2002).

Together, these agreements represent a conceptual and philosophical shift in thinking about development, and the role of aid in achieving it, from an instrument of foreign policy to an instrument of development. In this new vision, the donor-recipient relationship is replaced by a 'partnership' for development, which encompasses other instruments of international relations, such as trade, and in which partner countries take the lead. However, this new consensus is very much a Northern one: emerging donors such as China and India do not necessarily subscribe to it (Grimm *et al.* 2009). While it would be naïve to suggest that Northern donors no longer view aid as a means of achieving diplomatic and strategic goals, the overt politicisation of their aid is now held in check by international agreements such as the MDGs and the peer pressure exerted through aid watchdog mechanisms like those at the OECD/DAC (see below). So far, though, these mechanisms appear to have had less leverage over new donors (Woods 2008).

The emergence of a shared vision on the purpose of aid is mirrored by a narrowing of ideological differences within the multilateral system: between Bretton Woods' championing of economic growth and the free market on the one hand, and the UN's focus on social justice and the need for regulation, on the other. Today, both sides of this debate have shifted towards the centre, so the policies they advocate have more in common than they do differences. However (as Box 47.1 illustrates), this is a recent development, and may be more an indication of a broader global consensus on economic policy than an indication of the de-politicisation of aid.

Furthermore, even if there is common ground on the *development* intentions of aid, aid is provided for a variety of reasons. Indeed, one analysis suggests that only 37 per cent of total aid is available for *development* projects and programmes ('country programmable aid'), the rest being earmarked for special purposes such as humanitarian relief, debt relief, and food aid (Kharas 2007). The promotion of democracy, cultural exchange, and – importantly for health – the provision of global public goods, are examples of the diverse purposes of aid. This diversity pulls against the vision set out at Monterrey, which sees developing countries taking the lead in deciding how aid resources are spent. It is also at odds with the aid effectiveness agenda, which seeks to promote greater coherence between aid donors, and better targeting of aid resources to country priorities, as discussed in the next section.

How *should aid be provided and managed?*

As agreement on the *purpose* of development spending emerged, so did an understanding that all aspects of development – human and economic – are linked. This holistic vision gave birth to new aid instruments such as Poverty Reduction Strategies (PRS). In addition to being linked to debt relief (see Box 47.1), PRS were designed to tackle the full spectrum of development challenges. Similarly, budget support – whereby donors provide their aid directly to the Ministry of Finance or state bank, where it is mixed with the government's own revenues – aims to ensure that implementation is government-led and therefore sustainable. Equivalent approaches have developed at sector level. Sector-wide approaches (SWAps) seek to bring development partners and government together around a shared programme of sector development, pooling resources for this purpose and agreeing on joint mechanisms to assess progress.

Proponents of the new aid modalities draw on evidence of the inefficiencies of 'old ways of doing business' – high transaction costs for governments of managing multiple donors, all with their own procedures and reporting mechanisms; the difficulties of using aid strategically when it is programmed over the short term; and the risk of distortion towards donor rather than country priorities.

The aid effectiveness agenda, as set out in the Paris Declaration on Aid Effectiveness (OECD 2005) and illustrated in Figure 47.1, attempts to address these challenges. It argues that donors need to coordinate better with each other (harmonisation), support country priorities, use country systems to deliver their resources (alignment), and focus on overall development

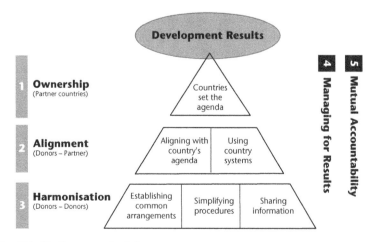

Figure 47.1 Aid effectiveness principles
Source: OECD/DAC.

progress rather than the outcome of particular aid projects (managing for results). While this is a conceptually persuasive approach, the complexity of forces influencing the provision of aid means it is likely to only ever be partially successful. Indeed, even with the Paris Declaration, the number of aid providers continues to increase, while the average size of donor activities in dollar terms continues to fall, suggesting that aid is becoming increasingly fragmented. The 'competitive aid world of many to many' (Picciotto 2007) is therefore likely to continue in the near future.

Does aid *achieve results*?

Being able to *show results* has an intuitive, persuasive power, both at a political level (for those setting aid budgets) and at a technical level (for those designing aid programmes). The question of whether aid has a positive influence on development outcomes has therefore been a prominent concern of policymakers and aid bureaucrats. Various studies (for example, Burnside and Dollar 1997) have attempted to provide empirical evidence, but findings are often contradictory or inconclusive.

In the age of globalisation, though, the question of whether aid 'works' may have become redundant. Aid is *one instrument* of international development, and in an era of interconnected trade, economic, and financial systems, it is more and more difficult to tease out aid's specific impact. Recognition of this difficulty has led many partners to the conclusion that attempting to attribute improvements in development outcomes to any particular donor, or even to aid in isolation from other financial flows or policy measures, is a lost cause. Rather, the focus should be overall development progress, not the outcomes of particular aid interventions.

This is a prominent aspect of aid effectiveness discussions, not least because a requirement to 'show impact' inevitably leads to a particular kind of aid modality – projects – which aid-effectiveness proponents are trying to move away from. Further, the quest for results may have the unintended consequence of weakening already-fragile accountability systems in recipient countries, as governments focus their attention on donor reporting needs rather than accounting to citizens.

Nevertheless, the political imperative to 'show results' remains, and the new aid modalities have been criticised for failing to do this. At one level, this is unfair: demonstrating progress on a national scale should be more meaningful than showing it in discrete project areas. However, the new aid instruments cannot link specific donor inputs to specific development outputs: each donor is only a *contributor* to overall progress, and when aid is mixed with government revenues it is almost impossible to disentangle the impact of aid. These issues may create political problems in donor capitals, and put pressure on aid agencies to spend their resources in more visible ways.

The politics of international health aid

Why do donors give health aid?

The mix of self-interest and altruistic motivations which characterise aid provision in general are also discernable in the provision of health aid, particularly in relation to bilateral donors. For example, Kassalow argues that 'improving the health of people in other countries makes both strategic and moral sense for the US government' (Kassalow 2001). This because it protects the US public from emerging infectious disease; because better health creates social cohesion, which in turn lessons the risk of political instability abroad; and because the provision of aid improves the US's international standing.

Unsurprisingly, in the post-9/11 world, 'realist' arguments became more common. Garrett, in advocating for greater investment in HIV/AIDS, claims: 'the nexus of poverty, HIV/AIDS and alienation from the West could provide fertile ground for anti-Western violence, possibly terrorism' (Garrett 2005). However, even as the realist arguments became more prominent, the moral case for investing in health in poor countries persisted, suggesting that, as in development more broadly, these two influences are always present.

As discussed above, bilateral donors are only one actor in the development arena. Civil society organisations, domestic lobby groups, and other non-state actors have a well-documented influence over aid allocations and donor policy, particularly in the US. For example, President Bush's domestic support base pushed him to fund HIV, but also to promote abstinence as the basis of HIV prevention – a policy direction that has more to do with domestic US politics than public health needs in poor countries. Similarly, CSOs have played a critical role in forcing HIV to the top of the health development agenda of bilateral agencies, in particular advocating for greater access to AIDS medicines (Shiffman 2008). While multilateral agencies and the new global partnerships do not have a domestic constituency as such, they too are subject to scrutiny from Northern lobby groups and globalised civil society networks such as the People's Health Movement (McCoy *et al.* 2006).

In health as in overall development, the emergence of new bilateral donors adds a further layer of complexity. Their approach is in part moral – representing the health interests of developing countries – but they are also interested in health issues that have strong foreign policy, economic, or trade links, and may use international development as an arena in which to make their foreign policy presence known. For example, Brazil championed a revision of international trade regulations to allow poor countries greater access to essential medicines still under patent. This was driven in part by an interest in preserving its own AIDS treatment programme, but the human rights aspects of this issue also featured very prominently. This intersection of development and foreign policy is a defining characteristic of global health issues (as opposed to health development issues), and is discussed further in the next section.

What is the purpose of health aid?

The ideological divisions which characterised development discourse in the 1980s and early 1990s also played out in health, resulting in major shifts in the health policies of large donors. The transitions from *Health for All* to a selective package of primary care, the demise of policies on community participation (Morgan 1990), and the move from free care to fee-for-service, are all examples.

As in overall development, major ideological and policy divisions in health have narrowed in recent years; the popularity of WHO's renewed focus on Primary Health Care (PHC) is one indication of this change. Presented both as a 'return to values' (after decades of privatisation and de-regulation), a means of strengthening health systems, and a way to protect investments in pro-poor aspects of care during times of financial crisis, PHC has attracted support from a wide constituency of civil society, developing countries, and donors. However, there are differences of opinion about how the PHC vision should be realised. In particular, old divisions between disease-specific and health systems approaches remain, not least because they compete for donor resources.

Global health

As discussed above, the world is moving from an international system (dominated by nation states) to a global one, in which non-state actors wield increasing power and influence. This has both positive and negative consequences for health. On the one hand, faster travel and increased communication associated with globalisation facilitates the spread of emerging diseases and new drug-resistant pathogens, which no state can address individually. On the other, the international community is now better placed than ever before to cooperate for the good of global public health, for example on medical research and lowering drug prices.

New structures have been developed to try to make the most of opportunities and minimise the threats. These include legal instruments such as the International Health Regulations and the Framework Convention on Tobacco Control, and new institutions such as Norway's Foreign Policy and Global Health initiative. Sovereign states retain the primary role in these structures – particularly in relation to health security – but non-state actors are also important. For example, the private sector will play an important role in the manufacture of any vaccine developed in response to a global pandemic, while academic centres will be involved in research and clinical trials.

As with health development, both self-interest and altruistic influences are present in debates around global health. Statements like: 'The collapse of an African country's health system could be the sign or symptom of a state failure with American security implications' (Malloch-Brown 2009) show that domestic as well as international politicians make the link between health development in poor countries health security in rich ones.

How is health aid provided?

As interest in health development has grown in foreign policy circles, so foreign policy experts have increasingly turned their attention to the ways in which health aid is delivered. Aid for health has more than doubled in recent years: from around US $6.8 billion in 2000 to $16.7 billion in 2008, taking into account official and non-official donors. This increase has been associated with a proliferation of health partners, fragmentation of aid channels, and distortion towards donor priorities. An analysis of ODA for health over the last decade found that countries with comparable health indicators receive remarkably different levels of aid (Piva and Dodd 2009). Furthermore, as shown in Figure 47.2, funding for HIV accounts for an

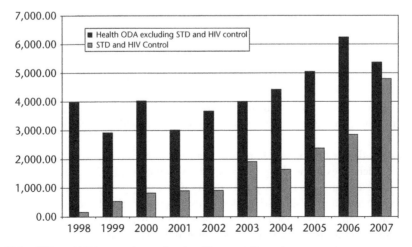

Figure 47.2 STD and HIV control vs. other health commitments
Source: WHO, adapted from OECD/DAC Statistics.

increasing share of health ODA, leaving many other health and health-related priorities insufficiently funded.

These challenges – and the problems they create for countries – have led to calls for the decentralisation of decision-making in aid from donor headquarters to their country offices. However, the influence of domestic constituencies in donor countries is likely to pull in the opposite direction – the more decentralised aid decisions become, the less influence domestic lobby groups have.

On the other hand, the health sector has one of the most active debates and some of the most advanced thinking on 'aid effectiveness' approaches. Indeed, some of the first practical applications of the SWAp mechanism were in the health sector. This push and pull – between those who seek to manage diversity, and the chaotic reality of multiple aid providers and channels – has been a prominent theme in international health over the last decade (Dodd and Hill 2007).

Does health aid achieve results?

As aid is only one influence on development outcomes, so health aid is only one contributor to health outcomes. In the majority of low-income countries, the bulk of health expenditure is 'out-of-pocket', that is, paid directly by individuals when they buy health services or medicines. Thus, the contribution of aid to total health expenditure is low. Further, many other aspects of development – education, income, water, and sanitation – have a determining impact on health outcomes. Finally, mortality indicators typically improve only very slowly – over a decade or more – making it even harder for donors, who normally plan over a short-term period, to influence them.

The aid effectiveness agenda acknowledges the political imperative to show results, but argues that the impact of donor resources should be judged collectively, and in terms of overall development progress. In this imagining, the role of partners is to move away from attempting to deliver results directly, towards an approach which tries to understand *why the existing health system does not deliver results*, and the role of aid in facilitating reform. Demonstrating progress is then a matter of demonstrating steady progress in the reform agenda – more a qualitative than a quantitative task – and arguing that this reform agenda has in turn contributed to overall development.

Conclusion

While scholars have long recognised that development assistance is subject to political influences, few analyses have attempted to describe how these forces play out in health. This gap is all the more surprising given that health development is intimately intertwined with global health issues such as health security, which – because they sit at the nexus of aid, foreign policy, and security – are among the most politically charged of all development issues.

The realist–idealist dichotomy, borrowed from international relations, is a useful starting point from which to examine the politics of international health. The framework highlights the self-interest of donors, but also points to the persuasive 'power of ideas', as exemplified by the persistence of a more altruistic vision of aid. However, the dichotomy also has limitations. The discussion in this chapter suggests that international health is in fact characterised by multiple inputs and agents – each with their own perspective and motivations – creating a complex interplay of heterogeneous influences. The web of actors, communication channels, and resource flows created by globalisation further complicates the picture, making it even more difficult to tease out the pathways of political influence. Nevertheless, these influences exist, and understanding them is key to understanding the *what, why, and how* of aid provision.

Note

1 Thanks to Andrew Cassels, Peter Hill, and Phyllida Travis for their valuable comments and inputs.

References

Burnside, C. and Dollar, D. (1997) *Aid, Policies and Growth*, World Bank, Policy Research Working Paper No. 1777, Washington, DC: The World Bank.

Dodd, R. and Hill, P.S. (2007) 'The Aid Effectiveness Agenda: Bringing Discipline to Diversity in Global Health', *Global Health Governance*, 1(2): 1–10.

Fidler, D. (2007) 'Architecture Amidst Anarchy: Global Health's Quest for Governance', *Global Health Governance*, 1(1): 1–17.

Garrett, L. (2005) *HIV and National Security: Where Are the Links?* New York: Council on Foreign Relations.

Grimm, S., Humphrey, J., Lundsgaarde, E., and de Sousa, S.-L. J. (2009) *European Development Cooperation to 2020: Challenges by New Actors in International Development*, European Commision, Working Paper No. 4, Brussels: European Commission.

Kassalow, J.S. (2001) *Why Health is Important to US Foreign Policy*, New York: Council on Foreign Relations.

Kharas, H. (2007) *Trends and Issues in Development Aid*, Working Paper No. 1, Washington, DC: Wolfensohn Center for Development.

Lancaster, C. (2007) *Foreign Aid: Diplomacy, Development, Domestic Politics*, Chicago: University of Chicago Press.

Lumsdaine, D.H. (1993) *Moral Vision in International Politics: The Foreign Aid Regime, 1949–1989*, Princeton, NJ: Princeton University Press.

McCoy, D., Narayan, R., Baum, F., Sanders, D., Serag, H., Salvage, J., Rowson, M., Schrecker, T., Woodward, D., Labonte, R., Sengupta, A., Qizphe, A., Schuftan, C., and People's Health Movement (2006) 'A New Director General for WHO: An Opportunity for Bold and Inspirational Leadership', *The Lancet*, 368(9,553): 2,179–83.

Malloch-Brown, M. (2009) Conference Keynote Address, Chatham House Conference on 'Rethinking Global Health: Political and Practical Challenges from Foreign and Security Policy', London, 10–11 March.

Morgan, L.M. (1990) 'International Politics and Primary Health Care in Costa Rica', *Social Science & Medicine*, 30(2): 211–9.

OECD (Organisation for Economic Co-operation and Development) (2005) *Paris Declaration on Aid Effectiveness*, Paris: OECD.

OECD (Organisation for Economic Co-operation and Development) (2009) *DAC Glossary of Key Terms and Concepts*, available at http://www.oecd.org/document/32/0,3343, en_2649_33721_42632800_1_1_1_1,00.html#ODA (accessed 19 November 2009).

Picciotto, R. (2007) Review of R. C. Riddell, *Does Foreign Aid Really Work?* and C. Lancaster, *Foreign Aid: Diplomacy, Development, Domestic Politics*, Annual Journal of the Carnegie Council on Ethics and International Affairs, 21(4): 477–80.

Piva, P. and R. Dodd (2009) 'Where Did All the Aid Go? An In-depth Analysis of Increased Health Aid Flows Over the Last 10 Years', *Bulletin of the World Health Organization*, 87(12): 930–9.

Shiffman, J. (2008) 'Has Donor Prioritization of HIV/AIDS Displaced Aid for Other Health Issues?', *Health Policy and Planning*, 23(2): 95–100.

UN (United Nations) (2002) *Monterrey Consensus of the International Conference on Financing for Development*, Monterrey, Mexico: UN.

Woods, N. (2008) 'Whose Aid? Whose Influence? China, Emerging Donors and the Silent Revolution in Development Assistance', *International Affairs*, 84(6): 1,205–221.

48

Developing Drugs for the Developing World

The Role of Product Development Partnerships[1]

Maria C. Freire

Estimated costs for the development of new therapeutics range from $800 million to $1.5 billion. It is not surprising, therefore, that pharmaceutical and biotechnology companies target their drug development activities to indications, such as cancer and Alzheimer's disease, for which the market can repay the outlay and ensure profits. In the case of diseases that disproportionately affect populations in developing countries, this equation is non-functional, suppressing the development of drugs and other interventions, such as diagnostics and vaccines, that are desperately needed for poor populations. A decade ago, a new paradigm for the development of these 'tools' emerged – the creation of the Product Development Public/Private Partnerships or PDPs, that leverage the resources and skills of the public sector, philanthropy, and industry to address these neglected health needs. This chapter discusses the development, evolution, and advances made by PDPs, the way they carry out their mission, and where they are today, using as a case study the Global Alliance for TB Drug Development.

Tuberculosis: disease of the poor

Mycobacterium tuberculosis, the bacillus that causes tuberculosis (TB), can be traced back thousands of years to Egyptian (Zink *et al.* 2003) and Peruvian mummies (Salo *et al.* 1994). The ancient scourge continues to this day – the World Health Organization (WHO) calls TB a 'worldwide pandemic' (WHO 2010). Numbers tell the deadly story: a third of the world, 2.2 billion people, is infected with TB and almost 5,000 people die every day, the vast majority (98 per cent) in developing countries.

Drug-susceptible TB is generally treated for six to nine months using a combination drug regimen that includes four first-line drugs: isoniazid, rifampin, pyrazinamide, and ethambutol. Multidrug-resistant tuberculosis (MDR-TB), TB resistant to rifampin and isoniazid, usually develops because of inappropriate treatment or failure to complete treatment (Iseman 1993), and is found in virtually all countries around the world. Treatment of MDR-TB requires individualised, prolonged therapy using second-line drugs (such as amikacin, kanamycin, or capreomycin), which are fewer in number, poorly tolerated, difficult to administer, and much more expensive than first-line drugs. The recently identified strains of extensively drug-resistant tuberculosis (XDR-TB), now documented in at least 50 countries, do not respond to the most powerful first-line and second-line drugs, making it dramatically clear that we are running out of treatments.

This precarious situation is the result of a 40-year gap in TB drug development. Contributing to the hiatus was the complacency of physicians and public health officials who felt secure because of the success of first-line treatments; the lack of foresight regarding the devastating speed and consequences of the emergence of drug resistance; and the inadequate economic incentives for the private sector to embark on the arduous process of drug development for an indication that primarily affects individuals in resource-poor countries.

The road to developing new drugs

Development of new medicines is complex, difficult, and expensive. It usually starts with the search for new chemical or biological molecules that, when tested *in vitro* (i.e. in the laboratory), show potential activity against a disease target or infectious agent (Nwaka and Ridley 2003). These basic research and discovery stages tap the knowledge generated by laboratory research and, in some instances, the experience and wisdom of traditional medicine. Once a compound (or 'lead') is identified and chemically modified to optimise its function, pre-clinical development ensues with extensive tests *in vitro* and *in vivo* (i.e. in living organisms, including in animal models of the disease). Only lead compounds that successfully meet these hurdles are approved to enter into human clinical trials.

Potential new drugs are first tested in a small number (20–100) of healthy human volunteers under strict standards set by regulatory authorities, such as the US Food and Drug Administration (FDA). The goal of the Phase I trials is to assess the safety of the potential drug, to determine how well it is tolerated, and to establish its metabolic path once inside the body. In Phase II clinical trials, which commence only if Phase I hurdles are met, the drug is administered to a larger group (100–500), usually limited to patients with the disease, to determine if the drug is effective, to find the therapeutic dosages, and to ascertain any toxicity. Most potential new drugs fail at this stage, either because they do not work as expected or because they have toxic effects. Phase III trials require the largest number of volunteers (1,000–5,000) and are the most difficult, time-consuming, and expensive trials in the drug development process. They are designed to show how well the new drug works and how it compares to current treatment. Phase III trials may take many years to complete, especially for chronic diseases. The time required to complete pre-clinical and clinical drug development is generally 10–12 years and, because of the hurdles that must be overcome, there is a high attrition rate of the compounds undergoing testing, resulting in very few approved drugs. The costs associated with traditional drug development are estimated by the pharmaceutical companies to be between $800 million and $1,500 million (DiMasi 2003; Adams 2006).

Traditionally, different actors have participated at specific stages of drug development (see Figure 48.1). Basic research, for example, is primarily the purview of academia and governments, with important contributions from pharmaceutical and biotechnology companies in the areas of their therapeutic interest. In contrast, clinical trials are mostly conducted by the private sector. Government organisations, including the US National Institutes of Health (NIH) and the US Centers for Disease Control and Prevention (CDC), however, fund and conduct clinical trials of public health importance, such as the CDC-supported Tuberculosis Trials Consortium (TBTC).

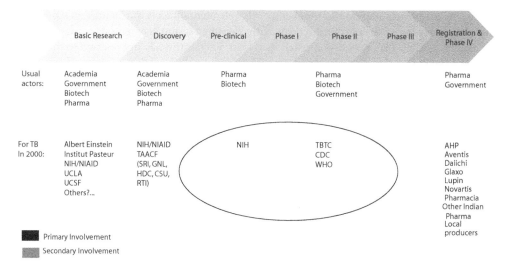

Figure 48.1 Drug development participation analysis: 2000
Source: Adapted from the Boston Consulting Group TB Landscape Analysts for the TB Alliance 2000.

In the late 1990s, the global health community began to recognise that the development of new tools (vaccines, drugs, and diagnostics) had been neglected for those diseases where market forces were unfavourable. The enormous disparity between the health afflictions in the developing world (particularly for diseases such as tuberculosis, malaria, dengue, etc.), and the commercial drivers for products to prevent or ameliorate them, led to the realisation that fighting and preventing these diseases requires novel, bold, and innovative strategies (Widdus 2005).

Public/private partnerships: a new way of doing business

A landscape analysis of TB drug development commissioned by the Rockefeller Foundation for the TB Alliance and conducted by the Boston Consulting Group (TB Alliance 2000) identified the development 'cliffs' that prevented translation of basic research findings into new drugs for TB. The data showed that while basic research in TB was being conducted, the information did not result in product development. If/when clinical trials were conducted, these were primarily to adjust or modify treatment regimens with existing TB drugs, rather than test potential new compounds; and, finally, drugs failed to reach patients due to lack of country-level health infrastructure, production facilities, high costs, or a combination of these and other factors. The analysis also provided evidence that there were no new TB drugs in the pipeline and that there was a demonstrable activity void from the pre-clinical through the clinical stages (Figure 48.1).

On 6–8 February 2000 in Cape Town, South Africa, a historic meeting of over 100 representatives from academia, industry, non-governmental organisations (NGOs), governments, and philanthropies was convened by the Rockefeller Foundation, hosted by the Medical Research Council of South Africa, and co-sponsored by the Stop TB Initiative,[2] the NIH, the Bill & Melinda Gates Foundation, the Wellcome Trust, and the UK Department of International Development. Reflecting the spirit of the participants, the resulting Cape Town Declaration called attention to the urgent need to accelerate the development of new drugs to shorten the treatment of TB with the aim of improving compliance and reducing the development of drug resistance, and to facilitate TB control in the poorest countries (Pablo-Mendez 2000).

Specifically, the participants pledged to work in concert with Stop TB for TB control, to lay out a scientific blueprint and economic analysis of TB drug development, to design a road-map for advocacy for the development of new TB drugs, and, importantly, to create a dedicated public/private partnership (PPP): the Global Alliance for TB Drug Development (TB Alliance).

The timing was propitious: the sequencing of the *Mycobacterium tuberculosis* genome had recently been completed, new sources of philanthropic and governmental funding were available, and there was a new urgency to address issues of health and poverty, as witnessed by the creation one month earlier of the WHO Commission on Macroeconomics and Health (WHO 2001).

Set up as a virtual drug research and development (R&D) organisation, the mission of the TB Alliance is to catalyse and streamline the development of new TB drugs. As part of a select group of not-for-profit PDPs, the TB Alliance's strategy is to optimise speed of development and reduce costs by combining the expertise of its staff with the skill and resources of collaborators and partners in the public and private sectors worldwide. To carry out its mission, the TB Alliance identifies and accesses promising drug candidates from myriad sources, spearheading their development from pre-clinical to clinical stages, and ultimately driving successful com-pounds through registration. Since its inception, the Alliance has funded the development of platform technologies, such as databases on clinical trial sites, and provided support for specialised evaluations, such as TB drug-combination testing, to benefit the field.

The target profile of the new TB drug(s) will: shorten the duration of treatment to two months; improve the treatment of drug-resistant disease; and halt TB infection in at-risk individuals, such as those living with HIV. The TB Alliance adheres to the 'AAA' strategy, which explicitly requires that resulting treatments must be affordable, available, and easily adopted in the field. After almost ten years of operation, the TB Alliance can report substantial, concrete progress in achieving this plan, having built the largest portfolio of potential TB compounds in the world (TB Alliance 2010), with three compounds currently in clinical trials.

One of these compounds, PA-824, along with its analogues and derivatives, was licensed in early February 2002 from Chiron Corporation (now Novartis). A novel nitroimidazole, PA-824 was brought into the portfolio at an early pre-clinical stage. The compound was of particular interest because in the mouse model it had shown sterilising activity that was as high as the combination of rifampin and isoniazid, two of the first-line drugs. Further, PA-824 and its analogues had demonstrated activity against drug-sensitive and drug-resistant forms of the TB bacillus. Development of PA-824 moved briskly and, in April 2005, having met all the required pre-clinical milestones, the TB Alliance filed an Investigational New Drug (IND) application with the FDA. Today, the drug is in Phase II clinical trials, and is primed to be tested in combination with other TB drugs for drug-sensitive and MDR/XDR-TB indications (TB Alliance 2009).

The licensing and development of PA-824 provides an excellent example of how PDPs operate, leveraging resources and expertise to achieve their technical and humanitarian goals. Specifically, it illustrates:

• Innovative intellectual property arrangements – the trailblazing agreement with Chiron demonstrated that it is possible to craft terms and conditions that meet industry standards and uphold the AAA mandate. As Tom Abate, a staff writer at the *San Francisco Chronicle*, put it:

> What a deal like this tells me is that biotech leaders, international health officials and philanthropic groups are trying to create mechanisms to address needs that would

otherwise fall through the cracks. I'm keeping my fingers crossed, both for the TB drug and the larger experiment in non-profit drug development.

–(Tom Abate, *San Francisco Chronicle*, 11 February 2002)

- Collaboration with industry – Chiron provided all the technical data in its possession, samples of the compounds and their analogues, and made their scientists available for consultation
- Assistance of government research organisations and CRO support – financing for the pre-clinical development stages was provided by the National Institute of Allergy and Infectious Diseases (NIAID) of NIH through their agreement with Research Triangle Institute (RTI) in North Carolina, to which the PA-824 development was outsourced
- Global participation – during the development process, the TB Alliance has involved over 24 organisations with every continent represented.

Because of their innovative business model and low overheads, PDPs act nimbly and can leverage investments. For example, PDPs can be opportunistic, advancing drugs approved for other indications if they show activity against the selected targets; they can develop a drug with single or multiple partners/collaborators, including industry, academia, governments, NGOs, and others; and PDPs can work jointly with companies to identify promising compounds in their libraries. The portfolios of PDPs and the speed of drug development in organisations like the TB Alliance, the Medicines for Malaria Ventures, and the Drugs for Neglected Diseases initiative are proof positive that the model is working.

Galvanising action

The TB Alliance was also charged with tracking the progress of global TB drug development efforts through its chairmanship of the Working Group on New TB Drugs, part of the Stop TB Partnership. In this role, the TB Alliance intervenes, as appropriate, when its efforts can help advance promising drug candidates. If a compound already has momentum, the organisation focuses its efforts and resources to spur advances elsewhere.

To help coordinate and catalyse TB drug development worldwide, the TB Alliance has worked to lower the scientific and regulatory hurdles for organisations interested in developing affordable drugs to treat TB. For example, the PDP provides support for screening potential anti-TB compounds, either directly or indirectly; assists in technical evaluations of third-party projects; and is working to streamline regulatory processes, which were essentially non-existent for TB given the lack of new compounds awaiting regulatory approval. Furthermore, the organisation invests in platform technologies, such as animal models and databases, which serve to harmonise standards and provide research tools to buttress the TB drug development process.

The galvanising effect of this PDP and of the commitment of the different actors in this global health field in helping bring new and unexpected actors to the TB drug development arena is seen in the landscape analysis shown in Figure 48.2.

As noted in the 2009 report of the Treatment Action Group (TAG) (Chou *et al.* 2009), there are currently five new compounds with novel mechanisms of action in clinical trials, making the TB drug pipeline 'the fullest' it has been in decades. From a broader perspective, the last ten years have shown that PDPs have opened new avenues for product development (Moran 2005) and brought with them expert, multidisciplinary teams to address health problems of global magnitude.

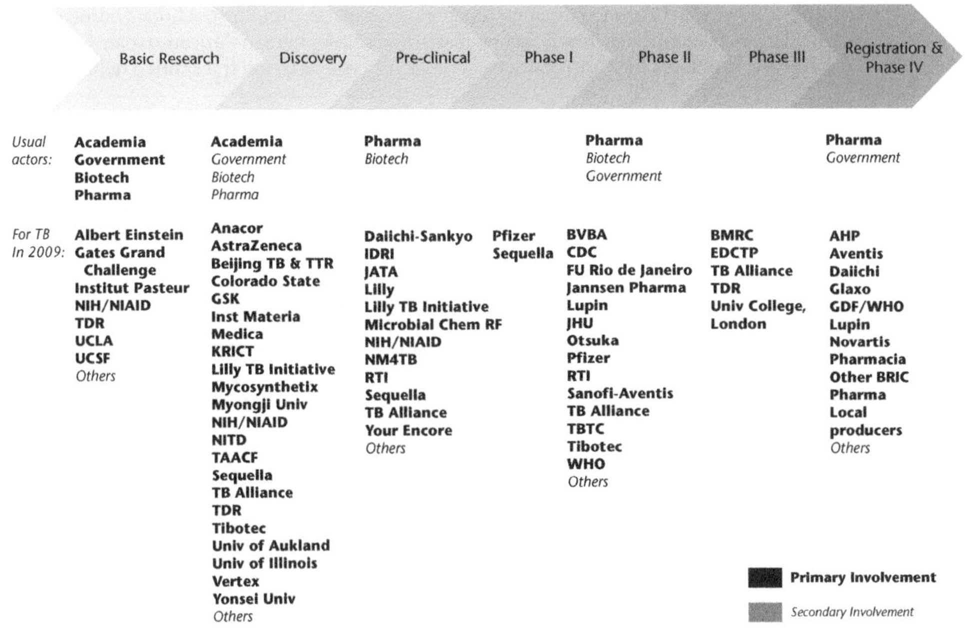

	Basic Research	Discovery	Pre-clinical	Phase I	Phase II	Phase III	Registration & Phase IV
Usual actors:	**Academia** **Government** Biotech Pharma	**Academia** Government Biotech Pharma	**Pharma** Biotech		**Pharma** Biotech Government		**Pharma** Government
For TB In 2009:	**Albert Einstein** **Gates Grand Challenge** **Institut Pasteur** **NIH/NIAID** **TDR** **UCLA** **UCSF** *Others*	**Anacor** **AstraZeneca** **Beijing TB & TTR** **Colorado State** **GSK** **Inst Materia Medica** **KRICT** **Lilly TB Initiative** **Mycosynthetix** **Myongji Univ** **NIH/NIAID** **NITD** **TAACF** **Sequella** **TB Alliance** **TDR** **Tibotec** **Univ of Aukland** **Univ of Illinois** **Vertex** **Yonsel Univ** *Others*	**Daiichi-Sankyo** **IDRI** **JATA** **Lilly** **Lilly TB Initiative** **Microbial Chem RF** **NIH/NIAID** **NM4TB** **RTI** **Sequella** **TB Alliance** **Your Encore** *Others*	**Pfizer** Sequella	**BVBA** **CDC** **FU Rio de Janeiro** **Jannsen Pharma** **Lupin** **JHU** **Otsuka** **Pfizer** **RTI** **Sanofi-Aventis** **TB Alliance** **TBTC** **Tibotec** **WHO** *Others*	**BMRC** **EDCTP** **TB Alliance** **TDR** **Univ College, London**	**AHP** **Aventis** **Daiichi** **Glaxo** **GDF/WHO** **Lupin** **Novartis** **Pharmacia** **Other BRIC Pharma** **Local producers** *Others*

■ **Primary Involvement**

▨ *Secondary Involvement*

Figure 48.2 TB drug development participation analysis: 2009
Source: Adapted from The Working Group on New TB Drugs, Stop TB Partnership and TAG 2009 Pipeline Report.

Conclusion

Despite the amazing progress, many hurdles lie ahead. In the case of TB, and increasingly in diseases like malaria, successful treatments are not based solely on the development of novel drugs. To have massive impact and prevent or minimise drug resistance, new medicines must be administered in the right combination (Ginsberg and Spigelman 2007). Combination therapy requires complex, lengthy, and, consequently, very expensive clinical trials in resource-limited settings to obtain the intricate data needed to gain regulatory approval.

Given the current world economic environment, it is unclear that the financial resources necessary to advance the global pipeline of drugs for neglected diseases,[3] including TB, to registration will be available. Indeed, financial sustainability of the public–private partnership models, including PDPs, has been a topic of discussion. With more than 60 drug development projects initiated by PDPs for neglected diseases, one estimate based on historical attrition rates indicates that at least $1 billion per year for ten years will be necessary to successfully register the compounds in the portfolio (Herrling 2009). Despite the economic barriers to action, the cost of inaction must be measured in millions of lives, and the further spread of these devastating diseases. We cannot and must not take that risk.

Notes

1 The author thanks Dr Doris Rouse and Mr David Keegan for their invaluable comments.
2 Now known as the Stop TB Partnership or Stop TB, this coalition brings together over 500 organisations in a global movement to stop the spread of TB, with the ultimate goal of achieving a TB-free world. Please see http://www.stoptb.org.

3 The FDA lists the following as neglected diseases: tuberculosis, malaria, blinding trachoma, buruli ulcer, cholera, dengue/dengue haemorrhagic fever, racunculiasis, fascioliasis, human African trypanosomiasis, leishmaniasis, leprosy, lymphatic filariasis, onchocerciasis, schistosomiasis, soil transmitted helmithiasis, and yaws.

References

Adams, C.P. (2006) 'Estimating the Cost of New Drug Development: Is it Really $802 Million?', *Health Affairs*, 25: 420.

Chou, L., Harrington, M., Huff, B., Jefferys, R., Syed, J. and Wingfield, C. (2009) *TAG 2009 Pipeline Report*, available at http://apps.who.int/tdr/diseases/tuberculosis/pdf/2009_pipeline_report.pdf (accessed 4 January 2010).

DiMasi, J.A. (2003) 'The Price of Innovation: New Estimates of Drug Development Costs', *Journal of Health Economics*, 22: 151.

Ginsberg, A.M. and Spigelman, M. (2007) 'Challenges in Tuberculosis Drug Research and Development', *Nature Medicine*, 13: 290–94.

Herrling, P. (2009) 'Financing R&D for Neglected Diseases', *Nature Reviews/Drug Discovery*, 8: 91.

Iseman, M. (1993) 'Treatment of Multidrug-resistant Tuberculosis', *New England Journal of Medicine*, 329(11): 784–91.

Moran, M. (2005) 'A Breakthrough in R&D for Neglected Diseases: New Ways to Get the Drugs We Need', *PLoS Medicine*, 2: 0828–32, e302.

Nwaka, S. and Ridley, R. (2003) 'Virtual Drug Discovery and Development for Neglected Diseases through Public–Private Partnerships', *Nature*, 2: 924.

Pablos-Mendez, A., for the Working Alliance for TB Drug Development (2000) 'The Declaration of Cape Town', *International Journal of Tuberculosis and Lung Disease*, 4(6): 489–90.

Salo, W.L., Aufderheide, A.C., Buikstra, J. and Holcomb, T.A. (1994) 'Identification of Mycobacterium Tuberculosis DNA in a Pre-Columbian Peruvian Mummy', *Proceedings of the National Academy of Sciences*, 91(6): 2,091–94.

TB Alliance (Global Alliance for TB Drug Development) (2000), *Report for Rockefeller Foundation*, Internal document (Personal communication, September 2001).

TB Alliance (Global Alliance for TB Drug Development) (2009) *Accelerating the Pace, 2009 Annual Report*, available at http://www.tballiance.org/downloads/publications/TBA%20Annual%202009.pdf (accessed 24 March 2010).

TB Alliance (Global Alliance for TB Drug Development) (2010) *TB Alliance Portfolio 2010*, available at http://www.tballiance.org/new/portfolio/html-portfolio (accessed 4 January 2010).

Widdus, R. (2005) 'Public-private Partnerships: An Overview', *Transactions of the Royal Society of Tropical Medicine and Hygiene*, 99S: S1–S8.

WHO (World Health Organization) (2001) *Macroeconomics and Health: Investing in Health for Economic Development. Report of the Commission on Macroeconomics and Health*, Geneva: WHO.

WHO (World Health Organization) (2010) *10 Facts about Tuberculosis*, available at http://www.who.int/features/factfiles/tb_facts/en/index5.html (accessed 4 January 2010).

Zink, A.R., Sola, C., Reischl, U., Graner, W., Rastogi, N., Wolf, H., and Nerlich, A.G. (2003) 'Characterization of *Mycobacterium tuberculosis* Complex DNAs from Egyptian Mummies by Spoligotyping', *Journal of Clinical Microbiology*, 41: 359–67.

49

Models of Cooperation, Capacity Building, and the Future of Global Health

Gerald T. Keusch

Introduction

If you listen carefully, you can almost hear the excitement on the campuses of universities in the United States (US) and in many other industrialised nations. Students are thinking and talking about global health, and asking what they can do to help to reduce the disparities that exist between rich and poor nations. They are being guided by faculty who are themselves committed to global health research, education and training, and service. Students are increasingly taking the plunge, finding ways to spend time in resource-limited developing nations, offering their best efforts to help (Merson and Chapman Page 2009). It has become a movement, not just of people, but of their hearts and their minds, and it has grown dramatically over the past several decades. Recently, the Consortium of Universities for Global Health surveyed 37 universities with well-established global health programmes (CUGH 2009). The results document a doubling in the number of students enrolled in global health programmes in these leading institutions over just the past three years, as well as an increase in the average number of student-led organisations focused on global health to over three per campus. More than 150 US universities are developing some sort of initiative in global health. There is considerable interest in the global epidemic of HIV and AIDS, but this is by no means the only problem driving student and institutional interest.

Whenever there is a movement, as global health can be characterised, it is important to know what it is about, why it began, what it is doing, and where it is going. The answers to these questions are essential prerequisites to any attempt to thoughtfully guide those involved to better achieve their goals, and to identify the changes necessary to accomplish it. Recently, a group of international experts defined global health as 'an area for study, research, and practice that places a priority on improving health and achieving equity in health for all people worldwide' (Koplan *et al.* 2009: 1,995). Much of this focuses on capacity-building, but other than the cost-effectiveness analyses of potential interventions recently published by the Disease Control Priorities in Developing Countries Project (Jamison *et al.* 2006) to identify 'best buys' to get the biggest bang for the buck, there has been little scholarly evaluation of the overall impact of such programmes on either those helping to build capacity or those at the receiving end. We do not know in any systematic way what has been accomplished, how to judge effectiveness, and whether or not there have been unintended consequences, and if so, what they are.

In this information vacuum, this chapter offers a perspective gained during the author's evolving professional career of 40 years devoted to global health. While the strength of the observations will inevitably suffer from their personal nature and from their grounding in efforts to build global health programmes at academic institutions in the US, the underlying intent is to identify the central issues that need to be more carefully and objectively evaluated in the future. The premise is that capacity-building for global health is inextricably linked to the future of the global health movement in developed nations, and the pace of development in the recipient nations.

Historical precedents

In the 1960s, the US had two major streams of support for research and capacity-building in 'tropical infectious diseases'. These included laboratories established and run by the US military and National Institutes of Health (NIH)-supported, university-run research centers in developing countries. The seventh cholera pandemic in the late 1950s had led the NIH intramural research programme to initiate studies on disease mechanisms, leading directly to the creation of the Pakistan-SEATO cholera research laboratory (the predecessor to the International Centre for Diarrhoeal Disease Research) in Dhaka, Bangladesh, and a companion capacity-building programme for US physicians under the International Research Career Development Program, which posted young scientists at the military or academic laboratories (van Heyningen and Seal 1983). Many of the current senior leadership in global health programmes in the US cut their teeth in this training programme, although no formal survey of subsequent career paths and contributions to science has ever been carried out. The goals were basic and clinical research as an agenda of importance to the US, and primarily infectious diseases such as cholera or malaria that troops or travellers might encounter. While these diseases were also important for developing countries, the host countries themselves did not have much say in the research agenda, nor, in general, was there a specific expectation of capacity-building within these countries as a result of the 'collaboration'. This was largely a one-way relationship, with the developed country doing the science and the developing countries providing the diseases and the affected populations.

In the mid-1970s, the World Health Organization (WHO) surprised many when it created the Tropical Diseases Research Programme (TDR) in partnership with the United Nations Development Programme (UNDP) and the World Bank, as an independent entity within WHO, supported through special funds provided by external donors specifically for TDR (WHO 2007). While TDR was limited to activities for which it could generate support, TDR itself, rather than the WHO leadership, determined how the funds were to be used. The first director was Adetokunbo Lucas, a Nigerian physician and public health expert, educated in the UK and the US, and Chair of the Department of Preventive and Social Medicine at the University of Ibadan. Under Lucas's leadership over the decade from 1976–86, TDR awarded 2,400 grants in 100 countries, trained local scientists through international academic programmes, and spurred the development of new products for tropical diseases. The new graduates, for the most part, returned home to continue to work and develop in the institutions from which they had come. Lucas proved that capacity-building involving disease-endemic country scientists could be led by a multinational organisation if funding was available, the necessary autonomy to act flexibly was in place, and there were training sites in developed countries where fellows could subsequently work.

Shortly afterwards, in 1978, Dr Kenneth Warren, then the head of Health Sciences at the Rockefeller Foundation, created a network of developed and developing country scientists called the Great Neglected Diseases of Mankind Biomedical Research Program, or the GND for short (Rockefeller Foundation 1979). The idea behind the GND was to attract the best scientists from the developed world in all relevant areas of basic research to focus on the neglected infectious diseases of interest to the Foundation, while training young scientists from developing countries within the research programme. Fourteen units in the US, Europe, Thailand, Egypt, and Mexico were ultimately established, involving 160 investigators, with support for a decade. Meeting yearly, they soon lowered the barriers to the communication of their work, pre-publication. The effort succeeded in attracting new talent from diverse scientific disciplines, and in rapidly bringing modern cellular and molecular biology and genetics into the study of tropical infectious diseases. Warren strongly promoted the back-and-forth travels of the developed country investigators from their laboratories to the field, and the training of 360 scientists, 150 from the developing world. The modest investments by the Foundation, $15 million over the duration of the programme, resulted in a five-fold leveraging of research funding from other sources, and a phenomenal scientific output, with over 1,800 peer-reviewed publications during the decade of support. Moreover, there was a life-long redirection of the scientific efforts of the participants to these global health challenges, continuing well beyond the end of the GND itself. The programme was, however, primarily unidirectional, from the developed country partner to the recipient, or what traditionally has been called capacity-building (Figure 49.1a).

In 1988, the Rockefeller Foundation launched a new programme, 'Health Sciences for the Tropics' (Rockefeller Foundation 1988), designed as the specific twinning of a developed world research group with a partner in the developing world, and now focused on a specific problem of mutual interest and major public health importance. The idea that scientific training efforts for developing country scientists could yield a group of effective scientists who would work in their own institutions, rather than move to the developed country institutions they trained in, had been demonstrated by TDR and GND. The next logical step in capacity-building was institutional twinning, through which infrastructure and support systems, in addition to individual scientist expertise, could be developed. Forty laboratories were supported under this programme, again for a decade, during which collaborative research, training, and faculty exchanges were highlighted. It ushered in an important change in philosophy, that funds were to be separately allocated to the two partner principle investigators, rather than to the developed country lead, thus ensuring that decisions – all of which required funding – were made by the two partners together. The model was now much more of a true partnership (Figure 49.1b).

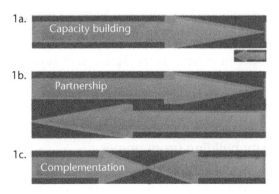

Figure 49.1   Models of collaboration

At the same time, the NIH's Fogarty International Center (FIC) created a new model for an institutional training programme – and reinvented itself – when it established and funded the AIDS International Training and Research Program (AITRP) under a new mechanism, which allowed federal training funds provided to a US university to be used to support developing country trainees who were neither citizens nor permanent residents of the US. The goal was to address the manpower shortage within the countries hardest hit by the HIV epidemic through training at institutions with NIH research grants on HIV/AIDS in those same countries. In 1999, a retrospective analysis of the first 1,500 trainees in the programme was undertaken. The response rate to a questionnaire was high (86 per cent), and it revealed that over 80 per cent of all the trainees were still in their country of origin, almost all still involved in HIV research or service provision. The factors identified as most important for trainees to remain in their own country were the chance to stay up-to-date through the work with their scientific partners, which also provided access to the National Library of Medicine, to the chance to attend and present at international meetings through project funding, and to be able to continually do research using the skills they had developed during their training. While these relationships were not yet representing equal inputs, it was clear that the collaboration was moving from a model of capacity-building (Figure 49.1a) to one of partnership (Figure 49.1b). The build-up of a critical mass of local investigators over time – which was dependent on continuous funding to the developed country partner – provided an opportunity for the partnership to mature into a more equal and complementary research relationship (Figure 49.1c).

Another model for capacity-building developed in the mid-1990s, when the NIH, under the leadership of Harold Varmus, convened the leaders of developed country research funding agencies and malaria researchers from sub-Saharan Africa to discuss the creation of a programme to accelerate the pace of malaria research and to build research capacity. The result was the Multilateral Initiative on Malaria (MIM), established in 1997 as a partnership of funders committed to improving research infrastructure in Africa and training African researchers. Through funds sent to TDR to support research projects and training fellowships, and the coordination of individual donor support through a secretariat, first at the Wellcome Trust, subsequently at FIC, then at Karolinska Institute, and currently at the AMANET Trust in Tanzania, it was possible to provide facilities and expertise to connect the African sites and investigators through the internet to one another and their developed country partners; to send data sets electronically to one another; to link with the National Library of Medicine at the NIH in order to access the world's literature; to create a reagent repository; and to organise the Pan-African Malaria Conference every three to four years to link the malaria research and control communities. These investments have continued for over a decade now, and the impact on capacity-building has been mirrored by the number of African scientists attending the MIM Conference, from 50 in 1997, to over 800 at the most recent meeting in Cameroon, with increasing organisational leadership from the African institutions (Heddini *et al.* 2004). The high level of complementary skills the partners now have is a third model of capacity-building, 'complementation' (Figure 49.1c). The Fifth MIM Conference took place in Nairobi, Kenya, in November 2009 and was organised by the African MIM secretariat.

Evaluating capacity-building programmes

Programmes often begin and continue on, secure in the belief they are meeting the mandate they started with, without the benefit of objective evaluation. In part, this is due to the failure to develop objective models for evaluation and criteria that would reflect the ultimate goal – capacity built and reflected by equity in collaboration. Rather, analyses tend to focus on the number of people trained, whether it is for an academic degree or for technical expertise, the number of grants obtained (without consideration of whose idea or who wrote the proposal), and the number of presentations made or papers published (without consideration of individual roles in the creation and delivery of a presentation or a published paper). There is also no serious consideration of the effects on institutional capacity development to address financial management, ethical review, or assume scientific leadership in priority-setting, grant applications, or implementation and evaluation of performance. This is in large part because agencies funding capacity-building do not require such evaluations, being satisfied with bibliometrics and an audit of the budget. During my tenure as Director of FIC, it proved impossible to target administrative and management capacity-building in international training grants because the mantra was that NIH supported research and research training, but not administrative and management infrastructure for foreign institutions.

A further complication affecting the evaluation of capacity-building programmes is that some developing country institutions have multiple partners, including university collaborators, funders such as NIH, CDC, the Wellcome Trust, the Gates Foundation, and different bilateral agencies, all of whom believe they are essential for institutional and individual scientist development. Actually, how do you separate out the contributions of each? How do you assess the negative impacts of some? How do they interact with one another? It can be awkward to ask these questions, and doing so may be hazardous to continued support. While which programme did what may not matter from the perspective of overall institutional capacity-building, it does matter when the question revolves around the cost and effectiveness of each of the capacity-building partners and their funders. However, capacity-building and its evaluation remains fragmented, essentially a project-by-project enterprise. Some funders may be more interested in how much corruption occurred than in how much leadership the local investigators assumed. Others may overlook the former if the latter outcome is favourable. At the same time, the personality and personal attributes of the individuals on both sides of the resource divide is a known critical factor in progress, and these qualities are difficult to assess and quantify. Similarly, the dynamics of the interactions between the leaders, and the nature of the peer-to-peer relationships among more junior scientists cannot be simply measured, yet are of fundamental importance to the long-term outcomes of capacity-building. In developing the Global Research Initiative Program to support re-entry of foreign scientists training or working in the US to their home country, FIC took specific steps to ensure the funds were under the control of the awardees themselves, in order to preclude the possibility that more senior staff at the international site would tap into the funds awarded to a more junior person.

The time has undoubtedly come for serious consideration of evaluation criteria, which in turn must be based on an acceptable definition of capacity-building, and a baseline assessment against which to compare progress. However, until external funders take steps to shift the power dynamic to the developing country partner, for example by directly funding them and/or running a grants competition among those in need of capacity-building so they define the problem to be addressed and, once awarded, pick an external partner, it will be difficult to tease out the infrastructural growth that has taken place. Perhaps the agencies, in collaboration with major developing country institutions, can come together on this and develop a set of useful criteria to assess capacity-building. Because successful capacity-building is not an instantaneous achievement, adequate time and investment must be factored in to the assessment. A Rockefeller Foundation Bellagio conference might be a way to begin the process and make some progress.

Personnel, staffing, and the two-way movement of faculty, students, and administrators

Research-intensive academic institutions in the developed world have relatively clear criteria for the academic advancement of faculty, and for the assessment of students. Faculty are often judged primarily on their research output (how many papers, in which journals, what was the role of the investigator in the research, and – of critical importance – how much direct research funding was generated and at what rate for indirect costs) and not their investment in building capacity through teaching at their own institution, let alone for their international partners. In such environments in the medical schools and science departments, applied research, particularly social science research, is often undervalued compared to basic or translational science, including clinical field trials, and is perceived as contributing minimally to academic advancement. There is little doubt of the chilling effect of this on the behaviour of the majority of faculty, except for those who are passionate about addressing global health problems. Like the latter faculty, and often modelled on them, students engage in applied research because they believe in the primary goals of global health – to reduce disparities – and ignore the many concerns about career paths. Changing these dynamics is perhaps more likely to be a bottom-up than a top-down process, although it obviously depends on who is at the top.

The two-way movement across the globe of faculty researchers, teachers, and students, is an inherently good thing. Those from developed countries can more readily understand the local circumstances and challenges. Those from developing countries can learn the possibilities that resources provide. On the other hand, they may think how much more they could accomplish if they were to migrate to the richer partner institution, the essential underpinning of the brain drain phenomenon. There are almost always more individuals from the developed world who want to and can spend time in a developing country, largely due to limited access to higher education in developing countries, which reduces the number who are academically qualified, on top of the costs for travel, tuition, and expenses to study in developed countries. Regardless of how much these costs are reduced by waivers or scholarships, someone has to pay real money.

These considerations are much less relevant to the movement of students towards developing countries, and we are already seeing increasing numbers of students, from undergraduates to professional school students, who want to work in global health and development, in many cases before they have many skills – other than enthusiasm and concern – to contribute.

As the number of such students going to developing country sites increases, the burden on the host institution and its faculty and staff grows in a progressive non-linear manner. More and more local staff attention is focused on these foreign students, leaving less time for their primary work-related responsibilities. This significant unintended consequence is very real, given that the rich institutions generally do not themselves make the investment needed to provide the full set of services needed by its students placed overseas. Local institutions are often asked to find housing, transportation, arrange student assignments, mentors, recreation, assure safety, security, and acculturation, respond to problems that inevitably arise, and also deal with whatever administrative requirements there may be in the first place, until such time that the programme is large enough to justify the richer institution's hiring of a programme administrator. At that point, the burden on local professionals may stabilise, or because of the sheer size of the programme, continue to increase. The scenario only becomes more problematic when there are multiple institutions sending students to the same local site, and to the same small number of internationally recognised local professionals, competing with one another and juggling for advantage. This is frequently the reality on the ground.

What is the future of global health?

While one can imagine a near-term future of increasing numbers of our faculty and students spending time at the partner's site, with all the bi-directional benefits of peer-to-peer relationships, it is also possible to imagine the displacement of local professionals and students by the visitors. If in the longer term the capacity-building strategy is handled extremely well, local scientists and institutional leaders and managers will grow in competence, confidence, and status, to the point where their counterparts become superfluous. This is the ideal outcome, when global health, as it currently means to us in developed countries, ceases to exist and a new paradigm is created. This does not necessarily imply relationships stop, but rather that they change, evolve, grow, and find new ways to enhance creative approaches to common problems, comparative studies, and promote the synergy of complementary skills applied to the same problem. It should coincide with a reduction in the disparities in access to health care and health status that is far greater than the relative change the economic indicators of the countries would suggest. It would also likely mean that the host country is now investing in the health security of its own people, and is building an effective health care system within indigenous institutions, which includes quality service, education, and research.

This may not mean that the sound of our students trekking to the partner institutions is in any way dampened. Instead, it can harmonise with the sound of students from the partners coming to our institutions. Faculty from both sides will work together to address the health problems affecting all populations – truly global health. What we now have for global health is instead largely a rebranding of what used to be called international health, a more bilateral and largely unidirectional effort to address the problems of the resource poor partner. Koplan and colleagues characterised the focus of international health as 'the health issues of countries other than one's own, especially those of low-income and middle-income'. Such programmes intend 'to help people of other nations' (2009: 1994). In contrast, they present global health programmes as ones that address 'issues that directly or indirectly affect health but that can transcend national boundaries' (2009: 1994). In a recent commentary, Peter Piot and Geoff Garnett called for a 'substantive new agenda and a new way of working' (2009: 1,122) for global health, but interestingly focused more on equity in relationships and partnerships 'mainly based in low-income and middle-income countries' (2009: 1,123), and did not highlight transnational problems which required transnational efforts to solve them.

A useful example is emerging infectious diseases, which may start in one part of the world but quickly spread everywhere. The most recent emergence, the novel H1N1 Influenza A (2009) strain, caused an outbreak in Mexico in spring 2009 and spread internationally with travellers even before it was identified. Emerging infections are now known to originate primarily from animals, having acquired the capacity to jump the usual species barriers for infection. They are more likely than not to be viruses that mutate rapidly. The drivers of emergence are also more commonly social, cultural, behavioural, ecological, and environmental rather than biological (Woolhouse and Gowtage-Sequeria 2005). This gives rise to the 'hotspot' concept, particular places where these drivers congregate, especially in developing countries because there are large, highly inter-mixed populations of animals, humans, vectors, and reservoir hosts (Jones *et al.* 2008). Early detection of these agents would allow a more rapid response, with the potential to limit spread and impact. To be most effective, there needs to be integrated surveillance in animal and human populations, especially in hotspot areas, establishing strong linkages between the human and animal health communities, and targeting high-risk human populations, such as animal health or food production workers in close contact with animals. This can only be accomplished by a complementation model of global health capacity (Figure 49.1c), and this depends first on human and institutional capacity-building in the hotspot countries, using global financial resources at the outset. It also requires widespread buy-in from the global community of nations and bi- and multi-national organisations so that political, economic, and trade considerations do not block the collection and dissemination of information for reaction and response.

Conclusions

There is little doubt that global health is receiving considerable and growing attention in our academic institutions, in our national priorities for humanitarian as well as pragmatic interests, and among celebrities in music and film, who help to capture media and public attention. The more resources devoted to capacity-building and the generation of new knowledge and evidence to identify best practices, followed by implementation, the more likely it is that health in the countries targeted, mainly low- and middle- income countries, will be favourably impacted.

At the same time, as the number of students with limited training and skills travelling to developing countries increases, there are a set of possible unintended negative consequences, such as the diversion of resources and effort of local health professionals from addressing the problems of the local population to catering to the needs of short-term visitors, or the displacement of local workers by the non-locals. Build-up of global health programmes must, therefore, be thoughtful, careful, selective, and mindful of the need to increase the benefits and reduce the adverse effects that may occur.

There needs to be particular attention to the paradigm being followed. Capacity-building must be targeted to achieve capacity built, with the relationship between the trainer and the trainee changing to one of full equity, which is called a 'complementation model' in this chapter. It requires that a set of evaluation criteria be available to judge success, where in the spectrum from 'building' to 'built' the programme is, and whether or not the relationship between the trainer and trainee has appropriately changed.

Finally, further attention needs to be given to the current stated objectives of global health, moving beyond the focus on fixing a problem in a recipient country, to working on truly transnational and global problems that require global cooperation and investment. Only then can we say that we have achieved a global health system that works, is sustainable, and is inclusive of all nations. After all, the definition of global generally denotes something universal, pertaining to the whole world and all nations.

References

CUGH (Consortium of Universities for Global Health) (2009) *CUGH Survey of University-based Global Health Programs: A Summary*, available at http://www.cugh.org/sites/default/files/survey-summary.pdf (accessed 20 October 2009).

Heddini, A., Keusch, G.T., and Davies, C.S. (2004) 'The multilateral initiative on malaria: past, present, and future', *American Journal of Tropical Medicine and Hygiene*, 71(Supplement 2): 279–82.

Jamison, D.T., Breman, J.G., Measham, A.R., Alleyne, G., Claeson, M, Evans, D.B., Jha, P., Mills, A., and Musgrove, P. (eds) (2006) *Disease Control Priorities in Developing Countries*, Washington, DC: The International Bank for Reconstruction and Development/The World Bank, available at http://dcp2.org/main/Home.html (accessed 20 October 2009).

Jones, K.E., Patel, N.G., Levy, M.A., Storeyguard, A., Balk, D., Gittleman, J.L., and Daszak, P. (2008) 'Global trends in emerging infectious diseases', *Nature*, 451: 990–93.

Koplan, J.P., Bond, C.T., Merson, M.H., Srinath Reddy, K., Rodriguez, M.H., Sewankambo, N.K., and Wasserheit, J.N. (2009) 'Towards a common definition of global health', *The Lancet*, 373: 1,993–5.

Merson, M.H. and Chapman Page, K. (2009) *The Dramatic Expansion of University Engagement in Global Health: Implications for US Policy*, Washington, DC: Center for Strategic and International Studies.

Piot, P. and Garnett, G. (2009) 'Health is global', *The Lancet*, 374: 1,122–3.

Rockefeller Foundation (1979) *The President's Review and Annual Report*, New York: The Rockefeller Foundation, available at http://www.rockfound.org/library/annual_reports/1970-1979/1979.pdf (accessed 20 October 2009).

Rockefeller Foundation (1988) *The President's Review and Annual Report*, New York: The Rockefeller Foundation, available at http://www.rockfound.org/library/annual_reports/1980-1989/1988.pdf (accessed 20 October 2009).

Van Heyningen, W.E. and Seal, J.R. (1983) *Cholera: The American Scientific Experience*, Boulder, CO: Westview Press.

Woolhouse, M.E.J. and Gowtage-Sequeria, S. (2005) 'Host Range and Emerging and Reemerging Pathogens', *Emerging Infectious Diseases*, available at http://www.cdc.gov/ncidod/EID/vol11no12/05-0997.htm (accessed 20 October 2009).

WHO/TDR (World Health Organization, Special Programme for Research and Training in Tropical Diseases) (2007) *Making a Difference: 30 Years of Research and Capacity Building in Tropical Disease*, Geneva: WHO, available at http://www.who.int/tdr/about/history_book/pdf/anniversary_book.pdf (accessed 20 October 2009).

50

Long-term Academic Partnerships for Capacity Building in Health in Developing Countries

Jeffrey D. Mulvihill and Haile T. Debas

Introduction

The provision of health care in developing countries, particularly those in sub-Saharan Africa, is grossly inadequate. Inadequacies exist in all aspects of the health system: the workforce, infrastructure (hospitals, clinics, equipment, and supplies), and in health system financing and administration. The combination of inadequate production of health care workers and brain drain has resulted in critical shortages of doctors and nurses throughout all the resource-poor countries (Anyangwe and Mtonga 2007; Sheldon 2006; UNESCO 2009). The World Health Organization (WHO) defines a critical shortage of doctors, nurses, and midwives as less than 2.3 per 100,000 of population. Of the 57 countries with critical health workforce shortages worldwide, 37 are in sub-Saharan Africa. Countries below this level fail to achieve an 80 per cent coverage rate for measles immunisation or for deliveries by skilled birth attendants (Chen *et al.* 2004). They are also unlikely to reach the Millennium Development Goals (MDGs) prescribed by the United Nations for completion by 2015 (WHO 2006). Lack of adequate investment in health and in higher education has resulted in dilapidated universities and teaching hospitals in many sub-Saharan African countries (Ishengoma 2003; Kariuki 2009; Polgreen 2007; Sawyerr 2004). In this chapter, we will focus on the problem of shortages of doctors, nurses, pharmacists, and dentists, and on the need to improve the quality of their training and the environment in which they train and work as one strategy to reinvigorate these universities and stem the brain drain.

The crisis in human resources in sub-Saharan Africa

Crisis in the healthcare workforce

Figure 50.1 shows the number of doctors, nurses, pharmacists, and dentists that provide care to the populations of seven sub-Saharan African countries. The stark reality is that the critical shortages are present not only in the numbers of doctors and nurses, but even more acutely in the numbers of pharmacists and dentists. As a consequence, health care in most district hospitals is provided by non-physician and non-nurse clinicians (NPCs) such as

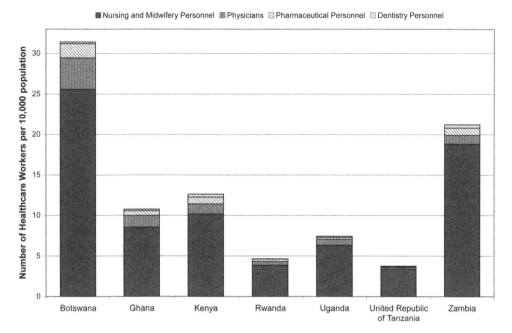

Figure 50.1 Human resources for health
Source: WHO (n.d.).

assistant medical officers (AMOs) and clinical officers (COs). Table 50.1 shows how some sub-Saharan African countries use NPCs to provide health care to their populations. By some estimates, AMOs are capable of performing 60 to 80 per cent of the clinical work that primary care physicians provide (Bryan *et al.* 2006). This makes them a necessary substitute for fully trained physicians, especially in resource-limited settings. This so-called 'task-shifting' is necessary for the foreseeable future, but what is lacking is proper licensure, quality control, and continuing education and skill improvement. Ministries of health in many countries lack the necessary higher-level workforce to create and maintain quality control and continuing skill improvement systems for these mid-level health care providers. It is unlikely that they will be able to do so until they produce their own doctors, nurses, pharmacists, and dentists in sufficient numbers and with the necessary skills.

Table 50.1 Comparing the numbers of non-physician clinicians (NPCs) and physicians in seven sub-Saharan African countries

Country	Total number of NPCs	NPCs per 10,000 people	Physicians per 10,000 people
Botswana	88	0.47	3.85
Ghana	432	0.19	1.41
Kenya	4,152	1.14	1.23
Rwanda	444	0.47	0.46
Uganda	6,000	2.01	0.74
United Republic of Tanzania	1,200	0.30	0.21
Zambia	1,000	0.85	1.08

Crisis in higher education

The funding shortage of African universities in the past two decades was caused, at least in part, by the 'Structural Adjustment Programmes' (SAPs) implemented by the International Monetary Fund (IMF) and the World Bank in the 1980s. The implementation of SAPs resulted in generally lower levels of spending on education in sub-Saharan Africa (Gupta *et al.* 1998), and the funding that remained was typically directed toward primary and secondary education and away from higher education. As a result, many universities in sub-Saharan African countries had faculty-hiring freezes imposed on them. This hiring freeze, combined with faculty attrition due to retirement and brain drain, on the one hand, and the demand on universities in recent years to double or even quadruple enrolment in professional schools on the other, has resulted in student: teacher ratios that are highly unfavourable. These circumstances have posed particularly severe challenges to medical and other professional schools.

From 1970 to 2007 in the United States, the student: teacher ratio at the university level decreased from about 14:1 in 1970, to about 13:1 in 2007, reaching its most imbalanced level of 16:1 in 1990 (Figure 50.2). This indicates the emphasis placed on improving this metric in the US in an effort to provide higher quality education. Over the same time period in sub-Saharan Africa, the number of students enrolled in universities has grown at nearly twice the rate of the number of professors teaching them (Figure 50.3). In 1970, there were 196,000 students enrolled in tertiary education in sub-Saharan Africa, and 18,000 professors. The resulting student: teacher ratio of about 12:1 was better (lower) than the ratio of 13:1 that we now see in the United States. Over the period from 1970 to 2007, however, the number of students enrolled exploded to 4,140,000, while the number of professors increased at a more modest rate to 174,000, creating the current student: teacher ratio of nearly 24:1. The figures in higher education in the health sciences are similar to these figures for higher education in general.

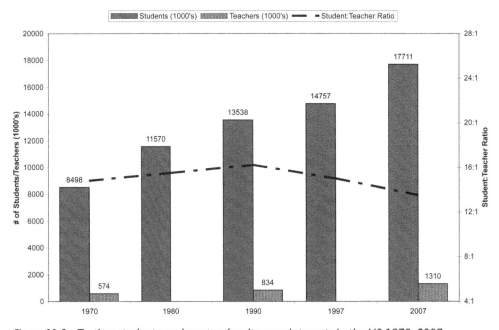

Figure 50.2 Tertiary student enrolment vs faculty appointments in the US 1970–2007

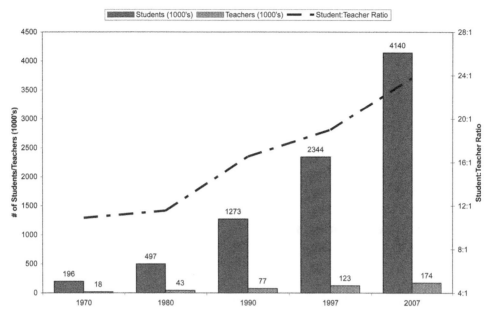

Figure 50.3 Tertiary student enrolment vs faculty appointments in sub-Saharan Africa 1970–2007

The compounding factor of brain drain

The shortages in human resources for health caused by insufficient production of new clinical professors are compounded by the persistent emigration of skilled health professionals from developing to developed countries. In most sub-Saharan African countries, emigrants are 20 to 50 times more likely to have tertiary or higher degrees than secondary education only (Carrington 1998). People with less education, such as non-physician, non-nurse clinicians, are less susceptible to brain drain, and represent a cadre of health providers more likely to locate themselves in district hospitals and clinics away from cities (Mullan and Frehywot 2007).

Brain drain is as prevalent today as it was 20 years ago. In Uganda in 1990, the rate of emigration for tertiary-educated individuals was estimated at 15.5–18.4 per cent (Carrington and Detragiache 1998). A survey of nursing students in Uganda conducted in 2006 showed that fully 92 per cent of them intended to leave the country and work elsewhere within five years of graduation (Nguyen *et al.* 2008). Emigration of nurses and doctors to foreign lands occurs primarily in search of a better quality of life and more fulfilling careers (Padarath *et al.* 2003). Although inadequate financial compensation is an important factor, as exemplified below, unsatisfactory working conditions with poor infrastructure, lack of career development, and lack of exciting academic environment and intellectual challenge are cited as equally important reasons. Other push factors cited are dangerous working conditions and lack of jobs in the home country (Nguyen *et al.* 2008), inability to utilise the skills and training acquired in patient care due to lack of equipment and supplies, and inefficient bureaucracy (Huddart and Picazo 2003).

Another form of brain drain is caused by the migration of health professionals from university and other public service jobs to higher-paying jobs within the developing countries themselves (Huddart and Picazo 2003). For example, jobs in non-governmental organisations (NGOs) and in multilateral and bilateral missions (e.g. WHO, the Centers for Disease Control and Prevention (CDC), the Global Fund to Fight AIDS, TB and Malaria (GFATM)) can pay twice as much or more than jobs in universities or ministries of health. In addition, the professionals that these in-country foreign organisations recruit away from the public sector tend to be the more qualified and more enterprising individuals.

The compensation gap is exemplified by nursing salaries, which are particularly skewed between developing and developed countries. While an experienced nurse in Malawi might earn about $3,312 per year (and a junior nurse might earn around $1,000 per year), entry-level nursing jobs in the UK typically pay about $33,290 per year (Record and Mohiddin 2006). The higher income earned abroad benefits not only the professional and his/her family in the adopted country, but also their families and relatives in the home country whose living conditions can be transformed because of regular remittances sent home.

Long-term academic partnerships

We believe academic institutions in high-income countries have great competitive advantages to help reverse the decline of the academic environment in their counterpart institutions in low-income countries, and, thereby, help to stem the brain drain. To realise this potential, two key ingredients are required. First, the partnerships must be long-term (greater than ten years), with signed affiliation agreements between the academic institutions. Second, to accomplish the goal of capacity building, these partnerships will require sustained funding. Unfortunately, private foundations, such as the Bill & Melinda Gates Foundation, appear reluctant to fund such long-term capacity building initiatives, believing instead that governments should fund them. However, without a jump-start from the international community, it is unlikely that the governments in poor countries will be able to successfully accomplish this goal. We are encouraged by the public comments of government officials that the Global Health Initiative of the US government is considering investing in capacity building projects in developing countries (Emanuel 2009).

If the long-term academic partnership is to be successful, it must have several attributes, including the following:

1. It must be long-term, spanning some 10–20 years. A long-term partnership provides stability in the institutional relationship and can help ensure that the focus is on sustainable capacity building initiatives rather than short-term, temporary projects or assistance
2. The partnership needs to be mutually advantageous to both parties. While the benefit to the institution in the developing country is obvious, that to the partnering richer institution should also be explicit, and includes opportunities for research collaborations, training sites for students, both at the undergraduate and graduate levels, and for learning new approaches and simple solutions to complex problems
3. The collaboration should be primarily based on the needs and priorities of the less-resourced party
4. The relationship must be one among equals and based on trust, and with respect for the customs and cultural and religious values of each party
5. All financial transactions must be transparent
6. From the beginning, there must be clear understanding and agreement on mechanisms of handling data, publications, specimens, and intellectual property
7. The work to be done must be based on previously agreed-upon principles for project development and for monitoring and evaluation

8. A mechanism for conflict resolution should be developed and agreed upon from the beginning

9. Long-term funding needs to be secured.

Value of long-term academic partnerships

There are many ways in which long-term academic partnerships can help reverse the decline in academic institutions. These include improving teaching, learning, research, and the infrastructure and technological innovations necessary to restore universities in sub-Saharan African countries to vital institutions of quality education. Table 50.2 illustrates four examples of successful long-term collaboration between US and African universities. Each partnership is different, and emphasises different scopes of work and the achievement of different outcomes. What they have in common is that they all deal with the institutional priorities of the less-resourced partner, and focus on strengthening academic programmes and institution-building.

Many academic institutions in developing countries are currently engaged in curricular reform and innovation. They are replacing outmoded, traditional curricula with new competence-based ones that emphasise active learning, small group sessions, team-based learning, and the use of instructional technology and wireless communication systems. They are also emphasising interdisciplinary teaching, learning, research, and clinical practice. Universities from more developed countries can support and ensure the success of this educational revolution through the exchange of faculty and students, through sharing technology, and through helping to improve the infrastructure for education and research.

Faculty and students in developing countries, like their counterparts in the developed countries, would like to see incentives and rewards for achievement and academic excellence. They want to see a clear pathway in their career development. These are routine practices that trainees in US and other Western institutions expect and experience. It will, however, require a change in institutional culture in many universities in developing countries: a change that is necessary if an academic environment is to be created to help minimise brain drain.

Conclusions

Universities and health professional schools in developing countries have experienced a decline in their quality and productivity in the past 20 years chiefly because of a lack of adequate investment in higher education and health. By contrast, the higher investment in elementary and secondary education has resulted in greater numbers of graduates seeking opportunities for higher education. Governments have responded by requiring universities and professional schools to double, triple, and sometimes even quadruple their enrolment without making the necessary resources available. There is great need to train faculty, improve teaching, and strengthen research in these universities to enable them to help solve the health workforce crises in their respective countries.

It is unlikely that the governments in these countries can muster the resources necessary to revitalise their universities in a timely fashion. We believe that, if given the necessary resources, US and Western universities are in a unique position to help their counterparts in developing countries to revitalise themselves. Several successful experiments exist that support this contention, and we have provided four examples. Modest investment is required to create many more similar long-term academic partnerships that will result in sustainable capacity building, in training the health workforce, and in strengthening academic institutions.

Table 50.2 Four examples of successful long-term academic partnerships

Indiana University and Moi University, Kenya (Indiana University 2008; Einterz et al. 2007)	University of Pennsylvania (UPenn) and the University of Botswana, Botswana (UPenn 2009)	University of California, San Francisco, and the Muhimbili University of Health and Allied Sciences, Tanzania (UCSF 2009; Taché et al. 2008)	Johns Hopkins University and Makerere University, Uganda (IOM 2009)
Partnership Duration			
Since 1989	Since 2006 (UPenn presence in Botswana since 2001)	Since 2005	Since 1988
Funding Source			
USAID	PEPFAR and other research grants	Bill & Melinda Gates Foundation	Multiple
Scope of Work			
Health care workforce capacity building, HIV/AIDS care and treatment, food and income security	Medical education, capacity building in response to HIV/AIDS epidemic, student exchange, AIDS research	Curricular innovation and reform, faculty development, student and faculty exchange, establishment of Center for Health Professions Education	Establishment of College of Health Sciences through joint planning, capacity building to improve health outcomes in Uganda
Outcomes			
• 70,000 HIV/AIDS patients treated at 18 sites in both urban and rural Kenya • High-production farms provide food assistance for 30,000 people per month • Income security provided through microfinance, skills training, and fair-trade-certified crafts workshops	• Several hundred Penn students, residents, researchers, and faculty travel to Botswana each year for educational and research experiences • Botswanan students and scholars visit UPenn reciprocally • 50 UPenn doctors and staff living full-time in Botswana • 22 ongoing research projects • Reversing the trend of brain drain of medical students	• Institution-wide faculty exchange programmes • Introduction of novel, interdisciplinary teaching methods • Development of competency-based curricula (in progress) • Establishment of the Center for Health Professions Education (CHPE) with laboratories for teaching, learning and clinical skills, simulation, and continuing professional education	• Restructuring to establish College of Health Sciences • Needs assessment plan written by Makerere students and led by Makerere and Johns Hopkins faculty members • Evaluation of how Makerere might most effectively promote local health initiatives • A strategic plan to be implemented over 8 years jointly by deans from Makerere and Johns Hopkins, and an advisory council drawn from Ugandan government and civil society

(continued on the next page)

Table 50.2 (continued)

Indiana University and Moi University, Kenya (Indiana University 2008; Einterz et al. 2007)	University of Pennsylvania (UPenn) and the University of Botswana, Botswana (UPenn 2009)	University of California, San Francisco, and the Muhimbili University of Health and Allied Sciences, Tanzania (UCSF 2009; Taché et al. 2008)	Johns Hopkins University and Makerere University, Uganda (IOM 2009)

Success Features

• Counterpart relationships at both individual and departmental levels	• Multifaceted partnership, involving multiple schools, programmes, and departments at both institutions	• Novel approach to cost-effective capacity building – working on an institutional scale	• Trust built on long-term partnership
• Collaboration among virtually all major disciplines at both schools	• Common unifying goal	• True coequal partnership through peer-to-peer relationships at both institutions	• Administrative transformation of Makerere into College of Health Sciences
• Mutual benefit achieved through equity, not equality	• Continual development of new projects to sustain and expand the partnership	• Resource-limited partner has strong influence on project objectives	• Strategic plan to enable Makerere to expand its impact on health outcomes in Uganda and East Africa

References

Anyangwe, S. and Mtonga, C. (2007) 'Inequities in the Global Health Workforce: The Greatest Impediment to Health in Sub-Saharan Africa', *International Journal of Environmental Research and Public Health*, 4: 93–100.

Bryan, L., Garg, R., Ramji, S., Silverman, A., Tagar, E. and Ware, I. (2006) *Investing in Tanzanian Human Resources for Health*, London: McKinsey & Co., Touch Foundation.

Carrington, W., and Detragiache, E. (1998) *How Big Is the Brain Drain?* International Monetary Fund Working Paper No. 98/107, Washington, DC: IMF, available at http://ssrn.com/abstract=882624 (accessed 4 November 2009).

Chen, L., Evans, T., Anand, S., Boufford, J., Brown, H., Chowdhury, M., Cueto, M., Dare, L., Dussault, G., Elzinga, G., Fee, E., Habte, D., Hanvoravongchai, P., Jacobs, M., Kurowski, C., Michael, S., Pablos-Mendez, A., Sewankambo, N., Solimano, G., Stilwell, B., de Waal, A., and Wibulpolprasert, S. (2004) 'Human Resources for Health: Overcoming the Crisis', *The Lancet*, 364(9,449): 1,984–90.

Einterz, R., Kimaiyo, S., Mengech, H., Khwa-Otsyula, B., Esamai, F., Quigley, F., and Mamlin, J. (2007) 'Responding to the HIV Pandemic: The Power of an Academic Medical Partnership', *Academic Medicine*, 82(8): 812–18.

Emanuel, Z. (2009) 'Global Health Initiative', presentation at the Consortium of Universities for Global Health meeting, Bethesda, MD, 14 September.

Gupta, S., Clements, B., and Tiongson, E. (1998) 'Public Spending on Human Development', *Finance and Development*, 35: 10–13.

Huddart, J. and Picazo, A. (2003) 'The Health Sector Human Resource Crisis in Africa: An Issues Paper', Washington, DC: United States Agency for International Development, Bureau for Africa, and the Office of Sustainable Development.

Indiana University (2008) *Indiana-Kenya Partnership*, available online at www.iukenya.org (accessed 28 January 2010).

IOM (Institute of Medicine) (2009) *The U.S. Commitment to Global Health: Recommendations for the Public and Private Sectors*, Washington, DC: The National Academies Press.

Ishengoma, J. (2003) 'The Myths and Realities of Higher Education Globalization: A View from the Southern Hemisphere', *In Focus Journal*, available at http://www.escotet.org/infocus/forum/2003/ishengoma.htm (accessed 4 November 2009).

Kariuki, K. (2009) 'The Challenges of Financing Research in Institutions of Higher Education in Africa', presentation at the 12th General Conference of the Association of African Universities, Abuja, Nigeria, 8 May.

Mullan, F. and Frehywot, S. (2007) 'Non-physician Clinicians in 47 sub-Saharan African Countries', *The Lancet*, 370(9,605): 2,158–63.

Nguyen, L., Ropers, S., Nderitu, E., Zuyderduin, A., Luboga, S., and Hagopian, A. (2008) 'Intent to Migrate among Nursing Students in Uganda: Measures of the Brain Drain in the Next Generation of Health Professionals', *Human Resources for Health*, 6: 5.

Padarath A., Chamberlain C., McCoy D., Ntuli A., Rowson M., and Loewenson R. (2003) 'Health Personnel in Southern Africa: Confronting Maldistribution and Brain Drain', Equinet Discussion Paper Series, 3, Durban: Regional Network for Equity in Health in Southern Africa, Health Systems Trust.

Polgreen, L. (2007) *Africa's Once-great Colleges are Overcrowded and Crumbling*, New York Times, 20 May, available at http://www.nytimes.com/2007/05/20/world/africa/20iht-africa.1.5785956.html (accessed 10 December 2009).

Record, R., and Mohiddin, A. (2006) 'An Economic Perspective on Malawi's Medical "Brain Drain"', *Globalization and Health*, 2: 12.

Sawyerr, A. (2004) 'Challenges Facing African Universities: Selected Issues', *African Studies Review*, 47(1): 1–59, available at http://www.jstor.org/stable/1514797 (accessed 4 November 2009).

Sheldon, G.F. (2006) 'Globalization and the Health Workforce Shortage', *Surgery*, 140: 354–8.

Taché, S., Kaaya, E., Omer, S., Mkony, C., Lyamuya, E., Pallangyo, K., Debas, H., and MacFarlane, S. (2008) 'University Partnership to Address the Shortage of Healthcare Professionals in Africa', *Global Public Health*, 3(2): 137–48.

UNESCO (United Nations Educational, Scientific and Cultural Organization) (2009) *Global Education Digest 2009: Comparing Education Statistics across the World*, Paris: UNESCO Institute for Statistics.

UNESCO (United Nations Educational, Scientific and Cultural Organization) Institute for Statistics (n.d.) Online Data Centre, available at http://stats.uis.unesco.org/unesco/TableViewer/document.aspx?ReportId=143&IF_Language=eng (accessed 20 October 2009).

UCSF (University of California, San Francisco) (2009) *MUHAS-UCSF Partnership*, available at http://globalhealthsciences.ucsf.edu/programmes/muhas-partnership/index.aspx (accessed 29 January 2010).

University of Pennsylvania (2009) *Botswana-UPenn Partnership*, available at www.upenn.edu/botswana (accessed 28 January 2010).

WHO (World Health Organization) (2006) *The Global Shortage of Health Workers and its Impact*, WHO Media Centre, available at http://www.who.int/mediacentre/factsheets/fs302/en/index.html (accessed 10 December 2009).

WHO (World Health Organization) (n.d.) *World Health Organization Statistical Information System*, available at http://www.who.int/whosis/en/ (accessed 29 January 2010).

Index

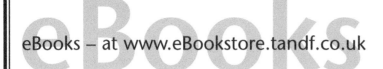

Printed and bound by CPI Group (UK) Ltd, Croydon, CR0 4YY

01/11/2024

01782610-0008